Ellis and Calne's
Lecture Notes in General Surgery

Ellis and Calne's
Lecture Notes in General Surgery

Edited by

Christopher Watson, MD BChir FRCS

Professor of Transplantation and Honorary Consultant Surgeon
Cambridge University Hospitals NHS Foundation Trust
Cambridge, UK

Justin Davies, MA MChir FRCS (Gen Surg) FEBS (Coloproctology)

Consultant Colorectal Surgeon
Cambridge University Hospitals NHS Foundation Trust

Affiliated Assistant Professor
University of Cambridge

Fellow in Clinical Medicine
Downing College, Cambridge, UK

Fourteenth Edition

WILEY Blackwell

Contents

Author affiliations

Hemantha Alawattegama
Consultant Anaesthetist
Cambridge University Hospitals NHS Foundation Trust

Anita Balakrishnan
Consultant HPB Surgeon
Cambridge University Hospitals NHS Foundation Trust

Peter A. Brennan
Consultant Maxillofacial Surgeon and Honorary
Professor of Surgery
Portsmouth Hospitals University Trust
Portsmouth

Alexandra J. Colquhoun
Consultant Urologist
Cambridge University Hospitals NHS Foundation Trust

Aman Singh Coonar
Consultant Thoracic Surgeon
Royal Papworth Hospital
Cambridge

Patrick Coughlin
Leeds Vascular Institute
Leeds

Justin Davies
Consultant Colorectal Surgeon
Cambridge University Hospitals NHS Foundation Trust

Affiliated Assistant Professor
University of Cambridge

Fellow in Clinical Medicine
Downing College, Cambridge

Amer J. Durrani
Consultant Plastic & Reconstructive Surgeon
Cambridge University Hospitals NHS Foundation Trust

Brian Fish
Consultant ENT/Head and Neck Surgeon
Cambridge University Hospitals NHS Foundation Trust

Manj Gohel
Consultant Vascular & Endovascular Surgeon
Cambridge University Hospitals NHS Foundation Trust

Honorary Senior Lecturer
Imperial College
London

Stavros Gourgiotis
Consultant Surgeon
Cambridge Oesophago-Gastric Centre
Cambridge University Hospitals NHS Foundation Trust

Ian Grant
Consultant Plastic Surgeon
Cambridge University Hospitals NHS Foundation Trust

Ekpemi Irune
Consultant Laryngology, Head & Neck Surgeon
Cambridge University Hospitals NHS Foundation Trust

David P. Jenkins
Consultant Cardiothoracic Surgeon
Royal Papworth Hospital
Cambridge

Eleftheria Kleidi
Consultant Oncoplastic Breast Surgeon
Cambridge University Hospitals NHS Foundation Trust

Vasilis Kosmoliaptsis
Honorary Consultant Abdominal Transplant, HPB
and Endocrine Surgeon

Associate Professor, Department of Surgery
University of Cambridge

Rodney J. C. Laing
Consultant Neurosurgeon
Cambridge University Hospitals NHS Foundation Trust

Arthur McPhee
Consultant Urologist
Cambridge University Hospitals NHS Foundation Trust

Kanwalraj Moar
Consultant Cleft and Maxillofacial Surgeon
Cambridge University Hospitals NHS Foundation Trust

Jonathan Morton
Consultant Colorectal Surgeon
Cambridge University Hospitals NHS Foundation Trust

Ioanna G. Panagiotopoulou
Consultant Colorectal Surgeon
Cambridge University Hospitals NHS Foundation Trust

Raaj Kumar Praseedom
Consultant HPB & Transplant Surgeon
Cambridge University Hospitals NHS Foundation Trust

Stephen Price
Honorary Consultant Neurosurgeon
Cambridge University Hospitals NHS Foundation Trust

Christopher Pring
Consultant Bariatric Surgeon
St Richard's Hospital
Chichester

Visiting Professor
University of Surrey

Peter Safranek
Consultant Surgeon
Cambridge Oesophago-Gastric Centre
Cambridge University Hospitals NHS Foundation Trust

Constantinos Simillis
Consultant Colorectal Surgeon
Cambridge University Hospitals NHS Foundation Trust

Lynsey Spillman
Hepatology and Liver Transplant Dietitian
Cambridge University Hospitals NHS Foundation Trust

Vijay Sujendran
Consultant Surgeon
Cambridge Oesophago-Gastric Centre
Cambridge University Hospitals NHS Foundation Trust

Elizabeth Tweedle
Consultant Colorectal Surgeon
Cambridge University Hospitals NHS Foundation Trust

Christopher Watson
Professor of Transplantation and Honorary
Consultant Surgeon
Cambridge University Hospitals NHS Foundation Trust

Preface

Many medical students will have effectively written their own textbook at the end of their clinical course – a digest of the lectures and tutorials assiduously attended and of the textbooks meticulously read. Unfortunately, students may approach the qualifying examinations burdened by the thought of many pages of excellent and exhaustive textbooks wherein lies the wisdom required of them by the examiners. Although the Internet is increasingly used as a source of information, we believe that there is still a serious need for a book that briefly sets out the important facts in General Surgery that are classified, analysed and, as far as possible, rationalized for the revision student. These lecture notes represent such a text; they are in no way a substitute for the standard textbooks, but they do draw together, in a logical way, the fundamentals of General Surgery and its subspecialties. As such we hope it will also be of use to the junior surgeon.

We wish to point the reader to the electronic resource accompanying the text, including case studies, radiographs and histology slides illustrating common conditions mentioned in the text, as well as a quiz to test the reader's knowledge.

The first edition of *Lecture Notes in General Surgery* was written by Harold Ellis and Sir Roy Calne and published in 1965. This is the first edition without their involvement, and we acknowledge their huge contribution to surgery and its teaching. Surgery has changed enormously since the days of that first edition, and each subsequent edition has tried to keep pace with surgical practice. Never has the pace of change been so great as it is today. The biggest changes have been seen in the development of specialist services, at the expense of the generalist, and the development of multidisciplinary teams to optimize management. Recognizing this, previous editions have relied heavily on colleagues from other specialties to keep chapters updated and relevant. For this edition we have taken this further, and each chapter now has a nominated expert author – who, for some chapters, has updated previous content; and, for others, has written completely new content – to ensure relevance for today's student.

Christopher Watson
Justin Davies

Acknowledgements

We are grateful to our colleagues – senior and junior doctors, and students – who have read and critiqued this text during its production, and to many readers and reviewers for their constructive criticisms. We are indebted to those colleagues in years gone by, too numerous to mention here, who have developed the text upon which the new chapter experts have built. We would also like to acknowledge the continued help give by the staff at Wiley for seeing this project through to publication, in particular James Watson, Catriona King, Mandy Collison, Ella Elliott, and Indirakumari Siva.

Abbreviations

ABPI	ankle brachial pressure index
ABG	arterial blood gas
ABLS	Advanced Burns Life Support
ACE	angiotensin-converting enzyme
ACTH	adrenocorticotrophic hormone
ADH	antidiuretic hormone
ADT	androgen deprivation therapy
AFP	α-fetoprotein
AIs	aromatase inhibitors
AIDS	acquired immune deficiency syndrome
AIN	anal intraepithelial neoplasia
AJCC	American Joint Committee on Cancer
ALK	anaplastic lymphoma kinase
ALP	alkaline phosphatase
ALT	alanine transaminase
ANC	axillary node clearance
ANS	axillary node sampling
ANUG	acute necrotizing ulcerative gingivitis
APFC	acute peripancreatic fluid collection
APACHE	Acute Physiology and Chronic Health Evaluation
APTT	activated partial thromboplastin time
APUD	amine precursor uptake and decarboxylation
ASA	American Society of Anesthesiologists
ASD	atrial septal defect
ASIA	American Spinal Injury Association
AST	aspartate transaminase
ATN	acute tubular necrosis
ATLS	Advanced Trauma Life Support
AXR	abdominal X-ray
β-HCG	β-human chorionic gonadotrophin
BCG	bacille Calmette–Guérin
BCS	breast conserving surgery
BMI	body mass index
BPH	benign prostatic hyperplasia
CABG	coronary artery bypass graft

CAPOX	capecitabine and oxaliplatin
CAR	chimeric antigen receptor
CaSR	calcium sensing receptor
CEA	carcinoembryonic antigen
CEAP	Clinical, Etiological, Anatomical and Pathophysiological
CHRPE	congenital hypertrophy of the retinal pigment epithelium
CMV	cytomegalovirus
CNS	central nervous system
COPD	chronic obstructive pulmonary disease
CPAP	continuous positive airways pressure
CPE	carbapenemase-producing enterobacteriaceae
CPPS	chronic pelvic pain syndrome
CRE	carbopenem-resistant enterobacteriaceae
CRP	C-reactive protein
CSF	cerebrospinal fluid
CT	computed tomography
CTLA4	cytotoxic lymphocyte–associated antigen 4
CTPA	computed tomographic pulmonary angiography
CVP	central venous pressure
CXR	chest X-ray
DBD	donation after brain-stem death
DCD	donation after circulatory death
DCIS	ductal carcinoma in situ
DCS	damage control surgery
DDAVP	deamino-D-arginine vasopressin
DHCA	deep hypothermic circulatory arrest
DIC	disseminated intravascular coagultion
DIOS	distal intestinal obstruction syndrome
DMSA	dimercaptosuccinic acid
DOPA	dihydroxyphenyl alanine
DST	dexamethasone suppression test
DTC	differentiated thyroid cancer
DTPA	diethylene triamine penta-acetic acid

DVT	deep venous thrombosis		GnRH	gonadotrophin-releasing hormone
EBV	Epstein-Barr virus		GORD	gastroesophageal reflux disease
ECG	electrocardiogram		GPA	granulomatosis with polyangiitis
ECST	European Carotid Surgery Trial		GTN	glyceryl trinitrate
EGFR	epidermal growth factor receptor		HAART	highly active antiretroviral treatment
EGC	early gastric cancer		HALO	haemorrhoidal artery ligation
EMG	electromyography		HALT	hungry, anxious/angry, late, tired
EMR	endoscopic mucosal resection		HAMN	high-grade appendiceal mucinous neoplasms
EMSB	Emergency Management of Severe Burns		HbA1c	glycosylated haemoglobin
ER	oestrogen receptor		HCl	hydrochloric acid
ERAS	Enhanced Recovery After Surgery		HCC	hepatocellular carcinoma
ERCP	endoscopic retrograde cholangiopancreatography		HER2	human epidermal growth factor receptor 2
ESBL	extended spectrum β-lactamase		HGD	high-grade dysplasia
ESD	endoscopic submucosal dissection		HHT	hereditary haemorrhagic telangiectasia
ESR	erythrocyte sedimentation rate		HHV	human herpes virus
ESWL	extracorporeal shock-wave lithotripsy		HIPEC	heated intraperitoneal chemotherapy
EUS	endoscopic or endoluminal ultrasound		HIV	human immunodeficiency virus
EVAR	Endovascular Aneurysm Repair		HLA	human leucocyte antigen
5-FU	5-fluorouracil		HNPCC	hereditary non-polyposis colon cancer
FAP	familial adenomatous polyposis		HoLEP	holmium laser prostatectomy
FAST	focused abdominal sonography for trauma		HPOA	hypertrophic pulmonary osteoarthropathy
FBC	full blood count		HPV	human papilloma virus
FDG	fluorodeoxyglucose		HQIP	Healthcare Quality Improvement Partnership
FEV_1	forced expiratory volume in 1 second		HRT	hormone replacement therapy
FFP	fresh frozen plasma		HSV	herpes simplex virus
FIT	faecal immunochemical test		HTIG	human tetanus immunoglobulin
FNAC	fine-needle aspiration cytology		IBD-U	inflammatory bowel disease unclassified
FOLFOX	folinic acid and oxaliplatin		ICC	interstitial cell of Cajal
FSH	follicle-stimulating hormone		ICP	intracranial pressure
GABA	γ-aminobutyric acid		ICSI	intracytoplasmic sperm injection
GANT	gastrointestinal autonomic nervous tumour		ICU	intensive care unit
GCS	Glasgow Coma Score		IFN	interferon
GEP-NETs	gastroenteropancreatic neuroendocrine tumours		IMA	inferior mesenteric artery
GFR	glomerular filtration rate		IMV	inferior mesenteric vein
GGT	γ-glutamyl transferase		INR	International normalized ratio
GI	gastrointestinal		IPMN	intraductal papillary mucinous neoplasm
GIM	gastrointestinal metaplasia		IPSS	International prostate symptom score
GIST	gastrointestinal stromal tumour		ITU	intensive therapy unit
GLA	γ-linolenic acid		IVC	inferior vena cava
GOJ	gastro-oesophageal junction		IVF	*in vitro* fertilization

IVU	intravenous urogram
JVP	jugular venous pressure
KSHV	Kaposi sarcoma herpes virus
KUB	kidneys, ureters and bladder
LAD	left anterior descending artery
LAMN	low-grade appendiceal mucinous neoplasms
LCIS	lobular carcinoma *in situ*
LDH	lactate dehydrogenase
LGD	low-grade dysplasia
LHRH	luteinizing hormone-releasing hormone
LIF	left iliac fossa
LiDCO	transpulmonary lithium dilution cardiac output
LMWH	low-molecular-weight heparin
LUTS	lower urinary tract symptoms
MAG3	*mercapto-acetyl triglycine*
MAMC	midarm muscle circumference
MCN	mucinous cystic neoplasm
MDT	multidisciplinary team
MELD	model for end-stage liver disease
MEN	multiple endocrine neoplasia
MHC	major histocompatibility complex
MIBG	meta-iodobenzylguanidine
MIBI	methoxyisobutylisonitrile
MOI	mechanism of injury
mpMRI	multiparametric MRI
MR	magnetic resonance
MRC	Medical Research Council
MRCP	magnetic resonance cholangiopancreatography
MRI	magnetic resonance imaging
MRSA	methicillin-resistant *Staphylococcus aureus*
mTOR	mechanistic target of rapamycin
MUST	Malnutrition Universal Screening Tool (ch 3)
NAFLD	non-alcoholic fatty liver disease
NASCET	North American Symptomatic Carotid Endarterectomy Trial
NCEPOD	National Confidential Enquiry into Perioperative Death
NELA	National Emergency Laparotomy Audit
NEWS	National Early Warning Score
NEN	neuroendocrine neoplasms

NHS	National Health Service
NICE	National Institute of Health and Care Excellence
NG	nasogastric
NOACs	novel oral anticoagulants
NPI	Nottingham Prognostic Index
NSAIDs	non-steroidal anti-inflammatory drugs
NSCLC	non-small cell lung cancer
NSGCT	non-seminomatous germ cell tumour
NST	no special type
OCP	oral contraceptive pill
OPG	orthopantomogram
OPSI	overwhelming post-splenectomy infection
PAC	plasma aldosterone concentration
PBC	primary biliary cholangitis
PCI	percutaneous coronary intervention
pcr	pathologic complete response
PDE5	phosphodiesterase type 5
PDGFA	platelet-derived growth factor receptor α
PDL	programmed death ligand
PE	pulmonary embolism
PEC	percutaneous endoscopic colostomy
PEG	polyethylene glycol
PEG	percutaneous endoscopic gastrostomy
PET	positron emission tomography
PI_RADS	prostate imaging reporting and data system
PICC	peripherally inserted central catheter
PN	parenteral nutrition
PNET	primitive neuroectodermal tumour
POEM	per oral endoscopic myotomy
POSSUM	Physiological and Operative Severity Score for the enUmeration of Mortality and Morbidity
PPE	personal protective equipment (ch 2)
PPGL	Phaeochromocytoma and paraganglioma
PPP	patient, procedure and people
PR	progesterone
PRA	plasma renin activity
PRC	plasma renin concentration
PSA	prostate-specific antigen
PSC	primary sclerosing cholangitis
PT	prothrombin time

PTA	percutaneous transluminal angioplasty		TCC	transitional cell carcinoma
PTC	percutaneous transhepatic cholangiography		TED	thromboembolism deterrent
			TEVAR	thoracic endovascular aortic repair
PTCA	percutaneous transluminal coronary angioplasty		TIA	transient ischaemic attack
			TIPS	transjugular intrahepatic portosystemic shunt
PTFE	polytetrafluoroethylene			
PTH	parathormone		TNF	tumour necrosis factor
PUJ	pelviureteric junction		TNM	tumour node metastasis
PV	portal vein		TOE	transoesophageal echocardiography
RIF	right iliac fossa		TPA	tissue plasminogen activator
SAH	subarachnoid haemorrhage		TPN	total parenteral nutrition
SBP	spontaneous bacterial peritonitis		TRAM	transverse rectus abdominis myocutaneous
SCLC	small-cell lung cancer		TRH	thyrotrophin-releasing hormone
SDHX	succinate dehydrogenase subunit genes		TRUS	transrectal ultrasound
SDM	shared decision-making		TSH	thyroid-stimulating hormone
SGA	Subjective Global Assessment		TUR	transurethral resection
SGOT	serum glutamic oxaloacetic transaminase (synonymous with AST)		UC	urothelial carcinoma
			UC	ulcerative colitis
SGPT	serum glutamic pyruvic transaminase (synonymous with ALT)		UFH	unfractionated heparin
			UKELD	United Kingdom Model for end-stage liver disease
SIADH	syndrome of inappropriate antidiuretic hormone			
			UW	University of Wisconsin
SLE	systemic lupus erythematosus		VAB	vacuum-assisted biopsy
SLN	sentinel lymph node		VAC	vacuum-assisted closure
SMA	superior mesenteric artery		VATS	video-assisted thoracoscopic surgery
SMV	superior mesenteric vein		VAWCM	vacuum-assisted wound closure device with mesh-mediated fascial traction
SORT	Surgical Outcome Risk Tool			
SSI	surgical site infection		VEGF	vascular endothelial growth factor
SV	splenic vein		VEGFR-3	vascular endothelial growth factor receptor 3
SVT	superficial vein thrombosis			
TAD	targeted axillary dissection		VET	venous thromboembolism
TB	tuberculosis		VIP	vasoactive intestinal polypeptide
T3	tri-iodothyronine		VISA	vancomycin-intermediate *Staphylococcus aureus*
T4	tetra-iodothyronine, thyroxine			
TACE	transarterial chemoembolization		VRE	vancomycin-resistant *Enterococcus*
TAE	tumour embolisation		VRSA	Vancomycin-resistant *Staphylococcus aureus*
TAP	transversus abdominus plane			
TAVI	transaortic valve implantation		WHO	World Health Organisation

About the companion website

This book is accompanied by a companion website.

www.wiley.com/go/Watson/GeneralSurgery14

The website features:
- Interactive multiple choice and short-answer questions
- Case Studies
- Extra images and photographs
- Biographies

Surgical strategy

Justin Davies

Learning objectives

✓ To understand the principles of taking a clear history, performing an appropriate examination, presenting the findings and formulating a management plan for diagnosis and subsequent investigations and treatment.

✓ To understand the common nomenclature used in surgery.

The principles of assessing patients referred to a surgical team has changed little in recent times. These include:

1 *Taking an accurate history.*
2 *Examination of the patient.*
3 *Accurate and contemporaneous documentation (written and/or electronic).*
4 *Constructing a differential diagnosis.* Ask the question 'What diagnoses would best explain this clinical picture?'
5 *Special investigations.* Which laboratory and imaging tests are required to confirm or refute the clinical diagnosis?
6 *Management.* Decide on the management of the patient, including provision of adequate analgesia. Remember that this will include reassurance, explanation, and good communication skills.

History and examination

Development of clinical skills is of paramount importance in all aspects of medicine and surgery. In some circumstances, excessive reliance on special

Ellis and Calne's Lecture Notes in General Surgery, Fourteenth Edition.
Edited by Christopher Watson and Justin Davies.
© 2023 John Wiley & Sons Ltd. Published 2023 by John Wiley & Sons Ltd.
Companion website: www.wiley.com/go/Watson/GeneralSurgery14

investigations and extensive imaging may be unnecessary. It is important to remember that the patient may be apprehensive and will often be in pain, especially when presenting as an emergency. Attending to these issues is an especially important aspect of good clinical care.

The history

The history should be an accurate reflection of what the patient has said. It is important to ask open questions such as 'When were you last well?' and 'What happened next?' rather than closed questions such as 'Do you have chest pain?' If you have a positive finding, it is important to explore this further with more directed questioning, for example, 'When did it start?' 'What makes it better, and what makes it worse?' 'Where did it start and where did it go?' 'Did it come and go, or was it constant?' If the symptom is characterized by bleeding, ask about what sort of blood (e.g. fresh, bright red, dark red), when it started, how much, whether there were clots, whether it was mixed in with food/faeces and whether it was associated with pain. Remember that most patients come to see a general surgeon, particularly in the emergency setting, because of abdominal pain or bleeding (Table 1.1). You will need to find out as much as you can about the presenting symptoms.

Keep in mind that the patient may have little accurate anatomical knowledge. They might say 'my stomach

Table 1.1 Examples of important facts to determine in patients with pain and rectal bleeding

Pain	Rectal bleeding
Exact site	Estimation of amount (often inaccurate)
Radiation	Timing of bleeding
Length of history	Colour – bright red, dark red, black
Periodicity	Accompanying symptoms – pain, vomiting (haematemesis)
Nature – constant/colicky	Associated features – fainting, shock, etc.
Severity	Blood mixed in stool, lying on surface, on toilet paper, in toilet bowl
Relieving and aggravating factors	
Accompanying features (e.g. jaundice, vomiting, haematuria)	

hurts', but this may be due to lower chest or periumbilical pain – it is important to ask them to point to the site of the pain. Bear in mind that they may be pointing to a site of referred pain, and a vague description such as 'back pain' will need further exploration and clarification as to where it is in the back – the sacrum or lumbar, thoracic or cervical spine, or possibly the loin or subscapular regions. Exploring pain outside of the abdomen is important, particularly shoulder pain. This may, for example, suggest referred pain from the diaphragm or gallbladder.

It is often useful to consider the viscera in terms of their embryology. Thus, epigastric pain is generally from foregut structures such as the stomach, duodenum, liver, gallbladder, spleen and pancreas; periumbilical pain is midgut pain from the small bowel and ascending colon, including the appendix; suprapubic pain is hindgut pain, originating in the colon, rectum and other structures of the cloaca such as the bladder,

uterus and Fallopian tubes (Figure 1.1). Testicular pain may also be periumbilical, reflecting the intra-abdominal origin of these organs before their descent into the scrotum – this is exemplified by the child with testicular torsion who initially complains of pain in the centre of their abdomen.

The examination

Remember the classic quartet in this order:

1   Inspection.
2   Palpation.
3   Percussion.
4   Auscultation.

Careful inspection is always time well spent. Inspect the patient generally, as to how they lie and breathe. Are they tachypnoeic because of a chest infection or in response to a metabolic acidosis? Look at the

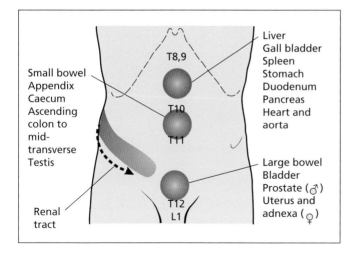

Figure 1.1 Location of referred pain for the abdominal organs.

patient's hands and feel the pulse. Asking the patient to walk may be revealing in someone with claudication or in assessment of general fitness.

Only after careful inspection should palpation start. If you are examining the abdomen in the emergency setting, it is important to ask the patient to cough. This is a surrogate test of rebound tenderness and indicates where the site of inflammation is within the peritoneal cavity. It is often helpful to examine the 'normal' or non-symptomatic side first, be it the abdomen, hand, leg or breast. Look carefully at the patient's face while you palpate, as this may provide subtle clues regarding discomfort or tenderness. If there is a lump, decide which anatomical plane it lies within. Is it in the skin, in the subcutaneous tissue, in the muscle layer or, in the case of the abdomen, in the underlying cavity? Is the lump pulsatile, expansile or mobile?

Documenting medical notes

We practice in an era where electronic patient records are becoming more commonplace, although currently the UK still has the majority of hospitals with paper-based medical records. The number with electronic records will continue to increase over time.

Always write or type your findings completely and accurately in a contemporaneous fashion. Start by recording the date and time of the assessment and check that you have the correct patient's notes open. Record all the negative as well as positive findings. Avoid abbreviations where possible since they may mean different things to different people; for example, PID – you may mean pelvic inflammatory disease, but the next person might interpret it as a prolapsed intervertebral disc. Use the appropriate surgical terminology (Table 1.2).

Table 1.2 Common prefixes and suffixes used in surgery

Prefix	Related organ/structure
angio-	blood vessels
arthro-	a joint
cardio-	heart
cholecysto-	gallbladder
coelio-	peritoneal cavity
colo- and colon-	colon
colpo-	vagina
cysto-	urinary bladder
gastro-	stomach
hepato-	liver
hystero-	uterus
laparo-	peritoneal cavity
mammo- and masto-	breast
nephro-	kidney
oophoro-	ovary
orchid-	testicle
rhino-	nose
thoraco-	chest
Suffix	**Procedure**
-centesis	surgical puncture, often accompanied by drainage, e.g. thoracocentesis
-desis	fusion, e.g. arthrodesis
-ectomy	surgical removal, e.g. colectomy
-oscopy	visual examination, usually through an endoscope, e.g. laparoscopy
-ostomy	creating a new opening (mouth) on the surface, e.g. colostomy
-otomy	surgical incision, e.g. laparotomy
-pexy	surgical fixation, e.g. orchidopexy
-plasty	to mould or reshape, e.g. angioplasty; also to replace with prosthesis, e.g. arthroplasty
-rrhaphy	surgically repair or reinforce, e.g. herniorrhaphy

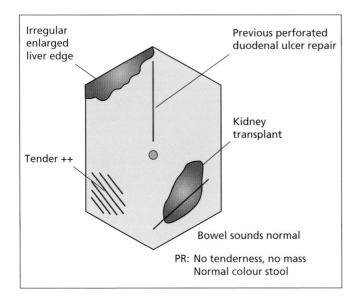

Figure 1.2 Example of how to record abdominal examination findings.

Illustrate your examination unambiguously with simple drawings when possible – use anatomical reference points and measure the diameter of any lumps accurately. When drawing abdominal findings, use a hexagonal representation (Figure 1.2). A continuous line implies an edge; shading can represent an area of tenderness or the site where pain is experienced. If you can feel all around a lump, draw a line to indicate this; if you can feel only the upper margin, show only this. Annotate the drawings with your findings (Figure 1.2). At the end of your notes, write a single paragraph summary and make a diagnosis or record a differential diagnosis. Outline a management plan and state what investigations should be done, indicating those which you have already arranged. Sign your notes and print your name, position and contact details, with the time and date recorded.

Case presentation

The purpose of presenting a case is to convey to your colleagues the salient clinical features, diagnosis or differential diagnosis, management, and investigations of the patient. The presentation should ideally be succinct and to the point, containing important positive and negative findings. At the end of a case presentation, the listening team should have an excellent word picture of the patient and their problems, what needs to be monitored and what plans you have for management.

2

Human factors in surgery

Peter A. Brennan

Learning objectives

✓ To understand the factors that can affect safe surgical practice.
✓ To know what measures to take to mitigate risks in surgery.

What are human factors?

There are many definitions of this term, but a simple one to remember is how we interact with each other (in teams), the systems in which we work, our variability and the factors that affect our performance and those of team members. In healthcare, human factors application can lead to improved patient safety, better team working and staff morale. Important elements of human factors also include situational awareness, effective team working, safe and effective communication, and good leadership. Furthermore, by recognizing how both physical and mental performance deteriorate over time helps to consolidate their importance.

As humans, we regularly make mistakes, with an average of five to seven simple errors affecting each of us every day. These might be something simple such as forgetting a wallet or a mobile phone when leaving for work because of a distraction. While these errors or omissions might be annoying, error in healthcare is a cause of significant patient harm and mortality. We can never completely eliminate error, and as the above-mentioned examples demonstrate, it is a familiar part of everyday life. The term 'never event' has been coined to describe occurrences that should not occur in a healthcare setting and includes wrong site surgery, retained instruments and swabs, and incorrect naso-gastric tube placement. A 'never event' is somewhat of a misnomer as error can never be completely eliminated, but the chances of error occurring can be minimized.

The Roman Philosopher Cicero (106–43 BC) wrote 'anyone is liable to err (make a mistake), but only a fool persists in error'. Learning from mistakes and sharing lessons widely with others is one of the most important elements to improving patient safety across healthcare.

Error in healthcare

The interplay of human error and human factors in clinical incidents (including factors that have their origins in hospitals where we work) is becoming more widely understood. It is often more than one issue (or layer) that leads to error, and this is readily demonstrated by the well-known Swiss cheese model (Figure 2.1).

Often, factors are multifactorial and take place simultaneously – recognizing this fact is the first step to understanding human factors in surgery. These multifactorial issues include ones that affect us as individuals, such as tiredness, repetition, stress, the effects of distraction and multi-tasking. Other factors can occur as part of team working, and these include poor communication or leadership, loss of situational awareness, and steep (or flat) authority gradients. The introduction of the World Health Organisation

Ellis and Calne's Lecture Notes in General Surgery, Fourteenth Edition.
Edited by Christopher Watson and Justin Davies.
© 2023 John Wiley & Sons Ltd. Published 2023 by John Wiley & Sons Ltd.
Companion website: www.wiley.com/go/Watson/GeneralSurgery14

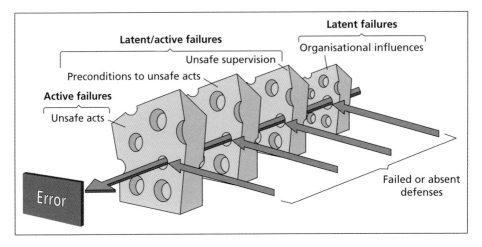

Figure 2.1 The Swiss cheese model of human error. Each slice can act as a barrier.

(WHO) surgical checklist (Figure 2.2) has improved attitudes towards pre-surgery briefing and patient safety, and the benefits of recognizing and applying these human factors principles in surgery are well known.

One in 20 hospital admissions has some form of error, and of these one in 20 are serious (i.e. one in 4,000 admissions). The operating theatre is known to be one of the most potentially error-prone places in the hospital as a result of high patient turnover, site-specific treatments, many heterogeneous surgical procedures, staff limitations and unfamiliar teams.

What are the different types of error and failure?

The Human Factors Analysis and Classification System (HFACS) categorizes failure across four broad domains:

1 Organizational influences.
2 Unsafe supervision.
3 Preconditions to unsafe acts.
4 Unsafe acts.

All four domains can be applied to the Swiss cheese model (Figure 2.1). Failures at each level may be active (decisions, actions or attitudes by individuals or surgical teams) or latent (results of deficiencies with the hospital or management team). Examples of failures in the clinical setting that can have their origin in the employing organization include pressures of overbooked clinics or operating theatre sessions, meeting clinical and hospital targets and prolonged working hours without breaks. Medical error may, therefore, begin to develop well before the actual event itself (such as wrong site surgery) as a result of institutional failure.

What human factors in surgery should we be thinking about?

Table 2.1 summarizes some important human factors that can contribute to and ultimately lead to surgical error, as categorized by the HFACS. These include factors that affect us as individuals, such as tiredness and fatigue; nutritional status; emotional states, including anger and stress; multi-tasking; and loss of situational awareness. These will now be considered further:

Tiredness and fatigue

Commercial aviation recognizes how tiredness and fatigue can influence personal performance and increase the likelihood of accidents, and as a result, rules are in place for maximum work hours. Tiredness (a state that can only be reversed by sleep) and fatigue (more complex in its aetiology and can be the result of chronic tiredness and/or physical or mental exhaustion) are both found in surgical team members. Both

Before induction of anaesthesia
Ask the patient to confirm his/her identity, procedure, site and consent.
Confirm the operating site has been marked, if applicable.
Confirm the anaesthetic machine and the medication checks are complete.
Confirm the pulse oximeter is working.
Check whether the patient has:
- A known allergy.
- A difficult airway.
- An aspiration risk.
Check the anticipated blood loss, noting particularly if >500 mL (>7 mL/kg for children).

Before skin incision
Team members to introduce themselves by their name and role.
Confirm the patient's procedure and where the incision will be made.
Confirm whether antibiotic prophylaxis has been given or prescribed.
Surgeon to identify:
- Critical or non-routine steps.
- How long the case will take.
- The anticipated blood loss.

Anaesthetist
- Identify any patient-specific concerns.

Nursing and wider theatre team
- Has sterility been confirmed?
- Are there any equipment issues or any concerns?

Imaging
- Has the essential imaging been reviewed, or is it displayed?

Before the patient leaves the operating room
Nurse confirms:
- The completion of instrument, swab and needle count.
- The correct labelling of specimens.
- The identification and reporting of any equipment problems.
Surgeon, anaesthetist and nurse identify key concerns for recovery and management of the patient.

Figure 2.2 The WHO surgical safety checklist.

can reduce complex cognitive tasks, decision-making and situational awareness as well as impairing our technical and physical performance. The value of taking regular short breaks, for example, during a long and complex 8-hour operation is not only beneficial for individuals and teams but may also prevent errors. Most of us would not drive for 8 hours non-stop, so why can it be deemed safe to do so for surgery? One useful fact to remember is that our cognitive function after being awake for 18 hours is like being twice over the UK legal alcohol limit for driving. Increasingly, employing hospitals recognize that tired clinicians are much more likely to make a mistake, not to mention the effects on mood and general well-being. No one else knows how an individual feels, and if they have been operating throughout the night and are expected to work the following day, the few words 'I don't feel safe' can be very powerful when discussing with managerial or other clinical colleagues.

Hydration and nutritional status

Hydration, nutrition and individual recovery are often overlooked human factors but are crucial in the operating theatre to maintain performance. Even small deficits in total body water can have a significant impact on cognitive function, resulting in poorer decision-making, causing sleepiness, apathy, headaches and impatience. For example, a 1–2 kg loss in body water in an average-build individual reduces cognitive function by 15–20%. This tends to happen slowly so that we are not aware our performance is deteriorating. Good

---

Table 2.1 Simplified Human Factors Analysis and Classification System (HFACS) relevant to surgery

The different levels are analogous to the holes in the Swiss cheese model lining up to cause an error.

Organizational influences within the hospital
- Hospital targets and pressures to deliver results (either perceived or real).
- Climate, process and resource management within the hospital.
- Communication, training and recognition by the senior management of human factors responsible for possible errors.

Unsafe supervision
- Inadequate supervision of trainees or other healthcare staff.
- Failure of briefings/complacency with the WHO checklist.
- Failure of the team to know what to do when things go wrong.
- Loss of situation awareness, especially if not recognized by the theatre team.

Preconditions to unsafe acts
- Fatigue, hunger and nutritional status.
- Emotional influences (anger and personal issues) and running late.
- Tiredness, boredom and communication issues, remember HALT – hungry, anxious/angry, late, tired.
- Environmental factors: background noise, distractions, lighting, ambient temperature and humidity.
- Panic.

Unsafe acts (less likely)
- Unfamiliar with changes from what is seen as a 'normal event'.
- Distracting and multi-tasking.
- Operating outside of one's area of expertise or following a long period of no operating (surgical currency).

---

hydration is particularly important if personal protective equipment (PPE) is being worn, as this can increase the rate of perspiration and loss of body water. Water requirements are unique to individuals, and while a multitude of factors, including body mass, ambient temperature, pregnancy and diet, play a role, the minimum requirement is approximately 2 L/ day.

Good and balanced nutrition when distributed over a sensible time period also helps optimize personal performance and supports complex mental and physical tasks over a sustained period. An example of this is a well-balanced, small-portioned meal consisting of complex carbohydrates, protein and healthy fats every 3–4 hours. In contrast, large meals eaten over erratic time periods consisting of simple sugars or processed foods are more likely to produce fluctuating energy levels, which can have a detrimental effect on our work. One only needs to look at athletes to realize how effective good nutrition can be on improving performance. Pre-planned breaks during long operating lists, clinics and on-call periods also ensure enough opportunity can be afforded for all team members to recover.

Emotion and stress

Mental perspective and its impact on work performance needs to be recognized. Powerful emotions such as anger or upset can easily interfere with decision-making while performing a task that requires intense concentration. The operating theatre can itself be an environment that can be stressful for members of the surgical team – many would have witnessed colleagues raise their voices or become angry – one of the reasons being a result of stress or other factors that align. During such times, error is far more likely, not to mention the potential effect of loss of civility on the wider team, which can lead to respect being lost, amongst other negative effects.

The value of pausing during an operation (if it is safe to do so) to address these underlying issues may reduce the likelihood of error. We recommend taking a short break, again if it is safe to do so. Bringing the aforementioned factors together, the easily remembered pneumonic HALT – hunger, anger/anxiety, lateness (or lonely), tiredness – is a powerful reminder of the factors that can lead to surgical error as well as recommending the importance of stopping when one or more of these factors arise. Recognizing the impact of stress and emotion not only helps reduce the risk of error but also benefits surgical training and more effective and happier team working, all of which ultimately improve overall patient management. 'Lonely' has also been included as this word introduces the idea of remembering the value of involving colleagues for complex cases or after

Table 2.2 Situations that might increase the chance of an error in the operating theatre environment

Being aware of the following risk factors for error can help improve situational awareness:
- High physical or mental workloads.
- Interruptions and distractions during key parts of an operation.
- Tasks requiring an 'out of normal' response and/or unanticipated new tasks.
- Multi-tasking.
- Changes in physical environment.

a prolonged period of no operating (during COVID-19, for example). Dual surgeon operating can be very useful in this regard, and not only can this give surgeons confidence, but it can also improve patient outcomes.

Situational awareness

A simple definition of situational awareness is being aware of what is going on around us. Awareness and appreciation of several factors that increase the risk of medical error (Table 2.2) can be used to help improve situational awareness for both individuals and the whole team. Situational awareness is dynamic and can change quickly.

An important concept to be aware of is how situational awareness can change or degrade over time in different circumstances and our ability (or not) to adapt to it. Scenarios in which a surgeon may become fixated on a task, develop tunnel vision and become blind to other factors may readily occur. Surgeons can lose their situational awareness, especially if they have confirmation bias in which they are looking for clues or information to confirm the direction they are following. This could include convincing oneself of an anatomical structure or location when it is something quite different. As a result, many errors have occurred, including, for example, cut bile ducts, ureters and important nerves.

Recognizing the value of situational awareness alongside a well-briefed and subsequently de-briefed team, all of whom feel safe and able to voice their concerns, provides the best environment to reduce the risk of medical error taking place. This way, team members are looking out for each other, thereby improving safety and more effective working. By actively thinking ahead (having the best situational awareness), an error can often be avoided. For example, the best drivers are those who anticipate problems early, thereby avoiding potentially hazardous situations. In a similar way, thinking and discussing with the team about any potential 'what if?' scenarios before an operation

commences can reduce the likelihood of a startle reaction and ensures the team is best prepared.

Patient, Procedure, People

The concept of Patient, Procedure, People (PPP) has recently been introduced. Essentially, it is an adaptation of the aviation mnemonic, aviate, navigate, communicate (ANC). This is a useful way of regaining situational awareness when something does not seem quite right. In some circumstances, it may be the procedure that needs re-discussing first, to help regain situational awareness. In most instances, stepping back from the acute situation (if safe to do so) and discussing with the team is the best way to understand the problem and decide the best course of action.

The team brief, lowering authority gradients and ensuring good communication

The team brief

Patient care is rarely, if ever, performed in isolation from other team members. The introduction of the WHO surgical safety checklist (Figure 2.2) and team brief has brought significant improvements to patient safety in theatre. It involves theatre staff standing together and introducing themselves and their roles. The lead surgeon describes the planned procedure, details any anticipated critical events and confirms that the necessary imaging has been reviewed; the anaesthetist identifies any patient-specific concerns; and the nursing staff ensure they know about any special equipment that may be required.

Enhancing team working, understanding, valuing and reducing hierarchy, all contribute towards safer patient outcomes. The way in which a briefing is conducted is important. It should not be rushed, and from the outset, all team members should feel valued equally and empowered to

Table 2.3 Items to consider during a team briefing
A well-prepared team is advantageous, in that every member knows their role and looks out for their colleagues. It can also help team members to feel valued.
Briefing
Introductions, open culture, 'Please speak up if concerned'.
Leadership, team working and decision-making.
Think about the 'what if?' scenarios that might occur during a procedure.
Identify the major steps and who will be doing what.
Ask 'What am I expected to do if and when something goes wrong?'
Situational awareness – how to intervene when something does not seem right.
Debriefing
A debrief is a powerful way to develop and enhance team working for future operating sessions.
• What went well?
• What should we do differently next time?
• What do you think about my performance today?
• Saying 'Thank you' to the team!

speak up if they have any concerns, without fear of retribution. Table 2.3 provides a summary of items that may be included in both briefing and debriefing sessions. The team brief should also stress the importance of looking out for each other to reduce the likelihood of losing situational awareness and highlighting when factors such as tiredness and stress are observed in others.

Tunnel vision

During periods of intense concentration, surgeons can become tunnel visioned and quickly lose track of time. Several hours can pass, and the reliance on others to keep an eye on the clock and suggest a short break perhaps after 3 hours is good practice.

Distraction

A distraction while you are concentrating can have a negative effect on performance. If there are safety-critical times during the operation, these should be raised at the team brief, and distractions should be kept to a minimum. The sterile cockpit approach (where pilots focus only on flying when below 10,000 ft, with no distractions) is a valuable technique to apply in theatre. A simple distraction such as a telephone call asking for advice during a complex part of an operation significantly raises the risk of error. It is far better to either limit distractions (including noise) during these times or stop and focus on one task at a time instead of multi-tasking.

Debrief

At the end of the operating list, it is good practice to conduct a short debrief. This does not necessarily have to be formal, but it gives an opportunity to discuss what went well and what could be improved next time. The power of saying thank you to the team cannot be emphasized enough. Gaining feedback from other team members on our own performance is also valuable and builds practice and non-technical skills.

Hierarchy

In aviation, the most junior airline pilot is actively encouraged to be able to question the most senior Captain without fear. Similarly, empowering all surgical team members, including medical students, trainees, nurses and non-clinical staff, to voice their concerns ensures a safe working environment for everyone. Of course, there has to be a team leader and hierarchy so that the wider team appreciates who is ultimately responsible. A flat hierarchy is as dangerous as a steep one as no one quite knows who is doing what as there is no leadership. However, what is most important is to know that any team member can speak up, if concerned, without fear and that their concern will be listened to.

Communication

Effective communication between team members is an essential element to good team working and interaction. Ninety percent of communication is non-verbal, so while wearing PPE, instructions may not be heard or understood due to the face being covered and voice being muffled. The regular use of open questions such as: 'What do you think we should do?' and 'What would you suggest here?' are good at bringing the team together. The use of pronouns (e.g. 'pass me *it* or *that*) should be avoided, especially at safety-critical times, and instead, usage of proper nouns to ensure clear instructions (such as the name of a required instrument) is much better. Finally, 'repeat back' is a useful tool to confirm that a message has been heard and understood by the receiver. Just because a team member has said something does not automatically mean that others have heard and understood the message or instruction.

In summary, human factors application is essential to ensure both individuals and teams are best optimized to care for patients. Some elements are just common sense, such as stopping for a short break regularly just as we would do while driving a long distance. However, it can be all too easy to leave common sense at the front door of the hospital when we come to work.

3

Fluid and nutrition management

Lynsey Spillman

Learning objectives

✓ To understand the distribution and composition of body fluids and how these may change following surgery.

✓ To understand the role of perioperative nutrition.

The management of a patient's fluid status is vital to a successful outcome in surgery. This requires preoperative assessment, with resuscitation if required, and postoperative replacement of normal and abnormal losses until the patient can resume a normal diet. This chapter will review the normal state and the mechanisms that maintain homeostasis and will then discuss the aberrations and their management.

Body fluid compartments

In an 'average' person, water contributes 60% to the total body weight: 42 L for a 70 kg man. Forty percent of the body weight is intracellular fluid, while the remaining 20% is extracellular. This extracellular fluid can be subdivided into intravascular (5%) and extravascular or interstitial (15%). Fluid may cross from compartment to compartment by osmosis, which depends on a solute gradient, and by filtration, which is the result of a hydrostatic pressure gradient.

The electrolyte composition of each compartment differs (Figure 3.1). Intracellular fluid has a low sodium

and a high potassium concentration. In contrast, extracellular fluid (intravascular and interstitial) has a high sodium and low potassium concentration. Only 2% of the total body potassium is in the extracellular fluid. There is also a difference in protein concentration within the extracellular compartment, with the interstitial fluid having a very low concentration compared with the high protein content of the intravascular compartment.

Knowledge of fluid compartments and their composition becomes important when considering fluid replacement. In order to fill the intravascular compartment rapidly, a plasma substitute or blood is the fluid of choice. Such fluids, with high colloid osmotic potential, remain within the intravascular space, in contrast to a crystalloid solution such as compound sodium lactate (Hartmann's[1]) solution, which will distribute over the entire extravascular compartment, which is four times as large as the intravascular compartment. Thus, of the original 1 L of Hartmann's solution, only 250 mL would remain in the intravascular compartment. Five percent

---

[1] Alexis Frank Hartmann (1898–1964), Professor of Paediatrics, St Louis Children's Hospital, St Louis, USA. Hartmann added sodium lactate to a physiological salt solution that was developed by Sydney Ringer (1834–1910), Professor of Materia Medica and Therapeutics, University College Hospital, London, and formerly also a physician at Great Ormond Street, London.

Ellis and Calne's Lecture Notes in General Surgery, Fourteenth Edition.
Edited by Christopher Watson and Justin Davies.
© 2023 John Wiley & Sons Ltd. Published 2023 by John Wiley & Sons Ltd.
Companion website: www.wiley.com/go/Watson/GeneralSurgery14

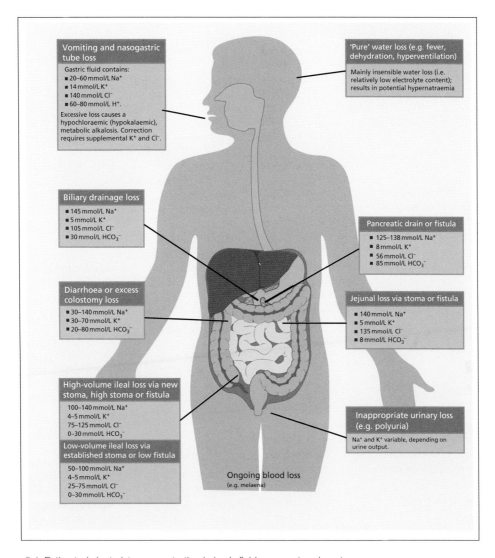

Figure 3.1 Estimated electrolyte concentration in body fluids encountered post surgery.

Source: From National Institute for Health and Care Excellence (NICE) https://www.nice.org.uk/guidance/cg174/chapter/1-recommendations

dextrose, which is water with 50 g of dextrose added to render it isotonic, will redistribute across both intracellular and extracellular spaces.

Fluid and electrolyte losses

In order to calculate the daily fluid and electrolyte requirements, the daily losses should be measured or estimated (Figure 3.1). Fluid is lost from four routes: the kidney, the gastrointestinal tract, the skin and the respiratory tract. Losses from the last two routes are termed insensible losses. In addition, losses from surgical drains should be accounted for. Weighing the patient daily can give a good indication of overall changes in fluid balance.

Normal fluid losses

The kidney

In the absence of intrinsic renal disease, fluid losses from the kidney are regulated by aldosterone and antidiuretic hormone (ADH). These two hormone

	Volume	Na$^+$	K$^+$
Fluid loss	**(mL)**	**(mmol)**	**(mmol)**
Urine	2,000	80–130	60
Faeces	300		
Insensible	400		
Total	2,700		

Table 3.1 Normal daily fluid losses

systems regulate the circulating volume and its osmolarity, and are thus crucial to homeostasis. Aldosterone responds to a fall in glomerular perfusion by salt retention. ADH responds to the increased solute concentration by retaining water in the renal tubules. Normal urinary losses are around 1,500–2,000 mL/day (Table 3.1). The kidneys control water and electrolyte balance closely and can function in spite of extensive renal disease. Damaged kidneys leave the patient exquisitely vulnerable to inappropriate water and electrolyte administration.

The gastrointestinal tract

The stomach, liver and pancreas secrete a large volume of electrolyte-rich fluid into the gut. After digestion and absorption, the waste material enters the colon, where the remaining water is reabsorbed. Approximately 300 mL is lost into the faeces each day.

Insensible losses

Inspired air is humidified in its passage to the alveoli, and much of this water is lost with expiration. Fluid is also lost from the skin, and the total of these insensible losses is around 700 mL/day. This may be balanced by insensible production of fluid, with around 300 mL of 'metabolic' water being produced endogenously.

Abnormal fluid losses

The kidney

Most of the water filtered by the glomeruli is reabsorbed in the renal tubules, so impaired tubular function will result in increased water loss. Resolving acute tubular necrosis (Chapter 43), diabetes insipidus and head injury may result in loss of several litres of dilute urine. In contrast, ectopic production

of ADH by tumours (the syndrome of inappropriate ADH, or SIADH) causes water retention and haemodilution.

The gastrointestinal tract

Loss of water by the gastrointestinal tract is increased in diarrhoea and in the presence of an ileostomy, where colonic water reabsorption is absent.

Vomiting, nasogastric aspiration and fistulous losses result in loss of electrolyte-rich fluid. Disturbance of the acid–base balance may also occur if predominantly acid or alkaline fluid is lost, as occurs with pyloric stenosis and with a pancreatic fistula, respectively.

Large occult losses occur in paralytic ileus and intestinal obstruction. Several litres of fluid may be sequestered in the gut, contributing to the hypovolaemia. Resolution of an ileus is marked by absorption of the fluid, and the resultant hypervolaemia produces a diuresis.

Insensible losses

Hyperventilation, as may happen with pain or chest infection, increases respiratory losses. Losses from the skin are increased by pyrexia and sweating, with up to 1 L of sweat per hour in extreme cases. Sweat contains a large amount of salt.

Effects of surgery

The stress response to surgery includes the release of ADH/vasopressin and catecholamines and activation of the renin–angiotensin system, resulting in oliguria and water retention. In spite of oliguria, the patient may be euvolaemic, hence the need to fully assess the state of hydration before prescribing postoperative fluids. Unnecessary administration of saline, for example, may expand the blood volume and thus reduce the haematocrit; overexpand the interstitial space, resulting in oedema; and provide a salt load that the patient cannot excrete.

Potassium is released by damaged tissues, and its concentration may be further increased by blood transfusion, each unit typically containing in excess of 10 mmol. If renal perfusion is poor and urine output sparse, this potassium will not be excreted and instead accumulates; the resultant hyperkalaemia causes life-threatening arrhythmias. This is the basis of the recommendation that supplementary potassium may not be necessary in the first 48 hours following surgery or trauma.

Prescribing fluids for the surgical patient

The majority of patients require fluid replacement for only a brief period postoperatively until they resume a normal diet. Some require resuscitation preoperatively, and others require replacement of specific losses such as those from a fistula. In severely ill patients, and those with impaired gastrointestinal function, long-term nutritional support is necessary.

Preoperative fluid management

Patients awaiting elective surgery can continue clear fluids up to 2 hours before surgery, unless they have a disorder affecting their gastric emptying (e.g. carcinoma of head of pancreas; diabetes mellitus). Preoperative carbohydrate drinks, 2–3 hours before surgery, have been shown to reduce preoperative anxiety and postoperative nausea and vomiting and are now routine adjuncts to preoperative care in elective surgery.

Intravenous fluid management

Assessment of fluid requirements

Assessment of fluid requirements involves history and examination.

History
- *Sensation of thirst:* implies at least 2% volume depleted
- *Fluid balance*: what were the previous fluid intake and losses?
- *Abnormal losses and their nature*, e.g. nasogastric output

Examination
- *Pulse* – Is there a tachycardia?
- *Jugular venous pressure* – Is the pressure wave visible, and if so, how high is it raised?
- *Capillary refill* – should be less than 2 seconds.
- *Skin turgor.*
- *Blood pressure* – Is there a postural fall?
- *Is there evidence of fluid overload*? Pulmonary oedema or peripheral oedema.
- *Weight,* useful to monitor losses. Minimum of twice a week.
- *Urine output* – hourly monitoring in early postoperative or shocked patients; daily outputs in maintained patients. Daily collections are often not accurate, hence daily weights may be preferred.

Special investigations
- *Full blood count* – a high haemoglobin may represent haemoconcentration.
- *Urea, creatinine and electrolytes* – important to ensure the correct electrolyte replacement to cover losses; raised urea may represent either renal impairment (creatinine also raised), dehydration or blood in the gut.
- *Urinary sodium* – useful in the presence of high volume gastrointestinal losses. Reduced urinary sodium excretion (<30 mmol/L) suggests total body sodium depletion. These measures are not reliable in the presence of renal impairment or diuretic usage.
- *Serum chloride* – useful in patients receiving a lot of normal saline to avoid hyperchloraemia. If present, saline needs to be switched to an alternative fluid with less chloride.
- *Drain fluid electrolytes* – where there are persistently high fluid losses, for example, from high fistulas, it may help to measure the electrolyte content to better judge the replacement fluid needs.

Resuscitation

Thirst, dry mucous membranes, loss of skin turgor, tachycardia and postural hypotension, together with a low jugular venous pressure, suggest a loss of between 5% and 15% of total body water. Fluid losses of under 5% body water are difficult to detect clinically; over 15%, there is marked circulatory collapse.

Fluid replacement in adults should comprise a crystalloid with a high sodium content (130–154 mmol/L, e.g. Hartmann's or 0.9% saline; Table 3.2), with a bolus of 500 mL over less than 15 minutes. Human albumin 4–5% solution may be considered for fluid resuscitation only in patients with severe sepsis. Following a fluid challenge, the patient should be reassessed – did the pulse fall and the jugular venous pressure (JVP) rise, and did the hourly urine output increase?

As an example, consider a 70 kg man presenting with a perforated peptic ulcer. On examination, he is noted to have dry mucous membranes, a tachycardia and slight postural fall in arterial blood pressure. If the loss is estimated at 10% of the total body water, itself 60% of the body weight, the volume deficit is 10% × 60% of 70 kg, or 10% of 42 L = 4.2 L. This loss is largely isotonic (gastric juices and the peritoneal inflammatory response), hence infusion of a balanced crystalloid solution (e.g. Hartmann's solution) is appropriate. A general rule of thumb is to replace half of the estimated loss quickly and then reassess before replacement of the rest.

Routine maintenance fluids

Table 3.1 shows the normal daily fluid losses. Replacement of this lost fluid in a typical adult is achieved by the administration of:

- 25–30 mL/kg/day of water
- 1 mmol/kg/day potassium, sodium and chloride
- 50–100 g/day glucose to limit starvation ketosis – N.B.: this does not meet nutritional needs. 5% dextrose only contains 50g/L dextrose.

Special considerations
- *Obese patients*: adjust the intravenous (IV) fluid prescription to their ideal body weight.
- *Renal failure*: adjust the volume to urine output plus insensible and special losses with care when prescribing potassium as this is not excreted in renal failure.
- *Cardiac failure and the elderly and frail*: these patients are prone to accumulate fluid in the lungs.
- *Malnourished* – see later. These patients are at risk of refeeding syndrome.

A typical prescription would be 25–30 mL/kg/day 0.18% saline in 4% dextrose with 1 mmol/kg potassium.

Therefore, for a 70 kg man, this may comprise 3 L of 4% dextrose/0.18% saline (31 mmol NaCl per litre), with 20 mmol potassium added to each 1 L bag (Table 3.2).

Excessive amounts of hypotonic crystalloid may cause hyponatraemia, particularly in children and the elderly. An alternative regimen involves the use of Hartmann's solution (Table 3.2). Adjustments to the fluid regimen should be based on regular clinical examination, measurement of losses (e.g. urine output), daily weights (to assess fluid changes) and regular blood samples for electrolyte determination. For example, if the patient is anuric, 1 L/day of 5% dextrose without potassium may suffice.

Replacement of special losses

Special losses include nasogastric aspirates, losses from fistulas, diarrhoea and stomas, and covert losses such as occur with an ileus (Figure 3.1). Loss of plasma in burns is considered elsewhere (Chapter 10). All fluid losses should be measured carefully when possible, and this volume added to the normal daily requirements. The composition of these special losses varies, but as a rough guide, replacement of excessive gastric fluid loss with an equal volume of normal

Table 3.2 Electrolyte content of intravenous fluids

Intravenous infusion	Human plasma	0.9% saline	4% dextrose* 0.18% saline	Hartmann's	Plasma-Lyte 148	4% gelatine	5% albumin
Osmolarity	275–295	308	283	278	295	290	300
pH	7.35–7.45	4.5–7.0	4.5	5.0–7.0	6.5–8.0		
Na$^+$ (mmol/L)	135–145	154	31	131	140	145	150
K$^+$ (mmol/L)	3.5–5			5	5		
Ca^{2+} (mmol/L)	2.2–2.6			2			
Mg^{2+} (mmol/L)	0.8–1.2				1.5		
Cl$^-$ (mmol/L)	95–105	154	31	111	98	145	150
Glucose (mmol/L)	3.5–5.5		222 (40g)				
Lactate (mmol/L)	1.0–2.0			29			
HCO$_3^-$ (mmol/L)	23–27						
Acetate (mmol/L)					27		
Gluconate (mmol/L)					23		

Note: Dextrose is the D-isomer of glucose, the only isomer that can be metabolized. Dextrose/saline combinations come in varying mixtures, including 4% dextrose, 0.18% saline, so the mixture must be specified clearly.

saline with extra potassium supplements should suffice; similarly, losses from diarrhoea, ileostomy, small bowel fistulas and ileus should be replaced with Hartmann's solution. Biochemical analysis of the electrolyte content of fistula drainage may be useful.

Nutrition

The catabolic response to surgery

Surgery elicits a stress and inflammatory response, which causes catabolism of glycogen, fat and protein. The stress response is proportional to the magnitude of surgical trauma and is necessary to achieve healing and recovery, but without sufficient nutritional reserve or support, poor outcomes are more likely. Measures to reduce the stress of surgery, such as enhanced recovery programs, have been shown to minimize catabolism, improve recovery and reduce complications of surgery.

Malnutrition and malnutrition risk

Many patients are well nourished and recover good dietary intake quickly after surgery and, therefore, do not require nutritional support. Some patients are malnourished prior to surgery or at risk of becoming malnourished following surgery.

Malnutrition is a state in which a deficiency of nutrients, such as energy, protein, vitamins and minerals, causes adverse effects on body composition, function or clinical outcome. Malnutrition lowers resistance to infections, impairs wound healing, delays functional recovery and increases postoperative mortality.

Risk factors for malnutrition

Patients at risk of malnutrition include those with health conditions that affect appetite, nutrient absorption and metabolism, such as Crohn's disease, gastrointestinal cancer, end-stage liver disease and cystic fibrosis. Dysphagia, social isolation, low income and older age are also risk factors for malnutrition. Surgery itself is a risk factor for malnutrition, particularly major or complicated surgery.

Screening for malnutrition

Identifying patients at risk of malnutrition

There are validated screening tools to identify patients *at risk of malnutrition*, such as the Malnutrition Universal Screening Tool (MUST[2]). All patients should be screened on admission to hospital and screening repeated weekly. Patients at risk of malnutrition must commence a nutrition treatment plan, which should include referral to a dietitian for those at high risk.

Diagnosing malnutrition

Tools *to diagnose malnutrition*, such as the Subjective Global Assessment (SGA[3]), can be used when malnutrition risk has been identified. Malnutrition may be less obvious in patients living with obesity but equally important to identify and treat as for patients with a lower body mass index (BMI).

Malnutrition can be diagnosed based on a combination of phenotypic and aetiologic criteria, for example:

- *Weight loss* of >5% within past 6 months, or >10% beyond 6 months.
- *BMI < 20 kg/m^2* in those under 70 years of age or <22 kg/m^2 aged 70 years or older.
- *Reduced muscle mass* based on body composition methods, including imaging, physical examination, or anthropometric measures such as mid-arm muscle circumference (MAMC). Functional assessment, such as handgrip strength, can support assessment as loss of muscle mass is often preceded or accompanied by reduced muscle function.
- *Reduced food intake or absorption.*
- *Disease burden and inflammation.*

Sarcopenia, cachexia and frailty

Sarcopenia, cachexia, frailty and malnutrition are overlapping syndromes that can present in the same surgical patient and are associated with worse postoperative outcomes. The definitions of these syndromes are debated and evolving.

- *Sarcopenia* has been defined as low muscle mass and function.
- *Cachexia* is a metabolic syndrome occurring with underlying illness and characterized by loss of muscle with or without loss of fat.

---

[2] http://www.bapen.org.uk/screening-and-must/must-calculator

[3] Described in the *Journal of Parenteral and Enteral Nutrition*, 1987;11:8-13.

- *Frailty* is characterized by loss of functional and cognitive reserves that increases vulnerability to adverse health outcomes.

Prehabilitation

Prehabilitation is the process of enhancing an individual's capacity to withstand surgery. It has a multimodal approach, including medical optimization, exercise, nutrition support, and stress and anxiety reduction prior to surgery. Benefits include reduced length of stay and postoperative pain with fewer postoperative complications. Prehabilitation may be included as part of the Enhanced Recovery After Surgery (ERAS) service (see below). Prehabilitation nutrition support may include dietary counselling, treatment of malnutrition, weight management and improved glycaemic control. There may be a standardized period of oral nutritional supplement drinks and carbohydrate loading.

Enhanced recovery after surgery (ERAS)

Enhanced recovery programs aim to optimize pre-, intra- and postoperative care to improve recovery and shorten length of hospital stay for surgical patients. ERAS protocols include multimodal, evidence-based processes that modify the physiological and psychological responses to major surgery. The key principles include:

- Preoperative counselling.
- Preoperative and early postoperative nutrition.
- Avoidance of prolonged fasting.
- Carbohydrate loading up to 2 hours preoperatively.
- Standardized anaesthetic and analgesic regimens (avoiding opiates where possible).
- Avoidance of surgical drains and tubes when possible.
- Avoidance of salt and water overload.
- Early, goal-orientated mobilization.

In addition, urinary catheters and nasogastric tubes (if used) are removed as soon as possible after surgery.

Postoperative nutrition

Early postoperative nutrition should be part of routine care. If the gastrointestinal tract is functioning satisfactorily, oral intake is the preferred route for nutritional support and can often be started as early as the first postoperative day. Early nutrition in abdominal surgery has been shown to enhance gastrointestinal function, reduce the risk of postoperative ileus and shorten length of stay, with no increased risk of postoperative complications.

Nutrition support is indicated for patients with malnutrition and those at risk of malnutrition. Artificial nutrition support should be initiated without delay for patients who are likely to be unable to eat for five days or who are anticipated to meet less than 50% of their nutritional requirements for seven days, for example, due to complications or prolonged intensive care unit (ICU) stay.

Nutrition support may be through a combination of food, oral nutritional supplements, fine bore nasogastric or nasojejunal tube, gastrostomy, jejunostomy or parenteral nutrition (PN), depending on the individual patient's need. The oral and/or enteral route is the preferred method of nutrition. Post-pyloric feeding may be indicated in the presence of delayed gastric emptying. Feeding tubes such as gastrostomies and jejunostomies may be indicated if long-term tube feeding is anticipated. Local policies for feeding, including feeding routes, may exist for certain patient groups such as patients undergoing surgery for head and neck cancer.

Energy and protein requirements are calculated on an individual basis, depending on the patient's gender, age, weight, BMI, weight changes, and stress and activity factors. Enteral feeding is usually started continuously over 20–24 hours and may be progressively weaned to support increasing oral intake of food. Formula is chosen based on individual patient requirements from a range, including standard whole protein formulas, with and without fibre, low volume, low electrolyte, high protein, elemental, high medium-chain triglycerides, and milk or lactose-free. Additional energy, protein and fibre boluses can be provided to help meet nutritional requirements.

Parenteral nutrition

PN is administered, with guidance from the intestinal failure team, when nutrition cannot be provided through the gastrointestinal tract, for example, with gastrointestinal obstruction, high-output fistula, prolonged ileus or malabsorption. Combinations of enteral and parenteral nutrition should be considered, when possible, to help maintain gut integrity.

PN is usually administered via a catheter in a central vein because of the high osmolarity of the solutions used; there is a high risk of phlebitis in smaller veins with lower blood flow. Usual timing is continuous infusion over 24 hours, with cyclical PN (e.g. 12- to 16-hour infusion) used more often for patients requiring long-term PN. Commonly, the protein:fat:carbohydrate calorie ratio approximates to 20:30:50%, but the glucose:fat calorie ratio may be increased, for example, due to hyperlipidemia and fatty liver, which is sometimes accompanied by cholestasis. Commercially available 'ready-made' nutrition mixtures are commonly used with trace elements and vitamins added. Non-standard formulations, known as 'scratch' or 'tailored' bags, can be made to exact specifications for amount of carbohydrate, fat, protein and electrolytes but vary according to physical and chemical stability, which is assessed by the PN pharmacist. PN is continued in the postoperative period until gastrointestinal function returns. Occasionally, parenteral feeding may be necessary on a long-term basis, and some patients require long-term or even lifelong PN at home.

Complications of PN

Complications of PN include:

- *Sepsis*: use of dedicated lines inserted using aseptic techniques, aseptic non-touch techniques when changing bags, and appropriate preparation and storage of feeds contribute to reducing rates of infection.
- *Thrombosis*: may occur on any indwelling venous catheter and in patients requiring long-term PN; this is a major cause of morbidity. If ongoing parenteral feeding access is required, anticoagulation should be lifelong after a first episode of thrombotic venous occlusion. Consideration should be given to anticoagulation for all patients fed parenterally if at risk.
- *Hyponatraemia*.
- *Hyperglycaemia* is common and nearly always requires insulin if the glucose infusion rate is to be maintained. If the calorie intake is not crucial, it may be possible to change the feed to one with lower glucose content.

- *Liver damage:* fatty liver. Encouraging enteral intake, reducing the lipid load, ensuring maximum carbohydrate oxidation is not exceeded and giving cyclical PN may help correct liver function or prevent further dysfunction.

Refeeding syndrome

Refeeding syndrome is a range of life-threatening clinical and biochemical abnormalities that arise in response to nutrition delivery, including cardiac failure, pulmonary oedema, dysrhythmias, acute circulatory fluid overload or depletion, electrolyte derangement and hyperglycaemia. Refeeding syndrome develops because of the biochemical shift from starvation metabolism to fed metabolism. During refeeding there is a switch in metabolism from fat to carbohydrate with consequent insulin release, stimulated by the glucose load. Insulin release stimulates the sodium potassium ATPase pump (which requires magnesium as a cofactor). This drives potassium into the cells and sodium out. Carbohydrate load and insulin release stimulate phosphate shifts into the cells. Phosphate depletion is associated with increased urinary magnesium excretion. These phenomena lead to low extracellular phosphate, magnesium and potassium concentrations.

Enteral and parenteral feeding are more likely to precipitate refeeding syndrome. Risk factors include low BMI; little or no nutritional intake for 5 or more days; weight loss; low potassium, phosphate or magnesium prior to feeding; a history of alcohol excess; and a drug history, including insulin, chemotherapy, antacids or diuretics. Refeeding syndrome is managed through gradual introduction of nutrition; monitoring and replacement of electrolytes; vitamin supplementation; and monitoring fluid balance, pulse rate and clinical status.

Nutrition: A multidisciplinary approach

Good nutritional care of the surgical patient requires a multidisciplinary approach. Referral to a dietitian is essential for patients with malnutrition or requiring nutrition support.

4

Preoperative assessment

Hemantha Alawattegama

Learning objectives

✓ To be aware of the principles of preoperative assessment.

✓ To be able to identify and manage likely complicating factors prior to surgery.

The pathway for patients from surgical consult to leaving hospital after their operation has changed significantly over time. The perioperative service now is a multi-disciplinary team (MDT) of surgery, anaesthesia, medicine (involving elderly care specialists and other medical specialties, as needed), pharmacy, specialist nurses and allied healthcare professionals, including physiotherapists and dieticians, with the emphasis on shared decision-making (SDM). This puts the patient at the centre of decision-making, who, with the clinicians, agrees on the optimal management based on evidence and the individual's wishes and values. The norm for centres is to provide a formalized route of pre-assessment with a nurse-led and doctor-supported service. The surgeon's role in this is imperative, as early identification, referral and intervention can significantly improve outcomes for patients. This involves taking a careful history, ensuring repeated assessment of patients while on a waiting list (for deterioration in health), reassessing the indication for surgery on the day of surgery admission and facilitating the patient to be as fit as possible for the procedure.

Fitness for a procedure needs to be balanced against urgency – the approach to a patient with an acute aortic rupture will be significantly different to an elective liver resection. Nevertheless, a careful assessment of the patient and identification of premorbid conditions provides the best and safest care, allowing focused improvement of pre-existing conditions (when possible), planning of the surgical procedure and the postoperative pathway the patient will follow.

As part of the preoperative programme, Surgery Schools are group sessions to inform patients of what to expect when they come to hospital for their procedure. This is an excellent way of managing patient expectations, alleviating anxieties, informing health changes/adaptation and familiarizing with the environment they will be entering. It also allows patients to prepare for their admission and start beneficial lifestyle changes. These are run as face-to-face group sessions and/or as online sessions.

All patients should complete a self-assessment screening, as a form of clinical triage, as soon as listed for a procedure, which will highlight those who require a greater in-depth assessment and referral to a multi-disciplinary pathway. This is aided by early referral to the Preoperative Assessment Service for patients who are thought to be high risk. All patients should undergo a nurse-led preoperative process with subsequent medical input, as required.

The surgical assessment process can be considered in terms of factors specific to the patient and to the operation.

Patient assessment

In assessing a patient's fitness for surgery, it is worth going through the clerking process with this in mind.

Ellis and Calne's Lecture Notes in General Surgery, Fourteenth Edition.
Edited by Christopher Watson and Justin Davies.
© 2023 John Wiley & Sons Ltd. Published 2023 by John Wiley & Sons Ltd.
Companion website: www.wiley.com/go/Watson/GeneralSurgery14

History of presenting complaint

An emergency presentation may warrant an emergency procedure, so the assessment aims to identify factors that may be a problem during or following surgery. Some problems may be readily identifiable and treated in advance; for example, a history of vomiting or intestinal obstruction would indicate that fluid replacement is necessary, and this can be done swiftly prior to surgery.

In contrast an elective operation, given sufficient time from listing to surgery, can permit much greater levels of optimization in readiness for the procedure.

Past medical history

- *Diabetes* – whether controlled by insulin, oral hypoglycaemics or diet, diabetes may be complicated by gastroparesis (gastric stasis), with a risk of aspiration on induction of anaesthesia despite a preoperative fast.
- *Respiratory disease* – what is the nature of the chest problem, and is the breathing as good as it can be or is the patient in the middle of an acute exacerbation? Does the patient have symptoms of sleep apnoea, and do they use continuous positive airways pressure (CPAP) at home? This may affect where the postoperative care can be delivered.
- *Cardiac disease* – does the patient have angina, and is this stable or unstable? Is there a history of a myocardial infarction, and what was the treatment? What is their exercise tolerance?
- *Rheumatoid arthritis* – may be associated with an unstable cervical spine, so a cervical spine X-ray is indicated.
- *Sickle cell disease* – homozygotes for haemoglobin S are prone to sickle crises under general anaesthetic and postoperatively if they become hypoxic and/or dehydrated – liaison with the local sickle cell service is advisable. Current national guidelines no longer require a routine screening test for patients, but a family history must be sought.

Perioperative care of the elderly

Increasingly, we are faced with an ageing population and pre-existing cognitive impairment, Alzheimer's and other neurological conditions (e.g. Parkinson's disease) that increase the risk of delirium in the postoperative period. It is, therefore, vital that patients are screened to assess their cognitive function and

potential for the postoperative confusional state. Many centres now run specific multi-disciplinary preoperative clinics for assessment of patients at risk, allowing planning for their care, which includes stratification of drugs, appropriate anaesthetic technique and appropriate postoperative environment.

Abrupt cessation of medication for Parkinson's disease in the perioperative period can result in a rapid deterioration in function. The Parkinson's disease specialist nurse should be informed of the admission allowing planning of the inpatient stay.

Frailty

Frailty is related to the ageing process by which multiple body systems lose their in-built reserves. Frail patients are vulnerable to adverse health outcomes, and understanding the challenges and modifying their perioperative course can result in significant improvements in outcomes. To assist this, there are several screening assessment tools developed that can be used, for example, the Clinical Frailty Scale. Referral to the perioperative MDT is essential for patients at risk.

Past surgical history

- *Nature of previous operations* – what has been done before? What is the current anatomy? What problems were encountered last time? Ensure a copy of the previous operation note(s) is available.
- *Complications of previous surgery*, for example, deep vein thrombosis, methicillin-resistant *Staphylococcus aureus* (MRSA) wound infection or wound dehiscence.

Past anaesthetic history

- *Difficult intubation* – usually recorded in the previous anaesthetic note, but the patient may also have been warned of previous problems.
- *Aspiration during anaesthesia* – may suggest delayed gastric emptying (e.g. due to diabetes), suggesting that a prolonged fast and airway protection (cricoid pressure) are indicated prior to induction.
- *Suxamethonium apnoea* – deficiency of pseudo-cholinesterase resulting in sustained paralysis following the 'short-acting' muscle relaxant suxamethonium (Scoline). It is usually inherited

(autosomal dominant), therefore there may be a family history.

- *Malignant hyperpyrexia* – a rapid excessive rise in temperature following exposure to anaesthetic drugs due to an uncontrolled increase in skeletal muscle oxidative metabolism and associated with muscular contractions and rigidity, sometimes progressing to rhabdomyolysis; it carries a high mortality (at least 10%). Most of the cases are due to a mutation in the ryanodine receptor on the sarcoplasmic reticulum, and susceptibility is inherited in an autosomal dominant pattern, so a family history should be sought.

Social history

- *Smoking* – ideally, patients should stop smoking before any general anaesthetic to improve their respiratory function and reduce their thrombogenic potential.
- *Alcohol* – a history suggestive of dependency should be sought, and management of the perioperative period instituted using chlordiazepoxide to avoid acute alcohol withdrawal syndrome.
- *Substance abuse* – in particular, a history of intravenous drug usage should be sought, and appropriate precautions taken.

Medication

Most medications should be continued on admission. Drugs acting on the cardiovascular system should usually be continued and given on the day of surgery. The following are examples of drugs that should give cause for concern and prompt discussion with and between the surgeon and anaesthetist.

- *Oral anticoagulants* (e.g. warfarin, dabigatran, apixaban, rivaroxaban) – this is a balance between the risk of a thromboembolic event and perioperative bleeding. Due to the latter, when possible, these should be stopped before surgery. The indication for anticoagulation is important: a brief period without anticoagulation for atrial fibrillation is reasonable but not for mitral valve prosthesis. If continued anticoagulation is required, then convert to a low molecular weight heparin (LMWH) or unfractionated heparin (UFH) infusion (bridging therapy). Further discussion with cardiology and haematology specialists is essential where doubt exists.

- *Aspirin and clopidogrel* cause increased bleeding by irreversibly blocking platelet activity and, therefore, need to be stopped 7–10 days prior to surgery to reverse their effect.
  - *The risk of bleeding with aspirin* (with the exception of high-risk cases such as intracranial and medullary canal surgery) is minimal, and the general guideline is to continue throughout the admission. Aspirin precludes neither the use of neuraxial blockade nor the timing of removal of neuraxial catheters in the postoperative period.
  - *Clopidogrel*, a $P2Y_{12}$ inhibitor, is used primarily in patients who have had a previous cerebrovascular incident, recent acute coronary syndrome or recent percutaneous coronary (or systemic) vascular intervention. Cessation of the drug will depend on the acuity of these events, the risk of an embolic or thrombotic event and the risk of surgical bleeding. Bridging therapy will allow some cover, but LMWH and UFH are not antiplatelet agents. If there is any doubt, a cardiology consultation is recommended.
  - *The combination of aspirin and clopidogrel* is a particular risk and is found primarily in patients within one year of percutaneous coronary intervention (PCI). After the initial year has passed, patients usually continue aspirin alone. The safety of discontinuing these should be discussed with the responsible cardiologist.
- *Oestrogen-containing oral contraceptive pill* is associated with an increased risk of deep vein thrombosis and pulmonary embolism; consideration should be given to stopping it at least 4 weeks before surgery. The patient should be counselled on appropriate alternative contraception since an early pregnancy risks the teratogenic effects of some of the drugs used in the perioperative period. Progesterone only contraceptives have no additional thromboembolic risk.
- *Steroids* – all glucocorticoid-dependent patients are at risk of adrenal crisis as a consequence of surgical stress or illness, and if left untreated, this can be fatal. Patients in this group fall into three categories:
  - *Primary adrenal insufficiency* – diseases of the adrenal gland (failure of the hormone-producing gland)
  - *Secondary adrenal insufficiency* – deficient adrenocorticotropin hormone secretion by the

pituitary gland or deficient corticotropin-releasing hormone secretion by the hypothalamus (failure of the regulatory centres)
- *Tertiary adrenal insufficiency* – chronic administration of steroids ($\geq$5 mg/day for >1 month) for other disease processes (This is by far the largest group of steroid-receiving patients.)
- All these patients require additional steroid support in addition to their background dosage. Hydrocortisone 100 mg by intravenous injection should be given at induction of anaesthesia in adult patients with adrenal insufficiency from any cause, followed by ongoing hydrocortisone replacement, until the patient can take double their usual oral glucocorticoid dose by mouth. This is then tapered back to their normal dose, depending on the complexity of surgery and gut function.
- *Immunosuppression* – patients are more prone to postoperative infection, and absorption of immunosuppression may be disturbed. Consideration for changing the medications during the perioperative period needs to be discussed with the supervising specialist team.
- *Diuretics* – both thiazide and loop diuretics cause hypokalaemia. It is important to measure the serum potassium in such patients and restore it to the normal range prior to surgery.
- *Monoamine oxidase inhibitors* are not widely used nowadays but do have important side effects such as hypotension when combined with general anaesthesia.

Allergies

It is important to determine clearly the nature of any allergy before condemning a potentially useful drug to the list of allergies. For example, diarrhoea following erythromycin usually reflects its action on the motilin receptor rather than a true allergy, but a skin rash does suggest an allergy such that its use should be avoided. In particular, consider allergies to the following:

- Anaesthetic agents.
- Antimicrobial drugs.
- Skin preparation substances, for example, iodine and chlorhexidine.
- Wound dressings, for example, sticking plaster.
- Latex, present in operating gloves and urinary catheters, for example. Such patients should be operated on with non-latex gloves, and silastic catheters should be used if necessary

Management of pre-existing medical conditions

Diabetes

The aim should always be to minimize alteration of the patient's normal medication pattern for diabetes, minimize the fasting period and maintain normoglycaemia (6–10 mmol/L). The following should be checked in a diabetic patient:

- HbA1c (<69 mmol/mol for elective cases).
- Urea and electrolytes.
- Electrocardiogram (ECG) prior to surgery.

Variable-dose insulin infusions are less commonly used nowadays to control patients' diabetes but may still be needed in emergency surgery, poorly controlled diabetes or where a prolonged postoperative period of 'nil by mouth' is anticipated.

When possible, diabetic patients should be first on an operating list and miss just one meal. Patients with diet-controlled diabetes require no special preoperative treatment, except glucose monitoring. With oral medications, the general rule is that those medications prone to causing hypoglycaemia (meglitinides and sulphonylurea) are omitted on the day of surgery (one dose), while most of the other preparations (e.g. metformin and pioglitazone) can be taken. The oral dose is recommended once normal diet resumes.

Patients on insulin require a more in-depth modification of their treatment, depending on whether they are on a short- or long-acting insulin (or both).

Respiratory disease
Asthma

The degree of respiratory compromise can be readily assessed with a peak flowmeter. Many asthmatic patients will revert to reasonable peak flows between exacerbations, and in the quiescent phases, this may not be indicative of the degree of potential bronchospasm. Documentation of triggers and potential medications to avoid (e.g. non-steroidal anti-inflammatory drugs) and how well controlled the asthma is at present will inform the management.

Other points of history are previous hospital admissions for exacerbation of asthma, previous episodes of ventilation for exacerbation (an indicator of severity) and the need for oral steroids to control symptoms – this may require steroid supplementation in the intra and postoperative period (see later). If time allows, modification of therapy with the addition of a short course of corticosteroids may be indicated – this should be discussed with the patient's respiratory team.

Obstructive pulmonary disease

This is often more of a problem, since there is less reversibility and, even at the patient's best, respiratory reserve might be poor. Consider whether regional anaesthesia is possible, and if not, whether the patient will require postoperative ventilation on an intensive care unit; consider whether the addition of epidural or spinal analgesia would allow better postoperative respiratory function by controlling pain and avoiding opiates. Optimization of therapy, cessation of smoking and physiotherapy both pre- and postoperatively have shown benefit.

Cardiac disease

Angina is not a contraindication to general anaesthesia provided it is stable. An indication of the severity of angina can be gauged by the frequency with which the patient uses glyceryl trinitrate (GTN) preparations for acute attacks, exercise tolerance and co-morbidities (e.g. diabetes). Scrutiny of the patient's cardiac history will guide further preoperative referral and investigations.

Coronary artery revascularization (surgery or stent)

Patients who have had successful coronary artery bypass graft (CABG) or stents for ischaemic heart disease should have better cardiac function than they had prior to this. If CABG surgery or stenting was done some time previously, ascertain whether the patient's symptoms have changed, particularly whether there is any recurrence of angina or breathlessness, suggesting that the graft(s) or stent may have thrombosed or the disease progressed.

Routine ECG may detect abnormalities at rest. To rule out significant cardiac disease, consider stressing the heart, such as with an exercise ECG, stress echocardiogram or radionuclide myocardial perfusion scan.

Local anaesthesia should be considered in all patients with a history of cardiac or respiratory disease.

Other problems

Anaemia

There is increasing evidence that preoperative anaemia is associated with adverse outcomes. Trigger points for investigation and treatment are <120 g/L for women and <130 g/L in men. Treatment is dependent on several altered drug handling factors, not the least time between assessment and surgery (oral iron supplement or intravenous iron infusion), degree of blood loss potentially expected in surgery and co-morbidities.

Bleeding disorders

Patients should be managed in close collaboration with the haematology department. Patients with haemophilia A or B should be given the specific clotting factor replacement.

Obstructive jaundice

Patients with obstructive jaundice often have a prolonged prothrombin time and require vitamin K and either human prothrombin complex (e.g. Beriplex) or fresh frozen plasma (FFP) prior to surgery to correct the abnormality. Any intervention must be discussed with the appropriate clinical team looking after the patient for the condition.

Patients with jaundice are also more prone to infection and poor wound healing. Intraoperatively, it is important to maintain a diuresis with judicious fluid replacement and diuretics (such as mannitol) to prevent acute renal failure (hepatorenal syndrome) to which these patients are susceptible. In the presence of liver impairment, metabolism of some commonly used drugs may be impaired.

Chronic renal failure

Chronic renal failure carries many additional perioperative problems. Electrolyte disturbances are common, particularly hyperkalaemia, as well as anaemia, uraemia (associated impaired platelet function), altered drug handling and challenging vascular access. Impaired fluid handling is complex – if free water is restricted, the inability to concentrate urine results in hypernatraemia and hypertonicity. Conversely, this impaired ability to excrete a sodium load predisposes the patient to volume overload if overhydrated. Balancing fluid status with replacing losses equally is a reasonable starting point.

Venous access should be carefully chosen since such patients may have, or may in the future require, arteriovenous dialysis fistulas fashioned using their cephalic veins. In patients with chronic renal failure, avoid using the arm with an arteriovenous dialysis fistula *in situ* and avoid using cephalic veins.

Operative factors influencing preoperative management

Nature of the surgery

Some operations require special preparation of the patient, such as bowel preparation prior to colorectal surgery or preoperative localization of an impalpable mammographic abnormality prior to breast surgery. Different degrees of fitness are acceptable for different procedures. For example, a patient with severe angina might be a candidate for removal of a sebaceous cyst under a local anaesthetic but not for a complex incisional hernia repair under a general anaesthetic. When the surgery will correct the co-morbidity, different criteria apply; thus, the same patient with angina would be a candidate for a general anaesthetic if it was given to enable myocardial revascularization with aorto-coronary bypass grafts.

Urgency of the surgery

When patients present with life-threatening conditions, the risk–benefit balance often changes in favour of surgical intervention even if there is significant risk attached but where the alternative is probable death. A good example is a patient presenting with a ruptured abdominal aortic aneurysm, in whom death is often an immediate alternative to urgent surgery, and there is little time for preoperative preparation. In many settings, some time is available to make even the smallest of interventions that will help in improved outcomes, for example, nebulizers in patients with asthma, fluid resuscitation and anticoagulation reversal.

Auditing of outcomes in emergency patients is important to improve care and outcomes. The National Emergency Laparotomy Audit (NELA) was established by the Healthcare Quality Improvement Partnership (HQIP) to describe and compare inpatient care and outcomes of patients undergoing emergency laparotomy (in England and Wales). It is a national audit introduced to promote quality improvement, by collecting high-quality comparative data from all National Health Service (NHS) providers. It has significantly improved outcomes by assessing risk before surgery; guiding consent and SDM discussions, including Treatment Escalation Plans; and guiding the seniority of clinicians present for surgery as well as appropriate postoperative levels of care (e.g. intensive care unit immediately after surgery).

Objective operative risk assessment

The ability to have a useful prediction of 30-day mortality and morbidity following surgery allows clinicians the opportunity to better plan patient care. Is the risk too high, should alternative treatments be sought and what pathway should the perioperative period take? Most importantly, it informs the SDM process.

Various scores exist for risk stratification, taking type of surgery, urgency of intervention and patient factors into account. No individual risk predictive system is totally dependable and should not be used in isolation to direct clinical decision-making – this is illustrated by the number of scoring systems available.

Surgical risk assessment

The systems outlined below are an example of the most used.

Two surgical models are the Physiological and Operative Severity Score for the enUmeration of Mortality and Morbidity (POSSUM) and the Surgical Outcome Risk Tool (SORT).

- *POSSUM* (Table 4.1) was developed as a predictive scoring system for surgical mortality and combines information regarding the patient's physiological status and the operative procedure. A subsequent refinement from authors in Portsmouth resulted in P-POSSUM, which is now widely used as an audit tool to compare estimated mortality with actual mortality.

Table 4.1 Factors involved in the estimation of risk using P-POSSUM

Physiological parameters	Operative parameters
Age	Operation severity, e.g. minor, moderate and/or major
Cardiac disease, e.g. heart failure, angina, cardiomyopathy	Number of procedures
Respiratory disease, e.g. degree of exertional dyspnoea	Operative blood loss
ECG, e.g. presence of arrhythmia	Peritoneal soiling
Systolic blood pressure	Presence of malignancy
Heart rate	Urgency, e.g. elective, urgent and/or emergency
Leucocyte count	
Haemoglobin concentration	
Urea concentration	
Sodium concentration	
Potassium concentration	
Glasgow Coma Score	

ECG, electrocardiogram.

Table 4.2 The ASA grading system

ASA grade	Definition	Typical mortality (%)
I	Normal healthy person, no co-morbidity	<0.1
II	Mild systemic disease that does not limit activity, e.g. current smoker, obese, well-controlled hypertension or diabetes	0.3
III	Severe systemic disease that limits activity but is not incapacitating, e.g. poorly controlled diabetes or hypertension, chronic obstructive pulmonary disease (COPD), morbid obesity, alcohol dependence, dialysis-dependent renal failure	2–4
IV	Severe systemic disease that is a constant threat to life, e.g. recent (<3 months) myocardial infarction, stroke, transient ischaemic attack (TIA), severely reduced left ventricular function, shock, sepsis	20–40
V	A moribund patient who is not expected to survive without surgery, e.g. a ruptured abdominal aneurysm, massive trauma	>50

- *SORT*[1] was developed using data from the 2011 National Confidential Enquiry into Perioperative Death (NCEPOD) study, 'Knowing the Risk'. Adding a clinical assessment component, using an experienced clinician or an MDT, has been shown to increase its accuracy (SORT-clinical judgement model). It has an advantage over many existing prediction tools by consisting of solely preoperative variables and allowing rapid and easy data entry.

[1]http://www.sortsurgery.com

Anaesthetic risk assessment

The American Society of Anesthesiologists (ASA) has produced a grading scheme to estimate co-morbidity (Table 4.2). Half of all elective surgery will be in patients of grade I, that is, normal fit individuals with a minimal risk of death. As the patient's ASA grade increases, reflecting increased co-morbidity, the postoperative morbidity and mortality increase.

5

Postoperative complications

Elizabeth Tweedle

Learning objectives

✓ To know the common postoperative complications.

✓ To be aware of measures to prevent complications.

✓ To be familiar with the assessment and management of an acutely unwell surgical patient.

A complication of surgery can be defined as any deviation from the normal postoperative course; this definition also takes into account asymptomatic complications. True complications should be separated from other types of negative outcome following surgery, such as the need for a stoma in bowel surgery or failure to achieve cure in cancer surgery.

Classification

When assessing postoperative patients on the ward, it is essential to utilize a system to identify the most likely complication so that the patient can be managed effectively. The most common methods of classifying complications are according to when they occur and whether they relate directly to the operation or are remote from it.

Time of occurrence

- *Immediate* – within the first 24 hours.
- *Early* – within the first 30 days.

- *Late* – any subsequent period, often long after the patient has left hospital.

Aetiology

- *Local* – involving the operation site itself.
- *General* – affecting any of the other systems of the body, such as respiratory, urological or cardiovascular systems.

These two elements can be combined to categorize complications into a useful scheme such as the one in Table 5.1

Grading the severity of complications

The severity of a complication can be classified in terms of the operation (e.g. blood loss quantification post vascular surgery) or in terms of the effect on the patient. One such example of the latter scheme is that classification proposed by Clavien and Dindo,[1]

Ellis and Calne's Lecture Notes in General Surgery, Fourteenth Edition.
Edited by Christopher Watson and Justin Davies.
© 2023 John Wiley & Sons Ltd. Published 2023 by John Wiley & Sons Ltd.
Companion website: www.wiley.com/go/Watson/GeneralSurgery14

[1]Pierre-Alain Clavien and Daniel Dindo, Surgeons, University Hospital of Zurich.

Table 5.1 Postoperative complications following abdominal surgery

Time	Local	General
First 24 hours	Reactionary haemorrhage Anatomical injury, e.g. ligation of ureter during pelvic surgery	Asphyxia • Obstructed airway • Inhaled vomit
Second day to 3 weeks	Paralytic ileus Infection • Wound • Peritonitis • Pelvic • Subphrenic Secondary haemorrhage Dehiscence • Wound • Anastomosis Obstruction due to adhesions	Pulmonary • Collapse • Bronchopneumonia • Embolus Urinary • Retention • No production (acute tubular necrosis) Deep venous thrombosis Enterocolitis Bed sores
Late	Obstruction due to adhesions	After extensive resections or gastrectomy • Anaemia • Vitamin deficiency • Steatorrhoea and/or diarrhoea • Dumping syndrome • Osteoporosis

which is now widely used. It can be summarized as follows:

- *Grade I:* Any deviation from the normal postoperative course without the need for surgical, endoscopic, or radiological intervention but with simple treatment measures such as antiemetics, analgesia, diuretics, together with physiotherapy and bedside attention to wounds.
- *Grade II:* A complication requiring pharmacological treatment other than allowed for grade I complications, e.g. blood transfusion or parental nutrition.
- *Grade III:* A complication requiring surgical, endoscopic or radiological intervention (a) not requiring or (b) requiring general anaesthetic.
- *Grade IV:* A life-threatening complication requiring intensive care management, involving (a) single organ (e.g. renal failure) or (b) multiple organ dysfunction.
- *Grade V:* Death of the patient.

Predisposing factors

Assessing a patient's risk of complications and then taking measures to reduce the complications is a vital part of the surgical process. It is helpful to think about these three areas:

- *Preoperative* – factors already existing before the operation is carried out.
- *Operative* – factors that come into play during the operation itself.
- *Postoperative* – factors introduced after the patient's return to the ward. Consider the following sections covering surgical site infection (SSI) and thromboembolic disease as examples of this.

Surgical site infection (SSI)

Preoperative risk factors

- *Diabetes* impairs neutrophil function and humoral immunity and is a risk factor for SSI. Optimization of glucose control should be carefully planned preoperatively, which may necessitate referral to the diabetes service (Chapter 4).
- *Obesity* (BMI > 30 kg/m^2) is an independent risk factor for SSI. Patients should, where feasible, be encouraged to lose weight before surgery, best achieved with dietetic help and exercise.

- *Malnutrition and low BMI (<18 kg/m²)* are also risk factors for SSI.
- *Nasal and skin contamination* with *Staphylococcus aureus* predisposes to SSI. The risk is reduced by using nasal mupirocin in combination with a chlorhexidine body wash before high-risk procedures (such as joint replacements or paediatric surgery) and in patients who are carriers of methicillin-resistant *Staphylococcus aureus* (MRSA).
- *Surgical skin preparation.* Patients should shower but not shave prior to surgery as skin abrasions can increase the risk of SSI. If hair removal is required, this should be performed in theatre using single-use electric clippers. Aqueous or alcohol-based solutions of chlorhexidine or povidone iodine are routinely used.

Operative factors

The incidence of wound infection after surgical operations is related to the type of operation and the theatre environment. The common classification of risk groups is as follows:

1 *Clean* (e.g. hernia repair)– an uninfected operative wound without inflammation and where no viscera are opened. Infection rate is 1% or less.
2 *Clean contaminated* – where respiratory, alimentary or genitourinary tract is opened but with little or no spillage. Infection rate is less than 10%.
3 *Contaminated* – where there is a major break in sterile technique or obvious spillage or obvious inflammatory disease, for example, a gangrenous appendix. Infection rate is 15–20%.
4 *Dirty or infected* – where there is gross contamination (e.g. a gunshot wound with devitalized tissue) or in the presence of frank pus or gross soiling (e.g. a perforated large bowel). Infection rates of 40% or more.

Good theatre etiquette should reduce the incidence of nosocomial infection. This should include:

- theatre wear, used in the theatre suite, and not while walking elsewhere in the hospital;
- minimizing movement of staff in and out of the operating room;
- removal of hand jewellery;
- appropriate handwashing technique with an aqueous antiseptic, and nail brushing, prior to donning sterile gowns and gloves.

Operation sites and risk of SSI

Elective surgery to the liver, bile duct or pancreas has the highest risk of SSI (9.1%), followed by large bowel surgery (8.3%), as would be expected from the degree of contamination in the surgical field. In contrast, hip and knee replacement surgery, where prostheses are implanted, has the lowest risk of SSI (0.5%).[2]

Antibiotic prophylaxis

Antibiotic prophylaxis is used to prevent wound infections in certain procedures, but its use must be balanced with the risk of adverse effects. These include the risk of *Clostridium difficile*–associated disease and increased prevalence of antibiotic-resistant bacteria. For this reason, antibiotic prophylaxis should not be used routinely for clean uncomplicated surgery where no prostheses are used.

The prophylactic antibiotic should cover the organisms most likely to cause infection at the particular surgical site and be guided by the local antibiotic protocol avoiding broad-spectrum agents where possible. Dosing should be repeated intraoperatively if the duration of surgery exceeds the half-life of the antibiotic to maintain prophylactic cover.

Antibiotic prophylaxis is indicated as follows:

Surgical indications

- *Clean surgery* involving the placement of a prosthesis or implant, e.g. a vascular prosthesis, prosthetic hip or heart valve
- *Clean-contaminated surgery* such as resection in prepared bowel
- *Contaminated surgery* and surgery on a dirty or infected wound, where antibiotic treatment is required in addition to prophylaxis.

Additional indications

- *Valvular heart disease.* In patients with valvular heart disease, commonly rheumatic mitral valve disease, prophylaxis is given against haematogenous bacterial colonization of the valve, resulting in infective endocarditis.

[2]Figures from the Public Health England Surveillance of Surgical Site Infections in NHS Hospitals in England (2019–2020).

- *Amputation of an ischaemic limb*, where the risk of gas gangrene is high, particularly with above-knee amputations due to their proximity to the perineum and faecal organisms.
- *Organ transplant surgery*. Prophylaxis should be given against not only wound infection but also opportunist viral, fungal and protozoan infections occurring as a consequence of initial high-dose immunosuppression.

Postoperative factors

- *Wound care*. Wounds should be cleaned with sterile saline for the first 48 hours. After that, non-sterile water can be used and the patient can safely shower.
- *Dressings*. Dressing type is important, with some incorporating a transparent window so that wounds can be inspected for SSI without removing them. Tissue glue is now commonly used and applied over the closed incision in place of a formal dressing.
- *Open wounds*. Leaving wounds open instead of closing them is a traditional and highly effective way of managing contaminated wounds or cavities, including the peritoneal cavity, and minimizing the risk of invasive infection.
- *Negative pressure wound therapy* systems. These devices apply gentle suction to wounds, evacuating exudate and promoting healing. They can be used two ways:
  - *on closed wounds* (e.g. PICO™) where they have been shown to reduce wound infection and breakdown in high-risk patients;
  - *on open wounds* (e.g. Vacuum Assist Closure (VAC) devices), where healing is accelerated and granulation promoted. This may be combined with irrigation of the wound undergoing suction.

Causative organisms

Analysis of hospitals in England suggests that Gram-negative Enterobacterales (most commonly *Escherichia coli*) and *Staph. aureus* are the most prevalent organisms causing SSI. Methicillin sensitive *Staph. Aureus* (MSSA) is the most common organism in joint replacement surgery, whereas Enterobacterales are the most common cause of SSI in bowel surgery. Polymicrobial infection, where more than one infecting bacterial species is identified, is more common after bowel surgery, but it is also common after coronary artery bypass grafting (CABG).

Fungal infections such as candida are generally rare (<1%) in most surgery groups with the exception of colonic procedures with rates of 4%; they can also be significant causes of morbidity in the immunosuppressed.

Clinical features

Some wound infections are asymptomatic. If symptoms are present, there is often localized pain and swelling, or the general effects of infection (malaise, anorexia and vomiting).

Typically, there is a swinging pyrexia, and the wound is erythematous and swollen. Pus may be seen leaking from the wound. Removal of sutures or probing of the wound with a sterile swab releases some of the contained pus.

Treatment

The mainstay of SSI management is drainage of the infection. The wound is opened to release the pus, and necrotic tissue debrided. Large wounds may require operative debridement, but usually the wound can be opened at the bedside. The pus should be swabbed and the infecting organism identified.

The infected wound is left open to heal by secondary intention, aided by a negative pressure wound therapy device.

Systemic antibiotics are indicated in the presence of cellulitis, with initial choice of antibiotic governed by the likely organism, and then reviewed once bacterial sensitivities are obtained from culture of pus.

Complications of antibiotic therapy

Antibiotic-associated colitis: *Clostridium difficile*

Broad-spectrum antibiotics disrupt the normal commensal organisms in the gut, selecting out resistant forms, such as the toxin-producing strains of *C. difficile*, a Gram-positive, spore-forming bacillus. The patient experiences severe watery diarrhoea due to extensive colitis, and the bowel shows mucosal inflammation with superficial whitish yellow plaques, which may coalesce to form pseudomembranes – pseudomembranous colitis.

Risk factors for *C. difficile* colitis include antibiotics (especially cephalosporins and quinolones), proton pump inhibitors, as well as large bowel surgery. With postoperative rates of approximately 1%, *C. difficile* remains the most common cause of diarrhoea in hospitalized patients.

Clinical features

Mild cases present simply with watery diarrhoea. Severe cases have a cholera-like picture with a sudden onset of profuse, watery diarrhoea with excess mucus, abdominal pain and distension, and shock due to the profound fluid loss. Occasionally, *C. difficile* infection may present with a toxic dilation of the colon. Definitive diagnosis is made by identification of the *C. difficile* toxins (A and B) in the stool. The glutamate dehydrogenase (GDH) enzyme can also be identified in the stool and is a sensitive test but does not discriminate between toxigenic and non-toxigenic strains (about 20% of the *C. difficile* population).

Treatment

The patient is at risk of both hypovolaemia and sepsis; ABCDE assessment (see later) is crucial with delivery of intravenous (IV) fluid and electrolyte replacement. Broad-spectrum antibiotics are stopped when possible. Proton pump inhibitors should also be discontinued when possible as they allow spores to evade gastric acid and increase transmission.

Antibiotic therapy is indicated for symptomatic cases with a positive *C. difficile* toxin result. Initial treatment is with oral metronidazole for 10 days, while oral and/or rectal vancomycin and oral fidaxomicin are reserved for second-line therapy, with immunoglobulin therapy as third line, if necessary. Subtotal colectomy and ileostomy should be considered in medically resistant cases.

C. difficile is highly contagious, so in order to prevent further spread on the ward, scrupulous hand hygiene should be practiced and the patient placed in isolation until diarrhoea resolves (defined as 48 hours of formed stool).

Methicillin-resistant *Staphylococcus aureus*, MRSA

Pathology

Most community-acquired species of *Staph. aureus* are sensitive to flucloxacillin and methicillin (MSSA), but increasingly in hospital, the organism is resistant to these and other antibiotics, including cephalosporins and gentamicin. *Staph. aureus* has a record of developing resistance to antibiotics. Most species already possess a β-lactamase that confers resistance to penicillin. MRSA strains have been increasing in incidence, and most remain sensitive to vancomycin, although MRSA species with reduced or no sensitivity to vancomycin (vancomycin-intermediate *Staph. aureus*, VISA, and vancomycin-resistant *Staph. aureus*, VRSA) are now rarely encountered.

Clinical features

Most MRSA species are colonizers and do not cause clinical infections. It can be difficult to eradicate in individuals with open wounds (such as ulcers) or indwelling catheters. MRSA spreads by contact, and scrupulous hand hygiene is a cheap and effective way to reduce colonization. Typically, the organism causes a local infection in the same way that non-MRSA species do. It is commonly found in unwell patients, particularly those on intensive care units who have been on broad-spectrum antibiotics and who are already severely debilitated.

Aggressive targeting of MRSA in UK hospitals with a combination of simple handwashing measures, isolation of colonized patients, and screening and eradication of MRSA in elective admissions has seen the incidence of MRSA-related infections fall, emphasizing the benefit of simple hygiene in controlling sepsis.

Treatment

Asymptomatic MRSA carriers in the community rarely require decolonization. Patients for planned admission to hospital in whom skin swabs are positive for MRSA should be managed with 5 days 4% chlorhexidine daily body wash plus mupirocin nasal cream to attempt to decolonize.

Clinical infections are treated with intravenous vancomycin.

Other multi-resistant organisms of significance

Extended spectrum β-lactamases (ESBL)

While MRSA is one of the most prevalent antibiotic-resistant bacteria, others exist. One such class of bacteria is the Gram-negative bacteria such as *Klebsiella* and *E. coli* that produce an ESBL, an enzyme that hydrolyses the β-lactam ring of β-lactam antibiotics, including second- and third-generation cephalosporins (e.g. cefotaxime). Most ESBL-producing bacteria are also exceptionally resistant to non-β-lactam antibiotics such as quinolones and aminoglycosides, the resistance for which is carried and spread to other bacteria by plasmids. As with other resistant organisms, they are commonly found in patients treated with prolonged courses of broad-spectrum antibiotics.

Vancomycin-resistant Enterococci (VRE)

Enterococci constitute a significant portion of the normal gut flora. The emergence of resistance of enterococci to vancomycin is an inevitable consequence of the increased usage of vancomycin for prophylaxis and treatment of MRSA, as well as the use of similar drugs in animal foodstuffs to enhance growth. VRE is commonly isolated in patients who have had prolonged hospital admissions with exposure to antibiotics, such as those on intensive care units, transplant units and haematology wards.

At present, there are a few antibiotics capable of treating VRE, and treatment is best delayed until microbiological sensitivities are known. As with MRSA and ESBL, VRE are best contained by appropriate infection control measures, such as handwashing and isolation.

Carbapenem-resistant Enterobacteriaceae (CRE)

First identified in the USA in 2001, Enterobacter that are resistant to carbapenem antimicrobials such as meropenem and imipenem have spread worldwide. Those affected have usually been subject to intensive medical care or are immunosuppressed by drug or disease.

While handwashing and isolation are important in controlling the spread of resistance, CRE have been shown to be particularly resistant to normal measures used for cleaning sinks; therefore, ironically, these have on occasions been themselves a source of infection if not properly disinfected.

Patients admitted from areas with a high prevalence of CRE should be isolated and swabbed until proven not to be carriers, in order to avoid incidental contamination.

Antimicrobial stewardship

The prevalence of bacteria with resistance to antibiotics poses an increasing healthcare challenge. In order to limit the development of multi-resistant organisms, prescribers are required to exhibit due diligence in the use of antibiotics. This includes:

- taking samples for microbiological assessment before commencing treatment;
- taking microbiological advice on the most appropriate antibiotic;
- delaying initiation of therapy, where it is safe to do so, until the organism and sensitivities are known;
- prescribing treatment for the shortest possible effective course;
- using the most appropriate dose;
- where intravenous antibiotics have been prescribed, considering stepping down to an oral formulation at 48 hours if the infection is responding.

Venous thromboembolism

Deep venous thrombosis (DVT) and pulmonary embolism (PE), a life-threatening complication of venous thrombosis, are relatively frequent following major surgery. Incidence rates are around 30% after orthopaedic surgery, 8% following thoracic surgery, 7% after abdominal surgery and 4% in gynaecologic surgery. The postoperative predisposition to thrombosis has three main components (Virchow's triad[3]).

1 *Increased thrombotic tendency*: Following blood loss and platelet consumption intraoperatively, more platelets are produced, with numbers peaking around 10 days after surgery. The new platelets have an increased tendency to aggregate. Fibrinogen levels also increase, predisposing to clot formation.
2 *Changes in blood flow (rheology)*. Increased stagnation within the veins occurs as a result of immobilization on the operating table and postoperatively in bed and with depression of respiration.
3 *Damage to the vein wall* prompts thrombus formation on the damaged endothelium. The damage may be due to an inflammatory process in the

[3]Rudolf Ludwig Carl Virchow (1821–1902), Pathologist at the Charité Hospital, Berlin. He made many notable discoveries, including describing Virchow's node.

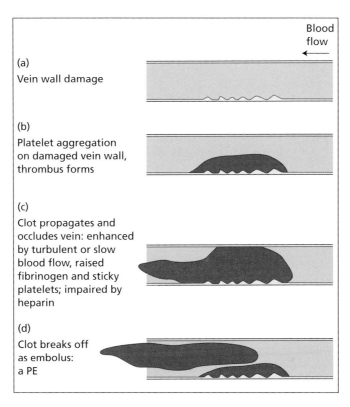

Figure 5.1 (a–d) Progression of deep vein thrombosis. PE, pulmonary embolus.

pelvis or may be produced by pressure of the mattress against the calf or direct damage at operation (particularly the pelvic veins during pelvic procedures) or by disease (e.g. pelvic sepsis).

Platelets deposit on the damaged endothelium, the vein is occluded by thrombus, and a propagated fibrin clot then develops, which may detach and embolize to the lung (a pulmonary embolus, above seen; Figure 5.1).

Risk factors

All patients admitted into a hospital setting should have an assessment of their risk of venous thromboembolism (VTE) performed within 24 hours and again if the clinical situation changes. For surgical patients, this will include risks related to the type of surgery planned. Many tools exist for the assessment of risk of VTE, which screen for factors associated with increased risk. The National Institute for Health and Care Excellence (NICE) has produced a VTE risk assessment tool, which is recommended for use in NHS hospitals. The three components of the assessment are as follows:

1 *Mobility factors* – anticipated reduction in mobility during admission
2 *Thrombosis risk factors*:
   a *Patient-related factors*, such as age over 60 years, obesity, cancer treatment, previous DVT, prothrombotic tendencies (e.g. Factor V Leiden[4]), oestrogen-containing contraceptive or hormone replacement
   b *Admission-related factors*, such as nature of surgery (hip/knee replacements and pelvic surgery), sepsis and prolonged surgery
3 *Bleeding risk assessment*:
   a *Patient related:* active bleeding, bleeding disorders, thrombocytopaenia (platelet count $<75 \times 10^9/L$), anticoagulant therapy and/or acute stroke
   b *Admission related:* surgery to the brain, spine, or eye; use of lumbar puncture, epidural or spinal anaesthetic

[4]Factor V Leiden is a G to A substitution at nucleotide 1691 of the factor V gene first described in the Dutch city of Leiden in 1994; there is also a thrombophilic prothrombin mutation, G to A at nucleotide 20210 in the factor II gene (*F2*).

Synthesis of the assessment answers allows the thrombosis and bleeding risks to be evaluated and an appropriate recommendation made for prophylaxis.

Thromboprophylaxis

NICE guidelines exist for different therapeutic areas. For abdominal surgery, they recommend a combination of both mechanical and pharmacological prophylaxis. Women should stop oestrogen-containing oral contraceptives 4 weeks before elective surgery.

1 *Mechanical VTE prophylaxis*
   a Anti-embolism stockings (graded compression stockings), correctly measured and worn from admission. They should not be given to patients with peripheral arterial disease, peripheral artery bypass graft, peripheral neuropathy, severe leg oedema or any other condition preventing their atraumatic fit
   b Intermittent pneumatic compression (e.g. Flotron boots)
2 *Pharmacological VTE prophylaxis* for a minimum of 7 days where VTE risk outweighs the risk of bleeding
   a Subcutaneous low molecular weight heparin (LMWH) injections, such as dalteparin.
   b Fondaparinux sodium. This medication binds to antithrombin III, which potentiates the neutralization Factor Xa by antithrombin.
   c Direct acting oral anticoagulants (DOACs), such as rivaroxaban. This oral medication is a selective direct Factor Xa inhibitor. Neither this nor fondaparinux are commonly used for prophylaxis in general surgery.

In addition, patients should be well hydrated and encouraged to mobilize as early as possible after surgery. Pharmacological prophylaxis should continue for at least 7 days post-surgery or until the patient has regained their normal mobility. Extended prophylaxis for 28 days postoperatively is recommended for people who have had major cancer surgery in the abdomen.

Monitoring heparin therapy in renal failure

LMWHs are eliminated by the kidneys, and in case of renal failure, levels of activated Factor X (Factor Xa) rise, leading to inadvertent over-anticoagulation. Factor Xa is responsible for cleaving prothrombin into thrombin, and it is this factor that heparin inhibits.

Patients with renal failure should have Factor Xa levels measured regularly while on treatment and may require dose adjustment.

Deep vein thrombosis

DVT is a major cause of morbidity and mortality among postoperative patients. An incidence of up to 40% has been reported in general surgery patients and may be as high as 60% among orthopaedic patients and patients undergoing amputation for peripheral vascular disease.

Clinical features

In over 90% of patients, occurrence of DVT is 'silent' and presents no symptoms. If symptoms and signs do develop, these typically appear during the second postoperative week, although they may appear earlier or later.

The patient complains of pain in the calf, and on examination, the calf is tender and warm, with swelling of the foot, often with oedema, raised skin temperature and dilation of the superficial veins of the leg. This may be accompanied by a mild pyrexia. If the pelvic veins or the femoral veins are affected, there is massive swelling of the whole lower limb.

DVT of the upper limbs is increasingly common and accounts for a small proportion of DVTs. Most of these events are precipitated by the use of peripherally inserted central catheters (PICCs) or central venous pressure (CVP) lines. Upper arm DVTs are much less likely to cause pulmonary emboli than lower limb DVTs. The detection and management remain the same.

Special investigations

- *Duplex scanning.* The course of large veins can be scanned and filling defects due to thrombi detected. In skilled hands, duplex scanning can detect thrombi in all the major veins at and above the knee or elbow but is less reliable below these levels. It has the advantage that it is simple and non-invasive.
- *Magnetic resonance imaging (MRI) scan* is sensitive for diagnosis of pelvic or intra-abdominal venous thrombosis, as is contrast-enhanced computed tomography (CT).
- *Venography and ^{125}I-labelled fibrinogen.* These sensitive tests are usually confined to research studies.

Table 5.2 The Two-Level Wells score for estimating the clinical probability of a pulmonary embolism

Clinical Feature	Points
Clinical signs and symptoms of DVT (minimum of leg swelling and pain with palpation of the deep veins)	3
An alternative diagnosis is less likely than PE	3
Tachycardia >100 bpm	1.5
Immobilization for > 3 days or surgery in the previous 4 weeks	1.5
History of DVT or PE	1.5
Haemoptysis	1
Cancer, either undergoing treatment or treated in the last 6 months, or palliated	1

Management

- *LMWH* should be commenced immediately while diagnosis is confirmed.
- *DOACs* are an alternative treatment option in ambulatory patients.
- *Mechanical compression stockings* – once anticoagulation has been started, patients should be encouraged to mobilize and to wear mechanical compression stockings, such as Thrombo-Embolus Deterrent (TED) stockings.

Pulmonary embolism

This occurs when a clot, usually originating in a femoral vein or a pelvic vein (and occasionally in a calf vein), detaches and travels to the heart to become lodged in the pulmonary arterial tree.

Clinical features

Pulmonary emboli classically occur around the 10th postoperative day but may occur sooner or later. The clinical features of PE may vary from dyspnoea, or mild pleuritic chest pain, to sudden death due to occlusion of the pulmonary artery trunk. Minor symptoms include pleuritic chest pain, dyspnoea and haemoptysis. Severe dyspnoea may occur with cyanosis and shock, and larger emboli may prompt acute right heart failure and death.

It is important to appreciate that pulmonary embolus may occur without any preceding warning signs of thrombosis in the leg. Indeed, once there are obvious clinical features of deep vein thrombosis, detachment of an organized and adherent clot from this limb is unlikely, especially if anticoagulant therapy has been commenced so that fresh clot formation is inhibited. The great majority of fatal pulmonary emboli are unheralded.

On examination, the patient has tachypnoea, often with a spike of fever. There is a tachycardia and a raised jugular venous pressure (JVP) reflecting the pulmonary hypertension. A pleural rub may be audible if the emboli are small and peripheral. Oxygen saturations on ambulation are frequently reduced.

Risk prediction of a pulmonary embolus

Risk factors for PE, and their relative importance, are illustrated by the two-level PE Wells score[5] illustrated in Table 5.2 and recommended by NICE. The Wells score also permits triage of patients:

- Score ≥4: PE likely - investigate with CT pulmonary angiography (CTPA)
- Score <4: PE unlikely - initial investigation with D-dimer

Special investigations

- *Arterial blood gases* may confirm hypoxaemia; hypocapnia (low CO_2) may also be present secondary to tachypnoea.
- *Chest radiograph* is often normal initially, but patchy shadowing of the affected segment may be present. It is more useful in identifying alternative causes such as pneumonia.
- D-*Dimer:* A degradation product of fibrin present in the blood of patients with intravascular thrombi. A negative result effectively rules out thromboembolism in patients with a two-level PE Wells score <4.
- *CT pulmonary angiography (CTPA)* is the definitive diagnostic test used when pulmonary emboli are suspected and is particularly useful when pulmonary disease is present.

[5]Philip Steven Wells, contemporary, Haematologist and Professor of Medicine, University of Ottawa, Ontario

- *Ventilation-perfusion (V/Q) scans* can be considered where it is preferable to minimize the radiation dose exposure (such as pregnant patients).
- *Electrocardiogram (ECG)* findings include rhythm changes (e.g. atrial fibrillation, heart block) or features of right heart strain (ST segment depression in leads V1 to V3, III and aVF, with right axis deviation), as the heart pumps against the obstructed pulmonary arterial tree. The oft-mentioned 'S1–Q3–T3' pattern (S wave in lead I, with a Q wave and an inverted T wave in lead III) is seldom present.
- *Echocardiogram* is most useful in patients with a confirmed massive PE to detect signs of right heart failure and pulmonary hypertension.

Treatment

1 *Oxygen* should be commenced if hypoxic.
2 *LMWH* at a therapeutic dose should be commenced immediately a PE is suspected pending the formal diagnosis.
3 *DOAC therapy* is commenced once a PE is confirmed, assuming it is safe to do so, and the likelihood of bleeding complications is minimal. It is continued for at least 3 months.
4 *Inferior vena cava (IVC) filters* are designed to trap fragmented thromboemboli from the deep leg veins *en route* to the pulmonary circulation (while preserving blood flow in the IVC). They are indicated in patients where anticoagulation is contraindicated or where emboli recur in spite of anticoagulation.
5 *Thrombolysis* may be indicated in the first 48 hours after PE if there is evidence of haemodynamic compromise. Thrombolysis can either be given into a peripheral vein (systemic thrombolysis) or directly into the pulmonary arteries via a catheter (catheter-directed thrombolysis). Recent surgery (within 14 days) is a contraindication to systemic thrombolysis due to risk of bleeding.
6 *Surgical pulmonary embolectomy*, with the patient on cardiopulmonary bypass (Chapter 13), is indicated in patients with massive pulmonary embolus who have a high risk of bleeding with thrombolysis and of dying without treatment.

Management of the unwell postoperative patient

Between 2% and 4% of postoperative patients will have a severe complication. The evaluation of a critically unwell patient is the same irrespective of the setting and applies equally to a surgical patient. It is important to have a simple scheme to follow in each case. The ABCDE approach discussed next follows guidance from Resuscitation Council UK. It occurs in two phases, an initial rapid assessment followed by a more detailed assessment.

Initial assessment

The initial rapid assessment determines whether the patient *looks* unwell, whether they are able to communicate or whether they are unresponsive and require cardiopulmonary resuscitation. Surgical drains should be inspected for evidence of bleeding. Measurement of vital signs (pulse and blood pressure) and pulse oximetry are important, with ECG monitoring if available. Where possible venous access through a peripheral cannula should be obtained and can be combined with taking bloods.

ABCDE assessment

Following the initial assessment, a systematic ABCDE assessment takes place.

A: Airway

- *Airway obstruction:* Is the airway clear, or does it require clearing/suctioning? The presence of stridor or wheeze imply partial airway obstruction. If wheeze is present, nebulized salbutamol may help.
- *Airway maintenance:* Physical manoeuvres such as chin lift and jaw thrust lift the tongue from the oropharynx and allow airflow. A number of devices are available to maintain an airway:
  - nasopharyngeal airway;
  - oropharyngeal airway (e.g. a Guedel airway);
  - supraglottic airway device (e.g. an I-Gel), which sits over the laryngeal inlet.
- *Endotracheal intubation:* This may be required if an airway cannot otherwise be maintained. In extreme circumstances, a cricothyroid membrane puncture may be necessary, or a formal tracheostomy if circumstance and time permit.
- *Oxygen* should be given at high concentration, aiming for an oxygen saturation of >94% (88%–92% if at risk of hypercapnic respiratory failure, such as in some patients with chronic obstructive pulmonary disease [COPD]).

B: Breathing

During the assessment of breathing, it is important to diagnose and treat conditions that are an immediate threat to life, such as a tension pneumothorax and massive haemothorax. In addition, non-surgical conditions such as acute asthma and pulmonary oedema may need to be treated.

- *Signs of respiratory distress:* the use of accessory muscles of respiration, abdominal breathing and sweating.
- *Respiratory rate and depth:* shallow and/or rapid breaths (>25 bpm) are adverse signs.
- *Chest wall:* Is the chest deformed? Is the trachea deviated? Is there paradoxical movement or movement of only one hemithorax? Is surgical emphysema present suggesting pneumothorax?
- *Auscultation:* may reveal features of pneumothorax or pneumonia.

Investigations include measurement of oxygen saturations and arterial blood gases help to establish the extent of respiratory compromise and the effects of treatment. A chest radiograph is important if chest pathology is suspected. If fluid overload is suspected, then diuretics or dialysis may be indicated, depending on renal function.

C: Circulation

Shock is discussed in Chapter 8. Hypovolaemia is the most likely cause of shock post operatively, but cardiac (e.g. myocardial infarction) and pulmonary (e.g. tension pneumothorax, PE) causes are also common. In assessing a surgical patient, the following should be considered:

- *Peripheral skin colour:* Pallor, cyanosis and mottling of hands or fingers suggest hypoperfusion.
- *Capillary refill time* over 2 seconds suggests poor perfusion but may also be present in the elderly or a cold environment.
- *Heart rate and pulse strength:* Tachycardia and a weak, thready pulse are common in shock.
- *Blood pressure.* In young patients, the blood pressure may be maintained in spite of significant fluid loss; the elderly tend not to be able to compensate for haemodynamic insults.
- *Auscultation of the heart* may reveal a new murmur or pericardial rub or heart sounds may be inaudible in cardiac tamponade.

- *Urine output* reflects end organ perfusion. Oliguria (<30 mL/h) suggests renal hypoperfusion.
- *The operative site and surgical drains,* with particular reference to features of peritonitis after abdominal surgery and blood in the drains. Note that significant intrabdominal or intrathoracic bleeding may occur with little or no blood appearing in the drains if the drains are blocked by clot.

An ECG and troponin levels should be checked to rule out an acute coronary syndrome. If bleeding is suspected, blood should be cross-matched and an assessment should be made as to whether an immediate return to theatre or urgent imaging is appropriate.

D: Disability

Disability refers to the patient's inability to follow commands, usually as a result of loss of consciousness. It may be a consequence of hypoxia or impaired perfusion of the brain, drugs (e.g. opiates, sedatives) or metabolic disorders (e.g. hypoglycaemia)

- *Assess the level of consciousness* using the Glasgow Coma Scale (Chapter 17).
- *Check the capillary blood glucose* level and treat hypoglycaemia (glucose <4 mmol/L) with a glucose infusion (50 mL of 10% glucose, repeated as necessary).
- *Seizures* require initial treatment with benzodiazepines.
- *Exclude drug causes, including*:
  - *Opiates:* small, pinpoint pupils, slow respiration give naloxone (often requires repeated doses)
  - *Benzodiazepine:* give flumazenil
- *Exclude metabolic causes,* such as hyponatraemia.

E: Exposure

Having gone through the aforementioned screening process, it is important that a full examination exposing the whole body is undertaken to ensure nothing has been missed.

At the end of the assessment, it should be clear what immediate investigations are required, their urgency, and where the patient is best nursed (ICU, high dependency unit or ward). Repeated observation and reassessment are important adjuncts to achieving the correct diagnosis.

Postoperative haemorrhage

Surgical bleeding may be divided into primary bleeding at the time of surgery; reactionary (or early) bleeding, which occurs within 24 hours of surgery; and secondary (or delayed) bleeding, which has a peak incidence between 7 and 10 days. The consequences of bleeding may be hypovolaemia presenting with hypotension and tachycardia, or in closed spaces like the cranium, it may present with pressure effects (loss of consciousness).

Reactionary bleeding

Reactionary bleeding from the operative field may be a consequence of several things, such as:

- a blood vessel that was in spasm, or minimally bleeding intraoperatively but that opens up with restoration of normal blood pressure and patient warming;
- a vessel from which a ligature or laparoscopic clip has slipped;
- unnoticed damage to an abdominal wall blood vessel as a drain was placed while closing – commonly the inferior epigastric artery in abdominal surgery, an intercostal artery in thoracic surgery;
- a raw surgical bed following resection where haemostasis is difficult;
- an underlying bleeding disorder, or anticoagulation, or in patients taking aspirin or clopidogrel.

Secondary haemorrhage

Secondary haemorrhage is usually a consequence of infection in the operative field, possibly related to leakage of enteric contents or pancreatic juice. It is particularly common following resection of the head of pancreas when an enzyme leak may often present with catastrophic haemorrhage. It may also manifest with intraluminal bleeding from the site of an intestinal anastomosis, or haemorrhage from an infected vascular anastomosis.

Clinical features

Bleeding may be overt or concealed. Overt bleeding, where there is visible blood loss, is readily appreciated. In concealed bleeding there may be intracavity or intraluminal bleeding which does not manifest immediately. This may occur in spite of the placement of drains. In this setting, the diagnosis is suggested by a patient becoming tachycardic and hypotensive, cold, sweaty and an appearance of pallor, all reflecting sympathetic nervous system stimulation shutting down the peripheral circulation. Chapter 8 discusses hypovolemic shock. It should be remembered that the young tend to maintain their blood pressure by peripheral vasoconstriction in spite of significant haemorrhage, making the initial diagnosis difficult without a high index of suspicion.

Management

Initial management follows the ABCDE principles outlined previously. Further management of postoperative bleeding depends on the manner of its presentation.

- *Reactionary haemorrhage* often requires an immediate return to theatre, with little role for imaging.
- *Secondary haemorrhage* may also require urgent re-exploration, but there is often a short period where investigations may take place. In some cases, radiological intervention, embolizing a bleeding vessel identified on a prior CT scan, may be the treatment of choice.

Postoperative fever

Postoperative fever may be defined as a temperature over 38 °C on two consecutive postoperative days or a single reading over 39 °C on any postoperative day. While it may be a manifestation of the inflammatory response to surgery, it may signify a serious postoperative complication.

There are many possible causes of pyrexia, which can either be considered in terms of the timing postoperatively (Table 5.3) or by considering local and general causes both infectious and non-infectious:

Local causes
- Infectious: wound infection, anastomotic leak
- Non-infectious: post-surgical inflammatory response

General causes
- Infectious: aspiration, pneumonia, urinary tract infection

Table 5.3 Causes of postoperative fever according to postoperative day

Phase	Postoperative day	Causes
Immediate	0–1	Blood transfusion reaction Anaesthetic reaction (such as malignant hyperthermia) Bacteraemia from instrumentation of infected viscus Gas gangrene of dirty wound
Acute	0–3	Basal atelectasis Urinary tract infection
	3–5	Pneumonia or aspiration Deep venous thrombosis Surgical site infection Early anastomotic leak
	5–10	Surgical site infection Pneumonia or aspiration Line infection (e.g. central venous catheter) Pulmonary Embolus
Early	10–28	Intra-abdominal collection
Delayed	>28	Viral infections Partially treated deep space infection

- Non-infectious: blood transfusion reaction, anaesthetic reaction, drug reaction, DVT, PE, basal atelectasis and thyroid crisis

Patients who are immunosuppressed have a reduced inflammatory response and may lack fever and have minimal physical signs in spite of serious infection.

Assessment

A systemic approach is required in assessing the patient:

1 The ABCDE approach to evaluate severity
2 The operation notes should be reviewed, looking in particular for any anastomoses or gastrointestinal (GI) tract sutures placed to repair bowel and any other operative concerns that may result in postoperative problems.
3 Examine systems, in turn, and in particular:
   a *Inspect the wound*: superficial wound infection or haematoma
   b *Inspect venous cannula sites*: thrombophlebitis is common when a cannula has remained *in situ* for a few days or when irritant infusions have passed through it
   c *Examine the chest clinically,* considering pulmonary collapse, infection, infarction and subphrenic abscess
   d *Examine the legs*: deep vein thrombosis
   e *Rectal examination*: pelvic abscess
   f *Urine culture*: urinary infection
   g *Stool culture*: for *C. difficile* toxin to exclude enterocolitis
   h Consider the possibility of *drug sensitivity*

Following this, investigations should be initiated according to the most likely diagnosis or diagnoses. These may include:

- *Cultures* of blood, lines, urine, sputum and stool (where appropriate)
- *Chest radiograph*
- *Duplex* of the deep veins if DVT is suspected
- *Contrast-enhanced CT scan* if intra-abdominal cause is suspected
- *CTPA* for suspected pulmonary embolus

In patients who are very unwell, it may be necessary to commence antibiotics before the initial assessment has been completed, in which case it is important to ensure that relevant cultures have been taken. The antibiotic most likely to treat the probable infective cause should be selected.

Postoperative respiratory problems

Respiratory problems are common after surgery, being particularly common following open upper abdominal surgery. Causes can be divided into those presenting with shortness of breath and those where respiration is suppressed.

Aetiology

A useful classification of causes by system is:

1 Respiratory
   a Atelectasis
   b Pneumonia, often secondary to aspiration
   c Pneumothorax, e.g. from central line placement
   d Exacerbation of underlying COPD or asthma
2 Cardiovascular
   a Left ventricular failure due to fluid overload
   b Myocardial infarction
   c PE
3 General
   a Metabolic acidosis, with compensatory hyperventilation giving the impression of breathlessness
   b Anaemia
4 Suppressed respiration
   a Neuromuscular blockade, due to incomplete anaesthetic reversal postoperatively
   b Opiates causing respiratory depression, especially in the presence of renal failure
   c Sleep apnoea

ABCDE assessment and management should be undertaken. Oxygen should be administered, and the underlying cause investigated, which usually requires arterial blood gases, chest radiograph and 12-lead ECG.

Opiates, renal failure, and respiratory depression

Opiates are partially eliminated through the kidneys, therefore clearance is impaired by renal failure. Naloxone will reverse the effects of the opiates but may require repeated doses because the half-life of naloxone (60–90 minutes) is much shorter than that of most opiates. An infusion of naloxone is usually required in patients with renal failure if a delayed respiratory arrest is to be avoided.

Pulmonary collapse and infection

Some degree of pulmonary collapse, also called atelectasis, occurs after almost every abdominal or transthoracic procedure within the first 48 hours of surgery. Mucus is retained in the bronchial tree, blocking the smaller bronchi; the alveolar air is then absorbed, with collapse of the supplied lung segments (usually the basal lobes). The collapsed segment or entire lung continues to be perfused and acts as a shunt, which reduces oxygenation. The lung segment may become secondarily infected by inhaled or aspirated organisms, and, rarely, abscess formation may occur.

Aetiology

Preoperative factors

- chronic obstructive airway disease;
- smoking;
- asthma (which increases the amount of bronchial secretion);
- chest wall disease, such as ankylosing spondylitis, which restricts ventilation and makes coughing difficult;
- poor mobility;
- obesity.

Operative factors

- anaesthetic drugs, such as atropine, which increases the viscosity of secretions;
- surgery in the upper abdomen or thorax;
- long operative time;
- excessive fluid replacement (goal-directed replacement – the gold standard using cardiac output monitoring).

Postoperative factors

- insufficient analgesia to permit full inspiration opening all alveoli and expectoration;
- abdominal distension causing diaphragmatic splinting.

Clinical features

The patient is dyspnoeic with a rapid pulse and elevated temperature. There may be cyanosis. The patient attempts to cough, but this is painful and, unless encouraged, may fail to expectorate. The sputum is at first frothy and clear but may become purulent later, diagnostic of secondary infection. The chest movements are diminished, particularly on the affected side; there may be basal dullness with reduced air entry and coarse crackles.

The haemoglobin oxygen saturation on pulse oximetry may fall, and chest radiograph may reveal an opacity of the involved segment(s) (usually basal or midzone), together with mediastinal shift to the affected side if a significant portion of one lung is affected.

Treatment

Preoperatively

Breathing exercises are given, and smoking is discouraged. Any prior chest infection is treated, and surgery delayed, if possible, until the chest is optimized.

Operatively

The surgical approach associated with the least respiratory compromise should be considered where appropriate; laparoscopic surgery is preferable to open surgery. Epidural or spinal anaesthesia is used where possible and continued postoperatively. Intercostal nerve blocks may be used for thoracic or upper abdominal surgery and continued postoperatively. Transversus abdominus plane (TAP) anaesthetic blocks or catheters may be placed alongside abdominal wounds to minimize immediate postoperative pain.

Postoperatively

The patient is encouraged to take deep breaths and cough while supporting any abdominal wound with their hands. Chest physiotherapy, saline/salbutamol nebulizers and incentive spirometry are initiated. Incentive spirometry encourages patients to take slow, deep breaths and uses devices that provide visual cues to the patients to confirm that the desired flow or volume has been achieved.

In the event of development of shortness of breath or low oxygen saturations, a full ABCDE assessment should take place to resuscitate the patient and confirm the diagnosis of chest infection with chest radiograph. Sputum cultures are sent, and antibiotic treatment begun.

It is important to recognize adverse clinical features that suggest that increased levels of respiratory support may be required, ranging from increased inspired oxygen to non-invasive ventilation (e.g. continuous positive airways pressure [CPAP]) to intubation and ventilation on an intensive care unit. Recognizing these can allow pre-emptive treatment. A number of early warning scores have developed to aid nurses and doctors in recognizing such patients, such as the National Early Warning Score (NEWS) 2 used in the UK. Features suggesting respiratory support may be required include:

- use of accessory muscles, intercostal recession;
- respiratory rate >25 bpm, which may be followed by exhaustion and respiratory failure;
- respiratory rate <8 bpm;
- decreasing vital capacity (shallow breathing);
- tachycardia and sweating (reflecting sympathetic activity);
- agitation and restlessness;
- sitting up, unwilling to lie flat;
- hypoxaemia, with $pO_2 < 11$ kPa when the FiO_2 is 40%, or <8 kPa on air;
- HbO_2 saturations $\leq 90\%$;
- hypercapnia;
- impaired level of consciousness.

Postoperative ileus

This is discussed in Chapter 30.

Abdominal wound dehiscence

Wound dehiscence is an uncommon complication of surgery, being more common after emergency than elective surgery. It may be divided into superficial and full-thickness dehiscence:

- *Superficial dehiscence* is a failure of the skin closure such that subcutaneous tissue and even rectus sheath become exposed.
- *Full-thickness dehiscence* occurs when all layers of the wound fail such that some of the abdominal contents (usually small bowel) prolapse out. This is often termed a 'burst abdomen', a term that reflects the shock of patient and staff alike when they encounter bowel in the bed.

Risk factors

Predisposing factors can be divided into preoperative, operative and postoperative as follows:

Preoperative

Malnutrition (common with some cancers and emergency conditions), diabetes, COPD, obesity, smoking, liver and renal failure, steroids and mTOR inhibitors (everolimus and sirolimus). Previous radiotherapy may compromise the vascularity of a wound, rendering it more prone to break down.

Operative

Emergency surgery, intra-abdominal sepsis, long operations (increased incidence of wound infection), early reoperations where the fascia becomes friable, poor suture choice (insufficient strength or rapidly absorbed) and poor operative technique. Midline incisions are more likely to dehisce than paramedian or grid iron appendix incisions.

One recommended technique for abdominal closure uses a continuous suture that is four times the length of the wound, with individual 'bites' placed 1 cm apart (Jenkins' rule[6]). Some researchers have proposed even smaller bites of 5 mm. The key is to place the suture into healthy fascia without tension either laterally or longitudinally to avoid a 'cheese wire' effect cutting through the fascia.

Postoperative

Excessive coughing (such as with COPD or chest infection), abdominal distension due to prolonged ileus or obstruction, wound infection, wound haematoma and delayed introduction of nutrition. Prolonged periods in intensive care have also been cited as a cause.

Clinical features

Signs usually develop approximately 10 days after surgery. Overt wound infection may precede dehiscence, but often, there is a small defect in the skin where pink fluid discharges. This represents the blood-stained serous effusion, which is always present during the first week or two within the abdomi-

[6]Terence PN Jenkins, Surgeon, St Luke's Hospital and Royal Surrey County Hospital, Guildford.

nal cavity after operation and which seeps through the wound breakdown.

The wound may open slightly, at which point loose suture material and the smooth pink surface of small bowel may be seen in its depths, or a more extensive dehiscence may occur, especially after coughing or straining, with intestine and omentum prolapsing through.

Management

Depends on the clinical presentation. In both types of dehiscence, wound swabs are taken to determine the nature of any infecting organism.

- *Superficial dehiscence* should be explored to confirm the integrity of the deep fascia and then managed expectantly with wound dressings or negative pressure dressings.
- *Full-thickness dehiscence* is a shocking and psychologically disturbing occurrence for the patient who will need strong reassurance. The bowel is covered with a sterile dressing soaked in saline, and the patient returned to theatre. The abdomen is explored, and wound edges debrided. If there is no distension, the wound is closed primarily once again. In the presence of distension such that the wound edges will not oppose, the abdomen may be left open as a laparostomy or a vacuum-assisted wound closure device with mesh-mediated fascial traction may be considered. This technique involves suturing a polypropylene mesh across the wound to bridge the gap in the fascial closure. The mesh is gradually tightened over several days under general anaesthetic to draw the muscles together and aid delayed closure.

Following closure of superficial or full-thickness dehiscence, there is a high incidence of subsequent incisional hernia.

Anastomotic leak

An anastomosis is a join between two luminal structures, such as bowel, bile duct, pancreatic duct, ureter or blood vessel. It may be hand sewn or stapled, the latter being most common in bowel anastomoses. An anastomotic leak results in luminal contents passing through the suture or staple line into the extra-luminal space.

Risk factors

There are several factors that increase the risk of an anastomotic leak. A classification for an anastomotic leak following a bowel anastomosis is given below, although many of the factors apply to anastomoses of other luminal structures:

- *Preoperative:* Medication (such as corticosteroids), smoking, diabetes, obesity, malnutrition, intra-abdominal sepsis, liver disease and cirrhosis, neoadjuvant chemotherapy or radiotherapy for cancer
- *Operative*: emergency surgery, long intra-operative time, peritoneal contamination (pus or faeces), site of anastomosis (e.g. in the rectum, oesophagus or pancreas), poor blood supply to the cut ends of bowel, and distal obstruction. Operative technique is important, to avoid poor blood supply, tension across the anastomosis, malignancy at the anastomosis (i.e. inadequate resection) and incorrect orientation (e.g. a twist of the bowel)
- *Postoperative:* hypotension, inotropic support (vasoconstriction reducing blood supply to the anastomosis) and respiratory failure

Clinical features

Anastomotic leaks are important to recognize early. The consequences of a leak depend on the luminal contents. In the case of a vascular anastomosis, it is associated with haemorrhage, which is usually brisk with arterial anastomoses. Bile and urine cause a sterile chemical peritonitis. In contrast, a pancreatic duct leak causes release of digestive enzymes, which may result in necrosis of neighbouring tissues, causing bowel perforation or haemorrhage. A leak from a bowel anastomosis causes peritoneal soiling and sepsis. The remainder of this section considers bowel anastomotic leaks, but similar principles apply to other anastomoses.

Early diagnosis and treatment are important. Delay leads to prolonged contamination of the abdomen or chest by the luminal contents, leading to the development of severe sepsis and progression to multi-organ failure and death.

Leaks from a bowel anastomosis classically present with abdominal pain combined with high fever, a leucocytosis and raised CRP. It can present without localizing abdominal signs, or with cardiovascular instability, atrial fibrillation or even myocardial infarction. For this reason, it should be considered whenever a patient's recovery is not progressing as normal. On examination, patients may be pyrexial and tachycardic and may have signs of peritonism. There may be faeculant material in the wound or drains.

Early postoperatively, a leak will drain freely into the peritoneal cavity. Later, by day 10, the anastomosis tends to be walled off by inflammatory tissue and surrounding bowel and omentum so the leak may be 'contained'.

Special investigations

- *CT scan* will demonstrate free gas and fluid in the peritoneal cavity. Oral contrast such as gastrografin will be seen to leak outside of the bowel lumen.
- *Endoscopy*, usually under anaesthetic, to directly inspect an oesophago-gastric or rectal anastomosis will reveal a defect.

Management

The definitive management varies depending on the site of the leak, its extent, the amount of contamination and the physiological status of the patient. It also depends on whether the anastomosis was in a defunctioned segment of bowel, that is, one for which a proximal stoma was fashioned to divert the faecal stream to permit healing.

Contained leaks

Contained leaks are generally managed by drainage. This usually involves a radiologically placed drain into the infected cavity. It is particularly effective where the faecal stream has been diverted by a proximal stoma during the initial surgery. An alternative for oesophago-gastric and low rectal anastomotic leaks is to pass an endoluminal vacuum therapy device such as the Endo-SPONGE® via the bowel lumen into the cavity. This is a sponge through which negative pressure is applied, which prompts granulation tissue and healing. The sponge needs changing every 2 to 3 days, usually under general anaesthetic.

Uncontained ('free') leaks

Surgery is required for an uncontained leak, to wash out the infected material. This may be performed laparoscopically if the original surgery was minimally invasive but is more commonly performed via an open laparotomy approach. The anastomosis usually requires resection with formation of a proximal end stoma. Repair of an anastomosis is seldom successful because of local sepsis, poor vascularity and suboptimal condition of the patient.

Whether a contained or uncontained leak, optimizing the patient's nutrition is important and parenteral nutrition is usually required.

Postoperative fistula

A fistula is as an abnormal connection between two epithelial surfaces; an enterocutaneous fistula is a communication between the bowel and the skin. Most enterocutaneous fistulae are a consequence of anastomotic leaks or inadvertent injury to the bowel during surgery or following trauma. Spontaneous enterocutaneous fistulae may occur from Crohn's disease, malignancy, diverticulitis or radiotherapy.

Similar factors are responsible for postoperative fistulas and anastomotic leaks. An alternative classification is to consider them in terms of general factors and local factors.

General factors include uraemia, anaemia, jaundice, protein deficiency or cachexia from malignant disease.

Local factors include factors affecting anastomotic healing (e.g. blood supply and tension), local sepsis before or during surgery, a distal obstruction or the presence of local malignancy or chronic inflammation such as Crohn's disease.

Clinical features

Diagnosis of a fistula is usually obvious, with bowel contents or bile leaking from the wound or drain site, usually between 10 and 14 days post-surgery. If the diagnosis is in doubt, the fluid can be tested for bilirubin to diagnose a biliary leak and creatinine for a urinary tract leak, while the fluid from a pancreatic or small bowel leak is rich in amylase. Water-soluble contrast or methylene blue can be given by mouth and the fistula imaged or observed for the presence of dye.

The patient is typically pyrexial with localized abdominal pain. The enzyme-rich fluid of the upper alimentary tract and of a pancreatic fistula produces rapid excoriation of the surrounding skin. This is less marked in a faecal fistula, as the contents of the colon are relatively poor in proteolytic enzymes.

Classification

Fistulas are usually classified by the volume of output and the area of the GI tract involved in the fistula.

- *Output:* High output (>500 mL over 24 hours), moderate output (between 200 and 500 mL over 24 hours) and low output (<200 mL over 24 hours).
- *Site of origin of fistula:* oesophageal, gastroduodenal, small bowel, large bowel. A fistula occurring from bowel exposed in an open wound is termed an enteroatmospheric fistula.

Treatment

The management has four aims, which can be considered to form the acronym *SNAP*:

1 **Skin and Sepsis control**
   a *Local control to protect the skin around the fistula*: The edges of the wound are covered by Stomahesive® (which adheres even to moist surfaces) or aluminium paste or silicone barrier cream. It may be possible to collect the effluent by means of a stoma appliance and thus reduce skin soiling. If the mouth of the fistula is large, continuous suction may be necessary.
   b *Antibiotics and radiological drainage of purulent collections*: Repeated drainage may be necessary.
2 *Nutritional support*: In a high alimentary fistula, gastric and pancreatic secretions, which are stimulated when feeding enterally, are lost through the fistula. Instead, the patient is kept 'nil by mouth' and parenteral nutrition commenced (Chapter 3). A low fistula, occurring in the distal alimentary tract, may be managed with an elemental diet given by mouth. This is rapidly absorbed in the upper intestine and is thus not lost through the fistula. Regular monitoring of nutritional state is important.
3 *Anatomical delineation of the fistula:* A CT scan with water-soluble contrast either by mouth or via the fistula tract will identify the site of leakage, assess the likelihood of spontaneous closure and facilitate planning of any future intervention.
4 *Procedure for definitive control:* Whether closure of the fistula tract is required depends on the likelihood of spontaneous closure. Good nutritional support, eradication of sepsis, no distal obstruction, low fistula output and small bowel fistulas are associated

with spontaneous healing. Where surgical control is required, ideally re-operation should not be attempted until sepsis is eradicated and nutrition optimized, which may take several months.

Localized intraperitoneal collections

Following peritonitis, pus may collect in localized pockets within the peritoneum. These may be dependent anatomical spaces in the abdomen when the patient lies supine, such subphrenic spaces and pelvis or non-anatomical, where pus exists walled off by loops of bowel and omentum.

Risk factors

- *Preoperative:* perforated viscus or peritonitis at presentation, obesity, immunocompromised by drugs or disease, for example, corticosteroid use, diabetes, malnutrition
- *Operative*: peritonitis, soiling with luminal contents during surgery, inadequate intra-operative lavage, retained infected material (such as faecolith from perforated appendix and gallstones following cholecystectomy)
- *Postoperative*: presence of an organism resistant to the antibiotics used

Clinical features

The patient may present with a swinging pyrexia or a pyrexia that has persisted since surgery. There is malaise, weight loss, anaemia and leucocytosis. If antibiotics have been given without a diagnosis, the presentation of an abscess may be disguised and may only manifest weeks or even months after the original episode

Special investigations

- *Full blood count:* A polymorph leucocytosis is common, with a white cell count typically 15–20 × 10^9 /L.
- *CRP* is raised.
- *CT scan* will confirm the diagnosis and anatomical site of the collection and determine whether it is drainable by a radiologically guided percutaneous approach.

Subphrenic abscess

Anatomy

The subphrenic region lies between the diaphragm above and the transverse colon with mesocolon below and is divided further by the liver and its ligaments (Figure 5.2). The right and left *subphrenic*

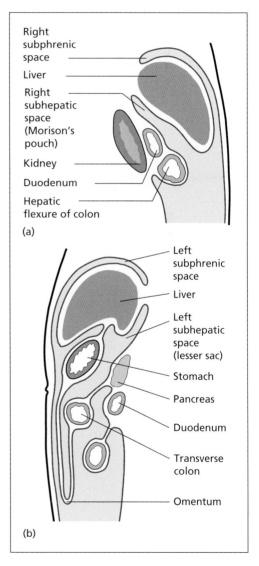

Figure 5.2 The anatomy of the subphrenic spaces (sagittal views): (a) right and (b) left.

spaces lie between the diaphragm and the liver and are separated from each other by the falciform ligament. The right and left *subhepatic spaces* are below the liver, the right forming Morison's pouch[7] and the left being the lesser sac, which communicates with the former through the foramen of Winslow.[8] The right *extraperitoneal space* lies between the bare area of the liver and the diaphragm. About two-thirds of subphrenic abscesses occur on the right side. Rarely they may be bilateral.

Aetiology

The underlying cause is a peritonitis involving the upper abdomen – leakage following biliary or gastric surgery or a perforated peptic ulcer. Rarely, infection occurs from haematogenous spread or from direct spread from a primary chest lesion, for example, empyema.

Clinical features

In addition to the features of a localized collection of pus (see previous sections), there may be right upper quadrant pain and pain referred to the shoulder tip with localized upper abdominal or chest wall tenderness. There may be signs of fluid or collapse at the lung base. In late cases, a swelling may be detected over the lower chest wall or upper abdomen. In many cases, there are no localizing features.

Special investigations

- *Chest X-ray* may show the following:
  - elevation of the diaphragm on the affected side;
  - pleural effusion and/or collapse of the lung base;
  - gas and a fluid level below the diaphragm.
- *CT scan* will demonstrate an abscess.

Treatment

In early cases, where there is absence of gas and free fluid on X-ray, the patient is placed on broad-spectrum antibiotic therapy. If there is clinical or radiological evidence of a localized abscess, or if resolution fails to occur on antimicrobial chemotherapy, percutaneous drainage may be carried out under ultrasound or CT guidance. If this fails, or the abscess is loculated, surgical drainage is performed.

Pelvic abscess

A pelvic abscess may follow any general peritonitis, but it is particularly common after acute appendicitis (75%) or after gynaecological infections. In men, the abscess lies between the bladder and the rectum; in women, it lies between the uterus and posterior fornix of the vagina anteriorly and the rectum posteriorly (pouch of Douglas[9]).

Left untreated, the abscess may burst into the rectum or vagina or may discharge onto the abdominal wall, particularly if there has been a previous laparotomy incision at the time of the original episode of peritonitis. Occasionally, the abscess may rupture into the peritoneal cavity.

Clinical features

- *General features of intraperitoneal pus* (see above).
- *Local*: diarrhoea, mucus discharge per rectum and the presence of a tender extrinsic mass felt on rectal or vaginal examination. Rarely, this may be large enough to be palpated abdominally.

Treatment

- *Broad-spectrum antibiotic therapy* adjusted according to microbiological sensitivities when available. Anti-fungal agents may be added in certain cases (e.g. immunosuppressed and chronic infection).
- *Percutaneous radiologically guided drainage* using ultrasound or CT. This carries a risk of vascular and hollow viscus injury.
- *Internal drainage* is possible when the abscess points into the vagina or rectum.

[7]James Rutherford Morison (1853–1939), Professor of Surgery, University of Durham, Durham, UK.

[8]Jacob Winslow (1669–1760), Danish; became the Professor of Anatomy and Surgery in Paris, France.

[9]James Douglas (1675–1742), Obstetrician and Anatomist, London, UK.

Delirium

Delirium is an 'acute confusional state', which presents as an altered state of consciousness, cognitive function and behaviour. Typically, it develops over 1 to 2 days and is common in, but not confined to, elderly patients undergoing major surgery. Patients may develop visual or auditory hallucinations; become restless, agitated and aggressive, or lethargic; have disturbed sleep; and lack cooperation with simple requests. It is associated with poorer surgical outcomes, in part as a consequence of the delirium and in part the underlying condition that prompted the state of delirium.

Risk factors

- *Preoperative:* the elderly, past or current cognitive impairment or dementia, other comorbidity, metabolic derangement, alcohol and other substance abuse, and sleep deprivation.
- *Operative*: type of surgery (more common in major surgery); opiate and benzodiazepine use, especially benzodiazepine premedication; surgical blood loss and requirement for transfusion. The use of spinal anaesthesia for hip surgery, for example, is associated with less delirium than a general anaesthetic. Ketamine and dexmedetomidine as part of the anaesthetic regimen are associated with less delirium.
- *Postoperative*: inadequate pain relief, opiates, electrolyte imbalance, anaemia, infection, sensory deprivation (such as loss of glasses or hearing aids), and malnutrition.

Management

Management usually involves assistance from Care of the Elderly or psychiatric teams. Initial management requires careful review of history and repeat examination for any new signs, such as pyrexia, new murmurs and neurological deficits (suggesting a new cerebral event). Investigations should aim to exclude other possible causes:

- *Pain*: A common cause of confusion, but its treatment may also cause confusion. Use of blocks in preference to drugs to reduce immediate postoperative pain helps.
- *Hypoxia*: Haemoglobin saturations should be checked, and oxygen administered if necessary; a CT pulmonary angiogram may be necessary to exclude a PE.
- *Sepsis*: Common (urinary tract and/or chest) and uncommon sources should be considered, and urine, sputum and any drain fluids cultured. CT imaging may be required to exclude a complication of the surgery such as an anastomotic leak.
- *Electrolyte disturbance*, especially hyponatremia.
- *Myocardial infarction*: Troponin and serial ECGs.
- *Arrhythmia*: An ECG is necessary to exclude a change in rhythm, for example, new atrial fibrillation.
- *D-dimers* will exclude a thrombo-embolic event if negative.
- *Medication review* to check:
  - critical preoperative drugs have not been omitted inadvertently;
  - currently prescribed drugs for any that may be responsible, such as pain killers, sedatives and GABAergic drugs (benzodiazepines).
- Drips, drains and catheters can prompt confusion: These should be avoided or removed as soon as possible.

Complications of minimally invasive surgery

Minimally invasive operative techniques have become commonplace for many surgical procedures. The use of such techniques is associated with their own complications, some of which are listed later. Management follows standard surgical principles, but early diagnosis, achieved by an awareness of what might go wrong, is important.

Radiological intervention

The interventional radiologist has taken on many procedures that used to be the preserve of the surgeon, but it is often the surgeon who is left to diagnose and manage the complications. Typical complications of radiological intervention include the following.

1 **Imaging 'guided' needle core biopsy of mass or lesion**

   General: bleeding; perforation of viscus; inadvertent puncture of other organs or vessels; and arteriovenous malformation (especially in liver and kidney).

Cancer: seeding of tumour along the biopsy track, thereby disseminating it

2 **Transarterial procedure**

General: arterial dissection; distal embolization; thrombosis; loss of guidewire; false aneurysm

Angioplasty: vessel rupture

Embolization of a bleeding bowel: infarction and/or perforation

3 **Transvenous procedure (e.g. caval filter placement)**

General: bleeding, thrombosis, thromboembolism and loss of guidewire

4 **Transcoelomic procedure (e.g. abscess drainage)**

General: bleeding, bowel injury and bladder injury

Endoluminal surgery

Upper and lower GI endoscopy, together with any procedures performed, carry their own risks, the most common of which is perforation.

1 *Upper GI endoscopy*: oesophageal perforation; haemorrhage from varices or from peptic ulcer if clot displaced

2 *Endoscopic retrograde cholangiopancreatography (ERCP)*: perforation, cholangitis and pancreatitis

3 *Lower GI endoscopy*: perforation, especially if snaring polyp or stenting stricture

Laparoscopic surgery

1 *Port insertion*: perforation of viscus; perforation of bladder; puncture of the aorta (especially if aneurysmal), vena cava or iliac vessels; and puncture of the uterus

2 *Insufflation*: vagal stimulation causing profound bradycardia, CO_2 retention and embolism.

3 *Collateral damage*: unseen collateral visceral or vascular damage by surgical instruments; trauma due to excess force applied by instruments (which act as levers magnifying the exerted force), for example, causing avulsion of vessels; mis-identification of structures (e.g. aorta divided instead of renal artery during nephrectomy).

4 *Port closure*: visceral perforation; inadequate closure, leading to hernia

◉ Additional resources

6

Acute infections

Christopher Watson

Learning objectives

✓ To know the common surgical infections and their management.

✓ To be particularly cognisant of tetanus and gas gangrene, including prophylaxis and treatment.

There is an important general principle in treating acute infection anywhere in the body; antibiotics are invaluable when the infection is spreading through the tissues (e.g. cellulitis, peritonitis, pneumonia), but drainage is essential when abscess formation occurs.

Diabetic patients are very prone to infection; anyone presenting with an infection should have their blood tested for glucose, and an HbA1c checked if doubt exists.

Cellulitis

Cellulitis is a spreading inflammation of connective tissues. It usually affects the skin and subcutaneous tissue, but the term may also be applied to pelvic, perinephric, pharyngeal and other connective tissue infections. There is usually a prior breach of the skin, usually of a limb, which admits the infecting organism. The common causative agent is the β-haemolytic Group A *streptococcus (Strep. pyogenes) in around two-thirds of cases*, with *staph. aureus involved in most of the other cases*. The invasiveness of *streptococcus* is due to the production of hyaluronidase and streptokinase, which dissolve the intercellular matrix and the fibrin inflammatory barrier, respectively.

Ellis and Calne's Lecture Notes in General Surgery, Fourteenth Edition.
Edited by Christopher Watson and Justin Davies.
© 2023 John Wiley & Sons Ltd. Published 2023 by John Wiley & Sons Ltd.
Companion website: www.wiley.com/go/Watson/GeneralSurgery14

Predisposing factors include diabetes, venous insufficiency, eczema and obesity. It is also more common in those immunosuppressed by drugs or disease.

Characteristically, the skin is dark red with local oedema (peau d'orange) and hot; it blanches on pressure. There may be blistering and, in severe cases, cutaneous gangrene. Cellulitis is often accompanied by lymphangitis and lymphadenitis, and there may be an associated septicaemia.

Treatment

Any pustules, ulcers or areas of skin breakdown are swabbed, and the margin of the inflammation is marked so that progression or regression of infection can be readily assessed. The limb is immobilized, elevated, and antibiotics begun. Typically, the first-line antibiotics will be flucloxacillin, with co-amoxiclav if the infection is near the eyes. Second choice, in case of allergy, would be clarithromycin, erythromycin or doxycycline. If methicillin-resistant *staph. aureus* (MRSA) infection is possible, then vancomycin is added. Careful observation is necessary to ensure necrotizing fasciitis does not ensue (see later in this chapter).

Erysipelas

Erysipelas is a superficial form of cellulitis affecting the upper dermis and superficial cutaneous lymphatics.

The culprit is nearly always a Group A beta-haemolytic streptococcus.

Abscess

An abscess is a localized collection of pus, usually, but not invariably, produced by pyogenic organisms. They typically occur under the arms, complicating pilonidal disease, and around the anus and genitals. Occasionally, a sterile abscess results from the injection of irritants into soft tissues (e.g. a corticosteroid injection).

An abscess commences as a hard, red, painful swelling, which then softens and becomes fluctuant. If not drained, it may discharge spontaneously onto the surface or into an adjacent viscus or body cavity. There are the associated features of bacterial infection, namely a swinging fever, malaise, anorexia and sweating with a polymorph leucocytosis.

Treatment

An established abscess, in any situation, requires drainage. Antimicrobial agents cannot diffuse in sufficient quantity to sterilize an abscess completely. Pus left undrained continues to act as a source of toxaemia and becomes surrounded by dense, fibrous tissue.[1]

The technique of abscess drainage depends on the site. The classic method, which is applicable to a superficial abscess, is to wait until there is fluctuation and to insert the tip of a scalpel blade at this point. The track is widened by means of sinus forceps, which can be inserted without fear of damaging adjacent structures. If there is room, the surgeon's finger can be used to explore the abscess cavity and break down undrained loculi. Drainage is then maintained until the abscess cavity heals – from below outwards, since otherwise the superficial layers can close over, with recurrence of the abscess. Occasionally, the abscess may be kept open with use of a drain, and the drain is gradually withdrawn until complete healing is achieved. Packing of most abscesses after drainage can generally be avoided.

[1] An old surgical aphorism states that the sun should never set on undrained pus, something that is still relevant today.

Deep abscesses can be localized and drained percutaneously using ultrasound or computed tomography (CT) guidance.

Boil

A boil (furuncle) is an abscess that involves a hair follicle and its associated glands. It is, therefore, not found on the hairless palm or sole but is usually encountered where the skin is hairy, injured by friction or is dirty and macerated by sweat; thus, it occurs particularly on the neck, axilla and the perianal region. It is usually due to the *staphylococcus aureus*, and like cellulitis, occurs more commonly in patients with diabetes or other immune compromise.

Occasionally, a furuncle may be the primary source of a staphylococcal septicaemia and may be responsible for osteomyelitis, perinephric abscess or empyema, particularly in debilitated patients. A boil on the face may be complicated by a septic phlebitis spreading along the facial veins, resulting in thrombosis of the cavernous sinus.

Differential diagnosis

Hidradenitis suppurativa: Multiple infected foci in the axillae or groins due to infection of the apocrine sweat glands of these regions are usually misdiagnosed as boils. They generally do not respond to antimicrobial therapy, but some will respond to treatment with a monoclonal antibody against tumour necrosis factor (TNF) (e.g. adalimumab). Excision of the affected skin is often necessary; if this is extensive, the defect may require skin grafting.

Treatment

When pus is visible, the boil should be incised. Recurrent crops of boils should be treated by improving the general hygiene of the patient and by the use of ultraviolet light and hexachlorophene baths, but systemic antibiotic therapy is seldom indicated.

Carbuncle

A carbuncle is an area of subcutaneous necrosis that discharges onto the surface through multiple sinuses. It is usually staphylococcal in origin. The subcutaneous tissues become honeycombed by small abscesses separated by fibrous strands. The condition is often associated with general debility, and diabetes, in particular, must be considered.

Treatment

Surgery is rarely indicated initially. Antibiotic therapy is given, and the carbuncle merely protected with sterile dressings. Occasionally, a large sloughing area eventually requires excision and a skin graft. Diabetes, if present, must be controlled.

Specific infections

Tetanus

Tetanus is now a rare disease in the Western world, thanks to a comprehensive immunization policy. In the developing world, it remains prevalent with a high mortality.

Pathology

Tetanus is caused by *Clostridium tetani*, an anaerobic, exotoxin-secreting, Gram-positive bacillus. It is characterized by formation of a terminal spore ('drumstick') and is a normal inhabitant of soil and faeces. The bacillus remains at the site of inoculation and produces a powerful exotoxin, tetanospasmin. Tetanospasmin principally affects inhibitory neurones that secrete γ-aminobutyric acid (GABA) and glycine. By blocking the inhibitory effects of these neurones, there is unopposed excitatory activity from motor and autonomic neurones. Motor effects include increase in muscle tone, with rigidity and reflex spasms; autonomic effects include sympathetic overactivity with tachycardia, increased cardiac output and reduced vascular tone.

Tetanus follows the implantation of spores into a deep, devitalized wound where anaerobic conditions occur. Infection is related less to the severity of the wound than to its nature; thus, an extensive injury that has received early and adequate wound toilet is far less risky than a contaminated puncture wound that has been neglected.

Clinical features

The incubation time is 24 hours to 24 days, the initial injury often being trivial and forgotten. Muscle spasm first develops at the site of inoculation and then involves the facial muscles and the muscles of the neck and spine. As a rule, it is the trismus of the facial spasm (producing the typical '*risus sardonicus*') that is the first reliable indication of developing tetanus. This may be so severe that it becomes impossible for the patient to open his or her mouth ('lockjaw'). The period of spasm is followed, except in mild cases, by violent and extremely painful convulsions, which occur within 24–72 hours of the onset of symptoms and may be precipitated by some trivial stimulus, such as a sudden noise. The convulsions, like the muscle spasm, affect the muscles of the neck, face and trunk. Characteristically, the muscles remain in spasm between the convulsions. The temperature is a little elevated, but the pulse is rapid and weak.

In favourable cases, the convulsions, if present at all, become less frequent and then cease and the tonic spasm gradually lessens. It may, however, be some weeks before muscle tone returns to normal and the *risus sardonicus* disappears. In fatal cases, paroxysms become more severe and frequent; death occurs from asphyxia due to involvement of the respiratory muscles or from exhaustion, inhalation of vomit or pneumonia.

Poor prognostic features are a short incubation period from the time of injury to the onset of spasm (under 5 days) and the occurrence of convulsions within 48 hours of the onset of muscle spasm.

Differential diagnosis

- *Hypocalcaemic tetany*: characteristically affects the limbs, producing carpopedal spasm (Chapter 40).
- *Strychnine poisoning*: flaccidity occurs between convulsions, whereas in tetanus, the spasm persists.
- *Meningitis*: neck stiffness.
- *Epilepsy*.
- *Conversion disorder (previously known as hysteria)*.

Treatment

Prophylaxis

Active immunization

This comprises two initial injections of tetanus toxoid (formalin-treated exotoxin) at an interval of 6 weeks. Booster doses are given at intervals of 10 years or at the time of any injury. Toxoid should be given to any population at risk of injury, particularly the elderly in whom cover may have lapsed.

Wound toilet

The risk of tetanus can be reduced almost to zero if penetrating and contaminated wounds are adequately excised to remove all dead tissue and a course of prophylactic penicillin (or erythromycin for penicillin-sensitive patients) is given. Antibiotic therapy is no substitute for thorough wound debridement.

Passive immunization

This is done to neutralize the toxin. Patients who have previously received toxoid should be given a booster dose. If toxoid has not been given in the past, human tetanus immunoglobulin (HTIG), prepared from fully immunized subjects, should be given if the wound is heavily contaminated or is a puncture wound, and more than 6 hours have elapsed before treatment is received. HTIG is *not* sufficient to confer long-term immunity; therefore, a course of toxoid immunization should also be given.

Curative treatment

Control of convulsions

The patient is nursed in isolation, quiet and darkness, and is heavily sedated. In severe cases, pharmacological paralysis with tracheostomy and mechanical ventilation is required, and this may have to be continued for several weeks. It is terminated when the spasms and rigidity are absent during a trial period without muscle relaxants.

Control of the local infection

Excision and drainage of any wound is carried out under a general anaesthetic. High-dose penicillin (or erythromycin if the patient is penicillin sensitive) is administered.

Nutrition

Feeding via a fine-bore nasogastric tube may be needed to maintain the general condition and electrolyte balance.

Necrotizing soft tissue infections

These are bacterial infections characterized by rapidly progressive tissue destruction, systemic toxicity and high mortality. The three main types of necrotizing soft tissue infections are:

- *Polymicrobial infection*, with multiple organisms present
- *Single organism infection*, usually a haemolytic Group A streptococcal infection but may also be *staph. aureus* (including MRSA)
- *Gas gangrene,* typically due to *Clostridium perfringens*

Clinical features

Although there are three main sorts of necrotizing infection, in reality, presentation and treatment are similar. An often-overlooked initial breach in the skin, whether accidental or surgical, is followed by infection with a bacterium producing powerful exotoxins, which result in tissue destruction.

Around the wound, an area of rapidly spreading cellulitis appears. At the same time, the patient develops intense pain at the site of infection out of proportion to the initial external appearance of the skin. This is followed by rapid features of systemic sepsis and confusion. The local manifestations progress, with swelling of the tissues, skin discolouration, blistering and the appearance of black (necrotic) spots; these features may be delayed if the infection is more deeply seated.

Risk factors

As with the other infections described in this chapter, patients at risk of necrotizing infections include those who are immunosuppressed by drugs or disease, such as diabetes mellitus or malignancy, as well as the elderly and the obese. In addition, surgery or infections around the perineum are prone to develop into necrotizing infections.

Investigation

- *Skin swabs* are often negative, but blistered or ulcerated areas may be more revealing.
- *Blood cultures.*
- *CT and magnetic resonance imaging (MRI) scans* will identify gas within soft tissues.
- *Creatine kinase* may be risen due to myonecrosis.

Treatment

Treatment involves a high index of suspicion, with cellulitis often being the initial differential diagnosis.

Skin and blood cultures are obtained and high-dose, broad-spectrum antibiotics are commenced immediately, but the mainstay of treatment is a radical debridement of all the affected area.

The infection spreads extensively along fascial planes, so the true extent of spread may not be apparent until surgery. Wounds are widely debrided and left open, which allows them to be reassessed twice a day with further debridement performed until all the affected area is cleared. The resulting defect may require covering with skin or a composite tissue graft, which can only be performed after the infection has settled.

Mortality from necrotizing infections is high.

Polymicrobial infection: 'Synergistic gangrene'

Polymicrobial infection, also known as synergistic gangrene, progressive bacterial gangrene and Meleney's gangrene,[2] is caused by the synergistic action of two or more organisms, commonly aerobic haemolytic *staphylococcus* and microaerophilic non-haemolytic *streptococcus*. Where it affects the scrotum and perineum, it has been termed Fournier's gangrene.[3]

Group A streptococcal infection

Necrotizing fasciitis was the term used historically to describe the necrotizing soft tissue infection caused by Group A *streptococcus* (*strep. pyogenes*), the 'flesh-eating bug' of media fame. *Streptococcus* is a common skin commensal, and infection follows entry of the bacteria through an often-trivial break in the skin, such as a cut, graze, insect bite or puncture wound.

Gas gangrene
Pathology

Gas gangrene results from infection by *Clostridium perfringens* (*welchii*) and other *Clostridium* species. The organism, a Gram-positive, anaerobic spore-forming bacillus like *Clostridium tetani*, also pro-

duces powerful exotoxins. The toxins have various activities, including phospholipase, collagenase, proteinase and hyaluronidase, which facilitate aggressive local spread of infection along tissue planes, with liberation of CO_2, H_2S and NH_3 by protein destruction. The organisms are found in soil and faeces.

Gas gangrene is a typical infection of deep penetrating wounds, particularly of war, but sometimes involvement of the abdominal wall or cavity may follow operations upon the alimentary system. Occasionally, gas gangrene complicates amputation of an ischaemic lower limb or follows abortion or puerperal infection. It may also arise in drug addicts giving themselves subcutaneous injections of contaminated heroin.

Clinical features

The incubation period is about 24 hours. Severe sudden onset of pain is characteristic, together with severe toxaemia with tachycardia, shock and vomiting. The temperature is first elevated and then becomes subnormal. The affected tissues are swollen, and crepitus is palpable due to gas in the tissues. The skin becomes gangrenous, and the infection spreads along the muscle planes, producing at first dark red swollen muscle and then frank gangrene. The gas imparts a typical foul smell.

Treatment
Prophylaxis
Debridement

Adequate excision of wounds removes both the organisms and the dead tissues that are essential for their anaerobic growth. Seriously contused wounds (such as those produced by a gunshot) or contaminated wounds are left open and lightly packed with gauze; primary closure should be avoided. Delayed primary suture can then safely be performed after 5–6 days, by which time the wound is usually healthy and granulating.

Antimicrobial therapy

Penicillin is given in all heavily contaminated wounds and to patients undergoing amputation of an ischaemic leg.

[2] Frank L Meleney (1889–1963), Professor of Clinical Surgery, Columbia University, OH, USA.

[3] Jean Alfred Fournier (1832–1914), 'Professeur des maladies cutanées et syphilitiques', Hôpital St Louis, Paris, France.

Curative treatment

In the established case, all involved tissue must be excised. Involvement of all muscle groups in a limb is an indication for amputation, which in the lower limb may mean a disarticulation at the hip. High-dose penicillin is given, and other supportive measures as required. Hyperbaric oxygen therapy, to eliminate the anaerobic environment, has been used with varying degrees of success.

Anthrax

Anthrax is caused by *Bacillus anthracis*, a Gram-positive, aerobic spore-forming bacillus that lives in the soil. It may manifest in one of three ways:

1 *Cutaneous anthrax* – infection through a break in the skin.
2 *Gastrointestinal anthrax* – spore entry through the gut mucosa.
3 *Inhalational anthrax* – inhalation of spores causing pulmonary disease.

It is an occupational disease of people working with wool ('wool sorter's disease') and the hides from infected animals.

Cutaneous anthrax is the most common manifestation and presents as a painless, pruritic papule that develops into a vesicle 1–2 cm in diameter. The vesicle ruptures, undergoes necrosis and enlarges to form a black eschar with surrounding oedema. Associated features include lymphangitis and regional lymphadenopathy as well as general manifestations of sepsis.

Gastrointestinal anthrax manifests as nausea, vomiting, fever and abdominal pain, with bloody diarrhoea and features suggestive of an acute abdomen. Symptoms first appear 2–5 days after the ingestion of contaminated food. Haemorrhagic mesenteric adenitis and ascites are late features, and mortality is around 50%.

Prophylaxis and treatment of anthrax are with ciprofloxacin.

Botulism

Botulism is caused by an exotoxin of *Clostridium botulinum* and is associated with ingestion of contaminated food, originally described with contaminated sausages (*botulus* is Latin for sausage). The botulinum toxin is a heat-labile toxin (hence destroyed by cooking) that penetrates cholinergic neurones and prevents neurotransmitter (acetylcholine) release at the neuromuscular junction, thus inhibiting muscular contraction. While botulism is itself a condition more familiar to infectious disease units, the toxin is widely used in surgery for conditions as diverse as fissure *in ano*, achalasia and hyperhidrosis (excess sweating, especially of the palms).

Actinomycosis

Actinomyces are Gram-positive anaerobic bacteria that commonly colonize the mouths of cattle in whom they cause a condition called lumpy jaw, a manifestation of abscesses in the jaw; if an abscess discharges through the skin as a sinus, the resultant pus is said to have a characteristic appearance of sulphur granules.

Actinomyces species, most commonly *Actinomyces israelii*, can cause human disease (actinomycosis). They are commensals in human mouths and may cause infection particularly in the presence of poor dental hygiene or previous irradiation (Chapter 20). In addition to the mouth, *A. israelii* is a commensal of the female genital tract and the gastrointestinal tract. Actinomycosis may follow perforated appendicitis or colonic surgery, or may present as chronic pelvic pain in women, associated with weight loss and vaginal discharge, especially in the presence of an intrauterine device. It is characterized by an indolent infection, often with a palpable mass and presence of discharging sinuses. While the diagnosis may be difficult to make, the treatment is less challenging since the organism responds to penicillin.

Additional resources

7

Tumours

Christopher Watson

Learning objectives

✓ To know the pathology and clinical features of tumours, as well as the ways in which a tumour might present and the histological features that influence prognosis.

✓ To understand the principles of tumour staging.

✓ To know the treatment options, including the principles of cytotoxic chemotherapy and the broad classes of agents available.

Cancers are so common and widespread that their consideration must at least pass through the mind in most clinical situations. It, therefore, behoves the student, both for examinations and, still more importantly, for the future practice of medicine, to have a standard scheme with which to tabulate the pathology, diagnosis, treatment and prognosis of neoplastic disease.

Pathology

When considering the tumours affecting any organ, this simple classification should be used.

1 Benign
2 Malignant:
   a primary;
   b secondary.

For each particular tumour, the following headings should be used:

- Incidence.
- Age distribution.
- Sex distribution.

Ellis and Calne's Lecture Notes in General Surgery, Fourteenth Edition.
Edited by Christopher Watson and Justin Davies.
© 2023 John Wiley & Sons Ltd. Published 2023 by John Wiley & Sons Ltd.
Companion website: www.wiley.com/go/Watson/GeneralSurgery14

- Geographical distribution (where relevant).
- Predisposing factors.
- Macroscopic appearances.
- Microscopic appearances.
- Pathways of spread of the tumour.
- Treatment options.
- Prognosis.

Clinical features and diagnosis

A malignant tumour may manifest itself in any or all of four ways:

1 The effects of the *primary tumour* itself.
2 The effects produced by *secondary deposits (metastases)*.
3 The general effects of *malignant disease*.
4 *Paraneoplastic syndromes*. These are remote effects caused by hormones or other tumour cell products, which are most common in carcinoma of the lung, particularly small cell tumours. For example, production of ectopic adrenocorticotrophic hormone (ACTH) may present like Cushing's syndrome, and production of ectopic parathormone (PTH) may present with hypercalcaemia and its symptoms.

Table 7.1 The 10 most common cancer killers in the UK in 2018

	Cancers in males		Cancers in females	
	Cancer site	**Mortality per 100,000**	**Cancer site**	**Mortality per 100,000**
1	Lung	65.9	Lung	47.0
2	Prostate	45.9	Breast	33.3
3	Colorectal	32.8	Colorectal	21.4
4	Oesophagus	19.6	Pancreas	13.3
5	Pancreas	17.5	Ovary	12.5
6	Bladder	14.0	Brain, other CNS and intracranial tumours	7.3
7	Liver	12.6	Uterus	7.3
8	Brain, other CNS and intracranial tumours	10.5	Oesophagus	7.1
9	Kidney	10.5	Liver	6.3
10	Non-Hodgkin's lymphoma	10.1	Non-Hodgkin's lymphoma	6.2

Data for 2018 obtained from Cancer Research UK, January 2022.
CNS, central nervous system.

The only common exceptions to this scheme are primary tumours of the central nervous system (CNS), which seldom produce secondary deposits.

Diagnosis is always made by history, clinical examination and, where necessary, special investigations.

Let us now, as an example, apply this scheme to carcinoma of the lung – the most common lethal cancer in the UK, accounting for 21% of all deaths from cancer; bowel (10%), breast (7%), prostate (7%), pancreas (6%) and oesophagus (5%) follow lung cancer in this comparison of cancer frequency by site (Table 7.1).

History

- *The primary tumour* may present with cough, haemoptysis, dyspnoea and pneumonia (sometimes recurrent pneumonia due to partial bronchial obstruction).
- *Secondary deposits* in bone may produce pathological fracture or bone pains; cerebral metastases may produce headaches or drowsiness; liver metastases may result in jaundice.

- *General effects of malignant disease*: the patient may present with malaise, lassitude, poor appetite or loss of weight.
- *Paraneoplastic syndromes*, such as:
  - ectopic hormone production (e.g. PTH, ACTH);
  - myasthenia-like syndrome (Eaton–Lambert syndrome[1]);
  - hypertrophic pulmonary osteoarthropathy (HPOA) and finger clubbing.

Examination

- *The primary tumour* may produce signs in the chest.
- *Secondary deposits* may produce cervical lymph node enlargement hepatomegaly or obvious bony deposits (e.g. in the skull).
- *The general effects of malignancy* may be suggested by pallor or weight loss.

[1]Lealdes M Eaton (1905–1958), Professor of Neurology, Mayo Clinic, Rochester, MN, USA. Edward Lambert (1915–2003), Professor of Physiology and Neurology, Mayo Clinic, Rochester, MN, USA.

Special investigations

- *The primary tumour*: chest X-ray, computed tomography (CT) scan, bronchoscopy, cytology of sputum and needle core biopsy.
- *Secondary deposits*: CT scan and isotope bone scan.
- *General manifestations of malignancy*: a blood count may reveal anaemia. The erythrocyte sedimentation rate (ESR) may be raised.
- *Paraneoplastic hormone production*: hormone assay.

This simple scheme applied to any of the principal malignant tumours will enable presentation of a full clinical picture of the disease.

Tumour markers

These are blood chemicals (often fetal proteins) produced by the malignant cells. Some tumours have a characteristic marker associated with them, such as α-fetoprotein (AFP) in hepatoma and teratoma and prostate-specific antigen (PSA) in carcinoma of the prostate (Table 7.2). Tumour markers may indicate malignant change in a benign condition and are useful in postoperative monitoring. If a marker was raised before treatment, it should fall when the disease is controlled but will rise again if recurrence occurs. Some tumours produce excess amounts of the appropriate hormone, such as medullary carcinoma of the thyroid producing calcitonin, in which case hormone assay may be used to detect tumour activity.

Table 7.2 Tumour markers

Marker	Nature of marker	Malignant disease associated with rise in marker	Benign disease associated with rise in marker
α-Fetoprotein (AFP)	Protein secreted by fetal liver	Hepatocellular carcinoma and testicular teratoma	Viral hepatitis (e.g. hepatitis C) and cirrhosis; pregnancy esp. if spinal cord abnormality
β-Human chorionic gonadotrophin (β-HCG)	Protein normally produced by placenta	Testicular teratoma and chorion carcinoma	Pregnancy
Ca 15.3	Oncofetal antigen	Breast carcinoma	Hepatitis, cirrhosis, autoimmune diseases, benign lung disease
Ca 27.29	Glycoprotein mucin 1 (MUC1) on epithelial cells	Breast carcinoma	Benign breast disease, ovarian cysts, liver and kidney disease
Ca 19.9	Intracellular adhesion molecule related to Lewis blood group	Hepatocellular and cholangiocarcinoma. Also colorectal and ovarian carcinoma	Pancreatitis, cholestasis, cholangitis, cirrhosis
Ca 125	Glycoprotein on coelomic epithelium during fetal development	Ovarian carcinoma	Pregnancy, ovarian cysts, pelvic inflammation, ascites, cirrhosis, hepatitis, pancreatitis
Carcinoembryonic antigen (CEA)	Oncofetal protein (protein secreted by fetal gut)	Advanced colorectal, breast and lung carcinomas	Peptic ulcer, inflammatory bowel disease, pancreatitis
Prostate-specific antigen (PSA)	Glycoprotein produced by epithelium of prostatic duct	Prostatic carcinoma	Prostatitis, benign prostatic hypertrophy and prostatic trauma

Prognosis

The prognosis of any tumour depends on four main features:

1 Extent of spread.
2 Microscopic appearance.
3 Anatomical situation.
4 General condition of the patient.

Extent of spread (staging)

The extent of the tumour (its staging) on clinical examination, on radiological imaging, at operation and on studying the excised surgical specimen is of great prognostic importance. Obviously, the clinical findings of palpable distant secondaries or gross fixation of the primary tumour are serious. Similarly, the local invasiveness of the tumour at operation and evidence of distant spread are of great significance. Finally, histological study may reveal involvement of the lymph nodes that had not been detected clinically or radiologically, or microscopic extension of the growth to (and by inference beyond) the edges of the resected specimen with consequent worsening of the outlook for the patient.

The TNM classification

The TNM classification is an international system for tumour staging. Tumours are staged by scoring them according to the following.

- *T*umour characteristics – size and degree of invasion.
- *N*ode involvement – regional nodes and distant nodes.
- *M*etastases – presence or absence.

An example of TNM staging as it relates to breast cancer is illustrated in Table 37.2. Tumours are most accurately staged by pathological criteria (i.e. measurement of size, invasion and nodal involvement on the excised specimen) rather than based on clinical examination, although the latter gives an immediate idea of spread. Use of pathological criteria when referring to tumour stage is denoted by the prefix 'p', hence pT1 for a pathologically proven T1 tumour.

Some tumours have additional classifications that are more familiar to the clinician. Examples are Breslow's staging of local invasion of malignant melanoma (Table 11.2) and Dukes' staging of rectal carcinoma (Figure 28.4).

Microscopic appearance (histological differentiation)

As a general principle, the prognosis of a tumour is related to its degree of histological differentiation (its grading) on the spectrum between well differentiated (low grade) and poorly differentiated (anaplastic).

The spread of the tumour and its histological differentiation should be considered in conjunction with each other. A small tumour with no apparent spread at the time of operation may still have a poor prognosis if it is poorly differentiated, whereas an extensive tumour is not incompatible with long survival of the patient after operation if the microscopic examination reveals a high degree of differentiation.

Anatomical situation

The site of the tumour may preclude its adequate removal and thus seriously affect the prognosis. For example, a tumour at the lower end of the oesophagus may be easily removable, whereas an exactly similar tumour situated behind the arch of the aorta may be technically inoperable; a brain tumour located in the frontal lobe may be resected, whereas a similar tumour in the brain stem will be a desperate surgical proposition.

General condition of the patient

A patient apparently curable from the point of view of the local condition may be inoperable because of poor general health. For example, gross congestive cardiac failure may convert what is technically an operable carcinoma of the rectum into an unacceptable anaesthetic risk.

Treatment

The treatment of malignant disease should be discussed in a multidisciplinary team setting, involving review of histopathology and radiology, with surgical and oncological expertise. Treatment options should then be discussed with the patient before a treatment plan is pursued. Treatment could be considered under two headings.

1 *Curative*: an attempt is made to ablate the disease completely.
2 *Best supportive/palliative*: although the disease is incurable or has recurred after treatment,

measures can still be taken to ease the symptoms of the patient and provide best supportive care.

In this section, we will summarize the possible lines of treatment for malignant disease in general; in subsequent chapters, the management of specific tumours will be considered in more detail. Treatment given after surgery to reduce the risk of recurrence is often referred to as *adjuvant therapy* (Latin *adiuvare*, to help); treatment given before surgery with the intention of shrinking a tumour and making it easier to resect is known as *neoadjuvant therapy*.

Curative treatment

1 *Surgical resection* (e.g. carcinoma of the lung or colon).
2 *Radiotherapy* alone (e.g. tumours of the mouth and pharynx).
3 *Cytotoxic chemotherapy* when the tumour is especially sensitive to particular agents, such as teratoma of the testis to platinum compounds.
4 *A combination of treatment modalities* including surgery and/or radiotherapy and/or cytotoxic chemotherapy.

Best Supportive/Palliative treatment

1 *Operative intervention*
   a *Surgical resection*. The palliative excision of a primary lesion may be indicated, although secondary deposits may be present. For example, a carcinoma of the ascending colon may be excised to prevent recurrent bleeding and pain, although secondary deposits may already be present in the liver.
   b *Prevent obstruction:* Obstructing cancers in the large bowel may be stented. Inoperable obstructing tumours of the oesophagus or cardia of the stomach may also be stented so that dysphagia can be relieved. The bile duct may be stented endoscopically via the duodenal papilla for the relief of jaundice and pruritus in patients with inoperable carcinomas of the head of pancreas.
2 *Radiotherapy*. Palliative treatment may be given to localized secondary deposits in bone, irremovable breast tumours, inoperable lymph node deposits and some symptomatic primary tumours, for example. It is particularly indicated for localized irremovable disease, such as bleeding, pain and mucus from a low rectal cancer.
3 *Hormone therapy*. Applicable in carcinoma of the breast and prostate.
4 *Radiofrequency ablation* is a treatment for primary or secondary tumours of the liver, lung and kidney. It involves a needle-like probe being passed percutaneously into the tumour through which a radiofrequency current is passed, causing a thermal injury that destroys the tumour cells
5 *Tumour embolization (TAE):* Some tumours, such as small primary or secondary cancers in the liver, may be treated by embolizing the feeding artery with a chemotherapy agent, or beads coated with a slow-release chemotherapy agent, to reduce growth (transarterial chemoembolization, TACE), or simply embolizing the tumour deposit to deprive it of its blood supply completely. Radioactive beads, typically yttrium-90, may also be used which cause local irradiation to tissue around the bead.
6 *Cytotoxic chemotherapy*. A wide range of drugs have anti-cancer action, but this action is not specific; all the drugs damage normal dividing cells, especially those of the bone marrow, gut, skin and gonads.
7 *Non-chemotherapy drugs*. These are administered for pain relief (e.g. non-steroidal analgesics, opiates), hypnotics, tranquillizers and anti-emetics (e.g. chlorpromazine).
8 *Nerve blocks*, with phenol or alcohol for relief of pain.
9 *Psychological support*. This is often impossible but might be improved by a cheerful and kindly attitude of medical and nursing staff, and sometimes with formal psychological input. The surgeon must also deal with the psychological effect of not being able to cure the patient, or that their treatment has failed, and not lose sight of the patient in need of psychological support.

Anti-neoplastic agents

The chemical therapy of cancer can be divided into four classes of agent:

- Cell cycle chemotherapy, typically targeting cell proliferation pathways. Cancers with very rapid growth are particularly susceptible.

- Targeted chemotherapy, utilizing specific properties of cancer.
- Hormone therapy, used commonly for the treatment of hormone sensitive prostate, breast, ovarian and uterine cancer.
- Immunotherapy, utilizing immune system components to fight cancer.

Some drugs may fall into more than one class, such as the CD20 monoclonal antibody rituximab, which targets the CD20 epitope on B cells and is used for the treatment of B cell lymphoma.

Cell cycle chemotherapy classification

Chemotherapy agents that target the cell cycle are particularly suited to the treatment of rapidly dividing tumours, which are, therefore, affected more than non-cancer cells. Non-cancer cells that turn over rapidly may be affected and manifest with side effects, such as bone marrow suppression and mucositis.

There is no standard classification of such agents, but a useful classification is as follows:

- *Alkylating agents* bind to DNA or RNA, interrupting synthesis of DNA, RNA or proteins, e.g. cyclophosphamide, chlorambucil, busulphan, and the platinum compounds cisplatin, carboplatin and oxaliplatin.
- *Antimetabolites.* Structural analogues of substrates of DNA and RNA synthesis, which they interrupt:
  - Pyrimidine analogues: 5-fluorouracil, cytarabine and gemcitabine;
  - Purine analogues, e.g. 6-mercaptopurine, thioguanine;
  - Folate analogues, e.g. methotrexate.
- *Anti-microtubule agents.* Inhibit mitosis by interfering with microtubule formation or function:
  - Plant alkaloids, e.g. vincristine and vinblastine
  - Taxanes, e.g. paclitaxel, docetaxel
- *Topoisomerase inhibitors.* Cause DNA strand breaks by disrupting action of topoisomerase enzymes:
  - Topoisomerase I inhibitors, e.g. irinotecan, topotecan;
  - Topoisomerase II inhibitors, e.g. etoposide; anthracyclines (e.g. daunorubicin).
- *Cytotoxic antibiotics.* Interfere at different points of cell cycle division: e.g. bleomycin and mitomycin.

Immunotherapy

Immunotherapy involves harnessing elements of the immune system for anti-cancer therapy. The list below gives some examples, although there may be overlap between them; for example, some monoclonal antibodies may act as checkpoint inhibitors.

- *Monoclonal antibodies* – targeting specific cell surface protein or cytokine
- *Checkpoint inhibitors* – molecules on the cell surface that keep the immune response in check, preventing immune activation against self. Checkpoint molecules are highly expressed on some tumour cell types.
- *Cytokines*, such as interferon, used to enhance an immune response, although less commonly used nowadays.
- *Vaccine therapy*, which can utilize a historic vaccine response. For example, using an immune response to *Bacille Calmette-Guérin* (BCG) in immunized individuals to stimulate a local immune response in bladder cancer. Alternatively, the vaccine may be a protein or nucleic acid fragment of the cancer cell, stimulating an immune response to the cancer.
- *Chimeric antigen receptor (CAR)-T cell therapy* – T cells are removed from the patient's blood, then engineered to express a receptor for a protein expressed by the cancer, after which they are cultured in volume before reinfusing into the patient.

Targeted drugs

Some tumours have characteristic metabolic pathways that can be targeted, or histological or genetic analysis of individual tumours may identify such pathways or pathological cell surface protein expression. Targeting may be either with small molecules, which usually act within the tumour cell, or monoclonal antibodies to cell surface proteins or products. Examples are:

1 *Checkpoint inhibitors* block the mechanisms by which cancer cells evade the immune response, by targeting specific cell surface proteins/receptors on leucocytes
   a Programme cell death-1 receptor, blocked by pembrolizumab and nivolumab, for example.
   b Programme cell death-1 ligand, blocked by atezolizumab and avelumab.
   c Cytotoxic T-lymphocyte–associated antigen 4 (CTLA4), such as ipilimumab.

2 *Angiogenesis inhibitors*, targeting tumour-produced vascular endothelial growth factor (VEGF)

  a VEGF inhibition: monoclonal antibodies to VEGF, e.g. bevacizumab.

  b VEGF receptor blockade: monoclonals in development.

  c VEGF receptor signal transduction: small molecule tyrosine kinase inhibition by sorafenib and sunitinib.

  d VEGF signal translation: mTOR inhibitors, e.g. everolimus and temsirolimus.

3 *Proliferation signal inhibition*

  a Blockade of epidermal growth factor receptor (EGFR), e.g. cetuximab and panitumumab.

  b Blockade of human epidermal growth factor receptor 2 (HER2), which is overexpressed on the cells of some cancers, especially breast, e.g. trastuzumab.

Combination chemotherapy

Multiple drugs with different modes of action and different toxicity profiles may be used to increase the efficacy of treatment. A balance must be made between the chances of regression of the tumour in relatively fit patients with tumours likely to be sensitive (e.g. breast, ovary and testis) and the toxic effects of the drug regimen.

Radiotherapy

Radiotherapy involves administering ionizing radiation that causes DNA damage and thus prevents tumour cell proliferation. It can be divided into:

- *External radiotherapy*, where the irradiating source is outside of the body.
- *Internal radiotherapy*:
  a *Systemic radioisotope therapy* where the radioactive source is within the body and is taken up preferentially by the tumour cells, such as *iodine-131* for thyroid cancer.
  b *Selective internal radioisotope therapy*, such as *yttrium-90 beads* injected via the hepatic artery into the arteries feeding liver metastases.
  c *Brachytherapy* where the irradiation is from an implanted radioactive source placed inside or adjacent the tumour, used for cancers of the prostate, cervix and uterus.

External radiotherapy

There are many different ways external radiotherapy may be administered, but the principles are similar:

- *Total dose* is different for different tumours and given either as a curative or as a palliative treatment;
- *Fractionation*, applying a total dose over several sessions, thus allowing adjacent tissue to recover and also to treat tumour cells that were in a relatively resistant phase of the cell cycle at one session but are actively dividing at a subsequent session;
- *Stereotactic targeting* using cross-sectional imaging to define the tumour, which is then subjected to a total dose of irradiation applied as beams from different directions, which come to a focus on the tumour, minimizing the exposure of healthy tissue. There are several advanced types of radiation delivery using such principles.

Cancer screening

Screening is the process of testing asymptomatic individuals for a specific condition. It is commonly performed for tumours but may be used in other contexts such as abdominal aortic aneurysm and hypertension. Effective screening for a given condition using a particular test has several prerequisites:

- The condition, if untreated, is sufficiently serious to warrant its prevention.
- The natural history of the condition should be understood.
- The condition has a recognizable early stage.
- Effective treatment is available.
- Treatment at an early stage could improve the prognosis and is of more benefit than treatment started later in the disease.
- The screening test is simple, reliable and acceptable to the patient.
- The screening test should have minimal false-positive and false-negative outcomes (i.e. it should be both sensitive and specific). Incorrect diagnosis can have serious consequences.

In reality, cost-effective screening requires restricting the testing to those groups at highest risk of a condition. This may involve large-scale population screening or screening of families where a genetic predisposition exists.

Population screening

Examples of population screening include breast cancer screening by mammography, which is restricted to older women (over 50 years) and cervical cancer screening for women over 25 years. In cervical cancer, for example, a distinct progression exists from dysplasia to invasive cancer. This progression may take 10 years. Hence, screening the population every 3–5 years by cervical smear cytology is cost-effective. However, the advent of immunization of females with a vaccine against human papilloma virus may reduce the need for such frequent population screening for that cancer.

Screening for high-risk individuals

A number of cancer syndromes exist in which there is an inherited predisposition (e.g. familial adenomatous polyposis [FAP]) or a familial risk (e.g. breast and ovarian cancer).

Inherited cancer syndromes

Like FAP, most inherited cancers are autosomal dominantly inherited. In at-risk families, early identification may be possible through either genetic mapping of the cancer or early recognition of a component of the syndrome. In FAP, early colonoscopy may identify adenomas (polyps) while they are still dysplastic and before they become malignant, at which stage prophylactic colectomy is indicated. In addition, identification of the *APC* gene (located on chromosome 5q21) will also signify carriage.

Familial clustering

Many of the familial cancers are now being associated with mutations of specific genes. Incomplete expression of the gene may account for the sporadic incidence of the tumour. For breast cancer, many genes associated with increased susceptibility have been identified, the most important of which are *BRCA1* (chromosome 17q21) and *BRCA2* (chromosome 13q12). Mutations of either gene confer an 80% risk of breast cancer by the age of 70 years, together with an increased risk of ovarian cancer. Screening tests based on the detection of these genes differ from the other screening tests mentioned above, as they identify a tendency to malignancy and not premalignant change or early curable malignancy. There is no consensus at present as to the best management of such patients.

8

Shock

Vijay Sujendran

Learning objective

✓ To understand what shock is, what causes it and how it is best managed according to the cause.

Shock is characterized by inadequate perfusion with consequent inadequate oxygen delivery to the vital organs, principally the heart and brain, leading to cellular hypoxia and death.

Aetiology

Tissue perfusion requires adequate blood pressure, which is dependent upon the systemic vascular resistance and cardiac output. The cardiac output is a function of the heart rate and stroke volume. These may be expressed in mathematical terms:

$$CO = HR \times SV$$
$$BP = CO \times SVR$$
$$\text{Mean Arterial Pressure} = SV \times HR \times SVR$$

where CO is cardiac output, SV is stroke volume, HR is heart rate, BP is mean arterial blood pressure and SVR is systemic vascular resistance. Stroke volume is determined by preload, contractility and afterload.

Normal regulation of tissue perfusion

The autonomic nervous system is able to alter heart rate and peripheral vascular resistance in response to changes in blood pressure detected by the carotid sinus and aortic arch baroreceptors. Changes in systemic vascular resistance may alter venous return by changing the amount of fluid circulating in the cutaneous and splanchnic vascular beds. Venous return determines the stroke volume; increasing venous return causes an increase in stroke volume, the heart acting as a permissive pump (Starling's law):[1] the output depends on the degree of stretch of the heart muscle at the end of diastole (Figure 8.1).

Volume regulation is achieved by the kidney, in particular by the regulation of sodium loss by the renin–angiotensin–aldosterone system and antidiuretic hormone (ADH) produced by the posterior pituitary, which controls water loss in the renal tubules and collecting ducts. In addition, a fall in circulating volume prompts the sensation of thirst, stimulating increased fluid intake.

Abnormal regulation of tissue perfusion

Inadequate tissue perfusion (shock) may result from factors related to the pump (the heart) and/or the systemic circulation. The causes of shock may be classified accordingly, as follows:

Ellis and Calne's Lecture Notes in General Surgery, Fourteenth Edition. Edited by Christopher Watson and Justin Davies.
© 2023 John Wiley & Sons Ltd. Published 2023 by John Wiley & Sons Ltd.
Companion website: www.wiley.com/go/Watson/GeneralSurgery14

[1]Ernest Henry Starling (1866–1927), Professor of Physiology, University College, London, UK. Also described capillary flow dynamics and discovered secretin (with Bayliss).

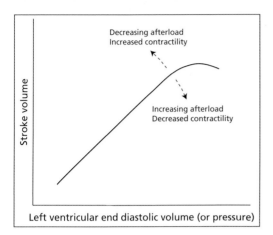

Figure 8.1 Starling law.

1 *Cardiogenic shock*. A primary failure of cardiac output in which the heart is unable to maintain adequate stroke volume in spite of satisfactory filling. Compensation involves an increase in heart rate and systemic vascular resistance, manifested clinically by a tachycardia, sweating (due to sympathetic nervous system outflow), pallor and coldness (due to cutaneous vasoconstriction). Causes of cardiogenic shock include the following:

 a massive myocardial infarction;
 b acute ventriculoseptal defect following myocardial infarction affecting the septum;
 c mitral or aortic valve rupture;
 d arrhythmia;
 e cardiomyopathy and viral myocarditis.

2 *Circulatory obstruction*. The heart continues to pump, but there is an obstruction to outflow or impairment of filling. Cardiogenic and obstructive causes of shock are characterized by a raised venous pressure; the other causes are characterized by a low venous pressure. Causes include:

 a outflow obstruction, e.g. pulmonary embolism;
 b obstruction to venous return, e.g. tension pneumothorax, acute cardiac tamponade.

3 *Hypovolaemia*. Reduction in circulating volume results in a reduction in stroke volume and cardiac output. Blood pressure is initially maintained as in cardiogenic shock, with increased sympathetic activity raising the peripheral vascular resistance leading to the clinical picture of a cold, clammy patient with a tachycardia. As volume losses increase,

the blood pressure falls. In severe cases, the patient is confused or semi-conscious. Causes include:

 a *haemorrhage*, revealed or internal (e.g. ruptured aneurysm; bleeding into the bowel or around a closed fracture);
 b *burns*, with massive loss of plasma and electrolytes;
 c *severe diarrhoea and/or vomiting*, with fluid and electrolyte loss, particularly in colitis or pyloric stenosis;
 d *bowel obstruction*, in which large amounts of fluid are sequestered into the gut, in addition to the losses due to vomiting;
 e *peritonitis*, with large fluid losses into the abdomen as a consequence of infection or chemical irritation;
 f *gastrointestinal fistulas*, with fluid and electrolyte loss;
 g *urinary losses*, for example, the osmotic diuresis of diabetic ketoacidosis, or polyuria in resolving acute tubular necrosis (Chapter 41).

4 *Reduction in systemic vascular resistance ('distributive shock')*. Reduction in systemic vascular resistance increases the size of the systemic vascular bed, producing a relative hypovolaemia, reduced diastolic filling, reduced stroke volume and thus a fall in blood pressure. Unlike the previous two causes, vasodilation occurs as part of the pathogenesis, so the patient appears warm ('hot shock'), not cold and peripherally shut down. The heart compensates with an increase in output. The principal causes are:

 a anaphylaxis;
 b sepsis;
 c spinal shock.

5 *Confounding factors*. Pre-existing medical conditions and medications may confuse the clinical picture. Consider a patient with hypertension and taking a β-blocker such as bisoprolol or atenolol. For that patient, a systolic blood pressure of 110 mmHg may be very low, and β-blockade prevents a compensatory tachycardia in response.

Special causes of shock

Adrenocortical failure

Loss of the hormones produced by the cortex of the adrenal gland may follow bilateral adrenal haemorrhage, adrenalectomy, Addison's disease[2], pituitary apoplexy (with loss of adrenocorticotrophic hormone, ACTH) or lack of corticosteroid replacement in patients who have been on long-term glucocorticoids.

Failure of aldosterone secretion results in volume depletion and glucocorticoid deficiency, which impairs autonomic responses. The ability to respond to minor stress is severely compromised and may provoke an Addisonian crisis characterized by bradycardia and postural hypotension, which is responsive to corticosteroid replacement. Adrenocortical failure should be considered, and a bolus of hydrocortisone given in all patients with unexplained hypotension.

Sympathetic interruption

This reduces the effective blood volume by widespread vasodilation. It follows transection of the spinal cord (spinal shock), but may also occur after a high spinal anaesthetic or thoracic epidural. It is not unusual for patients undergoing open oesophagectomy with thoracic epidural to have vasopressor support to help perfusion of the anastomosis while having epidural for analgesia.

The vasovagal syndrome (faint)

The vasovagal syndrome is produced by severe pain or emotional disturbance, leading to vagal stimulation. It is the result of reflex vasodilation together with cardiac slowing owing to vagal activity. Hypotension is caused by a fall in cardiac output due to both bradycardia and reduced venous return, the latter being the result of peripheral vasodilation. Clinically, it is recognized by the presence of a bradycardia and responds to the simple measure of laying the patient flat with elevation of the legs leading to less pooling and adequate preload.

Septic shock

Shock may be produced as the result of severe infection from either Gram-positive or, more commonly, Gram-negative organisms. The latter are seen particularly after colonic, biliary and urological surgery, and with infected severe burns. The principal effect of endotoxins is to cause vasodilation of the peripheral circulation together with increased capillary permeability. The effects are partly direct and partly due to activation of normal tissue inflammatory responses such as the complement system and release of cytokines such as tumour necrosis factor (TNF). If sepsis is identified, it is paramount to address this with the Sepsis 6 approach (oxygen, fluid, antibiotics, blood culture, blood tests including lactate and urine output) in the early stages in order to prevent clinical deterioration.

Disseminated intravascular coagulation (DIC) results from activation of the clotting cascade and may lead to blockage of the arterial microcirculation by microemboli. Fibrin and platelets are consumed excessively, with resultant spontaneous haemorrhages into the skin, gastrointestinal tract, lungs, mouth and nose.

Sequelae of shock

A continuous low blood pressure produces a series of irreversible changes such that the patient may die in spite of treatment. The lack of oxygen delivery affects all the vital organs. The features of hypoperfusion are as follows:

- *Cerebral hypoperfusion* results in confusion or coma.
- *Cutaneous hypoperfusion* in all except septic shock results in cold, clammy and pale skin.
- *Renal hypoperfusion* results in reduced glomerular filtration, with oliguria or anuria. As renal ischaemia progresses, tubular necrosis may occur, and profound ischaemia may lead to cortical necrosis (Chapter 43).
- *Coronary hypoperfusion* results in cardiac failure, arrhythmia and arrest.
- *Pulmonary capillaries* may reflect the changes in the systemic circulation with transudation of fluid, resulting in pulmonary oedema, hampering oxygen transfer and causing further arterial hypoxaemia and thus tissue hypoxia. Pulmonary capillary function may also be impaired following multiple blood transfusions (transfusion-related acute lung injury, TRALI) and contusions resulting from chest trauma, a condition known as acute lung injury (previously termed 'shock lung').
- *Raised lactate* occurs as a result of a switch to anaerobic metabolism in those tissues with impaired cellular oxygenation.

[2]Thomas Addison (1793–1860), Physician, Guy's Hospital, London, UK. His original specimens may still be seen in the Gordon Museum at Guy's Hospital.

Principles in the management of patients in shock

Assessment

The cause of shock may be clear from the history, such as overt blood loss from trauma. Following history taking, which of necessity may be rapid, a thorough clinical examination is required to fully appraise both the cause and degree of shock. This should include assessment of the skin colour and perfusion, heart rate and rhythm from the radial artery (or femoral/carotid if the radial is impalpable), blood pressure, jugular venous pulse (raised in cardiogenic and obstructive shock, seldom visible in hypovolaemia and sepsis), auscultation of the chest (is there a tension pneumothorax?), heart (quiet sounds of tamponade), and abdomen (peritonitis from diverticular perforation in septic shock; tender and distended with rupture aneurysm).

Immediate measures

Treatment is often started while the cause of shock is being determined. Initial measures and management should include assessing the airway, breathing and circulation. During airway assessment, 15 L of oxygen should be administered via a non-rebreathing mask and fluid resuscitation commenced by giving a litre of crystalloid or 20 mL/kg immediately (Stat) (Figure 8.2). Once the cause of shock is identified, it should be reversed as quickly as possible.

Ventilatory support

Emphasis should always be on delivering oxygen to tissues when managing shock. In most cases of shock, supplementary oxygen improves tissue oxygenation. The efficacy of this should be assessed by blood gas monitoring, and severe breathlessness, persistent hypoxaemia and worsening acidosis (pH<7.3) are indications to consider endotracheal intubation and ventilation.

Fluid resuscitation

Administration of fluids increases venous return and thus improves cardiac output, but they should be administered with caution in the presence of cardiogenic shock. The nature of the fluid used is discussed in Chapter 3, but crystalloid solutions are usually first choice unless the patient is actively bleeding, when blood is the most appropriate replacement fluid. The rate of fluid administration should be titrated against the desired response; in a patient who is shocked from fluid depletion rapid infusion of 1 L (or 20 mL/kg) should be given immediately with monitoring for response and titration of fluid thereafter. Over-infusion is undesirable; it may cause pulmonary oedema, and in patients who have been bleeding, raising the blood pressure may prompt further haemorrhage; permissive hypotension may be appropriate in such cases until the cause of bleeding is addressed. Emphasis should be on tissue perfusion, and if both the brain and heart are well perfused with a good Glasgow Coma Score (GCS) and good cardiac contractility after initial infusion, further fluid can be closely titrated accordingly.

Two causes of shock that merit mention for immediate treatment are bleeding and anaphylaxis.

Bleeding

Direct pressure should be applied to a bleeding wound. Immediate surgical exploration is indicated where continued bleeding is likely, such as in ruptured spleen, ruptured aortic aneurysm or ruptured ectopic pregnancy. In these cases, resuscitation cannot overcome the losses until the rate of blood loss is curtailed. While fluid replacement with crystalloid is helpful, replacement of blood loss with blood is what is required.

Anaphylaxis

In surgical practice, this may arise most commonly as an allergic reaction to an antibiotic or radiological contrast medium. In addition to hypotension (due to vasodilation), bronchospasm and laryngeal oedema may be present and warrant immediate therapy. The immediate treatment for anaphylaxis is the administration of adrenaline (epinephrine; 0.5 mL of 1:1,000 concentration) intramuscularly or subcutaneously, repeated every 10–30 minutes as required. Subsequently, hydrocortisone and antihistamine agents (e.g. chlorphenamine) may be given.

For milder reactions, aliquots of 1 mL of 1:10,000 adrenaline are given and titrated to effect.

Anatomy	Initial assessment	Treatment

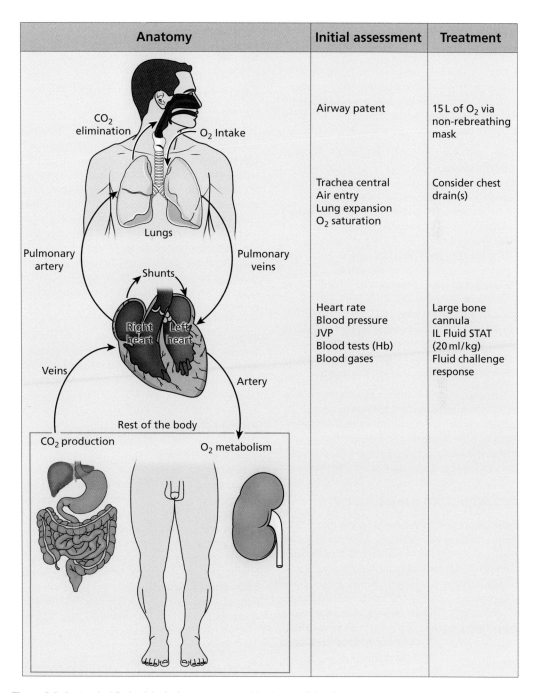

Initial assessment / Treatment entries:

Airway patent — 15 L of O_2 via non-rebreathing mask

Trachea central
Air entry
Lung expansion
O_2 saturation — Consider chest drain(s)

Heart rate
Blood pressure
JVP
Blood tests (Hb)
Blood gases — Large bone cannula
IL Fluid STAT
(20 ml/kg)
Fluid challenge response

Figure 8.2 Anatomical & physiological assessment and treatment of shock.

Monitoring and subsequent management

The severely shocked patient should be admitted to an intensive care unit where continuous supervision by specially trained nursing staff is available. Along with careful clinical surveillance, the following parameters need to be closely monitored:

- Core temperature, pulse, respiration rate and blood pressure.
- Hourly urine output (via a urinary catheter).
- Central venous pressure.
- Pulse oximetry. Oxygen is administered to ensure adequate oxygenation. Mechanical ventilation may be required.
- Electrocardiogram (ECG), looking at heart rate, rhythm and signs of cardiac ischaemia.
- Serum electrolytes, haemoglobin and white blood cell count.
- Arterial blood gases (PO_2, PCO_2, [H^+]).
- Blood lactate is raised in tissue hypoxia and also in septic shock through other mechanisms.
- The cardiac output, and left atrial and pulmonary arterial pressures (see later in this chapter).

The frequency of these measurements depends on the patient's condition and response to treatment. It is particularly important to remember that if the patient is conscious, he or she may well be terrified, in pain and acutely aware of all that is going on. Proper explanations and appropriate analgesia must be provided.

Cardiac output measurement

Cardiac output can be measured by the direct Fick[3] principle, indirect Fick principle, indicator dilution, transoesophageal ECHO and several less invasive procedures. Gold standard is the direct Fick principle, although indicator dilution techniques are less invasive in providing accurate results with minimal complications. Until the past decade, the Swan–Ganz catheter[4] was used in intensive care settings to measure cardiac output. Due to good accuracy, indicator dilution techniques like transpulmonary lithium dilution cardiac output (LiDCO™) measurement are now more commonly used in intensive care settings.

Swan–Ganz measurement of cardiac output

The Swan–Ganz technique involves passing a multiple-lumen catheter via a central vein into the right atrium. A small balloon on the end of the catheter is inflated, and the inflated balloon 'floats' with the blood returning to the heart across the tricuspid and pulmonary valves into the pulmonary artery. Once there, the catheter is advanced until it wedges itself in a small branch of the pulmonary arterial tree. The balloon is then deflated. During insertion, the position of the catheter can be monitored by the changing pressure waveform recorded by a transducer connected to the lumen. Along with measuring core temperature, a temperature probe at the tip of the catheter facilitates the measurement of cardiac output by the Fick principle: a bolus of cold is injected through the catheter and the change in temperature monitored. Importantly, the catheter also allows calculation of the systemic and pulmonary vascular resistances.

LiDCO measurement of cardiac output

Cardiac output is now more commonly measured using techniques like LiDCO: a very small amount of lithium is injected into a central or peripheral vein. An arterial line with a lithium sensor measures the lithium, and this measurement is subsequently used to calibrate pulse contour using software that provides continuous cardiac output data by analysing the arterial pressure waveform. This technique is minimally invasive, requiring only arterial and venous lines. A LiDCO monitor displays arterial pressure, stroke volume and cardiac output.

Prevention of hypothermia

Patients may cool down because of neglect, infusion of cold fluids, particularly unwarmed blood, and extracorporeal circulations such as haemodialysis or haemofiltration circuits. Allowing a patient to cool down to subnormal temperatures (35°C or below)

---

[3] Adolf Eugen Fick (1829–1901), German Physiologist working first in Zurich and then in Wurzburg.

[4] Harold J C Swan (1922–2005), Cardiologist, Cedars of Lebanon Hospital, Los Angeles, CA, USA. William Ganz (1919–2009), Professor of Medicine, UCLA, and Senior Research Scientist, Cedars of Lebanon Hospital, Los Angeles, CA, USA.

impairs the coagulation cascades and platelet aggregation, and promotes fibrinolysis. To prevent this, all infusions should be prewarmed, and the patient actively warmed using convective (forced air) warming (e.g. Bair Hugger™).

Pharmacological agents

The hypotensive patient may require significant vasopressor support. The principal drugs used are catecholamines or their derivatives, in addition to drugs to treat specific causes such as antimicrobial therapy for septicaemia. Patients in cardiogenic shock benefit from positive inotropic agents, whereas patients with low systemic vascular resistance due to sepsis require agents to increase vascular resistance. The drugs used in this context are sympathomimetics, with differing degrees of α (peripheral vasoconstriction), β_1 (inotropic and chronotropic) and β_2 (peripheral vasodilation) effects. Examples of such drugs include the following.

Noradrenaline (norepinephrine)

Noradrenaline has predominantly α effects, but with modest β activity. It is used to increase systemic vascular resistance through its vasoconstrictor α effects, while the β effects may help maintain cardiac output.

Metaraminol

Like noradrenaline, metaraminol has predominantly α receptor agonist actions causing vasoconstriction and inotropic effects on the heart increasing systemic blood pressure (both the systolic and diastolic blood pressure). It is weaker than noradrenaline but has a more prolonged duration of action (20–60 minutes).

Dopamine

Dopamine has three separate actions according to dose:

1 At *low doses* (2 µg/kg/min), dopaminergic actions dominate, causing increased renal perfusion. It

was thought to be useful in protecting the kidneys from acute kidney injury, but its value in this setting has been disproved.

2 At *moderate doses* (5 µg/kg/min), β_1 effects predominate with positive inotropic activity (increasing myocardial contractility and rate).

3 At *higher doses* (over 5 µg/kg/min), α effects predominate with vasoconstriction.

Dopamine was once commonly used in shock, but its lack of renal protective effect, increased incidence of arrhythmias and association with a higher mortality in cardiogenic shock have reduced its usefulness.

Adrenaline (epinephrine)

Adrenaline has strong α and β actions, and may be used to increase peripheral resistance while also increasing cardiac output. The powerful vasoconstrictor actions of both adrenaline and noradrenaline may result in ischaemia and infarction of peripheral tissues, most commonly fingers, toes and the tips of the nose and ears.

Vasopressin

Vasopressin (ADH) is a potent vasopressor, in addition to its effects on volume regulation in the kidney. Infusion of vasopressin has been shown to be a useful adjunct to noradrenaline in patients with septic shock. **Argipressin** is an analogue of vasopressin, with similar pressor properties.

Dobutamine

Dobutamine has predominantly β_1 actions, increasing myocardial contractility and rate, thus increasing cardiac output. It is used principally in cardiogenic shock.

Dopexamine

Dopexamine has predominantly β_2 actions, increasing myocardial contractility; it also acts on peripheral dopamine receptors, increasing renal perfusion.

9

Trauma surgery

Jonathan Morton

Learning objectives

✓ To understand the principles of initial trauma assessment.

✓ To understand the principles of damage control surgery.

✓ Gain knowledge of the trauma management of individual abdominal organs.

Trauma is the commonest cause of death for those under 40 years of age in the UK. Trauma networks have been associated with a reduction in mortality of between 10% and 40% for those severely injured. In 2012, as part of national trauma network systems, 27 designated major trauma centres were created in the UK. As a result, there has been a 19% increase in the odds of survival for trauma victims for those who reach secondary care alive.

Trauma types

- *Penetrating trauma* is defined as a foreign object penetrating the skin or mucosal membranes of the body.
- *Blunt trauma* may be associated with no breaks in the skin. However, it can result in deep tissue damage (including organs) depending on the forces involved with the initial event.

Generally, timelines for penetrating trauma are compressed, and physiology and injuries can evolve and change far more rapidly compared with those of blunt trauma. Management of time in the initial phase of assessment and intervention for trauma patients is critically important, especially for the team leader, as it is easy to lose situational awareness (Chapter 2).

Ellis and Calne's Lecture Notes in General Surgery, Fourteenth Edition.
Edited by Christopher Watson and Justin Davies.
© 2023 John Wiley & Sons Ltd. Published 2023 by John Wiley & Sons Ltd.
Companion website: www.wiley.com/go/Watson/GeneralSurgery14

Mechanisms of injury

The mechanism of injury is of great importance for trauma patients. Understanding the forces involved (and how these were transferred to the patient) can help anticipate injuries and injury patterns. For example, an unrestrained front seat passenger of a vehicle impacting the steering wheel at 50 mph may well have life-threatening injuries to their thorax and abdomen. In contrast, the same patient who was restrained with deployed airbags at the scene may have significantly less severity in their injury pattern(s).

Principles of trauma management

- Rapid assessment.
- Avoidance of secondary injuries.
- Interventions to stop the fatal triad of death in trauma.

The triad of death in trauma

A common pathway of eventual mortality has been described for critically injured trauma patients: the so-called trauma triad of death, which refers to the vicious cycle of evolving acidosis, hypothermia and coagulopathy (Figure 9.1).

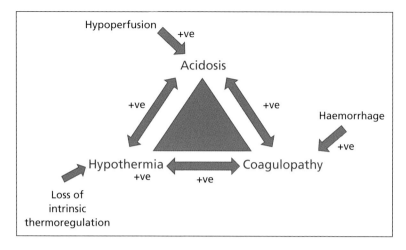

Figure 9.1 The triad of death in trauma care.

The positive feedback from each component of the triad promotes further worsening of physiology. Haemorrhage promotes loss/consumption of clotting factors and contributes to *hypothermia*. This also reduces oxygen delivery to tissues (hypoxia), with anaerobic respiration predominating. This results in lactic acid production and an increase in *acidosis*. This acidosis, together with hypothermia, adversely impacts the clotting cascade, further exacerbating *coagulopathy* and promoting further haemorrhage.

Most interventions and trauma objectives are directed at minimizing or stopping the propagation of the triad, and by so doing, minimizing secondary injuries and improving patient outcomes. The surgical approach used to stop this positive feedback loop is generally referred to as damage control surgery (see later).

For critically injured trauma patients, interventions to prevent worsening physiology are made at different stages of the patient pathway. Figure 9.2 summarizes a critically ill trauma patient's journey from the incident to definitive surgical intervention. During these different phases of care, interventions are made to arrest or reverse the effects of the triad of death.

advanced care teams for critically ill patients will be sent to the scene of incidents to initiate treatment interventions at the earliest opportunity. Some pre-hospital teams travel with blood products and other advanced medications to progress the early resuscitation of patients. These teams also assess where trauma patients should be transferred to minimize time to definitive management of injuries.

As part of the transfer process to definitive care, pre-alerts are given to the appropriate emergency centres to enable trauma teams to prepare appropriately for the imminent arrival of a critically ill patient. The acronym ATMIST (Table 9.1) is often used to standardize communication, summarizing the patient's situation. As part of this preparation of the receiving trauma centre, a team will be established (frequently utilizing a trauma call/page) and led by a team leader. A briefing will be given to the team on the mechanism of injury, understanding of current physiology and anticipated equipment needed. Roles within the team are established as different aspects of the primary survey (see below) are typically conducted simultaneously by various team members.

Phase 1: Pre-hospital trauma care and initial assessment

Care of the trauma patient starts from the time of the first call for help. Calls are screened, and the likely severity of traumatic injuries is assessed. Pre-hospital

Table 9.1 ATMIST Communication acronym

ATMIST
Age
Time of incident
Mechanism of injury
Injuries (top to toe)
Signs (vitals)
Treatment

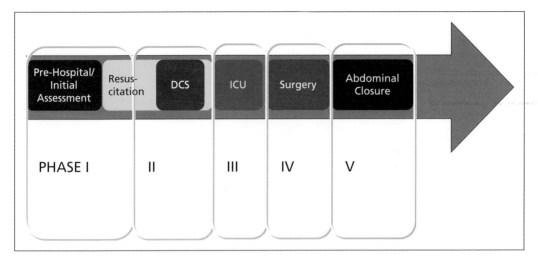

Figure 9.2 Phases of damage control. DCS: damage control surgery; ICU: intensive care unit.

Phase 2: Initial assessment with ongoing resuscitation

Assessment of trauma patients

The initial assessment of trauma victims as they arrive in the hospital is a critical aspect of trauma care. Great emphasis is on the mechanism of injury (MOI), which helps establish the transmitted forces involved with the accident/incident and enable the receiving hospital team to anticipate injuries and their severity. Upon arrival, there is a focused handover between the pre-hospital and trauma teams. An initial assessment of the trauma patient is performed: the *primary survey* (Table 9.2).

Table 9.2 The primary survey

Primary survey:

(C) Catastrophic haemorrhage control (not part of ATLS)
A Airway, with cervical spine control (hard collar or equivalent device/method)
B Breathing, with ventilation (oxygen application with a non-rebreathing mask)
C Circulation, with haemorrhage control (intravenous access and blood for analysis)
D Disability assessment (neurological assessment)
E Exposure, with environmental control

Advanced Trauma Life Support (ATLS)

Advanced Trauma Life Support is a training course and ethos in assessing trauma patients. In ATLS, an A to E assessment of patients is conducted in rigid sequential steps, simulating the worst-case scenario of an individual doctor alone looking after trauma patients. In most trauma centres, however, this initial assessment is conducted by multiple team members simultaneously while there is ongoing resuscitation.

Catastrophic haemorrhage control is listed at the top of the primary survey. While not part of the ATLS mantra, it has been added in recognition of the importance of haemorrhage control in the context of catastrophic haemorrhage (Table 9.2).

If at any stage interventions are required during the primary survey, or there is a significant change in the patient's physiology, repeated assessment(s) using this primary survey sequence are often performed. This ensures that no life-threatening conditions evolve unrecognized, requiring further intervention.

Catastrophic haemorrhage control

The principle of controlling catastrophic haemorrhage has evolved from recent military conflicts. For individuals who have lost limbs and are at risk of immediate exsanguination, temporizing haemorrhage control is required before starting the A to E assessment. This is typically achieved with either direct pressure or tourniquets. These will often be applied in the pre-hospital setting with a record of the time of when they were applied (either in medical notes or directly on the tourniquet). These are generally not removed until the patient is in the operating room environment. The same principle applies to any objects such as a knife that may still be in the patient on arrival to the hospital after an incident. These are also not removed until surgery/definitive management has either commenced or will do so imminently.

A: Airway with adequate cervical spine control

Before examining the patient, a simple question such as asking their name with an appropriate response confirms airway patency and indicates a good level of consciousness. In this scenario, a more formal airway assessment may not be required.

The airway should be inspected to exclude airway obstruction from foreign bodies (e.g. dentures). Signs that might suggest impending airway obstruction, such as evidence of inhalational injuries (carbonaceous material in the airways), often require pre-emptive/early intubation and ventilation. While controlling the cervical spine in recognition that there is often concurrent cervical spine trauma, simple airway manoeuvres can be performed to improve relative airway obstruction (e.g. jaw thrust / chin lift).

Adjuncts to airway control include oro/nasopharyngeal airways and, should the conscious level, as measured by the Glasgow Coma Score (GCS, Table 17.3), be 8 or below, a definitive airway is required. A *definitive airway* is defined as a secured, cuffed tube in the trachea.

Some penetrating injury patterns such as gunshot wounds to the face or complex facial fractures are also associated with significant difficulties in securing airways on occasion. It should be noted that there are specific anatomical differences between adults and children, and as such, different approaches and equipment to assist with the airway are required in the paediatric population.

B: Breathing with adequate ventilation

Combining these two aspects of 'B' alludes to the importance of the patient being able to breathe and the adequacy of that attempted ventilation/gas exchange. Supplemental oxygen should be placed on the patient at 100% unless the patient is already intubated and ventilated. A pulse oximeter should also be applied.

Life-threatening chest injuries such as massive haemothorax (IV access recommended before intervention), tension pneumothorax, tracheal or bronchial injuries should be identified, and treatment instigated/planned at this stage of the primary survey.

Tension pneumothorax is an immediate life-threatening clinical situation. The classical description of clinical presentation is the patient having a deviated trachea away from the side of the pneumothorax, distended neck veins (which can be hard to assess with a hard collar *in situ*) and the physiological state of shock. In reality, these are often quite late signs of a tension pneumothorax. Clinical examination should be sufficient to diagnose the condition as waiting for radiological confirmation is not appropriate from a time perspective. Treatment is rapid needle decompression. This is achieved by inserting a cannula into the fourth or fifth intercostal space (inferior to the pectoralis major muscle) just posterior to the anterior axillary line. The second intercostal space in the midclavicular line is advocated in paediatric populations.

C: Circulation with haemorrhage control

A rapid assessment of *circulation* can be achieved by assessing the patient's pulse, capillary refill time and level of consciousness. Blood pressure monitoring, if not already applied, should be commenced. Consideration needs to be given to the physiological state of shock for the individual and its cause while initiating resuscitation of the patient.

Intravenous access

Two large-bore intravenous catheters are typically placed in both antecubital fossae. If intravenous access is challenging, the trauma team may place either an interosseous needle or a long line (central line). Blood is taken and sent to the laboratory (Table 9.3) and rapidly analysed on a blood gas machine to obtain a lactate, which will indicate the degree of physiological shock. Once intravenous access has been successful, resuscitation can commence with either crystalloid (warmed normal saline or Hartmann's solution) or blood products.

Volume replacement

Consideration should be given to initiating the *major transfusion protocol* within the hospital. This protocol typically releases multiple resources within the hospital as well as blood products to help the trauma team. A 1:1 ratio for the various blood components, including red cells, fresh frozen plasma, platelets and cryoprecipitate, is typically delivered within the packs.

Haemorrhage control

Reversal of any anticoagulation should be considered as part of this phase of the primary survey. There is also evidence that tranexamic acid (an anti-fibrinolytic that stabilizes clot), given within 3 hours of injury, improves the long-term outcomes of trauma patients. As discussed above, tourniquets/splints/direct pressure can be used for peripheral limb haemorrhage control, and pelvic binders are frequently used to control bleeding from pelvic fractures.

D: Disability and neurological assessment

A rapid *neurological assessment* of the patient is made. This phase of the primary survey aims to establish the patient's conscious level, identify any potential spinal cord injuries and initiate the assessment of these. Pupillary size and blood glucose are also assessed at this stage. The conscious level is assessed using the GCS scale (Table 17.3), which divides assessment of consciousness into responses of the eyes, speech and movement. Each of the three domains of the GCS are added together to obtain a result out of 15. The maximum score is 15 and the minimum 3 (assuming all aspects can be tested).

Table 9.3 Blood tests for trauma patients
Typical blood tests for trauma patients
Full blood count (FBC)
Urea and Electrolytes (creatinine, potassium and sodium)
Metabolic/Endocrine tests (liver function and bone profile, including calcium)
Clotting studies
Beta-HCG
Group and save or cross-match samples
Amylase

E: Exposure with environmental control

Exposure has to be adequate so that additional injuries are identified, documented and assessed promptly is critical. This is particularly the case for penetrating trauma wounds, where exit wounds or other injuries can be hidden on the posterior aspect of the body.

Hypothermia has a profound adverse effect on coagulation; it inhibits the clotting cascade, impairs platelet aggregation and enhances fibrinolysis, resulting in a coagulopathy as well as an acidosis. Therefore, it is essential to maintain an adequate core temperature for the patient during this phase of the primary survey. In modern emergency rooms and operating theatres, it should be possible to rapidly increase the temperature of the rooms to facilitate adequate environmental control (minimizing the risk of hypothermia). Forced air warming devices (e.g. Bair huggers™) are frequently used to help maintain patients' core temperatures.

Submersion and exposure injuries

In submersion or exposure injuries, where the patient is profoundly hypothermic, more aggressive and/or controlled warming may be required either utilizing trans-vesical warming or, in extremes, cardiac or veno-venous bypass systems.

Spinal injury and thermoregulation

Patients with high spinal cord injuries often lose the ability to thermoregulate due to inappropriate vasodilation in the peripheries contributing to heat loss (with the loss of sympathetic tone).

The AMPLE history

Following the A to E assessment of the primary survey, a targeted medical history is taken, known as an ***AMPLE*** history. This involves

- **A**llergy history.
- **M**edical history.
- **P**ast medical history.
- **L**ast: ate / drank / menstrual period / tetanus injection.
- **E**vents leading to the trauma.

Special investigations

While the primary survey is conducted, *adjuncts* are utilized to improve the understanding of the patient's condition:

- *A **F**ocused **A**ssessment with **S**onography for **T**rauma (**FAST** scan):* a rapid targeted ultrasound scan giving real-time information on potential lung, pericardial and abdominal injuries.
- *X-rays:* Chest, pelvic and occasionally lateral C-spine X-rays may be performed at the bedside in the resuscitation department, although these have been largely replaced by rapid access to cross-sectional imaging.
- *Trauma CT scan from the head to the knees:* a contrast enhanced scan providing arterial and portal phase images of the chest and abdomen, and non-contrast images of the head and neck.
- *Arterial blood gas:* critical to providing a snapshot of the underlying physiology of the patient. Evidence of significant acidosis (low pH) or a raised lactate level indicates the urgency of definitive interventions.

Monitoring

Depending on the severity of injuries and time available before transfer to the operating room, additional lines, such as a central and arterial, may be placed. Consideration should be given to urinary catheter insertion, especially if the patient is to be transferred to a major trauma centre.

Relative contraindications to urinary catheterization in trauma patients include findings that might suggest urethral disruption, such as:

- blood at the urethral meatus;
- scrotal haematoma;
- high riding prostate;
- frank haematuria.

Secondary survey

Time permitting, a secondary survey is conducted by examining the patient head to toe. Important signs to consider *and record* include any bruising or disruption of the skin, previous surgical scars/injuries and areas of pain that may require further imaging. Specific signs/symptoms are considered below.

Head and neck

- *Basal skull fracture assessment:* any signs that might indicate a basal skull fracture should be recorded:
  - periorbital bruising (raccoon eyes);
  - cerebrospinal fluid (CSF) rhinorrhoea;
  - CSF otorrhoea;
  - Battle's sign (bruising over the mastoid process);
  - haemotympanum (blood behind the tympanic membrane);
  - cranial nerve palsy.
- *Scalp lacerations:* These can lead to significant blood loss. They should be addressed with direct pressure (bandages) or skin stapling devices as a temporizing measure if definitive management is not possible.
- *Assessment of the cervical spine:* This can also be performed in patients without distracting injuries. Any pain and/or neurological signs should be carefully recorded to determine if further assessments are required before removing the cervical spine protection.

Chest

- *Rib fractures:* These in isolation are a significant cause of pain, and patients often require admission for adequate analgesia. Without adequate analgesia, atelectasis is not uncommon, and if left untreated, progression to pneumonia may occur. In more severe trauma, a *flail segment* may be present (Chapter 14). This will compromise ventilation to a greater or lesser extent depending on the number and distribution of ribs involved. The vast majority of rib fractures are managed conservatively.
- *Contusions:* If significant force has been transmitted through the chest or thorax, pulmonary or cardiac contusions may exist, impairing oxygenation of the bloodstream or contributing to cardiovascular instability.

Transfer to the next phase of care

Once the primary survey has been completed, the team should understand how critically ill the patient is. The trauma team leader and surgical teams will need to consider the next step in the patient's journey. There will typically be options ranging from cross-sectional imaging, intensive care or moving directly to the operating theatre or interventional radiology suite. If in a small hospital or trauma unit, consideration will need to be given to transferring the patient for definitive care at a major trauma centre.

Indications for the immediate transfer to the operating theatre include:

- *evisceration;*
- *non-responders to resuscitation with hypovolaemic shock;*
- *impalement patients who are unstable.*

For patients not meeting the above-mentioned criteria, a judgement needs to be made about the patient's overall stability. Generally, patients who are either responders or transient responders to resuscitation are safe to be transferred to the cross-sectional imaging suite.

Damage control ethos

A damage control ethos is adopted for critically ill trauma patients and is included within the resuscitation phase of the patient's journey. The philosophy consists of different elements of care, including permissive hypotension and damage control surgery with balanced resuscitation (with appropriate blood products).

Permissive hypotension

Permissive hypotension (also known as hypovolaemic resuscitation) is a concept of accepting a lower-than-normal blood pressure (systolic 80–90 mmHg, mean arterial pressure around 50 mmHg), by avoiding aggressive resuscitation to 'normalize' blood pressure readings. This approach reduces blood loss by allowing vessels that have undergone vasospasm to continue to function in this manner rather than 'opening' them up with higher perfusion pressures.

Permissive hypertension is contraindicated in those with traumatic brain injuries where higher cerebral perfusion pressures (CPP) may be needed to maintain cerebral perfusion to prevent secondary brain injuries (Chapter 17). In trauma, the normal autoregulation of cerebral perfusion may be disrupted and, therefore, active management by maintaining a mean pressure of 80 mmHg may be required, or even higher in the elderly.

Damage control surgery

Research has shown that initial, short surgical procedures (typically 60 minutes or less) to 'control damage' were more successful than undertaking prolonged major surgery at the time of presentation. This surgical approach aims to control haemorrhage and contamination, and making specific organ interventions. The two main operative procedures are resuscitative/emergent thoracotomy and trauma laparotomy.

Resuscitative or emergent thoracotomy

A resuscitative or emergent thoracotomy may be required in the event of a loss of cardiac output in trauma patients or if intrathoracic pathology is suspected as the underlying cause for deterioration. This is generally performed by performing a left thoracotomy entering the chest typically in the fifth left intercostal space. Better exposure can be achieved by converting the incision into a 'clamshell' thoracotomy with the division of the sternum and right fifth intercostal space, facilitating excellent exposure of both left and right lungs as well as the heart itself. If this procedure is performed either in the pre-hospital setting or emergency department, thoracotomies are generally only performed as a clamshell.

Once in the adult thoracic cavity, a pericardial tamponade can be quickly evacuated through a vertical incision to avoid damage to the phrenic nerve as it runs over the anterolateral aspect of the pericardium. Once the pericardium has been evacuated, open direct current (DC) cardioversion shock can be administered if required.

Significant bleeding from lung parenchymal injuries can be controlled either temporarily using a clamp or more definitively using linear staplers and over-sewing the area of trauma. There may be a need to perform an emergent pneumonectomy, although this is quite rare.

Entering into the thoracic cavity gives the opportunity to control the descending thoracic aorta, with either manual manipulation or instrumentation. In order to avoid damage to the oesophagus, typically located immediately anterior to the descending thoracic aorta, many surgeons advocate manual compression rather than instrumentation.

Outcomes vary depending on the type of trauma (penetrating versus blunt) and indication for thoracotomy. Success rates for patients with penetrating traumatic injuries, leaving the hospital neurologically intact, range between 3% and 25%. This is only the case if the resuscitative thoracotomy is performed within 15 min of loss of signs of life. For blunt trauma, outcomes are significantly worse, with at best 1.5% of patients leaving the hospital alive and neurologically intact.

Indications for thoracotomy in the context of blunt trauma need to be considered carefully. The outcome in blunt trauma also depends on the location of the intervention (pre-hospital versus operative theatre) and the skill set of the team performing the procedure. Unless definitive treatment for the underlying cause of the blunt traumatic cardiac arrest is addressed rapidly, the outcome is unlikely to be successful.

Emergency laparotomy

There has been a significant fall in the number of patients undergoing emergency laparotomy for trauma due to improvements in cross-sectional imaging and changes in the management of specific organs. For example, splenectomy once was relatively commonly performed for traumatic indications; however, it is now much rarer with advancements in interventional radiology.

Preparation for an emergency laparotomy (if possible) includes a thorough team brief of the theatre staff before starting the case (Chapter 2). This ensures that all the required equipment is readily available and that potential unexpected steps have been planned for, such as an emergent thoracotomy or the need for particular stapling devices/energy devices. If the patient has not already been catheterized in the emergency room, this should be performed as soon they enter the operating theatre. Ongoing resuscitation will occur as the surgeons start the operation to try and correct the abnormal physiology. For critically ill patients, the theatre is often prepared similarly to that of a ruptured abdominal aortic aneurysm, with the patient often conscious while the skin preparation and draping is applied. Once the surgical team is ready to make the first incision, the anaesthetist will often induce the patient at that stage. The operation starts as soon as the anaesthetic team is prepared. Depending on the situation's urgency, a knife/scissors may be used rather than monopolar diathermy to expedite entry into the abdominal cavity.

Once the abdominal cavity has been opened, there is an immediate evacuation of any blood and the small bowel is delivered into the wound to enable packing of the abdomen. Using multiple large abdominal swabs, the abdominal cavity is then packed in quadrants, taking note of where most of the blood has originated from or where most of the injuries are suspected. Any damage or bleeding from the small bowel mesentery is addressed using sutures, but this is not the time to do anastomoses or other time-consuming interventions. In coordination with the anaesthetic team (dependant on the patient's stability), a systematic examination of the abdominal cavity is performed. This typically starts in the quadrant furthest away from suspected pathology. For example, if a shattered spleen has been the cause of the haemoperitoneum and the need for emergency laparotomy, packs will typically be removed from the right lower quadrant first and then removing swabs from successive quadrants until the final quadrant can be addressed safely.

Once all packs have been removed, and haemorrhage controlled, a more thorough assessment of the intra-abdominal organs can be performed. The primary objective is to control bleeding and any contamination from a hollow viscus.

Individual organ management

Spleen (see also Chapter 35)

Many splenic injuries are now managed conservatively or with interventional radiological techniques rather than splenectomy at open surgery. Splenic trauma can occur either as an isolated event or as part of a more complex multiple injury pattern in a trauma patient. Some predisposing pathological conditions of the spleen, such as splenomegaly, may result in splenic rupture with relatively minor force. Most assessments of potential splenic injury are performed using CT rather than ultrasound.

It is important to salvage the spleen if at all possible due to its role in protection against infection particularly from capsulated organisms. Most early stage splenic injuries can be treated conservatively (without intervention). More severe injuries may require radiological embolization if they result in cardiovascular instability. Severe splenic injury, such as a shattered spleen, often require a splenectomy to control the bleeding.

Liver (see also Chapter 32)

Most bleeding from liver injuries is a result of venous bleeding rather than arterial. As such, packing the liver by placing large abdominal swabs around the liver to re-approximate the tear in the liver capsule is usually sufficient to arrest the bleeding. Any further bleeding can be controlled using interventional radiological techniques with embolization.

Extrahepatic biliary tree

Injuries to the gall bladder are rare outside of the context of penetrating trauma. The treatment for most injuries is to perform a cholecystectomy with careful inspection of the porta hepatis.

Stomach, small bowel and colon

Primary repair of any isolated hollow viscus injury is usually performed in stable patients. In the context of damage control surgery, the mainstay of treatment is to control contamination and haemorrhage rather than definitive management of the injuries. This approach may include leaving the abdomen open (a laparostomy) and transferring the patient to the intensive care unit to normalize the abnormal physiology. In the context of damage control surgery, performing anastomoses or stomas would not be appropriate at this first laparotomy. Instead, stapling devices are typically used to close any defects in the hollow viscus to enable a rapid transfer to the intensive care unit. Consideration for anastomosis or a stoma can be made at a subsequent second look laparotomy 24–48 hours later.

Pancreas

Most pancreatic injuries are treated conservatively, especially when it is an isolated injury. Even in patients with multiple intra-abdominal pathologies, the pancreas often does not require surgical intervention outside of haemorrhage issues. Disruption of ducts, for example, can often be treated using stents and endoscopic retrograde cholangiopancreatography (ERCP) rather than open operative surgical techniques.

Diaphragmatic injuries

Diaphragmatic injuries are rare on the right side because of the bare area of the liver providing protection. The left diaphragm is more prone to injury from blunt force trauma or penetrating injuries. A surgical repair of such injuries is indicated. Typically, a strong non-absorbable suture is used to close such defects. Occasionally, small diagrammatic hernias can present late, some months or even years after the initial injury.

Abdominal closure

Temporary closure of the midline wound, or leaving it open as a laparostomy may be performed, with definitive closure some days later. Muscles left unopposed will contract over a period of days, making the eventual closure technically more challenging. For laparotomies in physiologically stable patients, definitive closure can be undertaken as part of the primary procedure.

Phases 3 to 5

After damage control surgery, the patients are taken to the *intensive care unit* where normalization of clotting and other physiological parameters are the main goals of therapy. Typically, patients with laparostomies will be reassessed in the operating theatre every 48 hours, although this is also dictated by the patient's response to treatment in the intensive care unit. Second look laparotomies can be used to definitively manage any hollow viscus injuries, with *anastomoses being performed or stomas* created at subsequent operations (Phase 4). Consideration is also given to the timing of *abdominal wall closure* (Phase 5), either with primary or secondary intention.

10

Burns

Ian Grant

Learning objectives

✓ To know the different types of burn.

✓ To be able to determine the extent of a burn injury as a percentage of the total body surface area and to understand how this affects treatment.

✓ To be able to assess the depth of a thermal burn.

✓ To know the principles of the initial management of the patient with burns.

Causes

- *Thermal burn*: the most common cause of a burn, due either to direct contact with a hot surface, flame or scalding liquid, or to hot vapour such as steam. The severity of the burn is related to the temperature of the surface, and the duration of exposure. The thermal burn from steam is due to both temperature of steam and latent heat released as it changes phase from vapour to liquid.
- *Electrical burn*: contact with a source of electricity. A voltage of more than 500 V is considered high voltage and likely to cause greater injury. The patient will often have burns at the site of entry and at the site of exit of the electricity, and internal organs, including muscle and nerve, can be injured.
- *Chemical burn*: inadvertent exposure to a strong acid or base (alkali). Most commonly, this is a commercially available product such as acid from a battery or alkali drain cleaner. Initial management of the wound includes prolonged irrigation for more than 10 minutes or until a neutral pH is achieved.

Ellis and Calne's Lecture Notes in General Surgery, Fourteenth Edition. Edited by Christopher Watson and Justin Davies.
© 2023 John Wiley & Sons Ltd. Published 2023 by John Wiley & Sons Ltd.
Companion website: www.wiley.com/go/Watson/GeneralSurgery14

- *Radiation burn*: exposure to radiation, such as radiotherapy treatment for cancer.

Severity

The severity of a burn is assessed based on the depth of burn and the amount of skin involved, together with other associated clinical features.

Depth of burn

Thermal burns can be subdivided according to the depth of thermal injury to the sequential layers of the skin (Figure 10.1). Burns of different depths exhibit different pathophysiology and require different treatment (Table 10.1).

Burns can be subdivided into:

- superficial/erythema;
- superficial partial thickness;
- deep partial thickness;
- full thickness burns.

Partial-thickness burns heal spontaneously, superficial partial-thickness wounds heal within 2–3 weeks without scarring, and deep partial-thickness wounds take longer than 3 weeks to heal and do so with scarring.

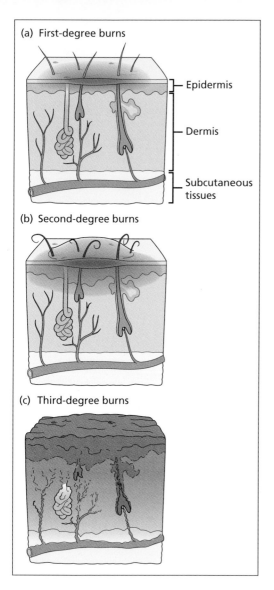

(a) First-degree burns

- Epidermis
- Dermis
- Subcutaneous tissues

(b) Second-degree burns

(c) Third-degree burns

Figure 10.1 A partial-thickness burn (a) leaves part or the whole of the germinal epithelium intact; complete healing takes place (b). A full thickness burn (c) destroys the germinal layer and, unless very small, can heal only by dense scar tissue.

Full thickness burns have no potential for spontaneous healing.

Area of the burn

Estimation of the area of a burn is critical. Burns of more than 20% of the patient's total body surface area (defined as a major burn injury) are associated with a systemic physiological change referred to as burns shock. A patient with a burn of this size requires immediate fluid resuscitation. The amount of fluid required by the patient can be calculated with knowledge of the weight of the patient, the burn area as a percentage of their total body surface area and the time of the injury.

Patients who have sustained major burn injuries and are best managed with the support of a specialist burns unit. Clinicians starting the initial management of these patients in peripheral locations are encouraged to liaise as quickly as possible with the local specialist burns unit in order to plan further care and urgent transfer of the patient.

The surface area of the burn area can be rapidly assessed using a 'Lund–Browder' chart (Figure 10.2). The chart takes into account differences in the body surface area with age. For example, an infant's head has a proportionately greater surface area than an adult's head. These charts are readily available in Emergency Departments. Areas of partial and full thickness burns are drawn on the chart to allow calculation of the burn area.

In the adult, a rough approximation of burn size can also be achieved using the rule of nines. The body is divided into zones of percentage of surface area (Figure 10.3). Alternatively, as a rough rule, the patient's hand is approximately 1% of the body surface area.

	Percentage surface area
Head and neck	9
Each arm	9
Each leg	$2 \times 9 = 18$
Front of the trunk	$2 \times 9 = 18$
Back of the trunk	$2 \times 9 = 18$
Perineum	1

The initial management of the severe burn injury patient

Urgent assessment, resuscitation and transfer to a specialist unit is likely to give the patient the best chance of recovery. Well-established protocols for the best management of these patients are documented in the Emergency Management of Severe Burns (EMSB) and Advanced Burns Life Support (ABLS) courses.

Table 10.1 Burn comparison

Thickness	Depth of thermal necrosis	Appearance	Pain/sensibility	Prognosis if untreated
Superficial/ erythema (historically called a first-degree burn)	Epidermis	Dry, blanching with pressure	Painful, and sensate to light touch	Heals without scars in 5–10 days
Superficial partial thickness (historically, this would be called a second-degree burn)	Upper (papillary) dermis, with preservation of the epidermal ridges of the dermo-epidermal junction	Blisters, wet, swollen, blanching with pressure	Painful, and sensate to light touch	Heals without scars in 14–21 days
Deep partial thickness (historically, this would also be called a second-degree burn)	Deep (reticular dermis) with necrosis of the dermo-epidermal junction but preservation of the hair follicles lined with epidermis	Blisters, does not blanch, colour can vary in patches from pale yellow to red	Painful, sensate to pressure but not to light touch	Heals with scarring in over 21 days, often requires tangential excision and then split skin grafting to accelerate healing and minimize scarring
Full thickness (historically called a 'third-degree burn')	The necrosis extends through the entire thickness of the skin	White, or brown, inelastic, dry	Painless, sensate only to deep pressure	Heals only by contraction. With the exception of small burns of less than 2% total body surface area; the burn requires excision and the application of a split skin graft

Airway management

A thermal injury to the upper airway should be suspected if the patient was in an enclosed space breathing in hot smoke. Examination of the patient might also reveal that he or she has a hoarse voice, stridor, burnt facial hair and soot around his/her mouth or nose. Dangerous narrowing of the airway can occur quickly due to oedema. The clinician with the greatest experience of airway management (most commonly an anaesthetist or emergency physician) should protect the patient's airway, possibly by urgent endotracheal intubation.

Breathing and ventilation

In rare circumstances, a patient may have circumferential full thickness burns of his/her chest, preventing normal respiratory movements. These patients require urgent bedside incision of the burn (termed an escharotomy) to allow the chest to expand.

Fluid resuscitation

A burn of >20% total body surface area initiates a dramatic release of pro-inflammatory cytokines, causing systemic changes that include an increase in capillary permeability with loss of proteins and fluid into the interstitial space. This starts at the time of injury and peaks at around 24 hours. It continues for approximately 72 hours. The effect of this loss of intravascular fluid is compounded by the toxic effect of the systemic response of the body to a major burn, which can reduce myocardial contractility, and the local response to the burn causing fluid loss from blistering and oedema.

Pain

Pain is severe in partial-thickness burns due to stimulation of numerous nerve endings in damaged skin; full thickness burns can be painless.

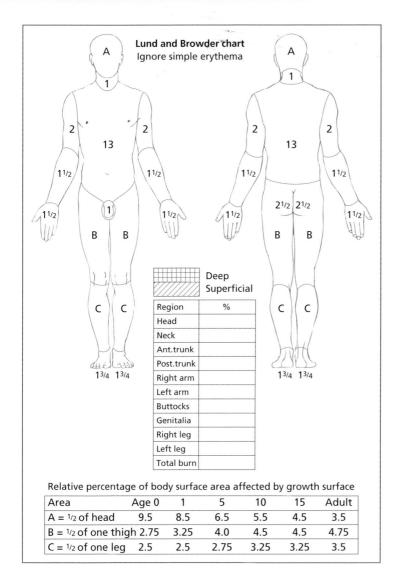

Lund and Browder chart
Ignore simple erythema

| | | | Deep |
| Superficial |

Region	%
Head	
Neck	
Ant.trunk	
Post.trunk	
Right arm	
Left arm	
Buttocks	
Genitalia	
Right leg	
Left leg	
Total burn	

Relative percentage of body surface area affected by growth surface

Area	Age 0	1	5	10	15	Adult
A = ½ of head	9.5	8.5	6.5	5.5	4.5	3.5
B = ½ of one thigh	2.75	3.25	4.0	4.5	4.5	4.75
C = ½ of one leg	2.5	2.5	2.75	3.25	3.25	3.5

Figure 10.2 The Lund and Browder chart allows more accurate estimation of burn surface area and is particularly useful in children. The extent of the burn is marked on the chart. The areas of burns on the head, thighs and lower legs (A, B and C on the chart) are calculated and multiplied by the age factor in the table.

Anaemia

Anaemia results partly from destruction of red blood cells within involved skin capillaries and partly from toxic inhibition of the bone marrow if infection of the burnt area occurs.

Stress reaction

Peptic ulceration (Curling's ulcers[1])can be seen in patients with major burns.

[1] Thomas Blizzard Curling (1811–1888), surgeon to the London Hospital; also wrote the first accurate description of cretinism in adults (myxoedema) in 1850.

Treatment

1 *Immediate first aid treatment.* The immediate treatment of any burn is to safely stop the process straight away. This can be achieved by removing the patient from the source of the burn and applying cold running water to cool the area to prevent continued damage. A temporary dressing such as 'cling film' can be applied to the wound during the transfer of the patient to an appropriate centre.

2 *Resuscitation.* The airway is checked for evidence of burns. If there is any suspicion of an inhalation injury urgent review and assessment of the patient by a clinician skilled in airway management is needed. Blood should be taken to assess the level

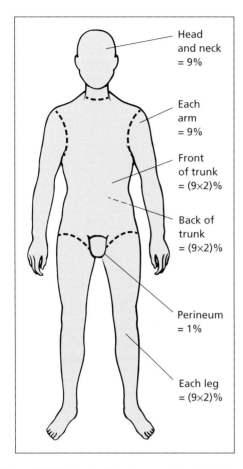

Head
and neck
= 9%

Each
arm
= 9%

Front
of trunk
= (9×2)%

Back of
trunk
= (9×2)%

Perineum
= 1%

Each leg
= (9×2)%

Figure 10.3 The 'rule of nines' – a useful guide to the estimation of the area of a burned surface. (Note also that a patient's hand represents 1% of the body surface area.)

of carboxyhaemoglobin (carbon monoxide has an affinity for haemoglobin over 200× that of oxygen). Patients suspected of having been exposed to carbon monoxide should be given oxygen through a re-breathing mask at a rate of 8–15 L/min for > 6 hours.

If the burn area is over 15% (or 10% if a child), admission and intravenous resuscitation are warranted; intravenous access with a large-bore cannula should be gained at a site remote from the burn, and fluid resuscitation started. Less extensive burns can be managed by oral replacement. Advice should be sought from a specialist burns unit.

3 *Assessment of burn severity.* The depth, extent and location of burn are assessed and documented using the Lund–Browder chart (Figure 10.2).

4 *Subsequent treatment.* Thereafter, the principles of the treatment of burns are as follows:
   a *local treatment* of the burn wound – minimizing fluid loss, prevention of infection, provision of an optimal environment for moist wound healing, avoidance of contracture.
   b *systemic treatment* – mitigating the systemic effects of severe burns.
   c *reconstruction and rehabilitation* of the patient.

Local treatment

Superficial partial-thickness burns

Superficial partial-thickness burns and very small deep partial-thickness burns are managed with simple non-adherent dressings such as paraffin-impregnated gauze under several layers of absorbent gauze; dressings are changed every 2–3 days. When the patient presents late, a topical antibiotic such as silver sulfadiazine cream (Flamazine) may be applied to the burn below the non-adherent dressings. When the hands are involved, the burn may be covered by sulfadiazine cream and placed in a sealed polythene bag. The wounds should heal with minimal scarring within approximately 2 weeks.

Full thickness burns

Full thickness burns, and more extensive deep partial-thickness burns, require excision of the burn wound. Early excision (within the first 2–7 days after injury) has been shown to produce better outcomes than delayed excision of the burn wound.

Full thickness burns can be excised by fascial excision (removal of the skin and fat to expose the fascia). Extensive (>2% TBSA) deep partial-thickness burns are likely to heal quicker and with less scarring if the burnt tissue is excised by tangential excision (the burnt skin is subject to progressively deeper tangential excision until healthy bleeding tissue is exposed).

The wounds are closed using meshed split skin grafts (usually from the patient's thighs or buttocks). The grafts take about 10–14 days to produce new skin. For burns that involve >50% of the total body surface area with limited donor sites, temporary closure of the burn wound can be achieved using cadaveric skin or commercial skin substitutes. These products are removed and replaced at approximately 2-week intervals with the patient's own skin (through repeated 'cropping' of the donor sites).

Facial burns

The deep sweat and sebaceous glands of the face facilitate the healing of most partial-thickness burns with only supportive topical dressings. Skin grafting is carried out if the eyelids are involved in order to prevent ectropion with the risk of corneal ulceration; an opaque cornea suggests a deep corneal burn requiring ophthalmic assessment.

Burns to hands

Burns to hands require careful management, as oedema and scarring can produce contractures across the joints. The palm skin will usually recover from most scalds, and deep partial-thickness burns and deeper injuries requiring burn excision and skin grafting are rare and are usually caused by prolonged contact burns. The skin on the back of the hand is thinner and more commonly requires surgery. Patients with hand burns often require hand therapy to maintain movement and splinting (usually with the metacarpophalangeal joints flexed and the interphalangeal joints extended as soon as the dressing requirements allow the application of a splint).

General treatment

Pain

Provide adequate pain relief; this may include intravenous opiates (e.g. morphine).

Hypovolaemic shock

Rapid fluid loss occurs, the rate of loss being quickest in the first 12 hours. Aggressive replacement of this fluid as soon as possible is essential. There are two underlying principles in this replacement: first, the correct amount of fluid should be replaced, and second, the correct type of fluid is important.

1 *Amount of fluid replacement.* This depends upon the extent of the burn as calculated from the Lund–Browder chart (Figure 10.2). The Parkland formula[2] is now the most accepted way of estimating the volume of fluid to be given in the first

[2] The Parkland Hospital, Southwestern University Medical Center, Dallas, TX, USA.

24 hours. Half the volume should be given in the first 8 hours, and the remainder over the next 16 hours.

$$\text{Fluid replacement (mL) in first 24 h after injury} = 2\text{–}4\,\text{mL} \times \text{weight (kg)} \times \%\text{burn area}$$

For example, a 70 kg patient with a 40% burn would, using this formula, require a figure of $4 \times 70 \times 40 = 11{,}200$ mL. Half of this (5,600 mL) is given in the first 8 hours, and the other half in the next 16 hours. In addition, the fluid regime should also include the daily maintenance fluid requirement (3 L in an adult).

During the resuscitation phase, clinical assessment of the patient should include monitoring the hourly urinary output, pulse, blood pressure, central venous pressure and core temperature. Fluid replacement may need to be adjusted according to these observations.

2 *Type of fluid used for replacement.* There is now consensus that a crystalloid solution is most appropriate for the first 24 hours after injury (most commonly this is Hartmann's solution). At the end of 24 hours, the fluid regimen can be augmented with colloids such albumin, fresh frozen plasma and blood.

Antimicrobial therapy

Burn wounds left untreated rapidly become colonized by bacteria. Burns presenting late are usually dressed with topical antimicrobial agents, with silver sulfadiazine most commonly used. Invasive infection requires the use of broad-spectrum antimicrobial treatment covering streptococcal and staphylococcal infection (including methicillin-resistant species, e.g. with vancomycin) as well as *Pseudomonas*; prophylaxis against fungal infection may also be appropriate in cases of extensive burns.

Nutrition

The patient's nutrition should be maintained, especially when burns are extensive. For major burns requiring resuscitation, enteral feeding should be started as soon as possible. The daily calorific requirement has been estimated at a minimum of 25 kcal/kg weight plus 40 kcal per percentage area burned.

Complications

Local

- Wound sepsis, usually with *Streptococcus pyogenes* or *Pseudomonas aeruginosa*.
- Scarring.
- Wound contractures.

General

- *Sepsis*, particularly chest infection in inhalational injury, urinary tract infection resulting from catheterization and septicaemia directly from wound invasion.
- *Acute peptic ulceration* (Curling's ulcer).
- *Seizures* in children, owing to electrolyte imbalance.
- *Acute kidney injury*, resulting from the initial hypovolaemia due to plasma loss, precipitation of haemoglobin or myoglobin, or nephrotoxic antimicrobial agents.
- *Psychological disturbance*. Burn injuries are disproportionately sustained by children, the elderly and patients with mental health conditions. Patients with severe burns require assessment by a psychiatric nurse or psychiatrist and often require psychological support and treatment.

Prognosis

The prognosis from a major burn is dependent upon the severity of the burn, total body surface area and physiological reserve of the patient. Young infants and the elderly carry a higher mortality than young adults. Refinements in the protocols used for severe burns, the organization of burn care to allow immediate access to expert advice and early transfer to a major burns unit has resulted in improvements in the survivability of major burns in younger patients (<50 years of age). Very few deaths occur during resuscitation, with most deaths now occurring due to later complications, including sepsis.

Additional resources

Case 8: Burnt thorax
Case 9: Burn treatment

11

The skin and its adnexae

Amer J. Durrani

Learning objectives

✓ To understand the general functions of the skin.

✓ To understand the anatomy and embryology of the skin.

✓ To recognize the range of benign lesions and conditions that may present in the skin.

✓ To distinguish between melanoma and non-melanoma skin cancers, and premalignant skin lesions, their presentation and management.

General functions of the skin

The skin can be considered as the largest organ in the body (16% total body weight in adults). It has multiple protective functions: as a barrier to mechanical trauma, chemical and thermal injury, and entry of microorganisms. It has a metabolic function in regard to vitamin D synthesis and a critical role in thermoregulation.

Skin anatomy and embryology

The skin has an outer epidermis, which is in a continuous state of regeneration. It is histologically divided into five layers (Figure 11.1). Cells mature from the basal layer to be shed as keratinocytes at the skin surface. The basal layer is the layer of origin of most skin cancers.

Below the epidermis, the dermis is subdivided into a superficial layer (papillary dermis) and deep layer (reticular dermis). The skin appendages are located in the dermis and extend into subcutaneous fat. They are structures from which tumours and inflammatory skin conditions can arise (hair follicles, sebaceous, eccrine and apocrine sweat glands, pain, temperature and pressure receptors). The distinction between the two layers of the dermis is also of importance when considering burn injury and healing (Chapter 10).

The dermis is a network of collagen that supports the neurovascular supply to the skin and dermal appendages. Elastin within the dermis provides stretch and elastic recoil, and loss of these fibres contributes to the ageing process seen in the skin. Hyaluronic acid and proteoglycans provide a gel to facilitate metabolite diffusion in the dermis.

The hypodermis is the layer beneath the skin and contains adipocytes, which provide insulation and can act as an energy source.

The epidermis is derived from ectoderm and dermis from mesoderm. Merkel cells and melanocytes originate from the neural crest (see later for malignant tumours derived from these cell types), and Langerhans cells are of mesenchymal origin (involved in cellular immunity).

Ellis and Calne's Lecture Notes in General Surgery, Fourteenth Edition.
Edited by Christopher Watson and Justin Davies.
© 2023 John Wiley & Sons Ltd. Published 2023 by John Wiley & Sons Ltd.
Companion website: www.wiley.com/go/Watson/GeneralSurgery14

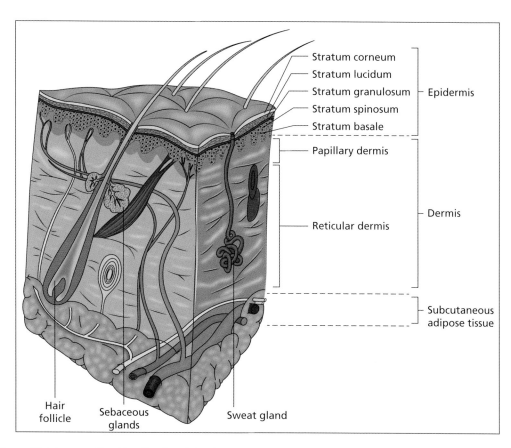

Stratum corneum
Stratum lucidum
Stratum granulosum ⎤ Epidermis
Stratum spinosum
Stratum basale

Papillary dermis

Reticular dermis ⎤ Dermis

Subcutaneous adipose tissue

Hair follicle   Sebaceous glands   Sweat gland

Figure 11.1 Layers of the skin with adnexal structures.

Epidermoid cyst

An epidermoid cyst (commonly referred to incorrectly as a sebaceous cyst) is a benign cyst that develops from the upper portion of a hair follicle. They are especially common on the scalp (pilar cyst), face, scrotum and vulva, and on the lobe of the ear. The cyst is fluctuant and cannot be moved separately from the overlying skin. There may be a typical central punctum (usually absent from a pilar cyst), and the contents are 'cheesy' with an unpleasant smell (keratin and cellular debris). The lining membrane consists of epidermis-like epithelium.

Epidermoid cysts may also result from traumatic implantation of epidermis into the subcutaneous tissue (inclusion cyst, sometimes referred to as an implantation dermoid cyst). Typically, these are on the pulps of fingers; there may be a healed scar overlying them.

Complications

- Infection.
- Calcification, producing a hard subcutaneous tumour misnamed a 'benign calcifying epithelioma'.
- Ulceration, which may then resemble a fungating carcinoma ('Cock's peculiar tumour'[1]).

Treatment

An uninfected sebaceous cyst can be considered for removal in order to prevent possible complications, particularly the risk of infection. A small elliptical skin incision is made around the punctum of the cyst under local anaesthetic; the capsule is identified and

[1] Edward Cock (1805–1892), Surgeon, Guy's Hospital, London, UK.

the cyst removed intact. Failure to remove the cyst in its entirety may lead to recurrence.

If the cyst is acutely inflamed and infected, incision and drainage may be required and the wound allowed to heal by secondary intention, with a course of oral antibiotics. This may be followed later by subsequent excision of the capsule wall if the cyst recurs.

Dermoid cyst

This is a congenital subcutaneous cystic swelling resulting from an embryological nest of epithelial cells along a line of fusion. The common sites are over the external angular process of the frontal bone (the external angular dermoid at the upper outer margin of the orbit), the root of the nose (internal angular dermoid) and in the midline. When in relation to the skull, the underlying bone is usually hollowed out around it. The possibility of communication with an intracranial dermoid or the meninges should be excluded by ultrasound and, if indicated, magnetic resonance imaging (MRI) scan prior to excision.

Verruca vulgaris (wart)

This is a well-localized horny projection that is common on the fingers, hands, feet and knees, particularly of children and young adults. Crops of warts may occur on the genitalia and perianal region, in many cases spread by sexual contact. Warts are often multiple and are due to a number of different strains of human papilloma virus.

Microscopically, there is a local hyperplasia of the prickle cell layer (stratum spinosum) of the skin (acanthosis) with marked surface cornification.

Treatment

Untreated, warts usually vanish spontaneously within 2 years, hence the apparent efficacy of folklore 'wart cures'. Often, reassurance that these lesions will disappear is all that is required, but if treatment is demanded, they can be treated with topical application of silver nitrate, podophyllin, frozen with liquid nitrogen or curetted under local or general anaesthesia.

Plantar warts

Otherwise known as verrucas, these occur on the weight-bearing areas of the foot. Pressure forces the wart into the deeper tissues, producing intense local pain on walking. They may occur in epidemics in schools and other such places where the hygiene of the communal bath or changing room is not of a high standard. They should be treated by topical podophyllin or curettage.

Ganglion

A ganglion presents as a cystic, subcutaneous swelling that transilluminates brilliantly. It most commonly occurs around the wrist and dorsum of the foot (joint capsule origin), or along the flexor aspect of the fingers and on the peroneal tendons (tendon sheath origin). Although ganglia are among the most common surgical lumps, their origin is uncertain. They may represent a benign myxoma of joint capsule or tendon sheath, a hamartoma or myxomatous degeneration due to trauma. They are thin-walled cysts with a synovial lining and contain clear colourless material with a jelly-like consistency.

Treatment

The patient may complain of discomfort or of the cosmetic appearance; if so, the cyst should be excised under a general anaesthetic using a bloodless field produced by a tourniquet. The old-fashioned treatment of hitting the ganglion with the family bible ruptures the cyst, but recurrence usually occurs after some time. Unfortunately, recurrence is also common after surgical excision.

Pilonidal sinus

The majority of pilonidal sinuses occur in the skin of the natal cleft. They may be solitary or appear as a row in the midline. Frequently, tufts of hair are found lying free within the sinus (Latin *pilus*, hair; *nidus*, nest).

Usually, young adults are affected, males more than females, and more often dark-haired individuals; the sinuses are rarely seen in children and do not present until adolescence. They are an uncommon occupational disease of hairdressers, in whom sinuses may occur in the clefts between the fingers. They are very occasionally found in the axilla, at the umbilicus, in the perineum and on the sole of the foot as well as on amputation stumps.

Aetiology

The occurrence of pilonidal sinuses remote from the natal cleft, and on the hands and feet of people working with cattle, where the contained hair is clearly of animal origin, supports the hypothesis that these sinuses occur by implantation of hair into the skin; these set up a foreign body reaction and produce a chronic infected sinus. It may be that, in some cases, postanal pits act as traps for loose hairs, thus combining both the congenital and acquired theories of origin. The hair enters the skin follicles from its distal end and works its way in due to tapered lateral hair extensions angled proximally, rather as a grass seed migrates up one's sleeve.

Clinical features

The pilonidal sinus is asymptomatic until it becomes infected; there is then a typical history of recurrent abscesses, which either require drainage or discharge spontaneously.

Treatment

1 *Acute abscess.* This is drained and allowed to heal by secondary intention.
2 *Quiescent sinus.* The track is excised, treated with injection of fibrin glue, or simply laid open and allowed to heal by secondary intention. Recurrence is diminished by keeping all incisions away from the midline and keeping the surrounding skin free from hair by shaving or the use of depilatory creams. Laser treatment can be effective in reducing hair growth in the area. Following excision of the sinus, particularly if it recurs after previous surgery, a local flap may be required with layered wound closure, to reduce the risk of recurrence.

Hidradenitis suppurativa

Hidradenitis suppurativa is a chronic inflammatory skin condition that affects apocrine gland-bearing skin in the axillae, groin, and under the breasts. Typically, patients present with persistent or recurrent abscesses, some of which may result in chronically discharging sinuses. Recurrent infections are common, as is the resultant scarring. It is more common in women, usually starting during puberty; there may be a family history (30–40% of patients) and it is associated with obesity and cigarette smoking.

Treatment

Management of hidradenitis suppurativa should include smoking cessation, weight control, wound care and pain management. Topical therapies may be effective in mild disease. Systemic antibiotics are frequently used for the control of acute infective episodes, often in conjunction with surgical incision and drainage. Medical therapy with biological agents may be of benefit.

Conditions affecting the nails

The nails are the site of some common and important surgical conditions.

Paronychia

Paronychia denotes bacterial infection of the lateral nail fold, usually of the finger, but it may complicate an ingrowing toenail (see later in this chapter). An acute paronychia is diagnosed when the nail fold is red, swollen and tender, and pus may be visible beneath the skin.

Treatment

If seen before pus has formed, while the nail fold is cellulitic, purulent infection may be aborted by a course of flucloxacillin or other appropriate anti-staphylococcal antibiotic together with immobilization by a splint to the finger and elevation of the arm in a sling. If pus is present, drainage is performed through an incision carried proximally through the nail fold, combined with removal of the base of the nail if pus has tracked beneath it.

Chronic paronychia is seen in those whose occupation requires constant soaking of the hands in water, but it may also occur as a result of fungal infection (*Candida*) of the nails and where the peripheral circulation is deficient, as in Raynaud's phenomenon (Chapter 12).

Ingrowing toenail

This is nearly always confined to the hallux and is usually due to a combination of tight shoes (particularly trainers) and the habit of paring the nail downwards into the lateral nail fold, rather than transversely; the sharp edge of the nail then grows into the side of the nail bed, producing ulceration and infection.

Treatment

If seen before infection has occurred, advice is given on correct cutting of the nails; advice is also given to avoid nylon socks and trainers. A small wick of cotton wool tucked daily into the side of the nail bed, after preliminary soaking of the feet in hot water to soften the nails, enables the nail to grow up out of the fold.

   If an acute paronychia is present, drainage will be required by means of removal of the side of the nail or avulsion of the whole nail. For recurrent cases when the infection has settled, the affected side may be excised together with the nail root (wedge excision), or the entire nail may be obliterated completely by excision of the nail root (Zadik's[2] operation) or by treating the nail bed with liquefied phenol, or a combination of the two techniques.

Onychogryphosis

The nail is coiled like a 'ram's horn'. It may affect any of the toes, although the hallux is the most common site. It may follow trauma to the nail bed and is usually found in elderly subjects.

Treatment

Relatively mild examples can be kept under control by trimming the nail with bone-cutting forceps. Merely avulsing the nail is invariably followed by recurrence, and the only adequate treatment is excision of the nail bed.

Lesions of the nail bed

It is convenient to list a number of relatively common conditions that affect the nail bed.

[2] Frank Raphael Zadik (1914–1995), Orthopaedic Surgeon, Leigh and Wigan, UK.

Subungual haematoma

As a result of crush injury to the terminal phalanx, with or without fracture of the underlying bone, a tense, painful haematoma may develop beneath the nail. Relief is afforded by evacuating the clot through a hole made by either a dental drill or a red-hot sterile needle; both procedures are painless. Occasionally, a small haematoma may develop after a trivial or forgotten injury and clinically may closely simulate a subungual melanoma.

Subungual exostosis

This is nearly always confined to the hallux and is especially found in adolescents and young adults. It appears as a reddish-brown area under the nail, which is tender on pressure. The exostosis may ulcerate through the overlying nail, producing an infected granulating mass. The diagnosis is confirmed by X-ray of the toe, and treatment is to remove the nail and excise the underlying exostosis.

Subungual melanoma

The nail bed is a common site for malignant melanoma (see later in this chapter). There is a long history of slow growth and often a misleading history of trauma. The lesion should be confirmed by removal of the nail plate and excision biopsy followed by multidisciplinary team discussion and management with the likely recommendation for wide local excision (which may involve amputation of the digit) with sentinel node biopsy.

Glomus tumour

The nail beds of the fingers and toes are a common site of this extremely painful lesion, which is a benign tumour arising in a subcutaneous glomus body (highly innervated arteriovenous anastomoses in dermis responsible for temperature regulation). It is considered later in this chapter.

Tumours of the skin and subcutaneous tissues

Classification

1 Epidermal.
   a *Benign*: skin tag, keratoacanthoma and seborrhoeic keratosis.

b *Premalignant*: Actinic keratosis, Bowen's disease and squamous cell carcinoma *in situ*.

c *Non-melanoma skin cancer*: squamous cell carcinoma, basal cell carcinoma and Marjolin's ulcer.

d *Secondary cutaneous deposits*, e.g. from carcinoma of breast, lung, kidney, leukaemia and Hodgkin's disease.

2 Pigmented skin lesions and malignant melanoma.
3 Tumours of sebaceous and sweat glands.
4 Dermal tumours from blood vessels, lymphatics, nerves, fibrous tissue or fat.

Epidermal tumours

Skin tag (acrochordon)

This is a common, benign, pedunculated tumour, often pigmented with melanin. Microscopically, it comprises a keratinized papillary tumour of squamous epithelium.

Keratoacanthoma (molluscum sebaceum)

This is a lesion that occurs in elderly patients, most commonly men, in sun-exposed areas such as the face and nose (75%), although it may occur on any skin surface. It appears as a rapidly growing nodule, which may reach 3 cm or more in diameter in a few weeks, with a characteristic central crater filled by a keratin plug. It closely resembles a squamous carcinoma or rodent ulcer in appearance, and it is only the history of very rapid growth that helps differentiate it from the latter.

Histologically, it consists of a central crater filled with keratin surrounded by hypertrophied squamous stratified epithelium. There is no invasion of the surrounding tissues.

If left untreated, the lesion disappears over a period of 4–5 months, leaving a faint white scar. It appears to be of hair follicle origin and may be associated with a minor injury.

Treatment

It is safest to remove the lesion to establish histological proof of the diagnosis.

Seborrhoeic keratosis (basal cell papilloma)

This is a common tumour occurring after the age of 40 years. It appears as a yellowish or brown raised lesion on the face, arms or trunk, and is often multiple.

Table 11.1 Fitzpatrick skin types

Skin type	Typical appearance	Response to sun exposure
I	Pale white skin, blue eyes, red or blond hair	Always burns, does not tan
II	Fair skin, blue eyes	Burns easily, does not tan
III	Darker white skin	Tans, after initial burn
IV	Light-brown skin	Burns minimally, tans easily
V	Brown skin	Rarely burns, tans darkly easily
VI	Dark brown or black skin	Never burns, always tans

It often appears greasy, and its surface is characterized by a network of crypts.

Microscopically, there is hyperkeratosis, proliferation of the basal cell layer and melanin pigmentation.

The lesion is entirely benign, but if there is diagnostic doubt on clinical examination and with a dermatoscope, the exclusion of skin cancer can only be made with certainty by incision or excision biopsy and histological examination.

Solar (actinic) keratosis

This is a small, hard, brown, scaly tumour on sun-exposed areas of skin (e.g. the forehead, ears and backs of hands) of the elderly. Keratoses are more common in individuals with fair skin (Fitzpatrick skin types I and II[3]; Table 11.1) usually associated with prolonged exposure to ultraviolet light.

Microscopically, hyperkeratosis is present, often with atypical dividing cells in the basal layer of the epidermis.

The lesions may be treated with liquid nitrogen cryotherapy or curettage; large areas may require topical chemotherapy (e.g. 5-fluorouracil). Imiquimod has also been used, and acts as an immune modifier, stimulating an immune response with resolution of the lesions.

[3] Thomas Fitzpatrick (1919–2003), Dermatologist, Massachusetts General Hospital, Boston. The Fitzpatrick scale is a 6-point scale describing how different skin types respond to sun exposure.

The importance of this lesion is that it may undergo change into a squamous cell carcinoma.

Bowen's disease[4]

Also known as intra-epidermal squamous cell carcinoma, this appears as a very slowly growing, red, scaly plaque, and represents squamous carcinoma *in situ*. It may be mistaken for a psoriatic plaque. Human papillomavirus (HPV) DNA (particularly HPV16, but also HPV2) has been found in some lesions.

Microscopically, atypical keratinocytes with vacuolization, mitoses and multinucleated giant cells are prominent in the epidermis, but the basal layer is intact.

Treatment is excision; if left untreated, eventually a squamous cell carcinoma will supervene.

Cutaneous squamous cell carcinoma

This is the commonest form of skin cancer after basal cell carcinoma, occurring on skin in areas exposed to sunshine, such as the face and backs of the hands. Like solar keratoses, it is relatively common in white subjects (Fitzpatrick skin type I), with cumulative lifetime sun exposure as the most significant risk factor. Incidence increases after the age of 40 years and the male:female ratio is 3:1.

Predisposing factors

These include the following.

- Solar keratosis.
- Bowen's disease.
- Exposure to sunshine or ultraviolet irradiation.
- Exposure to ionizing irradiation.
- Infection with human papilloma virus subtypes 6 and 11.
- Carcinogens, e.g. pitch, tar, soot and mineral oils.
- Chronic ulceration, particularly in burns scars (Marjolin's ulcer – see below).
- Immunosuppressive drugs, e.g. azathioprine and ciclosporin.

Pathology

Macroscopically, it presents as a typical malignant ulcer with indurated, raised, everted edges and a central scab.

Microscopically, there are solid columns of epithelial cells growing into the dermis with epithelial pearls of central keratin surrounded by prickle cells. Occasionally, anaplastic tumours are seen, in which these pearls are absent.

Spread occurs by local infiltration and then via lymphatics. Blood-borne spread occurs only in very advanced cases.

Treatment

A tissue diagnosis with either an incision or excision biopsy is mandatory. Subsequent treatment may consist of a wider excision, which may necessitate a reconstruction (skin graft and local flap) depending on the site and size of the lesion. Adjuvant radiotherapy may be required based on the histological characteristics of the primary tumour. If the regional lymph nodes are involved, block dissection is indicated.

Marjolin's ulcer[5]

This is the name applied to malignant change in a scar, ulcer or sinus, for example, a chronic venous ulcer, an unhealed burn or the sinus of chronic osteomyelitis. It has the following characteristics:

- *slow growth*, because the lesion is relatively avascular;
- *painless*, because the scar tissue does not contain cutaneous nerve fibres;
- *lymphatic spread is late*, because the scar tissue produces lymphatic obliteration.

Once the tumour reaches the normal tissues beyond the diseased area, rapid growth, pain and lymphatic involvement take place.

Basal cell carcinoma (rodent ulcer)

This is the most common form of skin cancer in white people (80% of non-melanoma skin cancers). It occurs usually in elderly subjects, in males twice as commonly as in females. Ninety percent are found on the face above a line joining the angle of the mouth to the external auditory meatus, particularly around the eye, the nasolabial folds and the hairline of the scalp. The tumour may, however, arise on any part of the

---

[4] John Templeton Bowen (1857–1941), Dermatologist, Harvard Medical School, Boston, MA, USA.

[5] Jean Nicholas Marjolin (1780–1850), Surgeon, Hôpital Sainte-Eugénie, Paris, France.

skin, including the anal margin. Predisposing factors are exposure to sunlight or irradiation.

Pathology

Macroscopically and on examination with a dermatoscope, the tumour has raised, rolled but not everted edges. It consists of pearly nodules over which fine blood vessels can be seen to course (telangiectasia). Starting as a small nodule, the tumour very slowly grows over the years with central ulceration and scabbing.

Microscopically, solid sheets of uniform, darkly staining cells arising from the basal layer of the skin are seen. Prickle cells and epithelial pearls are both absent.

Spread is by local infiltration, with slow but steady destruction of surrounding tissues; in advanced cases, the underlying skull may be eroded, or the face, nose and eye may be destroyed, hence the name 'rodent'. Lymphatic and blood-borne spread occur with extreme rarity.

Treatment

Treatment is by surgical excision, with an adequate measured margin, with reconstruction if required (skin graft or local flap). At anatomical sites where this may prove challenging, i.e. for high risk tumours at high risk sites (e.g. eyelid, periorbital and nasal areas), Mohs[6] micrographic surgery offers the lowest risk of tumour recurrence. It is also indicated in late cases where the tumour has recurred after irradiation or has invaded the underlying bone or cartilage.

Adjuvant radiotherapy may be required or used as a primary treatment depending on patient and tumour factors following a multidisciplinary discussion.

Pigmented skin lesions and malignant melanoma

Benign pigmented skin lesions

- Intradermal melanoma or naevus (the common mole).

[6] Frederic Edward Mohs (1910–2002), Surgeon, University of Wisconsin. Pioneered the concept of rapid histological examination at the time of tumour excision to ensure complete tumour excision while allowing maximal preservation of healthy tissue.

- Junctional melanoma or naevus.
- Compound melanoma or naevus.
- Spitz naevus.
- Malignant melanoma.

Nearly everyone possesses one or more moles; some have hundreds, although they may not become apparent until after puberty. Those moles that are entirely within the dermis remain benign, but a small percentage of the junctional naevi, so called because they are seen in the basal layer of the epidermis at its junction with the dermis, may undergo malignant change (Figure 11.2).

Intradermal melanoma or naevus

This is the most common variety of mole. The naevus may be light or dark in colour and may be flat or raised, hairy or hairless. A hairy mole is nearly always intradermal. They may be found in any place in the body except the palm of the hand, the sole of the foot or the scrotal skin.

Histologically, there is a nest of melanocytes situated entirely within the dermis where the cells form non-encapsulated masses. They never undergo malignant change, and need no treatment unless the diagnosis is uncertain.

Junctional melanoma or naevus

The junctional naevus is pigmented to a variable shade from light brown to almost black. It is nearly always flat, smooth and hairless. It may occur anywhere on the body and, unlike the intradermal naevus, may be found on the palm of the hand, sole of the foot and the genitalia.

Histologically, naevus cells are seen in the basal layers of the epidermis from which the cells may spread to the surface.

Only a small percentage of junctional naevi undergo malignant change, but it is from this group that the vast majority of malignant melanomas arise.

Compound melanoma or naevus

Clinically, this is indistinguishable from the intradermal naevus, but histologically, it has junctional elements that make it potentially malignant. It may be darker and palpable due to a raised border.

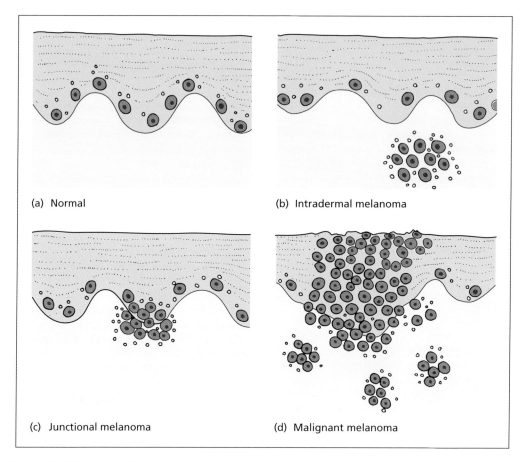

Figure 11.2 (a) The normal skin contains melanocytes (shown as cells) and melanin pigment shown as dots. The pigment increases in sunburn and freckles. (b) A benign intradermal naevus; the melanocytes are clumped together in the dermis to form a localized benign tumour. (c) A junctional naevus with melanocytes clumping together in the basal layer of the epidermis. (d) These are usually benign but may occasionally give rise to an invasive malignant melanoma.

Spitz naevus[7]

Spitz naevus is an uncommon type of mole (melanocytic naevus) that usually affects young people and children, hence it used to be known as a juvenile melanoma. It is a benign skin tumour, but it may resemble a malignant melanoma clinically and microscopically, so Spitz naevi are often excised as a precaution.

Malignant melanoma

Malignant melanomas develop from melanocytes, which are situated in the basal layer of the epidermis and originate from the neuroectoderm of the embryonic neural crest. Some melanomas contain no visible pigment (amelanotic melanoma). While most melanomas arise in the skin, they may also occur at other sites to which neural crest cells migrate, in particular the pigmented choroid layer of the eye.

Malignant melanomas can arise *de novo* or in preexisting naevi, either junctional naevi or compound naevi where there is a junctional component. They mainly occur in fair-skinned people on light-exposed

---

[7] Sophie Spitz (1910–1956), Pathologist, Memorial Sloan Kettering Cancer Centre, New York, NY, USA.

areas, hence the higher incidence on the legs of females. They are rarely found in the pigmented skin of non-Caucasians, tending to be found in the non-pigmented skin on the sole of the foot or, less commonly, the palm (acral lentiginous melanoma). A premalignant form, lentigo maligna, also exists.

Presentations

The two main presentations of malignant melanoma are the superficial spreading type and the nodular type.

- *Superficial spreading melanoma.* The most common presentation of malignant melanoma is of a previously dormant naevus starting to spread superficially. The surface has patches of deep pigmentation.
- *Nodular melanoma.* The naevus is nodular and deeply pigmented and may bleed or ulcerate. Such a nodule may occur on a pigmented background such as the lentigo maligna (see below). It tends to invade deeply rather than spread superficially and carries a poorer prognosis with earlier lymphatic involvement.

In addition to the common types of malignant melanoma above, less common forms include the following:

- *Lentigo maligna.* This is a brown pigmented patch with an irregular outline and is usually found on the cheeks of elderly patients, often called a Hutchinson's freckle.[8] The pale patch appears over several years; malignant change is indicated by darker, irregular pigmentation or nodule formation. Lentigo maligna has a small lifetime risk of malignant transformation into a melanoma, so complete excision should be considered.
- *Acral melanoma.* These are so called because they occur at the extremities, commonly on the palms and soles of the feet. It is this type that also occurs in dark-skinned races (Fitzpatrick skin types V and VI). Subungual melanoma is a variant of acral melanoma (see earlier in this chapter).
- *Mucosal melanoma.* Malignant melanoma may be found on the mucous membranes of the nose, mouth, anus and intestine.

[8] Sir Jonathan Hutchinson (1828–1913), Surgeon, The London Hospital, London, UK. Described numerous conditions and was the first to perform a successful operation for reduction of intussusception in a child.

- *Choroidal melanoma.* Melanomas may arise from melanocytes in the pigment layer of the retina. These are renowned for presenting many years after enucleation with hepatic metastases; hence, the aphorism 'beware the patient with the large liver and the glass eye.'
- *Amelanotic melanoma.* Paradoxically, melanomas are not always pigmented, but they remain dihydroxyphenylalanine (DOPA)-positive.

Signs of malignant change in a pigmented lesion – ABCDE

- **A**symmetry.
- **B**order is irregular.
- **C**olour – two or more colours of pigment.
- **D**iameter – >6 mm.
- **E**volution – change in size, shape, colour, development of a nodule.
- *Spread* of pigment from the edge of the naevus.
- *Itching or pain.*
- *Satellite pigmented nodules* (late change).
- *Palpable regional lymph nodes or evidence of distant spread* (often due to delayed presentation).

Pathology

Microscopically, pleomorphic cells are seen. These spread through the layers of the epidermis and are usually pigmented (occasionally the cells are amelanotic).

Spread

As well as local growth and ulceration, malignant melanoma can spread by local and regional lymphatics, which can produce cutaneous satellite or in-transit metastases by progressive proximal spread, and by lymphatic transit to regional lymph nodes. There is also a much smaller risk of haematogenous spread to distant organs, for example, brain, lungs and liver.

Staging

The prognosis of malignant melanoma depends upon its depth of invasion, according to its measured depth (Breslow depth[9]). Multidisciplinary discussion and management of melanoma are informed by the tumour stage (Table 11.2) and national treatment guidelines.

[9] Alexander Breslow (1928–1980), Pathologist, George Washington University Hospital, Washington, DC, USA.

Table 11.2 Ten-year survival according to Breslow depth				
Tumour thickness (mm)	Ulcerated or not	T	Stage	10-year melanoma specific survival
<0.8	No	T1a	1A	98%
<0.8	Yes	T1b	1A	96%
0.8–1.0	Either	T1b	1A	
>1.0–2.0	No	T2a	1B	92%
>1.0–2.0	Yes	T2b	2A	88%
>2.0–4.0	No	T3a	2A	
>2.0–4.0	Yes	T3b	2B	81%
>4.0	No	T4a	2B	83%
>4.0	Yes	T4b	2C	75%

American Joint Committee on Cancer staging system (2017) and melanoma specific survival for stage 1 and 2 melanomas (i.e. those without nodal spread)

Treatment of pigmented lesions

The following is a general guide to the management of pigmented lesions of the skin.

Prophylactic/diagnostic excision biopsy

Any pigmented tumour on the hand, sole or genitalia, or any that, in other situations, are subjected to trauma should be considered for excision; these are the most common among the small percentage of naevi to undergo malignant change. Such lesions are sent for histological examination and should always be removed in their entirety with a 2 mm measured margin.

Suspicious naevi

If the pigmented lesion shows any of the features already listed that suggest that malignant change has taken place, the naevus is first removed for urgent histological examination. If malignant melanoma is confirmed, a wide local excision of the area is then performed, with a margin of clearance (1–2 cm), as recommended at the multidisciplinary team discussion of the melanoma's pathology.

Wide local excision and sentinel lymph node biopsy for malignant melanoma

Wide local excision of the scar at the site of the primary melanoma can often be undertaken under local anaesthetic and is the minimum treatment recommended to minimize risk of local recurrence.

Wide local excision is usually undertaken in conjunction with sentinel lymph node biopsy for stage IB or greater stage, under a general anaesthetic. Sentinel lymph node biopsy offers additional prognostic information and informs further follow-up and management.

The primary lymphatic drainage of the tumour, known as the sentinel node, is identified and excised for histological examination. Identification of the sentinel node is by injection of patent blue dye around the scar at the site of initial excision biopsy of the primary melanoma, combined with preoperative lymphoscintigraphy to map the lymphatic drainage. If the sentinel node is involved, this upstages the melanoma (see American Joint Committee on Cancer, AJCC, Staging Classification, Table 11.2) and will inform the follow-up regimen and need for referral to the melanoma oncology team for consideration for adjuvant therapy.

Adjuvant therapy

Specific targeted and immunotherapy regimens are now available for stage 3 and stage 4 melanoma, with significant improvements in long-term outcomes for these patient groups. Their use is directed by melanoma oncologists as core members of the melanoma multidisciplinary team.

Prognosis

Prognosis depends on a large number of factors:

- *Breslow depth* of the primary lesion, measured vertically from the top of the granular layer to the deepest point of tumour invasion. This is the most important prognostic factor. Prognosis is good when this depth is less than 1.0 mm. The deeper the lesion, the greater the risk of lymph node metastasis and the worse the 10-year survival (Table 11.2).
- *Ulceration* of the lesion carries a poorer prognosis.
- *Type of lesion.* A superficial spreading melanoma has a better prognosis than a penetrating and ulcerating lesion.
- *The anatomical site.* Tumours on the trunk and scalp have a poorer prognosis.
- *Lymph node metastases.* They indicate poor prognosis, more so if there are cutaneous deposits. The presence of sentinel node involvement, or satellite lesions, reduces 5-year survival to under 30%.

Tumours of sweat glands and sebaceous glands

Benign and malignant tumours of these glandular adnexae of the skin are rare.

Sebaceous adenoma

These are more in the nature of a hyperplasia of the glands than true tumours. They occur as pink or yellow papules on the nose, cheek and forehead. Microscopically, they are merely overgrowths of sebaceous glands.

Adnexal-derived skin cancers

Sebaceous carcinoma

Found rarely on the face and scalp in elderly subjects, this is an uncommon but aggressive cancer, arising from the epithelium of the sebaceous gland. They may have a clinical appearance similar to a basal cell carcinoma.

Other rare adnexal-derived skin malignancies include trichilemmal carcinoma, porocarcinoma, eccrine carcinoma and apocrine carcinoma

Vascular anomalies

Tumours of blood vessels usually lie in the dermis, although the underlying muscles and soft tissues may be involved. The abdominal viscera, central nervous system and bone may also be the sites of these lesions. Vascular anomalies can be classified into tumours and malformations.

Vascular tumours

Vascular tumours are characterized by endothelial cell hyperproliferation. They tend to be rapid growing. Most are not present at birth.

Campbell de Morgan spots

Campbell de Morgan spots[10] are generally found on the trunk of middle-aged and elderly subjects. They are bright red aggregates of dilated capillaries, which can be emptied by pressing on them with the tip of a pencil. They are of no significance

Spider naevus

Spider naevus is another example of a capillary haemangioma. Isolated 'spiders' are present in normal people, but they are more common during pregnancy and in chronic liver disease. They comprise a central arteriole from which capillaries radiate. Pressure on the central arteriole with a pinhead causes the lesion to disappear while pressure is maintained.

Infantile haemangioma (strawberry naevus)

This is the most common benign tumour in children, appearing in the first weeks of life, usually on the head and neck, and affecting girls more commonly than boys. Preterm infants appear more susceptible, as do those where the mother suffered pre-eclampsia.

Most strawberry naevi increase in size over a period of 3 months, and then slowly regress over a period of years before disappearing spontaneously.

Cavernous haemangioma

These are made up of large blood spaces lined with endothelium. They occur on the skin and lip and, quite commonly, as multiple nodules in the liver. They are usually present at birth and grow to keep pace with normal body growth.

The lesions are blue, may be raised and may partly empty on pressure. They may infiltrate the underlying tissues and may be associated with unsightly overlying cutaneous thickening.

Treatment

This is often difficult. The condition may be disguised by the use of cosmetics, or thrombosis can be encouraged by injection of sclerosing agents. Very

[10] Campbell de Morgan (1811–1876), Surgeon, Middlesex Hospital, London, UK.

unsightly small lesions may be excised, and skin grafted if required.

Glomus tumour

Glomus bodies are found in the subcutaneous tissues of the limbs, particularly the fingers, toes and their nail beds. They are convoluted arteriovenous anastomoses with a cellular wall comprising a thick layer of cuboidal 'glomus' cells, which are modified plain muscles; between these cells are abundant nerve fibres. These structures are perhaps concerned with cutaneous heat regulation. Glomus tumours are blue or reddish, small, raised lesions, which occur in young adults at the common sites of glomus bodies. Their characteristic is exquisite tenderness, which makes the slightest touch agonizing.

Treatment

Treatment is by excision of the lesion and subsequent histological confirmation of the diagnosis.

Kaposi's sarcoma

This tumour has a multicentric origin. It used to be most common in the elderly in central Europe, particularly Ashkenazi Jews;[11] now, it is a more common tumour in patients with acquired immune deficiency syndrome (AIDS) and also occurs in immunosuppressed organ transplant recipients. DNA extracted from Kaposi's sarcoma[12] tissue has been found to contain human herpes virus type 8 (HHV8), now known as Kaposi sarcoma herpes virus (KSHV), indicating a significant aetiological role for this virus. It presents as a number of bluish red or dark blue nodules scattered over the extremities of one or more of the limbs. The nodules spread centrally along the limb, may ulcerate and can metastasize to the liver and lungs. In the aggressive form, which occurs in the immunosuppressed, visceral involvement occurs with bowel perforation, haemorrhage or intussusception.

Histologically, there are two components: blood vessels and fibroblasts. The latter show the malignant features, thus distinguishing this tumour from a haemangiosarcoma.

Treatment involves control of HIV infection with highly active antiretroviral treatment (HAART) or reduction of immunosuppression in transplant recipients, together with local radiotherapy or cytotoxic drugs.

Telangiectasia

Telangiectases, although not truly tumours, are conveniently mentioned in this section. They are dilations of normal capillaries and are seen in a number of circumstances, such as on the weather-beaten faces and legs of some people, who may complain of their cosmetic appearance.

Hereditary haemorrhagic telangiectasia (HHT; Osler–Weber–Rendu syndrome[13]) is an inherited autosomal dominant disease characterized by tiny capillary angiomas of the skin, lips and mucous membranes; they may give rise to repeated nosebleeds and gastrointestinal haemorrhage. The genetic abnormality is a mutation of either endoglin (HHT type 1) or activin receptor-like kinase (HHT type 2) genes. Occult arteriovenous malformations are common, such as within the liver and spleen.

Vascular malformations

A variety of types of congenital capillary malformation may be found in the skin, usually at birth:

- *Salmon pink patch* is a common blemish on the head or neck of a newborn child and rapidly disappears spontaneously.
- *Port-wine stain*, flush with the skin, usually on the face, lips and buccal mucosa, produces an extensive area of dark red, blue or purple discolouration. It is present from birth and shows no tendency to regress with age. Port-wine stains may respond to cutaneous laser therapy, but the simplest treatment remains camouflage with cosmetics.

Note that port-wine stains of the face may have a segmental distribution corresponding to the cutaneous branches of the trigeminal nerve and may be

---

[11] Ashkenazi Jews: contrast Sephardic and Oriental Jews. Migrated to Germany, Poland and Russia.

[12] Moriz Kaposi (1837–1902), Professor of Dermatology, Vienna, Austria.

[13] Sir William Osler (1849–1919), Professor of Medicine, successively at McGill University, Montreal, Canada; Johns Hopkins University, Baltimore, MD, USA; and the University of Oxford, Oxford, UK. Frederick Parkes Weber (1863–1962), Physician, London, UK. Henri Rendu (1844–1902), Physician, Hôpital Necker, Paris, France.

associated with angiomas of the cerebral pia-arachnoid, which may manifest themselves by focal epileptic attacks (the Sturge–Weber syndrome[14]).

Lymph vessel tumours

Lymphangiomas are congenital in origin and similar to haemangiomas; they are lined by endothelium but contain lymph. They are relatively uncommon, but occur mainly on the lips, tongue and cheek, resulting in macrocheilia or macroglossia.

Cystic hygroma

A form of lymphangioma, the aetiology of cystic hygromas is thought to be a combination of a failure of lymphatics to connect to the venous system, abnormal growth of embryonal lymphatics and sequestered lymphatic channels. Most occur in the neck, usually the left side, and are thought to be related to the embryonic precursor of the jugular part of the thoracic duct. They consist of a multilocular cystic mass, which is often present at birth or noticed in early infancy. Characteristically, they are supremely transilluminable. They may respond to injection of sclerosant agents such as alcohol or doxycycline. Surgical treatment consists of excision, but this is a difficult procedure as the cysts ramify throughout the structures of the neck.

Nerve tumours

Tumours of the peripheral nerves arise from the neurilemmal sheath of Schwann,[15] hence the terms neurilemmoma, neurofibroma or schwannoma. They push the fibres of the nerve to one side or actually grow within the substance of the nerve. The tumours may be solitary or multiple and may involve any peripheral nerve in the body. Of the cranial nerves, the eighth is most commonly involved, often as a solitary tumour (the vestibular schwannoma or acoustic neuroma; Chapter 16). Tumours may arise within the spinal canal, particularly from the dorsal nerve roots, resulting in an extramedullary, intrathecal, slow-growing spinal tumour (Chapter 18). Part of this tumour may protrude through the intervertebral foramen, producing a dumb-bell tumour, which projects into either the thoracic cavity or the abdominal cavity.

In the skin and subcutaneous tissues, there is a wide range of presentations, from a solitary tumour arising from a peripheral nerve to large tumour numbers involving the whole of the body (von Recklinghausen's disease;[16] his name is also applied to the osteitis fibrosa cystica of hyperparathyroidism – Chapter 40).

Clinical features

The tumours may appear in childhood, and there is often a family history. Three types of neurofibromatosis are recognized, and all are autosomal dominant. Von Recklinghausen's disease is type 1 neurofibromatosis[17] and results from a mutation in the neurofibromin gene. The cutaneous lesions are soft and often pedunculated. They are usually painless, although pressure may produce pain along the line of the nerve, particularly when larger nerve trunks are involved. The tumour is mobile from side to side but not longitudinally, in the line of the nerve to which it is attached. There may be associated café-au-lait patches of pigmentation. In some cases, there are disfiguring masses of neurofibromatous tissue over which the thickened skin hangs in ugly folds.

Treatment

Where the neurofibromas are solitary or few in number, removal can be performed, either by enucleation, if the nerve fibres are pushed to one side, or by resection with suture of the divided nerve. Incomplete removal must not be performed, as sarcomatous change may follow. Where the whole body is covered

---

[14] William Allen Sturge (1850–1919), Physician, Royal Free Hospital, London, UK, and Frederick Parkes Weber (1863–1962), Dermatologist, Mount Vernon Hospital, London, UK, with a lifelong interest in rare diseases.

[15] Theodor Schwann (1810–1882), Professor of Anatomy, Louvain and then Liège, Belgium.

[16] Friederich Daniel von Recklinghausen (1833–1910), Professor of Pathology, successively at Königsberg, Germany; Würzburg, Germany; and Strasbourg, France.

[17] Type II neurofibromatosis (mutation in neurofibromin 2 gene) is characterised by eighth nerve tumours, meningiomas and schwannomas of the dorsal roots of the spinal cord; type III neurofibromatosis has features of both type I and type II, with café-au-lait spots, cutaneous lesions and intracranial neurofibromas and meningiomas.

by these lesions, some cosmetic improvement can be affected by excising the more noticeable lesions from the face and hands.

Neurofibrosarcomas are uncommon. They may arise *de novo* or as malignant change in a neurofibroma. Clinical features are pain, rapid growth, and peripheral anaesthesia or paralysis. Treatment is by wide excision.

Fatty tumours

Lipoma

Lipomas are the most common benign tumours. They usually occur in adults, and the sex distribution is equal. Lipomas may arise in any connective tissue but especially in the subcutaneous fat, particularly around the shoulder and over the trunk. They do not occur in the palm, sole of the foot or scalp, because in these areas the fat is contained within dense fibrous septa. Occasionally, lipomas appear in large numbers subcutaneously and are tender (adiposis dolorosa or Dercum's disease,[18] a familial condition associated with obesity), and it is sometimes quite difficult to differentiate them from neurofibromas. Elsewhere, it is useful to remember that 'lipomas occur beneath everything'; thus, in addition to being subcutaneous, they may be subfascial, subperiosteal, subperitoneal, submucosal or subpleural.

[18] Francis Xavier Dercum (1856–1931), Professor of Clinical Neurology, Jefferson Medical College, Philadelphia, PA, USA.

Where diagnostic doubt exists, ultrasound may confirm the diagnosis and it may be further characterized by an MRI scan. Any rapidly growing, painful soft tissue tumour raises the concern of a soft tissue sarcoma and warrants urgent referral for multidisciplinary clinical and radiological assessment to exclude sarcoma.

Treatment

Treatment consists of excision if the lipoma is symptomatic or diagnostic doubt exists. If there is clinical concern regarding a soft tissue sarcoma, rapid referral to a specialist sarcoma centre is mandated.

Liposarcoma

A rare tumour, which probably arises as an unusual event in a pre-existing benign lipoma. The retroperitoneal site is most common, but it also commonly occurs around the thigh and should be suspected if the tumour is very large, firmer than usual, vascular or rapidly growing.

Additional resources

12

Arterial disease

Patrick Coughlin

Learning objectives

✓ To know the types of arterial trauma and their management.

✓ To know the causes of arterial aneurysms, their manifestation and treatment.

✓ To have knowledge of occlusive arterial disease (including thromboembolic disease), its risk factors, manifestations and treatment options.

Arterial trauma

Traumatic arterial injuries are due to either closed (blunt) trauma or open (penetrating) trauma.

Closed injuries

The artery is injured by extraneous compression such as a crush injury, fractures of adjacent bones with displacement of the artery (e.g. supracondylar fracture of the humerus in children) or joint dislocation.

Penetrating injuries

Penetrating arterial injuries may result from gunshot wounds, stabbing, penetration by bone spicules in fractures or iatrogenic injury.

Types of arterial injury

- *Mural contusion* with secondary spasm.
- *Intimal tear*. This injury is usually a result of distraction, in which the artery is stretched and the intimal layer tears, while the surrounding adventitia remains intact. The intima then buckles and causes a localized stenosis, which may or may not result in thrombosis or dissection.
- *Full-thickness tear*. All layers of the artery are divided, and this may be partial or complete. Partial tears bleed copiously, while complete division of the artery often results in contraction and spasm of the divided vessel with surprisingly little blood loss.

Consequences of injury

- *Haemorrhage*. This may be concealed or overt.
- *Thrombosis*. Immediate or delayed.
- *Arteriovenous fistula formation*.
- *False (pseudo-) aneurysm formation* (see later in this chapter).
- *Arterial dissection*.
- *Compartment syndrome*. Ischaemic muscle swells, and if the muscle is contained by a fibrous fascial compartment, such as in the forearm or in the lower leg, the swelling further exacerbates the ischaemia as the compartment pressure increases. Volkmann's[1] ischaemic contracture (Chapter 19) is a result of compartment syndrome.

Ellis and Calne's Lecture Notes in General Surgery, Fourteenth Edition. Edited by Christopher Watson and Justin Davies.
© 2023 John Wiley & Sons Ltd. Published 2023 by John Wiley & Sons Ltd.
Companion website: www.wiley.com/go/Watson/GeneralSurgery14

[1]Richard von Volkmann (1830–1889), Professor of Surgery, Halle, Germany.

Clinical features

The features of arterial injury may be those of acute ischaemia, haemorrhage or often both. Acute ischaemia is characterized by:

- pain (in the limb supplied, starting distally and progressing proximally);
- pallor;
- pulselessness;
- paraesthesia;
- paralysis;
- coldness.

Haemorrhage may be overt (bright red blood) or concealed (e.g. closed limb fractures). Symptoms are those of rapidly developing hypovolaemic shock (cold, clamminess, tachycardia, hypotension, loss of consciousness, oliguria progressing to anuria).

Treatment

Closed injuries

- *Treat causative factors*. If the cause of ischaemia is a tight plaster cast, remove or split the cast. If it is due to a supracondylar humeral fracture, the peripheral pulses should return when the fracture is reduced; if the radial pulse does not return rapidly, surgical exploration is indicated.
- *Angiography*. A computed tomography (CT) angiogram will reveal whether ischaemia is due to spasm, intimal tear or arterial disruption. Intra-arterial angiography may need to be performed in a radiology suite or intraoperatively. Partial tears in large vessels may be amenable to intravascular stenting.
- *Operative exploration*. If a limb fails to reperfuse after a fracture or dislocation is reduced, and angiography is unhelpful or shows a tear or block, exploration is mandatory. Either the affected vessel is repaired directly, or a segment of saphenous vein is interposed to replace the damaged area.
- *Fasciotomy*. Muscle ischaemia leads to swelling and compartment syndrome. The fascial compartments should be opened by splitting the deep fascia widely to relieve compartment pressure.

Open injuries

- *Direct compression*. Primary measures to staunch haemorrhage should include direct pressure. The use of a proximal tourniquet, properly applied, can limit blood loss but will render the limb ischaemic; therefore, prompt management is needed to deal with the arterial injury.
- *Resuscitation*. Replace blood loss.
- *Exploration*. Small vessels that are part of a large collateral supply may be sacrificed and ligated above the site of injury. Partial tears may be directly sutured or closed with a vein patch; complete division often requires interposition of reversed saphenous vein. The use of prosthetic material after trauma is avoided if possible, owing to the risk of contamination and graft infection.

Aneurysm

An aneurysm is an abnormal permanent dilation of an artery or part of an artery, or the wall of the heart. An arterial aneurysm is defined as having a diameter 1.5 times that of the normal arterial diameter. A true aneurysm is an aneurysm that incorporates all three layers of the arterial wall (intima, media and adventitia), whereas a false aneurysm (or pseudoaneurysm) is bounded only by the adventitial layer of the arterial wall and the surrounding tissue. False aneurysms are commonly caused by trauma, including iatrogenic trauma, and infection.

Aneurysm types (Figure 12.1)

Saccular aneurysms

A saccular aneurysm is a focal bulge of one side of the artery joined to the main arterial lumen by a narrow neck. Mycotic aneurysms are often of this sort, in which infection causes a local weakness of the wall, resulting in aneurysmal dilation. Saccular aneurysms may also develop from penetrating aortic ulcers, which are areas of irregularity of the aortic wall caused by plaque formation in atherosclerosis.

Fusiform aneurysm

A fusiform aneurysm is a more generalized dilation of the artery. This is the most common type of aneurysm to affect the abdominal aorta.

False (pseudo-) aneurysm

Blood leaks out of an artery and is contained by the adventitia and surrounding connective tissue lined with thrombus. The resultant blood collection communicates with the artery so it is pulsatile and

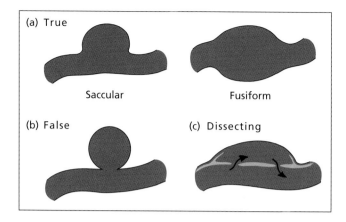

(a) True

Saccular   Fusiform

(b) False   (c) Dissecting

Figure 12.1 (a–c) Types of aneurysms.

expansile. It will either thrombose spontaneously or enlarge and rupture.

Aneurysm complicating arterial dissection

A dissection occurs where blood forces a passage through a break in the intima of a vessel, creating a separate 'false' channel between the layers of the arterial wall. This false channel creates a weakness in the arterial wall, which may predispose to rupture in the acute period or aneurysm formation more chronically.

Aetiology

Degenerative

Atheromatous degeneration of the vessel wall is the most common cause of a true aneurysm and is predominantly seen in older men with a smoking history.

Traumatic

Penetration or weakening of the arterial wall by a penetrating wound such as a bullet or knife, or iatrogenic injury during catheterization for angiography and angioplasty, may cause a pseudoaneurysm. If there has been concomitant injury of a neighbouring vein, this may lead to an arteriovenous fistula.

Inflammatory

Inflammatory aneurysms commonly affect the abdominal aorta and differ from the more common atherosclerotic aneurysms, in that there is an immune response to components in the aortic wall, resulting in a dense inflammatory response. Evidence suggests this inflammation may be mediated through an IgG4 pathway. Patients are typically younger than those with atherosclerotic aneurysms and tend to be symptomatic with back or abdominal pain. Investigation reveals a raised erythrocyte sedimentation rate (ESR) and C-reactive protein (CRP). Imaging usually reveals a rind of inflammatory tissue surrounding the aortic wall, which characteristically extends laterally into the retroperitoneum as retroperitoneal fibrosis when it may encase the ureters, causing bilateral hydronephrosis. The inflammatory component may subside with corticosteroid or other immunosuppressive treatment.

Mycotic

Mycotic aneurysms were historically seen in the thoracic aorta of patients with tertiary syphilis. They are now equally seen involving the abdominal aorta, typically as a consequence of salmonellosis, direct seeding from discitis or originating from infective endocarditis. Patients with immunodeficiency, whether resulting from immunosuppression for organ transplantation, chemotherapy or human immunodeficiency virus (HIV) infection, are prone to mycotic aneurysms from unusual bacteria and fungi.

Aortopathies

Aortopathies are a group of genetic conditions that are characterized by aneurysmal disease of the aorta. Such diseases can be syndromic, familial or sporadic, with common disorders being Marfan syndrome[2], Loeys-Dietz syndrome[3] and Ehlers-Danlos syndrome (vascular type, formerly called type 4)[4]. Such patients commonly develop arterial complications at a young age.

Clinical features of true aneurysms

The clinical features of an aneurysm depend on its location. It may present with symptoms due to local complications of the aneurysm or due to a more distal complication whose source is the aneurysm.

- *Rupture.* The likelihood of rupture increases as the diameter of the artery increases relative to its normal size.
- *Thrombosis.* Thrombus naturally lines the wall of the aneurysm. This may progress to cause complete occlusion of the artery with resultant distal ischaemia.
- *Embolism.* Lining thrombus may detach and embolize to distal circulation, either as small emboli, resulting in digital ischaemia, or as a large mass of thrombus threatening the entire limb.
- *Pressure.* Adjacent structures may be eroded or displaced. Hence, backache and sciatica are common in patients with large abdominal aortic aneurysms, and occlusion of the femoral vein is common with large femoral aneurysms.
- *Fistula.* An aneurysm may rupture into an adjacent vessel or viscus, causing a fistula, such as an aorto-caval fistula.

When examining an artery, an aneurysm will be felt as a dilation along the course of the artery. The aneurysm itself is both pulsatile and expansile. In smaller peripheral aneurysms, direct compression may empty the aneurysm sac or diminish its size, and pressure on the artery proximal to the aneurysm may reduce its pulsation. If the feeding vessel has a narrow

orifice, there may be a thrill and bruit, and if there is an arteriovenous communication, a machinery murmur is audible.

Aneurysms are most commonly an incidental finding in a patient undergoing imaging for something else or as a result of an aortic aneurysm screening protocol.

Special investigations

- *Abdominal X-ray.* This may show calcification in the wall of the aneurysm.
- *Computed tomography (CT), magnetic resonance (MR) and ultrasound scanning* may delineate the size and extent of an aneurysm, and its relationship to other structures, for example, the mesenteric and renal vessels in an abdominal aortic aneurysm. A CT scan will confirm if the aneurysm has ruptured.

Treatment

The treatment of an arterial aneurysm depends on its nature (true or false), location, size and symptoms. In asymptomatic patients with non-mycotic aneurysms, intervention is dictated by the size of the aneurysm since the risk of rupture increases with increasing size. Since elective aneurysm repair is done prophylactically to prevent rupture, the patient's concurrent health and the ease of treatment of the aneurysm need to be balanced against the benefit of the intervention.

False aneurysms and mycotic aneurysms are more prone to rupture and require more urgent attention often irrespective of size.

---

[2]Antoine Marfan (1858–1942), Agrégé of Paediatrics, University of Paris. Marfan syndrome is due to mutation in the fibrillin-1 gene

[3]Bart L Loeys (contemporary), Professor of Cardiogenomics, University of Antwerp, was a student of Harry (Hal) Dietz III (b1958), Professor of Genetic Medicine, Johns Hopkins University, Baltimore, MD, USA, when a mutation in the TGFBR2 gene was identified as the cause of this Marfan-like syndrome.

[4]Edvard Ehlers (1863–1937), Dermatologist, Frederiks Hospital, Copenhagen. Henri-Alexandre Danlos (1844–1912), Dermatologist and *chef de service*, Hôpital Tenon, Paris. The cause of the vascular type is a mutation in the COL3A1 gene coding for type III collagen.

Abdominal aortic aneurysm

Aneurysmal dilation of the abdominal aorta is a common finding in older men with a significant smoking history and in those with a positive family history. Around 10% will have a coincidental popliteal aneurysm. The speed at which an aneurysm grows is dependent on the size of the aorta, with a smaller aneurysm having a slower growth rate; on average, an aneurysm grows at 2 to 3 mm per year, size being measured in terms of the maximum antero-posterior diameter. The larger an aneurysm gets, the more likely it is to rupture.

The annual risk of rupture for an aneurysm with a maximum antero-posterior diameter of less than 5.5 cm is less than 1%, rising to 5% per annum for an aneurysm of 6 cm diameter, which is the point at which surgery is recommended for men. The threshold for women is slightly less, at 5.0 to 5.5 cm. The threshold for aneurysm repair is also dictated by the estimated operative mortality, which in a fit man is considered to be less than 5%.

Patients may present with abdominal and/or back pain but with no evidence of rupture on CT imaging. These patients are of concern as the pain may represent impending rupture, and in the absence of other causes of abdominal or back pain, urgent repair should be considered.

Management

Patients with small asymptomatic aortic aneurysms (defined as having a maximal diameter < 5.5 cm) are followed up by regular ultrasound scans to monitor the rate of growth. Once the threshold diameter is reached, or if the aneurysm becomes symptomatic then treatment is advised. Size and anatomy are then defined by CT angiograms. The options for intervention include:

- open surgical repair;
- standard endovascular repair with an infrarenal stent graft;
- complex endovascular repair (either a fenestrated or branched endovascular device);
- continue with non-operative management.

The decision-making process will involve assessment of the natural history of the aneurysm and associated risk of rupture, technical consideration and the fitness of the patient for surgery. Decision-making is commonly undertaken in a multi-disciplinary setting and needs to also involve the patient. The pre-operative cardiorespiratory assessment will vary between clinical settings, but if open surgical repair is to be undertaken, then a thorough objective evaluation of the cardiac and respiratory system is required.

Operative management
(Figure 12.2)
Open surgical repair

Open surgery involves replacement of the aneurysmal aorta with a synthetic graft, which is usually made of Dacron. The aneurysm sac is opened, any lumbar arteries oversewn, thrombus removed, and the graft sewn into healthy artery proximal and distal to the aneurysm. The operative mortality rate for such a procedure is between 3% and 5%.

Standard endovascular aneurysm repair (EVAR)

Suitability for an EVAR is determined by the anatomy of the aneurysm, iliac arteries and the infrarenal aortic neck. If suitable, the main body of the stent graft is inserted through a femoral artery and the stent positioned into place below the renal arteries. The stent is then deployed under fluoroscopy with the stent sealing against a normal infrarenal neck by radial force. The stent graft requires continuation into the iliac arteries (a bifurcated device) to allow the stent to seal appropriately into normal iliac arteries and prevent retrograde perfusion of the aneurysmal sac.

Complex endovascular repair

Complex endovascular repair of juxta-renal and supra-renal aneurysms is possible. The aim is still to provide an appropriate seal of the stent graft in normal artery above and below the aneurysm to prevent arterial flow into the aneurysmal sac. There is a subset of patients in whom standard EVAR is not possible as the proximal seal would be inadequate due to a short infrarenal neck. In such circumstances, it is possible to manufacture a custom-made device, created specific to the patient's anatomy, that has windows cut into the stent graft that align with the position of the visceral vessels (e.g. the superior mesenteric artery and renal arteries) to facilitate stenting of these vessels with covered stents from the aortic graft. These are known as fenestrated or branched devices.

Complications of surgery

Complications associated with abdominal aortic aneurysm surgery are similar for open and endovascular management but are more frequent in those patients undergoing open surgery. The complications include:

- *Haemorrhage.*
- *Myocardial infarction and arrhythmia* secondary to coronary artery disease, which is common in

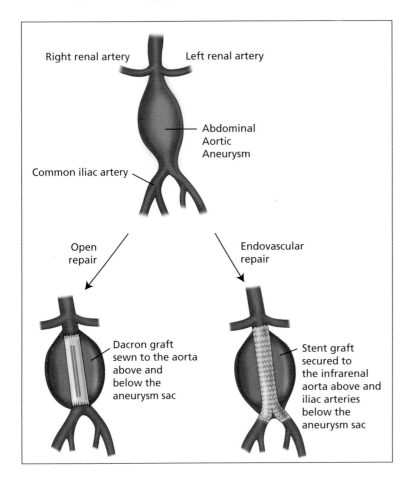

Figure 12.2 Aortic repairs.

patients who develop aneurysms. Cross-clamping the aorta during surgery and reperfusion of the legs cause additional myocardial stress.

- *Chest infection*, in relation to smoking-related pulmonary disease, post-operative pain on inspiration and prolonged anaesthesia.
- *Acute kidney injury*. In open surgery, this is related to clamping the aorta adjacent to the renal artery ostia and temporarily occluding them in open surgery. In endovascular surgery, this relates to the use of large amounts of radio-opaque contrast during stent grafting, and partial occlusion of the renal artery ostia by the proximal position of the stent. In both cases, hypotension exacerbates the renal injury.
- *Distal embolization* of thrombus displaced from the aortic sac or atheroma from arterial walls may block small vessels in the foot and lower leg, causing acute ischaemia.
- *Graft infection* occurs in around 1% and may result in an aorto-duodenal fistula.
- *Endoleaks*. There is a continued risk that the aneurysm sac may be reperfused with arterial blood, a complication known as an endoleak (Figure 12.3). Patients with a type 1 or 3 endoleak need urgent re-intervention to reduce the risk of rupture. Patients with other leaks can be carefully monitored with intervention required when there is associated sac enlargement. For this reason, patients undergoing any form of endovascular repair of an abdominal aortic aneurysm need to be enrolled into a lifelong surveillance programme, usually with a combination of ultrasound and plain abdominal X-ray.

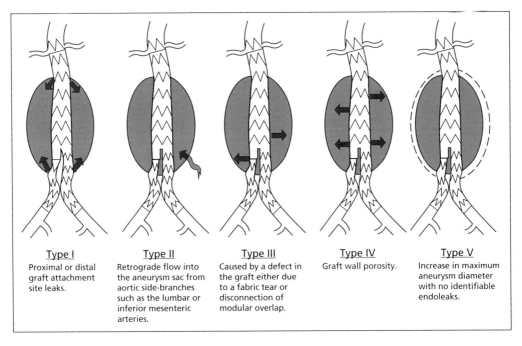

Type I
Proximal or distal graft attachment site leaks.

Type II
Retrograde flow into the aneurysm sac from aortic side-branches such as the lumbar or inferior mesenteric arteries.

Type III
Caused by a defect in the graft either due to a fabric tear or disconnection of modular overlap.

Type IV
Graft wall porosity.

Type V
Increase in maximum aneurysm diameter with no identifiable endoleaks.

Figure 12.3 Classification of endoleaks.

Ruptured abdominal aortic aneurysm

A patient with a ruptured aneurysm classically presents with severe back or abdominal pain, collapse and hypotension. Sometimes, the pain may radiate to the groin, mimicking renal colic. Occasionally, only groin or iliac fossa pain may be the presenting symptom, or the pain is confined to the epigastrium, leading to the mistaken diagnosis of myocardial infarction.

Fifty percent of patients die from the initial rupture and never reach hospital. Those patients who do make it to hospital usually have a rupture contained within the haematoma aided by the hypotension that follows rupture. The diagnosis is suggested by an ultrasound scan performed in the emergency department (a Focused Assessment with Sonography for Trauma [FAST] scan). If the patient is awake and alert and has a stable blood pressure (even if hypotensive), then it is appropriate to undertake a CT angiogram to (i) confirm the diagnosis and (ii) determine whether the anatomy would be suitable for an EVAR. If the anatomy is suitable and the patient continues to remain stable then an EVAR, ideally performed under local anaesthetic, is the most appropriate intervention. If the patient is unstable, then they need to proceed immediately for an open surgical repair.

Popliteal aneurysm

Popliteal aneurysms are the most common peripheral aneurysms. They are commonly associated with other aneurysms and are frequently bilateral.

Clinical features

Popliteal aneurysms are generally asymptomatic. When they do cause symptoms, this is usually due to distal embolization of the thrombus from within the aneurysm sac, leading to digital infarction or acute thrombosis of the aneurysm itself. Rupture or symptoms due to compression are less common. Examination confirms a prominent pulsation in the popliteal fossa, often extending proximally. Distal pulses should be sought for evidence of embolization.

The popliteal arteries should be examined in any patient with an abdominal aortic aneurysm.

Special investigations

- *Duplex ultrasonography.* Determines the size of the aneurysm.
- *CT or MR angiography.* Provides anatomical detail of the aneurysm and the arterial tree distal to the aneurysm.

Treatment

Symptomatic popliteal aneurysms

Acute limb ischaemia (see below) due to acute thrombosis of the aneurysm requires emergency treatment, usually in the form of a bypass from the distal superficial femoral artery to the distal below knee popliteal artery, with thrombectomy of the infra-popliteal arteries. Even with this, the amputation risk is approximately 50%. For symptomatic aneurysms without acute limb ischaemia, urgent treatment should be performed usually with a bypass with ligation of the aneurysm, but occasionally an endovascular procedure may be performed using a covered stent.

Asymptomatic popliteal aneurysms

Size is still the key factor that determines whether an asymptomatic popliteal aneurysm requires intervention. There is no definitive size threshold, but typically, a diameter of 2.5 to 3 cm is an indication for surgery. The presence of significant intraluminal thrombus, marked angulation or the occlusion of one or more infra-popliteal arteries may encourage earlier intervention. Open surgery or (covered) stent insertion may be considered when intervening on a popliteal aneurysm.

Assessing the patient with arterial disease

Arterial disease commonly causes impaired blood supply to the legs. The most common cause of such arterial disease is atherosclerosis. Given that atherosclerosis rarely localizes to the peripheries, involvement of other organs, particularly the heart, carotid arteries and abdominal viscera, must be kept in mind.

> **Box 12.1 Risk factors for atherosclerotic disease**
>
> - Smoking
> - Hyperlipidaemia
> - Hypertension
> - Diabetes mellitus
> - Male sex
> - Increasing age
> - Family history

Curiously, the upper limb vessels are commonly spared from atherosclerotic disease. Other conditions that may cause arterial disease include diabetic microangiopathy, thromboembolic disease, Buerger's disease, Raynaud's phenomenon and the vasculitides, together with arterial injury from trauma, cold or chemicals.

Risk factors for atherosclerosis (Box 12.1)

Many factors have been shown to contribute to atherosclerosis. While there is a familial tendency to the disease, the most common aetiological factors are smoking and diabetes followed by hyperlipidaemia/hypercholesterolaemia and hypertension. It is a disease that predominantly affects men, although, with increasing age, women become more susceptible.

Management of atherosclerotic disease involves optimization of modifiable cardiovascular risk factors. This includes smoking cessation, exercise and diet advice; lipid-lowering therapy, which will usually be high-dose statin therapy; and an antiplatelet agent. Co-existent diabetes mellitus and hypertension should be sought and treated. A chest X-ray will pick up an asymptomatic bronchial carcinoma, a common finding in patients with smoking-induced vascular disease.

Lower limb peripheral arterial disease

Patients with lower limb atherosclerotic disease most commonly present with intermittent claudication[5]. If

---

[5]Claudication, from the Latin *claudere*, to limp. The Roman emperor Claudius (10 BC to 54 AD) was afflicted with a limp from childhood.

the degree of atherosclerosis is more extensive, then patients may present with symptoms of critical limb-threatening ischaemia (gangrene / foot ulcer / rest pain). Some patients may have peripheral arterial disease yet display no symptoms – this is commonly because they do not walk far enough to elicit claudication-type symptoms.

Intermittent claudication

Intermittent claudication manifests as a gripping, tight, cramp-like pain in the muscles of the leg brought on by exercise and relieved by rest. It most commonly affects the calf but can affect the thigh and buttock. Pain that is present on standing and that requires the patient to sit down before it is relieved is more typical of cauda equina compression (spinal claudication) (Chapter 18).

Calf claudication is usually due to atherosclerosis within the superficial femoral artery, whereas buttock claudication is due to a reduced blood flow down the internal iliac arteries, owing to a lesion either there or higher up in the common iliac artery or the aorta. Bilateral buttock claudication is associated with impotence, as both internal iliac arteries are compromized (Leriche's syndrome[6]: absent femoral pulses, intermittent claudication of the buttock muscles, pale cold legs and impotence).

The natural history of the limb in claudication is relatively benign. In approximately 75% of patients, the symptoms will remain static or improve over time with no intervention. Patients with claudication have a higher risk of heart-related complications or stroke when compared to patients without peripheral arterial disease.

Critical limb-threatening ischaemia

Critical limb-threatening ischaemia may be defined as rest pain, ulceration or gangrene associated with absent pedal pulses. An ankle brachial pressure index (ABPI) of less than 0.5 also signifies critical ischaemia. Without revascularization, the natural history of a critically ischaemic leg is progression to major lower limb amputation. The five-year mortality in this group of patients is 50%.

[6]René Leriche (1879–1955), Professor of Surgery successively at Lyon, Strasbourg and Paris.

Rest pain

Rest pain occurs when the blood supply to the foot is insufficient. Initially, the pain occurs at night after the foot has been horizontal for a few hours in bed. The patient gains relief by sleeping with the leg hanging out of bed. As the disease progresses, the pain becomes continuous throughout the day.

Gangrene

The presence of gangrene indicates a severe degree of vascular impairment. Typically, it occurs in the toes or at pressure areas on the foot, particularly the heel or on the plantar aspect of the ball of the hallux. Gangrene results from infection of ischaemic tissues. Minimal trauma, such as a nick of the skin while cutting the toenails or an abrasion from a tight shoe, enables ingress of bacteria into the infarcted tissues; the combination of these two factors results in clinical gangrene.

Diabetic foot ulceration

Diabetic foot ulceration can be primarily neuropathic or neuro-ischaemic in nature. Neuropathy, caused by poorly controlled diabetes, can affect the sensory, motor and/or the autonomic nervous system. This causes limited sensation to the foot; abnormal shape of the foot, leading to a change in pressure areas; and reduced sweating, leading to dry skin and cracking, all of which predispose to ulceration. Patients with diabetes are also prone to atherosclerosis and small vessel disease. The atherosclerosis has a tendency to affect the infra-popliteal arteries, which makes revascularization more challenging and less successful.

Examination

Careful clinical examination will usually provide a very clear indication of the severity and nature of the ischaemic disease.

- *Heart rhythm.* The presence of atrial fibrillation or other cardiac arrhythmias should be noted, particularly if there is a history of acute limb ischaemia (see below).
- *Inspection of limbs.* Inspection of the legs may reveal marked skin pallor, an absence of hairs, ulcers (usually lateral malleolus and often in the interdigital clefts) and gangrene, all being evidence of impaired circulation.

- *Venous guttering.* The veins of the foot and leg in a patient with diminished arterial supply are often very inconspicuous compared with normal veins. Indeed, the veins may be so empty that they appear as shallow grooves or gutters, especially in the elevated limb.
- *Buerger's test*[7] involves raising the legs to 45° above the horizontal and keeping them there for a couple of minutes. A poor arterial supply is shown by rapid pallor. The legs are then allowed to hang dependent over the examination couch. The feet reperfuse with a dusky crimson colour in contrast to a normally perfused foot, which has no colour change. In severe cases, the foot may remain pale and some time may pass before the reactive hyperaemia appears.
- *Capillary return.* The speed of return of capillary circulation after the blanching produced by pressure on the nails is a very useful gauge of the peripheral circulation.
- *Skin temperature.* Skin temperature can be readily assessed by palpation, which is especially sensitive when the dorsum of the hand is used. A difference between the temperatures of one part of the leg and another or between the two legs can be readily ascertained. A clearly marked change of temperature may reveal the site of blockage of a main artery.
- *Peripheral pulses.* The peripheral pulses throughout the body should be examined. Whereas normal pulsation can be appreciated easily, palpation of weak pulsation requires practice, care and, above all, time. The presence of a weak pulse that is palpated is of considerable significance diagnostically and can be important prognostically, as even a weak pulse means the vessel is patent. Careful recording of the peripheral pulses will often clearly delineate a blockage in the arterial system. For instance, the presence of a good femoral pulse and absence of pulses distal to the femoral suggest a superficial femoral arterial block. Ischaemia of the digits in the presence of all pulses, including the radial and ulnar pulses, is a typical finding in Raynaud's phenomenon or small vessel disease.
- *Aneurysmal arteries.* The abdomen should be examined for any evidence of abnormal aortic

pulsation suggestive of an aneurysm; the popliteal and femoral arteries should also be examined with this in mind.
- *Auscultation of vessels.* In all areas where pulses are felt, auscultation should be performed. Partial blockage of arteries very often causes bruits, which are usually systolic in timing; they may even be felt as thrills. Arteriovenous communications will produce continuous bruits with systolic accentuation (machinery murmur) and pulsating dilated veins.
- *Ankle brachial pressure index.* The ABPI should be measured in each leg as part of the routine examination. A Doppler probe is held over the brachial artery and a blood pressure cuff inflated to occlude the blood flow. As the blood pressure cuff is deflated, a Doppler signal reappears and a systolic pressure can be recorded. Similar pressure readings are taken from the dorsalis pedis and posterior tibial arteries with a cuff just above the ankle. The ABPI is the ratio of pressure at the foot pulse to that at the brachial artery. A value between 0.9 and 1.1 is normal and values less than 0.5 indicate significant ('critical') ischaemia. Heavily calcified vessels, as are common in patients with diabetes, may be incompressible and give false normal or high readings.
- *Exercise test.* If it is difficult to obtain a clear history of the diagnosis of peripheral arterial disease in the context of exertional leg pain and a normal resting ABPI (common if spinal claudication is considered), then an exercise test is useful to perform. The patient should be exercised (corridor walking / treadmill test / heel-to-toe-tip exercise) with pre- and post-exercise ABPI measurements. A significant reduction in post-exercise ABPI indicates ischaemia.

Management

Intermittent claudication (Box 12.2)

Conservative treatment

If patients stop smoking and continue exercise or, better still, are enrolled into a programme of supervised exercise, over one-third will extend their claudication distance owing to the development of collateral vessels that bypass the blockage. Only one-third will deteriorate. In addition to cessation of smoking, the other risk factors for the development of arterial disease should be treated: diabetes should be sought

---

[7]Leo Buerger (1879–1943), born in Vienna, Surgeon and Urologist in various hospitals in New York and Los Angeles. Also described thromboangiitis obliterans in 1908.

Conservative

- Stop smoking
- Exercise to increase the collateral circulation
- Learn to live within a claudication distance, involving a change in lifestyle and perhaps employment
- Foot care, to prevent minor trauma which may lead to gangrene
- Treat co-existing conditions such as diabetes, hypertension and hyperlipidaemia

Interventional

- Angioplasty
- Endoluminal stenting
- Bypass surgery, but only if severely handicapped by symptoms

and treated aggressively, and all patients should be treated with intense lipid-lowering and antiplatelet therapy.

Interventional treatment

If claudication is a significant handicap to the patient and impacts their day-to-day quality of life, the possibility of reconstructive surgery or angiographic intervention may be considered, taking into account the natural history of the leg in patients with claudication alongside the short- and long-term risk of intervention (Figure 12.4).

Critical limb-threatening ischaemia.

Without revascularization, the leg will not be salvaged, and this will lead to either major lower limb amputation or palliation.

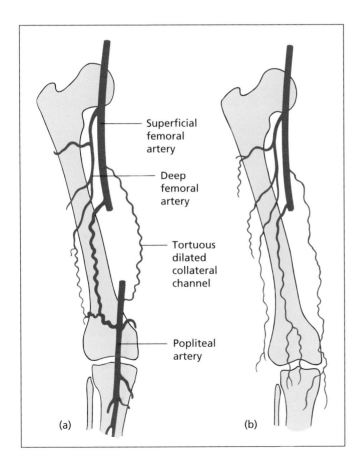

Superficial femoral artery

Deep femoral artery

Tortuous dilated collateral channel

Popliteal artery

(a)　(b)

Figure 12.4 Tracings of arteriograms. (a) An example of a good 'run-off' from the occluded superficial femoral artery, with a patent popliteal artery; this is suitable for reconstructive surgery. (b) The main arterial tree is obliterated, and reconstruction cannot be carried out.

- *Angioplasty* involves inflating a balloon within the vessel to open up a stenosis or occlusion to allow more blood to pass through. This is most successful with concentric stenoses or occlusions in the iliac system, and is less successful with longer occlusions over 10 cm, particularly in the distal femoral and popliteal arteries. An endovascular stent may be used to maintain patency. Angioplasty carries the risk of distal embolization and vessel perforation, and is prone to restenosis.
- *Bypass surgery.* Bypass surgery is reserved primarily for critical limb-threatening ischaemia. Successful surgical reconstruction demands four things:
  - *Inflow.* A good arterial supply up to the area of blockage is necessary to ensure that enough blood can be carried distally via the conduit to the ischaemic area.
  - *Outflow (run-off).* There should be good vessels below the area of disease onto which a conduit can be anastomosed. If there is nowhere for the blood to go, the conduit will occlude.
  - *The conduit.* Ideally, the saphenous vein, reversed or used *in situ* with valve destruction, should be used. If this is unavailable, then arm vein or an inert prosthetic material such as polytetrafluoroethylene (PTFE) may be used for the conduit. The conduit will take blood from the proximal to the distal segment of the artery beyond the blockage. In grafts that start and finish above the knee, there is little to choose between PTFE and vein in terms of long-term patency, but a graft that crosses the knee is much more likely to remain patent if it is saphenous vein rather than PTFE. Infection is less likely with autologous vein.
  - *The patient.* Critical ischaemia is often the first sign of the end-stage vascular disease that inevitably results in death. Surgery for critical ischaemia has a high mortality, reflecting this general deterioration.

Technical complications of surgery include intimal dissection, distal embolization and graft thrombosis, which worsen the initial situation.

- *Lumbar sympathectomy.* Palliation may be achieved by lumbar sympathectomy, which increases the blood supply to the skin and which can be performed percutaneously. The small increase in blood supply may make some clinical difference and is a relatively low-risk procedure.

- *Amputation.* Pain that is not controlled and ulceration or gangrene that is associated with life-threatening infection are indications for major lower limb amputation (defined as an above-ankle amputation). The general principle is to achieve a viable stump that heals primarily, and a secondary goal is to make the stump as distal as possible to facilitate rehabilitation on a prosthesis.

Acute limb ischaemia (Box 12.3)

Acute limb ischaemia is the sudden onset of pain in the leg / foot due to an abrupt deterioration in the circulation of the foot. It classically presents with the six Ps – pain, pallor, paraesthesia, paralysis, pulselessness and perishingly cold. The signs of paralysis and paraesthesia are important to determine as the presence of these are suggested of a threatened limb, and such patients require immediate revascularization.

The two main causes are (i) an embolus or (ii) *in situ* thrombosis due to atherosclerotic plaque rupture. Differentiating between the two is important as the management will differ. Other causes of acute limb ischaemia, which need to be borne in mind when assessing a patient, are a thrombosed popliteal aneurysm, aortic dissection and trauma.

Embolism

An embolus is abnormal undissolved material carried in the bloodstream from one part of the vascular system to impact in a distant part. While the embolus may comprise air, fat or tumour (including atrial myxoma), it is most commonly thrombus that becomes

---

Box 12.3 Acute limb ischaemia

- Pain
- Pallor
- Pulselessness
- Paraesthesia
- Paralysis
- Perishingly cold

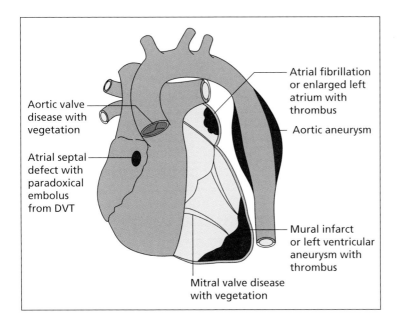

Aortic valve disease with vegetation

Atrial fibrillation or enlarged left atrium with thrombus

Aortic aneurysm

Atrial septal defect with paradoxical embolus from DVT

Mural infarct or left ventricular aneurysm with thrombus

Mitral valve disease with vegetation

Figure 12.5 Source of peripheral emboli. DVT, deep vein thrombosis.

dislodged from its source, usually the heart or major vessels (Figure 12.5).

Emboli tend to lodge at the bifurcation of vessels; their danger will depend upon the anatomical situation. Blockage of arteries of the central nervous system (CNS), retina and small intestine will produce dramatic effects. Emboli in the renal arteries will produce haematuria and pain in the loin. Emboli in the splenic artery will produce pain under the left costal margin. Large emboli straddling the aortic bifurcation (a saddle embolus) may cause bilateral signs.

Patients with an embolic cause of acute limb ischaemia will not have a previous history of claudication and are likely to have a normal set of palpable lower limb pulses on the contralateral leg. They will possibly have an evident source of the embolus:

- *Atrial fibrillation* is by far the most common cause of arterial emboli. Atrial fibrillation is most commonly due to myocardial ischaemia, but historically was due to rheumatic heart disease.
- A *mural thrombus*, typically forming following a myocardial infarction, may also dislodge and embolize. This typically occurs around 10 days after infarct.
- *Aortic dissection* is an uncommon differential diagnosis, when ischaemia may progress down the body, often with spontaneous recovery corresponding to the intimal flap dissecting away from the true lumen (Chapter 13).

- *Paradoxical emboli* are also uncommon. In patients with a patent foramen ovale or other septal defect, a clot originating in the veins may pass up towards the chest. In addition to impacting in the pulmonary arterial tree, the clot may pass across the septal defect and lodge in the arterial system. This is particularly likely after a pulmonary embolus, as the resultant raised pulmonary artery pressure results in increased shunting across a septal defect if present.
- An *atrial myxoma* is rare, but may present with distal embolization of adherent clot or tumour fragments.

Treatment

Limb ischaemia following an embolic event is usually profound due to the lack of development of collaterals.

1 *Anticoagulation.* As soon as the diagnosis is made, the patient should be systemically heparinized, to prevent propagation of clot from the site of blockage.
2 *Surgical embolectomy.* The approach to the involved vessel will depend on physical findings indicating the level of the block. The operative treatment is relatively simple: the vessel is exposed, opened and the clot removed. A special

balloon catheter (designed by Thomas Fogarty[8] when he was a medical student) is passed into the vessel with the balloon collapsed. The balloon is then inflated and pulled back, the clot being expelled by the balloon via the arteriotomy. Poor results will be due to propagation of clot beyond the embolus, particularly down the branches of the popliteal artery, and a popliteal embolectomy may also be required. Emboli in the upper limb vessels usually produce less disability than those in the lower limb, as a collateral circulation in the upper limb is better. Surgery is, therefore, indicated less often.

3 *Fasciotomy*. Patients requiring an emergency embolectomy commonly also require calf fasciotomy due to the high risk of compartment syndrome following reperfusion.

In situ thrombosis

Patients with *in situ* thrombosis associated with an atherosclerotic plaque rupture usually have less profound ischaemia due to the prior development of a collateral circulation that will still maintain some perfusion to the affected leg. They commonly give a history of claudication, will have atherosclerotic disease in other arterial beds and will likely have evidence of arterial disease in the contralateral leg evidenced by poorly palpable lower limb pulses. Revascularization in such patients is more complex.

Atherosclerotic occlusive arterial disease 🔘

Patients with lower limb arterial disease will commonly have atherosclerotic disease in other arterial beds. Occlusive disease results in ischaemia of the end organ or tissue that is supplied, and may manifest as exercise induced ischaemia progressing to rest pain, or acute ischaemia due to embolism or *in situ* thrombosis.

[8]Thomas Fogarty (b. 1934), medical student, Cincinnati, later surgeon, Stanford University Medical Center, California, and winery owner.

Coronary occlusive disease

Angina pectoris is the coronary circulation's equivalent of intermittent claudication, with pain on exertion as oxygen demand exceeds supply, and rest pain being analogous to unstable angina with resultant infarction if the coronary circulation is not revascularized by either thrombolysis or bypass surgery.

Mesenteric occlusive disease

Mesenteric angina occurs when the blood supply to the gut is impaired and classically is precipitated by eating. Patients present with central abdominal pain after meals, a history of marked weight loss and fear of eating because of pain. Loose motions or blood in the stool may be present. Typically, two of the three mesenteric vessels (coeliac trunk, superior and inferior mesenteric arteries) will be chronically diseased before symptoms of mesenteric ischaemia manifest. Diagnosis is usually late, and other causes of abdominal pain will need to be excluded.

Acute mesenteric arterial occlusion, usually secondary to embolus, results in bowel infarction (Chapter 29).

Carotid artery disease (Figure 12.6)

In the cerebral circulation, the most common symptoms are of transient ischaemic attack (TIA) or stroke. Atheroma usually affects the bifurcation of the carotid artery extending into the internal and external carotid arteries. Atheromatous plaques may ulcerate and thrombus forms on their surface. If this thrombus breaks off, it forms an embolus comprising platelet clumps or atheromatous debris. This may impact in the ipsilateral retinal artery, producing ipsilateral blindness, or the cerebral arteries of the ipsilateral hemisphere, producing *contralateral* paralysis. This is a medical emergency as patients with a significant stroke may benefit from early thrombolysis to improve cerebral perfusion.

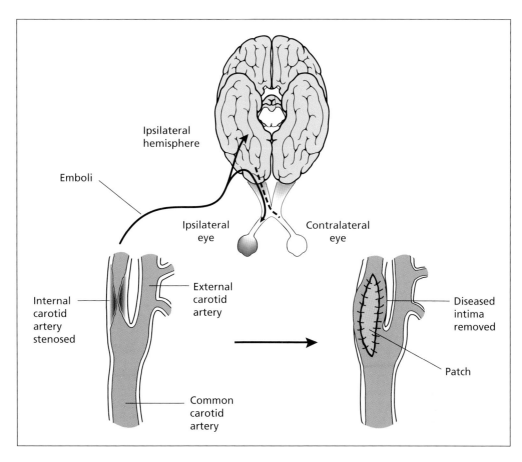

Figure 12.6 Consequences and treatment of carotid artery stenosis.

Clinical features

- *Amaurosis fugax.* The patient commonly complains of a loss of vision like a curtain coming down across their visual field. The blindness is unilateral, ipsilateral to the diseased carotid artery, and usually lasts a few minutes.
- *Cerebrovascular accidents (stroke).* Emboli in the carotid territory of the cerebral circulation of the ipsilateral hemisphere will result in symptoms affecting the contralateral side of the body, commonly loss of use of the arm. If the dominant hemisphere is involved, speech may be affected.
- *Transient ischaemic attack.* By definition, these mimic strokes, but last less than 24 hours.

Examination may reveal a bruit over the affected side (although very tight stenoses are often silent) and evidence of vascular disease elsewhere. During an attack, unilateral weakness affecting the arm or leg, dysphasia, and retinal emboli and infarction may be noted.

Differential diagnosis

Other causes of focal neurological deficits include hypoglycaemia, focal epilepsy, migraine, intracerebral neoplasm, and emboli secondary to cardiac arrhythmias and valve disease.

Special investigations

- *Duplex ultrasonography.* By measuring flow patterns, it is possible to quantify the degree of stenosis of a vessel because the blood velocity increases as it crosses a stenosis in order to maintain the same flow rate. This gives an accurate non-invasive assessment of the degree of stenosis and is useful to screen for the disease.

- *MR/CT angiography* can also give good images of the carotid vessels and allows good visualization of the vertebral system to assess the complete cerebral perfusion. It is less accurate in the measurement of the degree of stenosis.
- *CT of the brain* is indicated in any patient with a stroke or if any doubt over symptoms exists, since intracranial tumours may mimic carotid artery disease, and may co-exist.
- *MR of the brain*. A diffusion-weighted MRI scan will provide evidence of infarction.
- *ECG/echocardiography*. This may be necessary to exclude a cardiac cause of cerebral symptoms.

Treatment

Patients who have had a recent TIA, amaurosis fugax or stroke with full recovery in the presence of a significant internal carotid stenosis are at high risk of a subsequent stroke in the months following. The definition of a significant stenosis varies depending on the measurement parameters used (Figure 12.7). If the North American Symptomatic Carotid Endarterectomy Trial (NASCET) measurement is used, then a significant stenosis is defined as greater than 50%, and for the European Carotid Surgery Trial (ECST) measurement, it is greater than 70%, emphasizing the importance of understanding how a stenosis was defined. These patients benefit from carotid endarterectomy to remove the diseased intima and re-establish normal carotid flow. All patients should be started on antiplatelet therapy and a statin upon diagnosis, and this should be continued indefinitely as prophylaxis against further events. Surgery should ideally be undertaken within 2 weeks of symptoms. Patients with asymptomatic stenoses may also benefit from surgery, but here the risk/benefit ratio is not as favourable.

Carotid endarterectomy is performed as prophylaxis against future stroke. The diseased intima is removed. A shunt may be used during the surgery to preserve blood flow to the brain.

Complications of carotid endarterectomy

- *Disabling stroke*. Up to 3% of patients will suffer a stroke.
- *Death*, usually as a consequence of stroke, in up to 2%.
- *Haemorrhage*. Bleeding is common, as the patients are on antiplatelet therapy. Occasionally, post-operative haemorrhage requires wound re-exploration.
- *Hypoglossal neuropraxia*. The hypoglossal nerve crosses the upper part of the incision and may be damaged during surgery, resulting in a hypoglossal palsy, manifested by protrusion of the tongue to the ipsilateral side.
- *Reperfusion syndrome*. The sudden increase in blood flow to the brain may result in cerebral oedema and fitting or haemorrhage. Good postoperative blood pressure control is, therefore, vital.

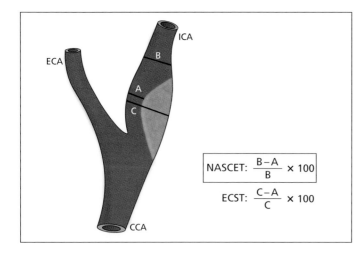

$$\text{NASCET: } \frac{B-A}{B} \times 100$$

$$\text{ECST: } \frac{C-A}{C} \times 100$$

Figure 12.7 Different measurement techniques for determining the degree of carotid stenosis. ECST: European Carotid Surgery Trial; NASCET: North American Symptomatic Carotid Endarterectomy Trial.

- *Restenosis*. The vessel may restenose at the site of the arteriotomy. To reduce this risk, a patch is usually used, made from saphenous vein or prosthetic material such as PTFE or Dacron.

Raynaud's disease and Raynaud's phenomenon[9]

Raynaud's disease is a vasospastic condition that affects the digital arteries within the hands and occasionally the feet.

Aetiology

This may be primary Raynaud's disease, almost invariably in women, or Raynaud's phenomenon, secondary to some other aetiology, particularly connective tissue disorders such as systemic sclerosis (scleroderma) and polyarteritis nodosa, the other symptoms of which it may precede by several years. It may occur in patients with cryoglobulinaemia, or it can result from working with vibrating tools. It is important to exclude other causes of cold, cyanosed hands, for instance, pressure on the subclavian artery from a cervical rib (sometimes complicated by multiple emboli arising from the damaged artery wall at the site of rib pressure), or blockage of a main artery in the upper limb due to atherosclerosis or Buerger's disease.

Clinical features

The syndrome occurs as a result of intermittent spasm of the small arteries and arterioles of the hands (and feet). Spasm is usually precipitated by cold exposure. During spasm, the hands go white. As the vasospasm resolves, the pallor changes to cyanosis and then crimson red as reperfusion and hyperaemia occur, the process commonly taking 30–45 min.

Treatment
Conservative

The management should initially be conservative. Patients should be urged to keep their hands and feet

warm, to wear gloves and fur-lined boots in the winter, and to make sure that the house, especially the bed, is warm at night. They should also avoid immersion of the limbs in cold water. Smoking must be stopped. Treatment with vasodilator drugs is usually tried, but the results are often disappointing.

Surgery

Sympathectomy almost invariably produces a dramatic improvement in the symptoms, but unfortunately may not be long-lasting in the upper limbs. Rarely, Raynaud's phenomenon or disease leads to actual necrosis of tissues and gangrene of the digits. If this occurs, local amputation may be necessary, but, as the circulation of the proximal part of the hand is usually satisfactory, major amputations are seldom required.

Buerger's disease

Buerger's disease (thromboangiitis obliterans) is a rather poorly defined entity, usually affecting men (90%), the salient features of which are similar to atherosclerosis, but the age incidence is much younger and the association with heavy smoking is almost invariable. Peripheral vessels tend to be affected earlier in Buerger's disease, and it is characterized by inflammation of small- and medium-sized arteries and veins, in contrast to atherosclerosis, although the symptoms of distal claudication and ischaemic ulceration of the toes are similar. It tends to affect the hands and fingers more commonly than atheroma. An autoimmune association has been proposed. Smoking cessation reduces but does not halt progression.

Cold injury

Frostbite may result from prolonged exposure to cold and is caused by a combination of ice crystal formation in the tissues, capillary sludging and thrombosis within small vessels of the exposed extremities. Treatment comprises gentle warming, anticoagulation with heparin to prevent further thrombosis and antibiotics to inhibit infection of necrotic tissues. Local amputation to remove necrotic digits is performed once clear demarcation develops. Raynaud's phenomenon may be experienced as a late complication.

[9]Maurice Raynaud (1834–1881), Physician, Paris. Described the condition in his doctoral dissertation.

⊙ Additional resources

13

The heart and thoracic aorta

David P. Jenkins

Learning objective

✓ To know the principal surgical conditions of the heart and thoracic aorta, and how they are treated.

Introduction

There are several unique features of cardiac surgery compared with other operations. The heart is continually beating to support life and, therefore, is a moving target; hence the use of cardiopulmonary bypass during surgery and the routine need for intensive care support following surgery.

Cardiopulmonary bypass

Background

If the circulation is temporarily stopped at normal body temperature, organs suffer ischaemic damage owing to lack of oxygen, the extent varying according to the metabolic demand of the organ. The brain is the most sensitive tissue in this respect and is liable to irreversible changes after 4 minutes of ischaemia. The spinal cord is next, followed by heart muscle, which will tolerate about 10 minutes of ischaemia at normal

Ellis and Calne's Lecture Notes in General Surgery, Fourteenth Edition.
Edited by Christopher Watson and Justin Davies.
© 2023 John Wiley & Sons Ltd. Published 2023 by John Wiley & Sons Ltd.
Companion website: www.wiley.com/go/Watson/GeneralSurgery14

temperature. The tolerance to ischaemia can be increased slightly by lowering the metabolic rate by hypothermia.

Prior to the development of cardiopulmonary bypass in the 1950s, surgery on the heart was limited to procedures that could be performed rapidly on a beating heart, such as mitral valvotomy to relieve mitral stenosis, where a finger is passed blindly through the left atrial appendage and through the stenotic mitral valve. Another alternative was to cool the whole patient, when periods of up to 10 minutes of absent circulation permitted very simple procedures to be performed relatively safely, such as closure of an atrial septal defect (ASD).

Following the development of cardiopulmonary bypass, it is now possible to operate on the heart for prolonged periods while the bypass machine is used to take over the function of the heart and lungs, and perfuse the body. Cardiopulmonary bypass has transformed the safety and reliability of cardiac surgery and led to the development of the specialty. The majority of heart operations performed today utilize cardiopulmonary bypass.

Technique

The heart is approached with a median sternotomy incision and the pericardium opened with an inverted 'T' incision. After full heparinization, cannulae are

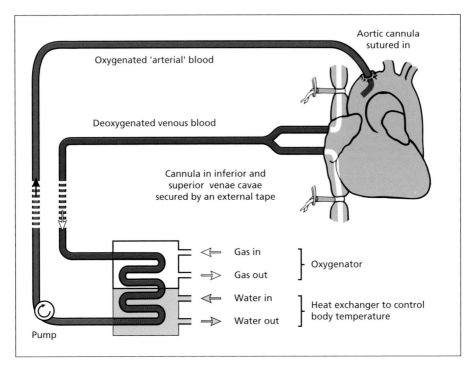

Oxygenated 'arterial' blood

Aortic cannula sutured in

Deoxygenated venous blood

Cannula in inferior and superior venae cavae secured by an external tape

Gas in

Gas out } Oxygenator

Water in

Water out } Heat exchanger to control body temperature

Pump

Figure 13.1 Cardiopulmonary bypass.

inserted into the venae cavae via the right atrium to syphon off the venous return from the systemic circulation. The blood is then pumped through an oxygenator, filter and a heat exchanger before returning to the systemic circulation via a cannula in the ascending aorta or occasionally a peripheral artery (femoral or axillary) (Figure 13.1). This form of bypass will perfuse the whole body with oxygenated blood at an adequate pressure while diverting it from the heart and lungs. The heart may now be stopped and the myocardium protected by 'cardioplegic' solution containing potassium to produce rapid cardiac arrest in diastole. The cardioplegia can be delivered antegrade into the aortic root or directly to the coronary ostia, or retrograde via the coronary sinus. With the aorta cross-clamped, the heart may be opened in a bloodless field with access to all chambers.

Cardiac intensive care

The nature of cardiac surgery means that patients are rarely woken and extubated immediately following surgery. They are usually managed in intensive care for the first night, with sedation and ventilation continued until they are warm and haemodynamically stable without excessive bleeding. Standard monitoring includes arterial and central venous lines, a urinary catheter, ventilator parameters and electrocardiograph.

Complications of cardiopulmonary bypass and cardiac surgery in general

- *Emboli*. Air entrapped during formation of the bypass circuit or entering during bypass, or thrombus forming in the bypass circuit, or atheroma from the aorta may embolize occasionally into the cerebral and peripheral circulation with catastrophic results, such as stroke and limb ischaemia.
- *Haemorrhage* postoperatively, which may result in cardiac tamponade and require re-exploration in up to 3%. Although heparinization is reversed after cardiopulmonary bypass is finished, the bypass circuit activates the clotting cascade and consumes platelets, thus increasing the risk of haemorrhage.

- *Infection.* Patients are at risk of all the potential complications of any surgical procedure, including wound infections (in up to 3%) and chest infections.
- *Low cardiac output.* This is the result of right or left heart failure post-surgery. It is usually managed with inotropic support.
- *Multi-organ failure.* This results if heart failure persists despite optimal management or if sepsis develops during prolonged intensive care. Although renal failure can be managed with haemofiltration, liver and gut failure are often fatal.
- *Death.* There are sophisticated risk stratification tools available to estimate risk of death (e.g. EuroSCORE[1]). The average risk of death for routine cardiac surgery is in the order of 1–3%.

Valvular disease

Valve repair and replacement

With the advent of cardiopulmonary bypass, it has become possible to remove diseased valves and replace them with artificial ones – mechanical, bioprosthetic or occasionally human allograft valves. In mitral valve regurgitation, repair is now usually undertaken in preference to replacement. In aortic valve regurgitation, valve repair may also be possible. For aortic valves, a minimal access option is also available to replace the valve with percutaneous access via peripheral arteries – transcatheter aortic valve insertion (TAVI). Similar procedures are under development for the mitral valve, but the access and anatomy is more complex.

Mechanical valves

Many examples exist, the most common in use today are bileaflet valves, where the valve comprises two semi-circular tilting leaflets made of pyrocarbon set in a sewing ring. Prosthetic valves may become obstructed by thrombus owing to turbulent flow across the non-biological valve leaflets; recipients must, therefore, be anticoagulated with warfarin indefinitely.

[1] The EUROpean System for Cardiac Operative Risk Estimation (http://www.euroscore.org).

Bioprosthetic valves

These are made from bovine pericardium or from pig heart valves. The valve is suspended on a prosthetic ring to allow it to be sewn in place. The bioprostheses are treated with glutaraldehyde and usually sewn onto a plastic frame. Once implanted, the recipient does not require anticoagulation, although antiplatelet therapy is recommended. The valves do not cause any immune reaction and are not rejected. The lifetime of such valves is generally shorter than prosthetic valves, but the avoidance of anticoagulation makes them the preferred choice in the elderly. Current guidelines recommend bioprostheses in the aortic position from 55 years and in the mitral position from 70 years.

Complications of valve replacement

- *Valve thrombosis* can cause embolus formation, especially if not on anticoagulation.
- *Mechanical structural failure* with embolism of valve fragments, or outflow obstruction or massive valve incompetence. This has become very rare with modern mechanical valves.
- *Haemorrhage,* especially when anticoagulated.
- *Paraprosthetic leaks,* where blood leaks between the artificial valve ring and the heart tissue, and can cause haemolysis.
- *Infection of the valve,* a situation akin to infective endocarditis of a native valve.

Aortic stenosis

Stenosis of the aortic valve is increasingly common in the elderly population. It may be as a result of:

- *Aortic sclerosis:* degenerative calcification of a standard three-leaflet valve.
- Calcification of congenitally bicuspid valves; 1% of the population have only two aortic valve leaflets owing to fusion of two adjacent valve cusps, and in these patients, stenosis can develop earlier in life.

No matter what the cause, the aortic valve, when stenosed, is usually grossly distorted and calcified and unsuitable for valve repair; replacement is the treatment of choice. Once calcification occurs, progression of the stenosis is inevitable. Aortic stenosis from rheumatic fever is now rare in the West, and usually coincides with mitral valve disease.

Clinical features

The three presenting symptoms of aortic stenosis are angina, dyspnoea on exertion and syncope (occasionally sudden death). Examination reveals a slow rising pulse and an ejection systolic murmur. Electrocardiogram (ECG) may show left ventricular hypertrophy and the echocardiogram is diagnostic. Computed tomography (CT) may show valve calcification and post-stenotic dilation of the aorta. Once the gradient across the valve exceeds 60 mmHg, or the patient is symptomatic, surgery is advised.

Treatment

Valve replacement on cardiopulmonary bypass remains the gold standard. Coincidental coronary artery disease may be treated at the same time. Percutaneous aortic valve replacement (TAVI), via the femoral artery, may be an alternative for some patients who are frail or the elderly and have relative contraindications to open surgery. This TAVI approach can also be placed into existing failing bioprostheses – the 'valve-in-valve' procedure.

Mitral regurgitation

This is now the most common lesion of the mitral valve. It is commonly due to myxomatous degeneration, typically of the posterior leaflet, but often affecting both valve leaflets. In severe form, with thickening and prolapse of both leaflets, it is termed Barlow's disease.[2]

Pathology

In degenerative disease, there is elongation of both leaflets but particularly of the *chordae tendinae*, which may proceed to rupture. The result is a prolapse of the leaflet into the left atrium during systole, with regurgitation of blood through the non-co-apting leaflets. This is followed by ventricular enlargement as a response to the volume load, and by annular

dilation. Later in the disease progression, there is left atrial enlargement and eventually loss of electrical co-ordination and the onset of atrial fibrillation. In some cases of 'functional' regurgitation, the regurgitation is due to dilatation and impairment of the left ventricle.

Clinical features

The patient may be asymptomatic for many years, with just a regurgitant murmur noted, until shortness of breath or atrial fibrillation occurs. The former may be of sudden onset, usually indicating a ruptured chord and abrupt increase of regurgitation into a still small left atrium. At a late stage, there may be secondary pulmonary hypertension and right heart failure.

Physical examination reveals an irregular pulse, a pansystolic murmur and perhaps lateral displacement of the apex beat.

Treatment

Symptomatic patients with severe regurgitation and preserved left ventricular function should have surgery. The regurgitant volume can be followed by surveillance echocardiography in the asymptomatic, as can the left ventricular size. Once the former reaches the classification 'severe', or if the left ventricle starts to enlarge, surgery is indicated.

For most patients, treatment can be valve repair; this option preserves the native valve, avoiding the need for replacement. It also optimizes left ventricular function, because the whole mitral valve apparatus – leaflet, chordae and papillary muscles – forms an integral part of the left ventricle.

The repair is performed on cardiopulmonary bypass, usually through a sternotomy. There is also a minimal access surgical approach, via a small right anterior thoracotomy and using telescopic vision and specially adapted instruments. The tricuspid valve may need to be repaired at the same time.

Mitral stenosis

With the great decline of rheumatic fever, mitral stenosis has almost disappeared in the West, but is still common in many parts of the world. At an early stage, when the leaflets are fused but mobile, the valve can be split open. This can be the conventional mitral

---

[2] John Bereton Barlow (1924–2008), Professor of Cardiology, Johannesburg, South Africa.

valvotomy, historically done with a finger, or increasingly with a balloon placed under radiological control.

When the valve is calcified, sophisticated repair techniques can be used, but are less successful than in the degenerative, regurgitant valves. Sometimes, valve replacement is required, using the same sort of valve options as discussed for the aortic valve.

Ischaemic heart disease

Angina, due to myocardial ischaemia, is caused by atherosclerosis in the coronary arteries and may be alleviated by increasing the arterial blood supply. Two treatment options exist: endoluminal intervention with balloon angioplasty and stenting, and surgical revascularization with coronary artery bypass grafts (CABGs).

Aetiology

The risk factors for coronary artery disease are those for atheroma in general (Box 12.1). In particular, raised serum cholesterol, hypertension and cigarette smoking, each double the risk of coronary artery disease. The presence of all three increases the risk eightfold.

Special investigations

- *Exercise ECG* shows whether there is myocardial ischaemia on exercise.
- *Myocardial perfusion imaging.* In patients unfit for treadmill exercise, myocardial stress can be induced pharmacologically using dobutamine or adenosine while imaging perfusion with magnetic resonance or methoxyisobutylisonitrile (MIBI).
- *Stress echocardiography* is an alternative to myocardial perfusion imaging. The contraction of different segments of the left ventricle is studied before and during pharmacologically induced stress.
- *CT coronary angiogram.* Modern high-resolution scans, with software algorithms and appropriate gating for heartbeat, can provide excellent definition of coronary anatomy and plaque disease, and is useful to exclude significant disease.
- *Coronary angiography* is performed in patients with ischaemic responses to exercise to determine

treatment options. It is important for accurate anatomical diagnosis and may be combined with endoluminal therapy.

Treatment

- *Angioplasty.* Isolated stenoses in proximal vessels are most appropriate for percutaneous coronary intervention (PCI) to reduce the symptoms of angina, with endoluminal stenting having an advantage over balloons alone to prolong patency.
- *Surgical revascularization* remains the procedure of choice for total occlusions or stenoses in multiple vessels and offers both symptomatic and prognostic benefits. It remains the guideline-recommended treatment for more complex coronary anatomy, especially triple-vessel disease and in patients with impaired left ventricular function and diabetes. This involves anastomosing an internal mammary (internal thoracic) artery to the diseased coronary artery distal to the blockage (usually the left to the left anterior descending coronary artery). For multiple grafts, autogenous reversed saphenous vein or radial artery can also be used as aortocoronary bypass conduits (Figure 13.2). Most CABG operations are performed on cardiopulmonary bypass, but surgery can be performed with the heart beating using special stabilizers and intracoronary shunts.

As with all arterial surgery for atherosclerosis, there is a tendency for recurrent disease with the passage of time. This may require repeat surgery or may be amenable to endoluminal procedures. Secondary prophylaxis with drug therapy, including statins, β-blockers and angiotensin-converting enzyme (ACE) inhibitors reduces the risk of further events, and antiplatelet therapy should be continued for life.

Surgery for the complications of myocardial infarction

1 *Acute ventriculoseptal defect.* When the infarcted ventricular muscle is part of the septum and undergoes necrosis, septal rupture may occur. This occurs 1–2 weeks after myocardial infarction in 0.5% of patients and requires urgent repair, which may be achieved surgically or via an endovascular approach. Mortality is high.
2 *Ventricular aneurysm.* If the infarcted ventricular wall is apical, it may necrose and rupture, leading

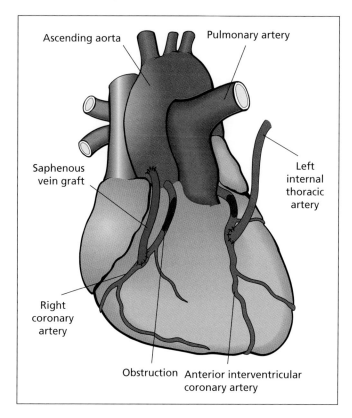

Figure 13.2 A saphenous vein graft from the aorta to the right coronary artery and a direct left internal mammary (thoracic) artery graft to the anterior interventricular coronary artery (also known as the left anterior descending [LAD] artery).

to rapid death by tamponade. Alternatively, it may heal with fibrosis, and subsequently a ventricular aneurysm may form. This may require excision if paradoxical movement or thrombus becomes symptomatic.

3 *Mitral regurgitation.* If the infarct involves a papillary muscle and it ruptures, then acute mitral regurgitation requires mitral valve replacement.

Heart transplantation

In patients with end-stage heart failure secondary to ischaemic heart disease, severe valve disease or dilated cardiomyopathy, heart transplantation is an option. Potential recipients require careful assessment and extensive comorbidity is often a contraindication. Donor matching is mainly based on blood group and size matching. The implant procedure is performed with anastomosis of the left atrial cuff, aorta, pulmonary artery, and finally inferior and superior venae cavae.

Thoracic aortic disease

As with other organs, disease of the thoracic aorta can be divided into congenital and acquired:

Congenital

- Persistent ductus arteriosus
- Coarctation of the aorta

Acquired

- Thoracic aortic aneurysm
- Thoracic aortic dissection

Persistent ductus arteriosus

Pathology

If the channel between the aorta and pulmonary artery fails to close at the time of birth, blood will be shunted from the systemic circulation with its higher pressure into the pulmonary circulation, resulting in pulmonary hypertension (Figure 13.3). In time, pulmonary vascular resistance increases and exceeds peripheral resistance, at which time the shunt reverses, deoxygenated blood from the pulmonary artery passes into the systemic circulation and the patient becomes cyanosed. It carries a risk of development of infective endocarditis and eventually right ventricular failure.

Clinical features

In neonates with a large duct, shunting may progress rapidly and cardiac failure may occur in infancy. A duct with moderate flow tends to present later with exertional dyspnoea. Most commonly, the patient is asymptomatic and the condition is diagnosed on finding the characteristic machinery-like continuous murmur, with systolic accentuation best heard over the second left space anteriorly. In infants, the bruit may be purely systolic.

Special investigations

- *Echocardiography and angiography* will demonstrate a persistent ductus, and indeed, the cardiac catheter can often be manipulated through the ductus into the aorta.

Treatment

Operative ligation and division of a persistent ductus should be undertaken on diagnosis, and before irreversible pulmonary hypertension or cardiac failure has occurred. Percutaneous endovascular insertion of an occlusive device into the ductus may achieve a cure without surgery.

Coarctation of the aorta

Pathology

This is a congenital narrowing of the aorta, which, in the majority of cases, occurs in the descending aorta just distal to the origin of the left subclavian artery

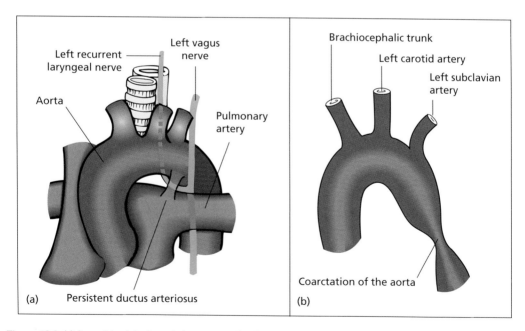

Figure 13.3 (a) A persistent ductus arteriosus – note its close relationship to the left recurrent laryngeal nerve. (b) Coarctation of the aorta. Reproduced from Ellis H, Mahadevan V (2019) *Clinical Anatomy*, 14th edn. Oxford: Wiley-Blackwell.

close to the obliterated ductus arteriosus. The pathogenesis of coarctation formation may be related to the presence of abnormal ductus tissue. Coarctation can rarely occur in other sites up and down the aorta. The stenosis is usually extreme, with only a pinpoint lumen remaining. There is sometimes a co-existent cardiac anomaly, most commonly a bicuspid aortic valve.

Blood reaches the distal aorta via collateral connections between branches of the subclavian, scapular and intercostal arteries, and by the anastomosis between the internal thoracic and inferior epigastric arteries. Although the blood supply to the lower part of the body is diminished, patients with coarctation seldom have peripheral gangrene, although occasionally they complain of intermittent claudication. The danger of coarctation is due to the effects of hypertension proximal to the coarctation. This is often severe and is likely to result in cerebral haemorrhage or left ventricular failure. The mechanism of the hypertension is probably due to the relatively poor blood supply to the kidneys, which results in release of renin and renal hypertension.

Clinical features

The diagnosis is considered in any child or young adult with hypertension. In addition to hypertension, the most characteristic physical sign, is absent, diminished or delayed femoral pulsations in relation to the radial pulse, and the condition is confirmed by a large difference in the blood pressure between the arm and leg. A systolic murmur is sometimes present posterior in the left chest, and large collateral blood vessels may be seen or felt in the subcutaneous tissues of the chest wall.

Special investigations

- *Chest X-ray* in an adult may show an enlarged heart, and often the ribs are notched by the large intercostal collateral blood vessels bypassing the stenotic area.
- *Echocardiography* in an infant is important to exclude co-existing cardiac anomalies.
- *Angiography and CT* will confirm the diagnosis.

Treatment

This is desirable before complications arise and consists of excision of the stenotic segment and either end-to-end anastomosis of the proximal and distal aorta or, if the gap to bridge is too great, an arterial graft interposed between the two aortic ends. Balloon angioplasty is an alternative treatment.

Thoracic aortic aneurysms

Aneurysms can occur in any place in the body (Chapter 12), but the aorta is particularly liable to be affected. Aneurysms of the arch of the aorta were once commonly syphilitic, but now are mainly due to atherosclerosis and sometimes connective tissue diseases, e.g. Marfan syndrome[3]. Aneurysms of the descending thoracic aorta are usually atherosclerotic. Once they have reached a sufficient threshold size, surgery is indicated to reduce the risk of rupture.

A thoracoabdominal aneurysm is an aneurysm extending across the diaphragm and involving the origins of the coeliac, superior mesenteric and renal arteries.

Clinical features

Aneurysms of the ascending aorta may be asymptomatic and discovered incidentally or present with chest pain, or breathlessness due to aortic valve disease.

Aneurysms of the arch of the aorta may compress the trachea or ulcerate into it; they are liable to stretch the left recurrent laryngeal nerve, leading to hoarseness, and may obstruct the left lower lobe bronchus, producing an area of collapse.

Aneurysms of the descending thoracic aorta may produce pain in the back or erosion of vertebrae or may press on the oesophagus, producing dysphagia, and even rupture into it. Not surprisingly, this is the most lethal cause of haematemesis.

Special investigations

- *Chest X-ray* may show the extent of the aneurysm due to calcification in its walls.
- *CT and magnetic resonance (MR) imaging* are useful in demonstrating the size and extent of the

[3] Antonine Marfan (1858–1942), Professor of Paediatrics, Hôpital des Enfants Malades, Paris, France. Marfan syndrome is due to a mutation in the fibrillin-1 gene on chromosome 15, and manifests with cardiovascular, skeletal and ocular abnormalities.

aneurysm and its relation to the major vessels of the neck.

- *Echocardiography* is important to diagnose associated aortic valve disease and assess heart function.

Treatment

Aneurysms of the ascending aorta and arch require cardiopulmonary bypass for adequate surgical treatment, which consists of partial excision of the aneurysm and insertion of a prosthetic graft with appropriate junction limbs to the main aortic branches. Whole-body cooling and deep hypothermic circulatory arrest (DHCA) is sometimes required to treat arch aneurysms.

Aneurysms of the descending thoracic aorta require a left heart bypass for their surgical treatment, which is similar in principle to those of the arch. More recently, endovascular stenting of descending thoracic aneurysms has proved to be a promising alternative.

Complications

- *Bleeding and the other complications of cardiac surgery in general (see above).*
- *Stroke* due to atherosclerotic embolism or malperfusion during surgery.
- *Spinal ischaemia* is due to loss of flow in the great radicular artery (of Adamkiewicz[4]), which arises from the aorta near T10 and supplies the lower part of the spinal cord. This results in paraplegia.

Aortic dissection

Pathology

An aortic dissection consists of a tear in the wall of the aorta, usually in the thoracic component, which allows blood to dissect along a plane of cleavage in the media and extend proximally and distally. The false passage thus formed may rupture internally into the true lumen, decompressing itself and resulting in an aorta with a double lumen. Such a patient may survive. More commonly, the dissected aorta ruptures externally into the pericardium, producing cardiac

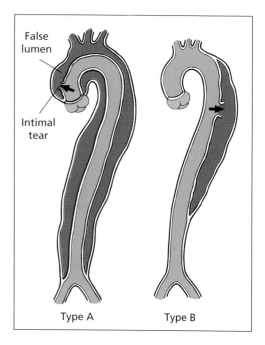

Figure 13.4 Stanford classification of aortic dissection.

tamponade, or into the thoracic or abdominal cavity with fatal haemorrhage.

Aetiology

Cystic medial degeneration weakens the wall of the aorta and enables the splitting to occur. It is usually found in atherosclerotic, hypertensive patients or those with connective tissue disease, e.g. Marfan or Ehlers-Danlos syndrome.

Classification

Aortic dissection has been classified into type A and type B (Stanford classification[5], Figure 13.4)

- *Type A dissection* affects the ascending aorta and occurs in two-thirds of cases.
- *Type B dissection* specifically excludes the ascending aorta but may involve the arch and/or descending aorta. It occurs in one-third of cases.

---

[4] Albert Adamkiewicz (1850–1921), Professor of Pathology, Cracow, Poland.

[5] Stanford University School of Medicine, Stanford, CA, USA. The Stanford classification was described in 1970 by Norman Shumway (1923--2006) and colleagues in the Division of Cardiovascular Surgery. Shumway has been described as the father of heart transplantation.

Clinical features

The patient usually presents with a sudden, severe pain in the chest, which may radiate to the arms, neck or abdomen, or with a tearing interscapular pain. In addition, there may be signs of shock, either from cardiac tamponade or from external rupture of the aneurysm. Patients with aortic dissection are sometimes initially diagnosed as suffering from a myocardial infarction, and an ECG may not help differentiate between the two conditions because if the coronary ostia are involved, coronary occlusion may have occurred. In type A dissections, the aortic valve may become incompetent as the root dilates.

As the dissection in the wall of the aorta progresses, the origins of the main arterial branches may become occluded, producing progression of symptoms and the disappearance and reappearance of peripheral pulses. If the renal vessels are involved, there may be haematuria or anuria. One or both femoral pulses may disappear with leg ischaemia. Mesenteric ischaemia is usually diagnosed late and carries a poor prognosis.

Neurological abnormalities may also occur, ranging from hemiparesis, as a result of occlusion of the carotid and subclavian artery origins, to paraesthesia, as a result of peripheral nerve ischaemia.

Special investigations

- *Chest X-ray* shows widening of the mediastinum in two-thirds of patients and a small left pleural effusion.
- *Contrast-enhanced CT* shows the diagnostic flap across the aortic lumen with true and false lumens, and is the key investigation to determine the classification and extent of disease.
- *Echocardiography* may also demonstrate a flap in the proximal aorta, a pericardial collection and aortic regurgitation.

Treatment

Once the diagnosis is made, treatment depends largely upon the type of dissection:

Type A dissections should be managed surgically as an emergency because of the risk of fatal mechanical complications. It is said that the risk of death is 1% per hour. The surgery aims to replace the ascending aorta with a prosthetic tube graft. The original tear should be excised if possible, and the aortic valve repaired or replaced if involved. *Deep hypothermic circulatory arrest* may be required to perform the distal anastomosis in the arch. The mortality risk is between 10% and 20%, but often nearer 100% without intervention.

Type B dissections are usually treated without surgery initially, and hypotensive drugs are used, reducing systolic pressure to 100–120 mmHg to prevent further extension of the dissection. The false lumen may then thrombose. Any complicating organ, limb or mesenteric ischaemia resulting from the dissection may require revascularization. An aneurysm resulting from a chronic dissection may require treatment if it enlarges or produces pressure symptoms. Treatment of the descending thoracic aorta is often delivered by vascular surgeons rather than cardiac surgeons in the UK, although some cases will require both specialist teams to provide their expertise. In cases where there is evidence of impending aortic rupture or non-perfusion of a visceral artery, endovascular placement of a covered stent (thoracic endovascular aortic repair [TEVAR]) is appropriate. The stent is placed to cover the proximal entry into the false lumen and to re-establish blood flow through the collapsed true lumen.

14

The chest and lungs

Aman Singh Coonar

Learning objectives

✓ To have knowledge of the types of chest injury and their management

✓ To have knowledge of pneumothorax and thoracic empyema, which are common conditions

✓ To know the steps of chest drain insertion

✓ To have knowledge of lung cancer and its management; this is particularly important as it is a common cause of cancer death in the UK

Thoracic surgery has undergone a revolution such that the majority of procedures are now conducted as video-assisted thoracic surgery (VATS). In the UK, lobectomy with lymph node dissection is performed more commonly as VATS than by open thoracotomy. A thoracoscopic approach is used from the simplest thoracoscopic inspection of the chest and pleural biopsies to complex anatomical resection. Pathways of care rely on a multidisciplinary team (MDT) approach with an emphasis on early mobilization and enhanced recovery.

Injury to the chest

Ventilation of the lungs depends on patent main airways and pulmonary alveoli, rigid bony skeleton of the thorax, and integrity of the nerves and muscles that control the movements of the ribs and diaphragm. Traumatic disruption of the chest wall can be lethal unless treatment is instituted rapidly. Dangerous complications of chest injury include:

- paradoxical breathing;
- pneumothorax;
- lung contusion;
- penetration of the lung (pulmonary laceration);
- haemothorax;
- cardiac contusion;
- cardiac tamponade due to laceration of the heart;
- large-vessel damage.

Serious harm can also result from blunt (crush) injuries that do not penetrate the chest; thus, the trachea or a main bronchus or the aorta may be ruptured, lung contused or torn, and papillary muscles of the heart or the coronary arteries may be damaged.

A common injury pattern is that seen in surviving occupants of a road traffic accident when the patient has been restrained by the seat belt and airbags. Characteristically, there is bruising in the seat belt pattern. Often, there are associated facial and neck injuries. There may be a mid-sternal fracture as well as broken ribs. There may be some lung and myocardial contusions. There may be a pneumothorax and haemothorax. In higher energy deceleration impact, there may be death due to transection of the aorta or airway rupture.

Ellis and Calne's Lecture Notes in General Surgery, Fourteenth Edition. Edited by Christopher Watson and Justin Davies.
© 2023 John Wiley & Sons Ltd. Published 2023 by John Wiley & Sons Ltd.
Companion website: www.wiley.com/go/Watson/GeneralSurgery14

Sternal fracture

Clinical features

A common site is mid-sternum. Usually, there is little displacement. There may be a retrosternal haematoma. Almost all such injuries will unite and heal without long-term problems. The patient is usually admitted for a period of cardiac monitoring as rhythm disturbances may occur.

Fractures of the ribs

Clinical features

A common injury to the chest is fracture of the ribs by a direct blow. The commonest pattern is that of fractures of the seventh, eighth and ninth ribs, in which the break usually occurs in the region of the mid-axillary line. The patient complains of pain in the chest overlying the fracture, and this pain is intensified by springing the ribs with gentle but sharp pressure on the sternum.

Special investigations

- *Chest X-ray* may confirm rib fractures and lung damage or haemorrhage that might not have been suspected from the patient's symptoms. A chest X-ray may not always demonstrate a fracture; if the patient has clinical signs of fractured ribs, they should be treated for this condition in spite of a negative X-ray. A repeat X-ray at 2 weeks may show fracture callus and confirm the diagnosis.
- *Computed tomography (CT) scan* is essential for assessing patients with complex chest injuries and penetrating injuries, and will demonstrate fractures and underlying visceral injury. Patients may go directly to CT as part of the trauma management protocol.
- *Echocardiography* can demonstrate a pericardial collection and cardiac tamponade.
- *Thoracic ultrasound* can also demonstrate pleural collections.

Complications

Flail chest

Crush injuries of the chest, in which the whole sternum is loosened by fractured ribs on either side or adjacent ribs are fractured in two places, result in the condition of flail chest (Figure 14.1). On inspiration, the flail part of the chest wall becomes indrawn by the negative intrathoracic pressure, as it is no longer in structural continuity with the bony/cartilaginous

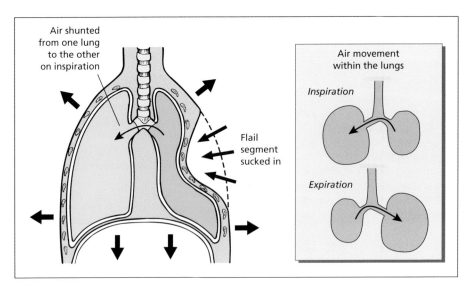

Figure 14.1 Flail chest. On inspiration, the detached segment of the chest wall is sucked inwards, producing paradoxical movement. The mechanics of breathing are impaired.

thoracic cage. Similarly, in expiration, the flail part of the chest is pushed out while the rest of the bony cage becomes contracted. This is termed *paradoxical movement*. With progressive ventilatory failure the patient becomes hypoxic due to failure of adequate expansion of the affected side. Hypercapnia can also occur as the patient tires.

Pneumothorax

If a bony spicule penetrates the lung, air escapes into the pleural cavity and will result in a pneumothorax.

A *tension pneumothorax* (Figure 14.2) results if the tear in the visceral pleural is valvular, allowing air to be sucked into the pleural cavity at each inspiration but preventing air returning to the bronchi on expiration. A tension pneumothorax produces rapidly increasing dyspnoea; the trachea and apex beat are displaced away from the side of the pneumothorax, and on the left side, cardiac dullness may be absent. The chest on the affected side gives a hyper-resonant percussion note, and there can even be bulging of the intercostal spaces.

This is an emergency, and decompression of the pleural space is needed by the careful insertion of a cannula or small incision.

Subcutaneous emphysema (surgical emphysema)

When a fractured rib tears the overlying soft tissue and allows air from the pneumothorax to enter the subcutaneous tissues, subcutaneous emphysema results. The skin over the trunk, neck and sometimes face gives a particular crackling feel to the examining fingers (*crepitation*), and in severe cases, the face and neck may become grossly swollen. The alternative name, 'surgical emphysema', is misleading as it is rarely caused by surgeons. Although distressing, subcutaneous emphysema almost never causes any lasting harm. Incisions in the skin may allow the air to escape more rapidly.

Sucking wound of the chest

A pneumothorax will also result from a penetrating wound of the chest wall produced, for example, by a knife stab or gunshot wound. The lips of the wound may also have a valvular effect so that air is sucked into the cavity at each inspiration but cannot escape on expiration, thus resulting in another variety of tension pneumothorax, which has been vividly named a 'sucking' wound of the chest.

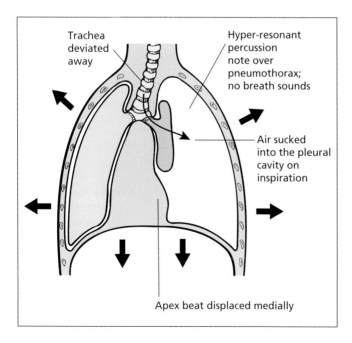

Trachea deviated away

Hyper-resonant percussion note over pneumothorax; no breath sounds

Air sucked into the pleural cavity on inspiration

Apex beat displaced medially

Figure 14.2 Tension pneumothorax produced by a valvular tear in the lung. Air is sucked into the pleural cavity on inspiration and cannot escape on expiration.

Haemothorax

A haemothorax often accompanies a chest injury and may be associated with a pneumothorax (*haemopneumothorax*). The bleeding is usually from an intercostal artery in the lacerated chest wall or from underlying contused lung, but on occasions may result from injury to the heart or a great vessel.

Traumatic asphyxia

With severe crush injuries of the chest, the sudden sharp rise in venous pressure produces extensive bruising and petechial haemorrhages over the head, neck and trunk. There are often subconjunctival haemorrhages and nasal bleeding. Any area of the skin that has been subject to compression at the time of injury (e.g. from a tight collar, braces or spectacles) is protected, and these areas remain mapped out on the body as strips of normal skin, giving a characteristic appearance to the patient.

Other visceral injury

It is important to remember that penetrating wounds of the chest may also injure the underlying diaphragm and thence the abdominal viscera. Thus, it is common for a knife or bullet wound of the left chest to penetrate the spleen or, on the right side, to damage the liver – incorrect placement of a chest drain may do the same!

Treatment

The priorities in the management of chest injuries are as follows.

- *Airway control*. This may involve the passage of an endotracheal tube, particularly where head injury co-exists with chest trauma. Aspiration of vomit is prevented by sucking out the oropharynx and passing a nasogastric tube to empty the stomach.
- *Breathing*. Ensure the patient is breathing and maintaining adequate oxygenation. A saturation monitor should be employed, and intubation and ventilation considered in the presence of hypoxaemia or hypercapnia.
- *Sucking wounds*. These should be closed. In an emergency, a dressing pad should be applied over the hole and secured in place.

- *Lung expansion*. This should be achieved by insertion of an intercostal chest drain with underwater drainage.
- *Stop bleeding*. Small haemothoraces, which do not interfere with the expansion of the lung, require only observation, but a large haemothorax should be drained, again with underwater seal as for a pneumothorax (Figure 14.3). Continued bleeding is an indication for an exploratory thoracotomy or thoracoscopy.

Simple rib fracture

- *Pain relief* may be achieved by paracetamol, non-steroidal anti-inflammatory drugs (NSAIDs), opiates or nerve modulating drugs (such as pregabalin or gabapentin). Local and regional blocks with local anaesthetic can also be used and are very effective.
- *Vigorous physiotherapy and mobilization* is administered to encourage deep breathing. The patient should be encouraged to be out of bed and walking as much as possible.
- *Strapping of the chest wall should be avoided* as it inhibits thoracic movement and encourages pulmonary collapse.

Flail chest

- *Support the flail segment* in the emergency situation by means of a firm pad held by short-term local strapping. This stops the paradoxical movement and air shunting.
- *Good pain control*, with paravertebral or even epidural anaesthetic blocks, *normovolaemia* and *antibiotics* are keys to successful management.
- *Rib fixation*, for which there are now a range of specialist devices, has an increasing role, particularly where there is displacement.
- *High-flow oxygen or non-invasive ventilation* with facemask or nasal continuous positive airway pressure (CPAP).
- *Endotracheal intubation and positive pressure ventilation* will stop the paradoxical movement, as the chest wall now moves as a single functional unit. The treatment is continued for a few days until stability of the chest wall occurs. This is only performed if other measures are ineffective or intubation is needed for other reasons.

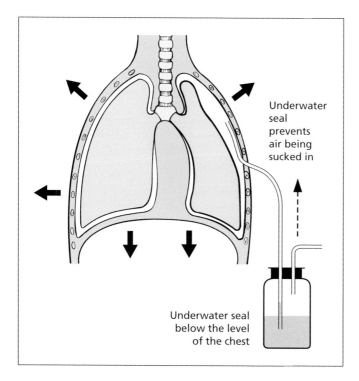

Figure 14.3 Underwater seal chest drain in the treatment of a pneumothorax. Air escapes from the pleural cavity on expiration but cannot be sucked back through the water seal on inspiration (as shown here). The water bottle is placed below the level of the chest to ensure fluid does not reflux into the thoracic cavity.

Pneumothorax

A traumatic pneumothorax requires insertion of a chest drain, in contrast to a spontaneous pneumothorax, which may resolve without intervention.

Tension pneumothorax

Emergency treatment is required by decompressing the chest with a cannula and then subsequently inserting an *intercostal chest drain*.

A *chest drain* is inserted into the pleural cavity via an intercostal space, the fifth space being preferred in between the mid-axillary and anterior axillary line. This should be clear of the heart and hilum. The overlying skin is cut, and then the remaining insertion is done by blunt dissection into the pleural cavity. It is very important that a fingertip is inserted to check that the lung has moved away. At this point, the drain is inserted. The insertion should be gentle. A pair of forceps, surgical clip or tracheal dilator can be used to guide the drain into the pleural cavity; this is usually done without the trocar within the drain. The drain is then secured, and the hole tightly closed. The drain is then connected to an underwater seal. When the pressure in the pleural space is increased on expiration, the air escapes through the water but cannot enter the chest at inspiration, as this is prevented by the water seal. This essential safety valve has been an important step in the development of safe thoracic surgery (Figure 14.3).

Re-expansion of the lung is assisted by attaching the drain to *low-pressure* suction.

A *bronchopleural fistula*, due to rupture of a bronchus into the pleural space, should be suspected if the pneumothorax persists, or if the lung remains collapsed despite suction on the drain bottle, and there is a large 'air leak'. It may require a minimally invasive VATS or thoracotomy to inspect and/or repair.

Penetrating wounds of the chest

Immediate application of a dressing is required in order to prevent suction of air into the pleural space. If the patient is unstable, emergency thoracotomy may be needed. In stable patients, significant penetrating wounds should be investigated with a CT scan. Minor cases require only wound toilet with an underwater intercostal chest drain to allow escape of any accumulated blood or air in the pleural space.

Wounds require exploration if there is continuous blood loss, suspicion of diaphragm damage or concern about injury to other organs. Remember that abdominal organs, the neck and spine can be injured from a chest wound.

Cardiac tamponade

This is suspected in any penetrating injury but particularly anteriorly between the mid-clavicular lines. It is characterized by a rise in venous pressure and a fall in arterial pressure. The heart sounds are distant, and the cardiac shadow enlarged on chest X-ray.

Urgent echocardiography is a definitive investigation, either identifying the problem or excluding tamponade as a cause of shock and diverting attention elsewhere; CT scan can also provide similar anatomical information. If present, treatment is emergency surgical exploration; the pericardium is opened, the blood is evacuated and the cardiac laceration sutured.

Lung abscess

Aetiology

- Central airway obstruction, such as a foreign body or slowly growing obstructive tumour; it is rarely seen with other malignant tumours because of the rapid progress of the disease.
- Inhalation pneumonitis, for example, inhaled vomit or pus.
- Inhaled foreign body, for example, at dental extraction.
- Infected cyst.
- Infected pulmonary infarct.

Clinical features

The history may suggest the primary cause. There is usually fever and other features of acute sepsis, although the disease may sometimes run a more chronic course. If the abscess ruptures into the bronchus, there is a foul productive cough and bad breath.

Complications

- Empyema (pus in the pleural cavity).
- Metastatic cerebral (a feared complication of all pulmonary sepsis) or embolic abscesses elsewhere.

Special investigations

- *Chest X-ray* shows a solid opacity or a fluid level if the abscess communicates with the bronchus.
- *Bronchoscopy* may demonstrate the primary cause if this is a foreign body or tumour.
- *CT scan* will accurately locate the abscess and confirm the diagnosis. *Percutaneous CT-guided drainage* may be possible and effective.

Treatment

The underlying cause may itself require treatment. The mainstay of therapy for lung abscess is antibiotics and chest physiotherapy. Sometimes percutaneous or bronchoscopic drainage is required. An obstructed airway should be opened if possible. Surgical excision is required only for the small percentage that fail to respond to this therapy, when some underlying cause needs to be treated or when, in a late case, there is a complicating empyema that requires drainage.

Empyema

An empyema (pyothorax) is a collection of pus in the pleural cavity.

Aetiology

- Underlying lung disease, such as pneumonia. A *parapneumonic* fluid collection becomes secondarily infected from the underlying lung.
- Bronchiectasis or carcinoma of the lung; tuberculous empyema is now uncommon.
- Penetrating wounds of the chest wall or infection following a transthoracic operation.
- Perforation or rupture of the oesophagus.
- Transdiaphragmatic infection from a subphrenic abscess.

Complications

- Progression to a thick-walled empyema cavity, which will not respond to simple drainage.
- Discharge through the chest wall (*empyema necessitans*).
- Cerebral abscess or abscess elsewhere from haematogenous spread.

Clinical features

There is usually a history of the underlying cause. The patient is febrile, toxic and may be anaemic. There are signs of fluid in the chest on the affected side. In chronic cases, finger clubbing may be present.

Special investigations

- *Full blood count* will reveal a leucocytosis. Inflammatory markers are elevated.
- *Chest X-ray* demonstrates an effusion, and there may be evidence of the underlying lung disease.
- *CT scan* will demonstrate the anatomy and magnitude of the problem.
- *Bronchoscopy* is useful in determining the primary pathology.
- *Aspiration* of the chest confirms the diagnosis and identifies the responsible bacteria. The infecting organisms are usually *Pneumococcus*, *Streptococcus* or *Staphylococcus*.

Treatment

An acute empyema may respond to drainage together with antibiotic therapy, based on the sensitivity of the responsible organism. Simple drainage with an adequately sized chest drain (ideally 28F or larger) may suffice. If this fails, intrapleural fibrinolytic therapy can be considered. If this fails, surgery should be considered. This is usually by VATS, but sometimes thoracotomy is needed.

After a few weeks, the cavity becomes thick walled and open removal (*decortication*) is required. The aim is to restore normal lung function.

Lung tumours

Classification

Benign

- Adenoma.
- Hamartoma.
- Haemangioma (rare).

Malignant

1 Primary:
  a small-cell lung cancer (SCLC);

  b non-small-cell lung cancer (NSCLC) includes the histological subdivisions of:
- squamous cell carcinoma;
- adenocarcinoma;
- large-cell carcinoma.

  c neuroendocrine (carcinoid) tumours.

2 Secondary:
  a carcinoma (especially breast, kidney);
  b sarcoma (especially bone);
  c melanoma.

Carcinoid tumours

These are a form of neuroendocrine carcinoma of which there are four types, all of which share the same neural crest origin:

- typical carcinoid;
- atypical carcinoid;
- large-cell neuroendocrine carcinoma;
- small-cell carcinoma.

Each has particular histological features along a spectrum from benign to malignant.

Typical carcinoid tumours

Nine out of 10 carcinoid tumours are 'typical carcinoids', and tend to follow a very benign course with metastases being rare and most other problems being due to local effects. Carcinoids presenting in central airways typically present with cough and dyspnoea, but rarely haemoptysis. Sometimes, it is thought to be late-onset asthma, which is a common condition. Any late 'asthma' that has no response to bronchodilators should be investigated. If the airway becomes obstructed, secretions can collect distally. These can then become infected and cause pneumonia.

Investigations

- *Chest X-ray* is often normal.
- *CT scan* usually reveals a mass, and evidence of spread (enlarged lymph nodes, distal metastases).
- *Biopsy,* either at bronchoscopy if a large central airway, or CT guided if peripheral.
- *CT-positron emission tomography (CT-PET) scan* and brain imaging if curative resection is planned, to exclude metastases.

Treatment

A patient who has presented with distal infection due to a proximal obstruction can have the lesion bronchoscopically debrided. The aim of this is to open the airway, relieve obstruction and reduce sepsis prior to definitive resection. Bronchoscopy can be repeated if the patient is too frail to undergo surgery.

Surgery consists of local removal, ensuring complete clearance. In central airways, it can almost always be done by lung-preserving techniques such as sleeve resection. Only occasionally is lung resection, such as lobectomy, required.

Lung cancer

This is the second most common cancer affecting men (after prostate) and in women is second only to breast cancer. In the period 2016–2018, there were 49,000 new cases per annum, with 35,000 deaths; the predicted long-term (10-year) survival for patients diagnosed in 2018 in England is just 10%. This is improving due to more cases being treated as a consequence of increased awareness and earlier presentation. When lung cancer is diagnosed early, survival is considerably improved with surgical resection.

The incidence of lung cancer in men has been falling since the late 1970s, reflecting a reduction in smoking. This fall is yet to be seen in women, although the rate of increase is slowing. Nine out of 10 cases occur in people 60 years and older.

Aetiology

In the UK, the main aetiological factor is smoking. Passive smoking; air pollution with diesel, petrol and other volatile hydrocarbon fumes; asbestos exposure; and exposure to radioactive gases such as radon in uranium mines are also predisposing factors. The incidence is higher in urban than in rural populations. There is also a familial element to lung cancer, with a 50% increase in risk if a first-degree relative has it. Although this could be due to similar environmental risks such as smoking, there are also genetic factors. Particular genotypes are associated with worse outcomes and also greater or lesser response to molecular therapy.

Carcinoma of the lung has a poor prognosis, and the gravity of this condition should be impressed on all patients who are smokers. The decision whether or not to continue smoking depends on the patient, but there is no doubt that the advice should be to stop smoking. There is an increased incidence of lung cancer even in patients who smoke only a few cigarettes a day, and this danger is greatly increased in patients smoking more than 20 cigarettes a day for a number of years.

Pathology

There are two main types of lung cancer, small-cell and non-small-cell lung cancer.

Macroscopic appearance

About half the tumours arise in the main bronchi (particularly squamous carcinoma), and 75% are visible at bronchoscopy. The growth may arise peripherally (particularly adenocarcinoma), and some appear to be multifocal.

The bronchial wall is narrowed and ulcerated. Surrounding lung tissue is invaded by a pale mass of tumour, which may undergo necrosis, haemorrhage or abscess formation. The lung segments distal to the occlusion may show collapse, bronchiectasis or abscess formation.

Microscopic appearance

1 *SCLC (15%)* (in the past called 'oat' cell). The tumour comprises small cells with little cytoplasm. It has neuroendocrine properties and can produce molecules giving rise to paraneoplastic syndromes. It has a poor prognosis, has generally spread by the time of diagnosis, and is best treated by chemotherapy and sometimes radiotherapy. It behaves very differently to typical carcinoid tumours.

2 *NSCLC* (85%).

   a *Squamous cell carcinoma.* Usually occurring in the main bronchi, it is mostly poorly differentiated and arises in an area of squamous metaplasia of bronchial epithelium.

   b *Adenocarcinoma.* This has glandular features and can be multifocal. It is the most common NSCLC.

   c *Large-cell carcinoma.* Large cells containing abundant cytoplasm and without evidence of squamous or glandular differentiation; this is also a rapidly growing cancer.

Spread

- *Local*: to pleura, left recurrent laryngeal nerve (hoarse voice), phrenic nerve, pericardium, oesophagus (broncho-oesophageal fistula), sympathetic chain (Horner's syndrome[1]) and brachial plexus (Pancoast's tumour[2] at lung apex).
- *Lymphatic*: to mediastinal and cervical nodes. Compression of the superior vena cava by massive mediastinal node involvement produces gross oedema and cyanosis of the face and upper limbs (*superior vena cava syndrome*).
- *Blood*: to bone, brain, liver and adrenals.
- *Transpleural*: pleural seedlings and effusion.

Clinical features

Carcinoma of the lung often presents late. Early cases are more commonly found at the time of investigation for other problems or by screening. Clinical presentation may be with one or more of the following:

- *Local features*, namely cough, dyspnoea, haemoptysis or lung infection. Chest pain suggests spread to pleural surface or a pleural effusion.
- *Secondaries (metastases)*, especially likely to occur in the brain, adrenal, liver and bones; thus, the patient may present with evidence of a space occupying lesion within the skull, pathological fracture, jaundice and hepatomegaly, or adrenocortical failure. Skin lesions may also occur and are readily biopsied.
- *Paraneoplastic syndromes* due to the remote effects of a hormone or cell product produced by the tumour. Small-cell carcinomas often produce adrenocorticotrophic hormone (ACTH), while squamous carcinomas may produce parathormone (PTH) and present with hypercalcaemia.
- *General effects of neoplasm*: loss of weight, anaemia, cachexia and endocrine disturbances. Patients may also present with bizarre neuropathies and myopathies.

Unfortunately, by the time lung cancer is diagnosed, most cases are incurable. About half the patients will be found to have inoperable tumours when they have had no symptoms at all, with a lesion discovered on routine chest X-ray. Any middle-aged or elderly person presenting with a respiratory infection or cough that has continued for more than 2 weeks should have a chest X-ray, and if the symptoms persist and nothing shows on the chest X-ray, a CT scan should be considered.

On examination, special attention should be paid to evidence of stridor or hoarseness of the voice due to recurrent laryngeal nerve involvement by the cancer. There may be clubbing of the fingers in addition to nicotine staining. The heart may be invaded, resulting in atrial fibrillation or a pericardial effusion. There may be enlarged lymph nodes, especially at the root of the neck, and signs in the chest of consolidation, fluid or collapse.

Special investigations

Investigation aims to confirm the presence of a cancer, and to identify its stage (spread) and histological type.

- *Chest X-ray* may show an opacity in the lung and enlargement of the hilar lymph nodes. The differential diagnosis of a mediastinal mass on radiological examination of the chest is listed in Box 14.1. There may be a raised hemidiaphragm due to paralysis secondary to involvement of the

> **Box 14.1 Abnormal opacity in the mediastinum**
>
> - Retrosternal thyroid
> - Aneurysm of the thoracic aorta
> - Thymic tumour and cysts
> - Lung cancer with a mediastinal mass
> - Heart enlargement: cardiac failure, valve incompetence, pericardial effusion, left–right shunts and cardiomyopathies
> - Enlarged lymph nodes: sarcoid, Hodgkin's disease, other lymphoma, leukaemia and secondary deposits
> - Oesophageal enlargement: tumour, hiatus hernia and mega-oesophagus in achalasia of the cardia
> - Paravertebral abscess, particularly due to tuberculosis
> - Scoliosis
> - Dumb-bell tumour of neurofibroma
> - Dermoid cyst or teratoma

[1]Johann Horner (1831–1886), Professor of Ophthalmology, Zurich, Switzerland.
[2]Henry Pancoast (1875–1939), Professor of Radiology, University of Pennsylvania, Philadelphia, PA, USA.

phrenic nerve. Abnormalities on chest X-ray should prompt a CT scan.

- *Contrast-enhanced CT scan* of the neck, chest and upper abdomen, including the whole chest, liver, adrenal glands and neck to base of skull, including the vocal cords, to assess the primary lung lesion and seek evidence of metastatic spread.
- *PET-CT scan* is an invaluable means of both confirming likely malignancy in peripheral lesions and identifying mediastinal spread. In conjunction with CT, it also permits diagnosis of, for instance, adrenal adenomas mimicking metastases.
- *Bronchoscopy and biopsy.* Bronchoscopy may reveal an ulcerating or exuberant growth, and involved lymph nodes may widen the carina. Brushings and washings may be taken for cytology in addition to biopsy of a visible tumour.
- *Percutaneous needle biopsy* of a peripherally placed lesion under imaging guidance.
- *Endobronchial/endo-oesophageal ultrasound guided biopsy.* Mediastinal lymph nodes can be sampled. Mediastinal spread is usually a contraindication to primary surgery.
- *Mediastinoscopy*, performed through a small suprasternal incision, may be indicated to remove lymph nodes from the region of the carina for histological examination to aid in staging. VATS may also be helpful.
- *Pulmonary function tests* to determine lung reserve and, hence, the capacity to withstand surgery. Chronic obstructive pulmonary disease is common in this patient group. Patients with a forced expiratory volume in 1 second (FEV_1) >2.0 L can usually tolerate pneumonectomy (removal of the whole lung); those with an FEV_1 >1 L can usually tolerate lobectomy (removal of one lobe of the lung). This should be coupled with a test of alveolar function (gas transfer), and in surgical candidates, a prediction of remaining function with a perfusion scan. Patients with impaired fitness must be carefully assessed to determine if surgery is appropriate.

Treatment

Surgery

Patient treatment will be determined in an MDT meeting. Surgery is undertaken in a subset of patients with sufficient respiratory reserve who have disease localized to one lobe or lung (T1, T2 tumours, and sometimes T3 and rarely T4) but with only intra-pulmonary or hilar (N1) lymphadenopathy. Mediastinal (N2) or more distal lymph node involvement is a marker of poorer prognosis, so generally such patients do not undergo resection. Sometimes, such patients will undergo induction treatment with chemotherapy and in selected cases radiotherapy to downstage the tumour before surgery. There is emerging evidence that molecular therapies can also downstage cancers, rendering them suitable for surgery.

The aim of surgery is complete resection of the tumour and the related local lymph nodes, together with extensive sampling of other ipsilateral mediastinal node stations. For many patients, this will require lobectomy with a mortality risk of 1–2%. Pneumonectomy is now performed relatively rarely – it is a major physiological insult, with a mortality risk of at least 4%.

When lung cancer is diagnosed early, survival is considerably improved with surgical resection. A patient with Stage 1 NSCLC (less than 4 cm, no nodal spread) that has been completely resected by lobectomy has at least a 60% five-year survival and in some groups even better. There is increasing interest in lesser lung resections (sub-lobar resections), particularly with smaller peripheral lesions. The outcomes of these resections appear similar to radical radiotherapy.

The majority of lung cancer resections in some countries, including the UK, are now performed by minimally invasive VATS, as long as appropriate oncological principles of surgical margin, gentle tissue handling and complete node clearance are adhered to. For patients with small tumours and limited reserve, *segmental* resections, following anatomical borders, give good long-term results.

Radiotherapy

Radiotherapy can be used with curative or palliative intent. In all such cases, there is careful assessment of the case by an oncologist who will determine a treatment plan. Radiotherapy may give useful palliation for inoperable cases. Although it may not prolong life, it may stop distressing haemoptysis, relieve the pain from bone secondaries and produce dramatic improvement in a patient with acute superior vena cava obstruction. It may also give some relief from the irritating cough and dyspnoea resulting from early bronchial obstruction.

Chemotherapy

Cyclical cytotoxic therapy combined with radiotherapy is the treatment of choice for small-cell tumours. Chemotherapy is also used in the adjuvant setting (post-surgery) if high-risk features are identified. This includes the presence of lymph node involvement. Sometimes, chemotherapy is used pre-operatively to 'downstage' tumours, with the aim of increasing the chance of successful surgery.

Targeted chemotherapy

Cancer specimens undergo sequencing to search for genetic mutations, usually involving pathways causing increased cell proliferation. These mutations are targets susceptible to particular inhibitors:

- Epidermal growth factor receptor (EGFR) mutations, targeted by gefitinib and afatinib, for example.
- Anaplastic lymphoma kinase (ALK), a tyrosine kinase. Mutation present in 5% of NSCLC, and is blocked by crizotinib and ceritinib, for example.
- ROS1, a tyrosine kinase similar to ALK.
- K-RAS gene, targeted by sotorasib.

Secondary tumours

The lung is second only to the liver as the site of metastases, which may be from carcinoma (especially breast, kidney and colorectal), sarcoma (especially bone) or melanoma. Spread may be as a result of either vascular deposits or lymphatic permeation from involved mediastinal nodes – *lymphangitis carcinomatosa*.

Pulmonary metastases are so common that it should be routine practice to image the chest by CT scan in every case of malignant disease to aid staging the primary cancer.

A low volume of metastatic disease to the chest may be treated by surgical excision, radiotherapy or radiofrequency ablation.

Additional resources

Case 19: A patient with a chest drain
Case 20: A fatal lung disease

15

Venous disorders of the lower limb

Manj Gohel

Learning objectives

✓ To understand the normal anatomy and physiology of the venous system.

✓ To know the causes and treatment of superficial and deep venous insufficiency of the lower limb.

Normal venous function

The venous system of the legs returns deoxygenated blood from the peripheries to the right heart via a network of low-resistance superficial and deep veins. Flow in the correct direction is maintained by a series of unidirectional valves in the peripheral veins, and flow is driven by muscle pumps, predominantly in the calf but also in the feet. As the calf and foot muscles contract, the deep veins within them are compressed and emptied, the blood passing upwards, directed towards the heart by the non-return valves. As the muscles relax, blood flows in from the superficial system via perforators, as well as from more distal segments of the vein, only to be forced upwards again by the next contraction of the calf muscles, which thus act as a pump.

Ellis and Calne's Lecture Notes in General Surgery, Fourteenth Edition.
Edited by Christopher Watson and Justin Davies.
© 2023 John Wiley & Sons Ltd. Published 2023 by John Wiley & Sons Ltd.
Companion website: www.wiley.com/go/Watson/GeneralSurgery14

Anatomy of the venous drainage of the lower limb

To understand venous disease in the leg, it is essential to understand the functional anatomy of the venous system. The venous system consists of a complex network of superficial veins, deep veins and perforating veins (Figure 15.1). Most of the venous flow is in the deep veins (around 90%), but both superficial and deep veins can cause disease.

The deep venous system

The deep veins of the leg usually accompany (and share the name of) the main arteries of the lower limb and are located deep to the fascia that envelops the muscular compartments. Crural veins in the calf (anterior tibial, posterior tibial and peroneal veins) drain into the popliteal vein behind the knee, which ascends as the femoral vein, becoming the common femoral vein in the groin and then the external iliac vein above the inguinal ligament. From there, blood flows up the common iliac vein, via the inferior vena cava, to the right atrium.

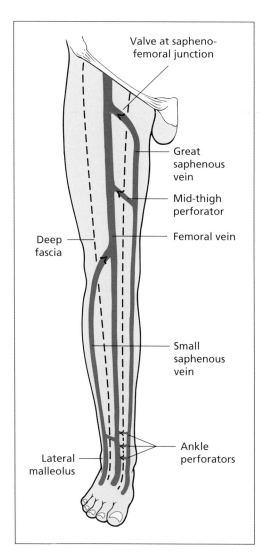

Figure 15.1 The venous system of the leg. Note that there are two main superficial veins, the great saphenous and small saphenous veins, each of which drains into the deep veins, at the saphenofemoral and saphenopopliteal junctions, respectively, but also via several perforating veins.

The superficial venous system

This comprises the medially placed great (long) saphenous vein, draining from the dorsum of the foot to the saphenofemoral junction in the groin, and the small (short) saphenous vein, which drains the lateral aspect of the lower limb into the popliteal vein behind the knee. There may also be accessory saphenous

veins (particularly the anterior accessory saphenous vein, in the territory of the great saphenous vein). These veins are located superficial to the deep fascia and drain the skin and superficial tissues.

Perforating veins

In addition to the saphenofemoral and saphenopopliteal junctions, there are numerous additional communications between superficial and deep veins. These are called perforating veins, or 'perforators', as they typically pierce the fascia to reach the deep veins. Although the anatomy of perforators is notoriously variable, there is typically a mid-thigh perforator (called the Hunterian perforator on account of its relationship to Hunter's canal[1]), and several calf perforators located on the medial aspect of the tibia from the ankle to the knee.

Aetiology of venous disease

The aetiology of venous disease may be classified as follows:

- Congenital;
- Primary, the most common;
- Secondary (post-thrombotic);
- Idiopathic, where no venous cause for disease is identified.

Primary venous disease

The underlying cause of venous disease is chronic venous hypertension. Persistent high pressure in the venous system of the leg can result in symptoms, clinical manifestations and complications of venous disease. A common cause of venous hypertension is damage or failure of the vein valves in superficial or deep veins, which can result in blood flow away from the heart, termed 'reflux' or 'incompetence' (Figure 15.2). The causes of valve incompetence are poorly understood, but there are likely to be genetic and acquired factors.

When trying to understand the development of varicose veins, some scientists favour the 'descending' theory, where superficial vein valve failure starts at the junctions and progresses down the leg. Alternatively,

[1] John Hunter (1728–1793), Surgeon, St George's Hospital, London, UK.

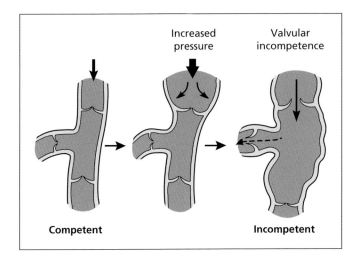

Figure 15.2 Normal veins and incompetent varicose veins. Note that the vein dilates under pressure and the valve becomes incompetent.

the 'ascending' theory suggests that varicose veins start distally and progress up the leg, and this is supported by the observation that varicose veins often exist with a competent saphenous junction. The development of varicose veins is likely to be multifactorial.

It was previously thought that superficial vein reflux causes only varicose veins, whereas venous skin changes and ulceration were caused by deep venous disease. Our understanding of venous pathophysiology has evolved, and it is now widely accepted that superficial venous reflux alone can (and often does) result in oedema, venous skin changes and ulceration. While the precise pathophysiological mechanisms linking venous hypertension and skin damage are debated, high capillary hydrostatic pressure results in diffusion of fluid, red cells and white cells into the soft tissues, resulting in chronic inflammation and skin changes.

Congenital venous disease

Dilated veins may be seen as part of a number of inherited syndromes, such as Klippel–Trenaunay syndrome[2]. The syndrome involves three elements: multiple congenital venous malformations producing varicose veins, hypertrophy of bones and soft tissues and extensive cutaneous haemangiomas. It usually affects the lower limbs.

[2] Maurice Klippel (1858–1942), Neurologist, Salpêtrière Hospital, Paris, France. Paul Trenaunay (b. 1875), Neurologist.

Secondary (post-thrombotic) venous disease

Previous deep vein thrombosis may result in chronic changes and damage to the vein, resulting in venous hypertension. There are several contributing factors:

- *Deep vein reflux*, secondary to valvular damage and inability to maintain the one-way flow after thrombosis.
- *Scarring of deep veins*, remodelling the vein wall.
- *Venous obstruction* may cause additional pressure on competent vein valves (in deep and superficial veins), causing further valve failure and compounding the clinical picture. There is a tendency for the condition to get worse as further valves are involved.

Tortuous, dilated veins may also be seen in patients with deep vein obstruction. These are important collateral veins providing an alternative route for venous return to the heart and should not be confused with varicose veins.

Clinical presentation

Patients with venous disease may seek help for a wide variety of reasons, including symptoms, complications or cosmetic concerns (or any combination of these). Typical symptoms include aching, throbbing or heaviness/tiredness in the legs as well as swelling of the ankles, particularly after long periods of standing. Patients with superficial or deep venous disorders may present with a range of overlapping symptoms and clinical signs. The CEAP classification[3] is the most widely accepted.

Thread veins / reticular veins

Also referred to as 'spider veins', or telangectasia, these are very small, superficial veins that can cause cosmetic concern. Treatment is not usually offered in public healthcare systems.

Leg swelling and skin changes

Peripheral oedema is a common manifestation of chronic venous disease, as the increased hydrostatic forces (Starling's forces[4]) result in increased volumes of interstitial fluid that the lymphatic system is unable to drain. Oedema may only affect the ankle after prolonged standing, but constant and extensive swelling may also be seen.

Often occurring on the medial lower calf (the medial gaiter area), there are several skin manifestations that are associated with venous disease, including:

- *Haemosiderinosis and pigmentation*: extravasation of red blood cells, which become deposited as haemosiderin in the skin and subcutaneous tissues.
- *Venous eczema / stasis dermatitis:* a common early skin complaint, characterized by dry, itchy and scaly skin.
- *Lipodermatosclerosis*: thickening and fibrosis of the skin and soft tissues, resulting in the '*inverted champagne bottle*' appearance, which occurs due to chronic inflammation secondary to venous hypertension.

Venous ulceration

A chronic leg ulcer is defined as a defect in the skin of the lower leg, remaining unhealed for more than 4 weeks. Chronic venous hypertension accounts for the vast majority of chronic leg ulcers and is recognized as an enormous cause of patient distress and health service resource use worldwide. Ulcers are usually superficial, can be very painful, and may start with minor trauma or without any obvious precipitant. Ulceration is considered the most extreme

presentation in the spectrum of venous disorders and patients usually have other signs of venous disease such as skin changes, varicose veins or oedema.

Venous ulcers either have an edge, which is ragged, or where the ulcer is healing, the margins will be shelving with a faint blue rim of advancing epithelium. Previous scarring appears as a white rim around the ulcer, known as *atrophie blanche*. Rarely, a squamous carcinoma can develop in the edge of a long-standing ulcer (Marjolin's ulcer[5]). Approximately 90% of all ulcers of the legs are venous in origin, but other, rarer, causes should always be considered (Box 15.1).

Other complications of varicose veins

In addition to the clinical presentations described above, patients may also present with specific complications of varicose veins.

1 *Bleeding*. Prominent, superficial dilated veins may bleed profusely if knocked. The high venous pressure in the incompetent vein can result in

> **Box 15.1 Differential diagnosis of leg ulcers**
>
> - *Chronic venous ulcer* due to venous hypertension.
> - *Ischaemic ulcer* due to impaired arterial blood supply; the peripheral pulses must always be examined and ankle-brachial pressure indexes checked.
> - *Mixed ulcers,* with ischaemic and venous contributions.
> - *Neuropathic ulcer*, particularly common in diabetics where they are often compounded by ischaemia due to diabetic microangiopathy.
> - *Malignant ulcer*, a basal cell carcinoma, or a squamous carcinoma (possibly arising in a pre-existing chronic venous ulcer) or an ulcerated malignant melanoma.
> - *Ulcer complicating systemic disease*, for example, acholuric jaundice, ulcerative colitis and rheumatoid arthritis.
> - *Repetitive self-inflicted injury* (factitious ulceration).

[3] Clinical, Etiological, Anatomical and Pathophysiological (CEAP) classification of venous disorders.
[4] Sir Ernest Starling (1866–1927), Professor of Physiology, University College, London, UK.

[5] Jean Nicholas Marjolin (1780–1850), Surgeon, Hôpital Sainte-Eugènie, Paris, France

life-threatening haemorrhage, particularly in elderly or frail patients who may be unable to apply pressure and elevate the leg.

2 *Superficial vein thrombosis (SVT)*. Formally referred to as 'thrombophlebitis' or 'phlebitis', SVT is a common clinical condition presenting as a hard, red, painful and engorged superficial vein. Virtually, all cases occur in patients with pre-existing varicose veins. Up to a quarter of patients presenting with SVT also have a co-existent deep vein thrombosis, indicating that there is likely to be a prothrombotic tendency in these patients.

Assessment of the patient with venous disease

History

A detailed history should include information about the presenting symptoms (including the severity and impact on the patient's quality of life). Patients should be specifically asked about the presence of skin discolouration or eczema and the current or past presence of leg ulcers. Other points to note are a history of deep vein thrombosis, or a history suggestive of thrombosis such as swelling and pain postoperatively, during pregnancy or after a long period of immobilization. Risk factors for venous thromboembolism (such as obesity, use of oestrogen-containing medication or thrombophilia) are important to ascertain, as this may direct the thromboprophylaxis plan after any intervention. Previous venous interventions should also be recorded as redo procedures are likely to be associated with greater risks.

Clinical examination

A patient with venous disease should be examined while standing, and the presence/extent of varicose veins should be carefully recorded. Photographic documentation may be of value. Examination of the legs should include inspection of the medial gaiter area for evidence of venous skin changes (eczema, haemosiderosis, lipodermatosclerosis and/or ulceration). The presence of scars should be noted. The arterial status of the leg (presence of peripheral pulses) should also be recorded.

A *saphena varix*, a prominent dilation of the great saphenous vein at the saphenofemoral junction, may be present. It gives a characteristic thrill to the examining fingers when the patient coughs, quite different from a femoral hernia. It disappears when the patient lies flat.

A *handheld Doppler* assessment can help identify venous incompetence in large or small saphenous veins but has also become largely obsolete due to the widespread availability of colour duplex ultrasound scanning

Special investigations

The aim of any venous investigations is to identify potentially treatable superficial or deep venous disease:

- *Duplex scan*[6]: The 'gold-standard' investigation, which is non-invasive, painless and can accurately map the superficial and deep veins in the leg to diagnose both valvular and perforator incompetence and deep venous occlusion. Guidelines suggest it should be performed before any venous intervention.
- *Ankle-brachial pressure index,* using a handheld Doppler, to assess the arterial supply to the leg in cases of ulceration and thus determine the appropriateness of compression therapy.
- *Cross-sectional imaging (CT or MR)* may be needed to assess proximal deep veins in the abdomen and pelvis.
- *Venography and intravascular ultrasound* may also be required to assess venous anatomy in some circumstances.

Treatment of venous disease

The main principle of management for patients with venous disease is to reduce venous hypertension, ideally by treating the underlying cause, in order to improve quality of life. Where it is not feasible or desirable to try and address the underlying superficial or deep venous problem, there are several general measures that may be used. Bed rest and leg

[6]Duplex is a combination of grey-scale ultrasound looking at physical structures and colour Doppler looking at flow in vessels. Doppler is named after Christian Doppler (1803–1853), an Austrian Physicist.

elevation are very effective at reducing venous hypertension but may not be very practical or acceptable to patients.

Compression therapy

A wide range of compression garments are available, including stockings, Velcro wraps and multilayer bandages. In patients with more advanced venous disease and ulceration, there is clear evidence that compression therapy is beneficial. The benefit is less clear in less severe venous disease (e.g. simple varicose veins), but stockings are commonly prescribed. It should be noted that compliance with compression therapy is often poor and generally worse for higher degrees of compression and for thigh-length (versus knee-level) stockings.

Compression therapy in venous ulceration

For patients with venous ulceration, healing can be accelerated by multicomponent compression bandaging that aims to deliver 40 mmHg of pressure at the ankle. Compression should be applied by a trained practitioner to ensure that the correct pressure is delivered. The firm pressure empties the dilated superficial veins and enables the calf muscle pump to act more efficiently. Once venous ulcers are healed, wearing compression stockings for the long term can reduce the risk of ulcer recurrence.

Treatment of superficial vein reflux

In patients with varicose veins or other manifestations of venous disease, treatment of refluxing superficial veins is often the most appropriate intervention as procedures are usually minimally invasive, low risk, and may be performed in an ambulatory setting under local anaesthesia. The principle of intervention for superficial venous reflux is to remove, obliterate or close the incompetent vein. Traditional operations have been superseded by several less invasive interventions in recent years. Consequently, there are many modalities and options available for treating incompetent saphenous veins, which will be summarized below.

[7]Friedrich Trendelenburg (1844–1924), Professor of Surgery, successively at Rostock, Bonn and Leipzig, Germany.

Traditional surgical 'stripping'

First described in the late 19th century by surgeons, including Trendelenburg[7], varicose vein surgery was one of the most performed elective surgical procedures in the UK. Surgery involves disconnection of the great saphenous vein at the saphenofemoral junction, after careful ligation of the terminal tributaries. The saphenous vein is then 'stripped' from groin to knee, and visible varicosities are treated by phlebectomy via small skin incisions over the veins. Although effective, recurrent varicose veins (often due to technical failure, *de novo* reflux or neovascularization at the saphenofemoral junction) were commonly seen. More importantly, complications after surgery were common (including venous thromboembolism) and recovery was often protracted due to pain and bruising.

Endovenous thermal ablation

Since 2000, endovenous treatments have increased in popularity and thermal ablation is widely accepted as the 'gold-standard' intervention for primary saphenous reflux, replacing traditional surgery. A variety of thermal ablation modalities are available, but laser and radiofrequency ablation are the most popular treatments.

The procedure involves cannulation of the vein to be ablated (usually the great or small saphenous veins) under ultrasound guidance. Once the vein is accessed, a laser or radiofrequency fibre is positioned 2 cm from the junction with the deep vein (saphenofemoral or saphenopopliteal junction). After infiltration of dilute anaesthesia (known as 'tumescent anaesthetic'), the fibre is used to deliver thermal energy to denature the vein wall and cause fibrotic vein occlusion. The fibre is withdrawn while delivering heat energy to ablate the entire incompetent vein. Procedures can be performed under local anaesthesia in an ambulatory setting, and patient recovery is quicker than after surgical stripping. Risks include venous thromboembolism (although lower than after surgical stripping) and thermal injury to nerves (such as the sural nerve near the short saphenous vein and the saphenous nerve near the great saphenous vein).

Endovenous ablation is particularly important in the treatment of patients with venous leg ulceration, where prompt treatment has been shown to accelerate ulcer healing, reduce the risk of ulcer recurrence and reduce costs.

Ultrasound-guided sclerotherapy

Sclerotherapy involves injection of a chemical sclerosant (such as sodium tetradecyl sulphate, or polidocanol) into the vein to be treated to cause a 'chemical ablation'. As there is no thermal component to the intervention, anaesthesia is not needed, and tortuous or superficial veins can also be treated. By mixing the sclerosant with air to create foam, blood in the vein is displaced during injection and larger veins can potentially be treated.

After injection, the treated vein is usually kept compressed with firm pressure bandaging for a period to enable fibrosis to take place. Treatments can be repeated easily, and complications include bruising, phlebitis with unsightly skin staining, ulceration and deep vein thrombosis. Foam sclerotherapy is the cheapest option for treating varicose veins and remains popular in many countries. Large clinical trials have shown that vein closure rates are probably inferior to thermal ablation techniques.

Non-thermal closure procedures

In recent years, non-thermal superficial vein closure procedures have been developed. Techniques such as cyanoacrylate glue closure (injection of medical cyanoacrylate glue into the vein to be ablated) or mechanochemical ablation (combination of mechanical damage to the vein and injection of sclerotherapy) aim to provide durable vein closure while avoiding potential risks of thermal ablation.

Treatment of deep venous disease

Despite efforts by many researchers over several decades, a reliable method to treat deep venous incompetence remains elusive. Attempted surgical repair of vein valves is not widely performed due to technical difficulty and poor outcomes, and vein valve implants or prostheses are in development, but not in clinical use.

In direct contrast to the lack of progress in the treatment of deep venous reflux, there have been dramatic advances in the diagnosis and management of deep venous obstruction. After previous deep vein thrombosis, particularly affecting the iliofemoral veins, residual scarring and obstruction are commonly seen and may be a significant contributing factor to venous hypertension. Modern endovascular techniques and stents allow effective recanalization of occluded veins. Long-term results are awaited, case selection is challenging and procedures may be technically difficult.

Deep vein thrombosis

The management of acute deep vein thrombosis is usually the domain of thrombosis teams and general physicians. There is some debate regarding the role of endovascular interventions to remove acute thrombus in extensive iliofemoral or iliocaval thrombosis. At present, early thrombus removal (using thrombolysis or thrombectomy) is usually reserved for patients with severe symptoms from the acute thrombosis. Deep vein thrombosis as a postoperative complication is covered in Chapter 5.

🖰 Additional resources

16

The brain and meninges

Stephen Price

Learning objectives

✓ To know the manifestations and causes of raised intracranial pressure, with particular reference to intracranial tumours.

✓ To know the presentations of pituitary adenomas.

Space-occupying intracranial lesions

Space-occupying lesions within the skull may be caused by the following:

1 Haemorrhage:
   a extradural;
   b subdural – acute or chronic (Chapter 17);
   c intracerebral.
2 Tumour.
3 Hydrocephalus.
4 Brain swelling (oedema), for example, head injury or encephalitis.
5 Cerebral abscess.

Other causes are rare and include hydatid cyst, tuberculoma and gumma.

Clinical features

A space-occupying lesion manifests itself by the general features of raised intracranial pressure and by localizing signs.

Raised intracranial pressure

A space-occupying lesion within the skull produces raised intracranial pressure not only by its actual volume within the closed box of the cranium but also by provoking oedema, and sometimes by impeding the circulation or absorption of cerebrospinal fluid (CSF), causing hydrocephalus (see later in this chapter). For example, a tumour in the posterior cranial fossa may present rapidly with severe symptoms of raised intracranial pressure secondary to hydrocephalus.

A slowly progressive rise in intracranial pressure may lead to the following presenting features:

- *Headache*: may be severe, often present when the patient wakes up and is aggravated by straining or coughing.
- *Vomiting*: often without preceding nausea.
- *Papilloedema*, which may be accompanied by blurring of vision and may progress to permanent blindness if prolonged due to optic atrophy.
- *Depressed conscious level.*
- *Neck stiffness*, particularly if the lesion is in the posterior fossa.
- *Diplopia.*
- *Ataxia.*
- *Enlargement of the head* in children before the sutures have fused.

A rapid rise in intracranial pressure results in a clinical picture of intense headache with rapid progression into coma.

Ellis and Calne's Lecture Notes in General Surgery, Fourteenth Edition. Edited by Christopher Watson and Justin Davies.
© 2023 John Wiley & Sons Ltd. Published 2023 by John Wiley & Sons Ltd.
Companion website: www.wiley.com/go/Watson/GeneralSurgery14

Localizing signs

Having diagnosed the presence of raised intracranial pressure, an attempt must be made to localize the lesion on the basis of the clinical findings; although in some cases, this is not possible. There may be upper motor neurone weakness, indicating a lesion of the pyramidal pathway; there may be cranial nerve signs, for example, a bitemporal hemianopia indicating pressure on the optic chiasm. A lesion of the postcentral cortex may produce loss of fine discrimination and of stereognosis. Cerebellar lesions may produce coarse ataxia, muscular hypotonia, incoordination and often nystagmus. A focal fit may provide valuable localizing data. Motor aphasia (the patient knows what he or she wishes to say but cannot do so) suggests a lesion in Broca's area[1] on the dominant side of the lower frontal cortex of the cerebrum. Pupillary dilation is a late sign and is caused by the uncus of the temporal lobe being displaced through the tentorial hiatus where it compresses the oculomotor nerve.

Special investigations

The following investigations are required in the study of a suspected space-occupying lesion:

- *Computed tomography (CT)*, with intravenous contrast enhancement, is a non-invasive and extremely accurate investigation for all cerebral tumours and other space-occupying lesions.
- *Magnetic resonance (MR) imaging* gives superb anatomical localization of intracerebral space-occupying lesions. Contrast enhancement is essential to characterize these lesions.
- *Positron emission tomography (PET)* further complements MR. The main use is to differentiate high-grade from low-grade tumours.
- *Imaging of the chest,* usually by CT scan, should always be performed if tumour is suspected to exclude a symptomless primary bronchogenic carcinoma; in the case of a cerebral abscess, it may reveal the source of infection.
- *Burr-hole biopsy* may be appropriate to establish a tissue diagnosis. This should be done using image guidance to improve accuracy.

---

[1] Pierre Broca (1826–1880), Professor of Clinical Surgery, Paris, France.

Intracranial tumours

Intracranial tumours can be divided into intrinsic tumours of the brain, arising usually from the supporting (glial) cells, and extracerebral tumours, which originate from the numerous structures surrounding the brain. In addition, 30% of patients with cerebral tumours presenting to neurosurgical units have tumours that are metastatic from distant sites, but many patients dying of widespread metastases have cerebral deposits and do not come under specialist care. The overall incidence of central nervous system (CNS) tumours is around 12 per 100,000 population. The only identified predisposing factors are previous cranial irradiation and certain genetic disorders (e.g. neurofibromatosis type 2).

Intracranial tumours cause generalized and focal symptoms. Generalized symptoms reflect a progressive increase in intracranial pressure and include headache (particularly in the early morning) that is characterized by progressively increasing severity, nausea and vomiting. Mental state changes and hemiparesis may also occur. Focal symptoms depend on the tumour location within the brain and are due to both the effect of the tumour on the brain and the associated oedema. Cerebellar tumours, therefore, lead to ataxia; occipital lobe tumours result in visual field disturbance; and tumours in the posterior aspect of the frontal lobe affecting the motor cortex will result in weakness. Seizures are common and may be focal; postictal neurological impairment may help localization. Investigation is outlined above.

Classification

Common tumours include the following:

Intracerebral

- Gliomas (45%), including astrocytoma, oligodendroglioma and ependymoma.
- Embryonal tumours, such as medulloblastoma.
- Lymphoma.
- Pineal gland tumour.
- Metastases (30%).

Extracerebral

- Meningioma (15%).
- Tumours of cranial nerves, for example, vestibular schwannoma (5%).

- Pituitary tumours (5%), including pituitary adenomas and craniopharyngioma.

Gliomas

Gliomas arise from the glial supporting cells and are usually supratentorial. They are classified according to the principal cell component, for example, astrocytes (astrocytomas), oligodendrocytes (oligodendroglioma) or a mixture of the two (oligoastrocytoma). A rarer fourth type, the ependymoma, arises from the ependymal lining of the brain and is commonly found in the ventricles – particularly the fourth ventricle in children.

These tumours are graded according to their aggressiveness:

- *Grade 1 gliomas – pilocytic astrocytomas*: These are slow-growing tumours that are most commonly found in children. Common sites include the fourth ventricle and the optic chiasm where they can be seen in patients with neurofibromatosis type 1. Surgical removal is usually all that is required. Transformation to more aggressive tumours is rare.
- *Grade 2 gliomas – diffuse astrocytomas and oligodendrogliomas*: These are slow-growing tumours that commonly present in younger patients and frequently present with seizures. These tumours commonly transform into higher grade tumours – 80% of astrocytomas will transform within 5 years, and 80% of oligodendrogliomas will have transformed in 8–9 years. Current treatment involves resection of the bulk of the tumour with radiotherapy reserved for progression.
- *Grade 3 gliomas – anaplastic gliomas*: Show evidence of cellular proliferation. They are aggressive tumours and are locally invasive. They are typically treated with surgical resection where possible, followed by radiotherapy. The median survival has improved to about 7 years with the combination of radiotherapy followed by chemotherapy. The exception is with anaplastic oligodendrogliomas where the loss of chromosomes 1p and 19q is a marker for significantly improved survival with chemotherapy (median survival not reached at 14 years).
- *Grade 4 gliomas – glioblastomas*: These account for 50% of gliomas and are the most aggressive. They are characterized by the presence of either necrosis or endothelial proliferation. They are locally invasive and frequently present with neurological deficits. This is commonly due to the associated oedema, and all patients are treated with dexamethasone to reduce this. Glioblastomas arise either *de novo* or from a pre-existing, low-grade tumour (secondary glioblastoma). The latter can be identified by the presence of a mutation of IDH-1. These IDH-1-mutated glioblastomas have a better prognosis. Treatment involves surgical resection of as much of the tumour as possible without causing neurological deficits, followed by radiotherapy and chemotherapy. Progression occurs in most patients, with a median survival of 18 months.

Medulloblastomas

These are rapidly growing small cell tumours generally affecting the cerebellum in children, usually boys. They may block the fourth ventricle, producing an obstructive hydrocephalus, and may spread via the CSF to seed over the surface of the spinal cord. The cells appear to be embryonal in origin, with elements of ependymomas and medulloblastoma in varying proportions, and are now more commonly called primitive neuroectodermal tumours (PNETs). Therapy involves treating any hydrocephalus followed by tumour resection. Radiotherapy is an effective treatment, but in young children, chemotherapy is used to reduce the risk of radiation-induced morbidity.

The differential diagnosis of a fourth ventricular mass in children includes medulloblastoma, pilocytic astrocytoma and ependymoma.

Cerebral lymphoma

Primary cerebral lymphoma is uncommon but is increasing in incidence. It occurs in two settings:

- Immunosuppressed patients, whether through disease (e.g. AIDS) or following organ transplantation, have a markedly increased risk of cerebral lymphoma.
- In non-immunosuppressed patients, the incidence peaks in the sixth and seventh decade, and is often multifocal.

Diagnosis is by stereotactic biopsy, and the treatment is chemotherapy and radiotherapy.

Meningioma

Meningiomas arise from arachnoid cells in the dura mater, to which they are almost invariably attached, and are typically found in middle-aged patients and are more common in females. Special sites are one or both sides of the superior sagittal sinus, lesser wing of the sphenoid, olfactory groove, parasellar region and within the spinal canal. The majority are slow growing and do not invade the brain tissue but involve it only by expansion and pressure, so they may become buried in the brain. The tumour may, however, invade the skull, producing a hyperostosis, which may occasionally be enormous. Most are benign; 8% atypical with features of increased proliferation and are more likely to recur; 2% are frankly malignant.

Treatment

Most meningiomas are surgically removable, with the aim of removing the tumour and dural margin. The incidence of recurrence in this setting for benign tumour is under 10%. Radiotherapy is used in recurrent tumours and malignant tumours. The role of radiotherapy at diagnosis in atypical tumours is debated. In some meningiomas that are inaccessible (e.g. in the cavernous sinus), radiosurgery (highly focused, high-dose radiotherapy) may be used.

Vestibular schwannomas

Vestibular schwannomas[2], previously inaccurately termed acoustic neuromas, are the most common cranial nerve tumour and are benign. They are usually found in adult patients between the ages of 30 and 60 years, and are occasionally associated with neurofibromatosis type 2, when they may be bilateral. They are characterized by unilateral sensorineural hearing loss. As the schwannoma slowly enlarges, it stretches the adjacent cranial nerves, VII and V anteriorly and IX, X and XII over its lower surface. It also presses on the cerebellum and the brain stem, and can produce the 'cerebellopontine angle syndrome' with the following features:

- unilateral nerve deafness often associated with tinnitus and giddiness (VIII) is the first symptom;
- facial numbness and weakness of the masticatory muscles (V);
- dysphagia, hoarseness and dysarthria (IX, X and XII);

- cerebellar hemisphere signs and, later, pyramidal tract involvement;
- eventually features of raised intracranial pressure;
- facial weakness with unilateral taste loss (VII) is very uncommon (<5%).

Treatment

Most vestibular schwannomas do not need any treatment and can be watched. Larger tumours or those that are shown to grow can be removed completely but with some risks to the facial nerve. Alternatively, stereotactic radiosurgery is now being used to treat some smaller tumours.

Pituitary tumours

Pituitary tumours have three special features.

1 Local mass effects:
   a *Visual field disturbance* (bitemporal hemianopia) due to compression of the optic chiasm.
   b *Headache* due to expansion of the pituitary fossa with dural stretching, erosion into the paranasal air sinus and/or haemorrhage within the tumour (pituitary apoplexy).
2 *Hormone deficiency* (hypopituitarism): as the tumour grows, it compresses the normal pituitary around the tumour, resulting in reduced production of anterior pituitary hormones. Deficiency tends to first suppress luteinizing and growth hormone production, followed in sequence by loss of thyroid-stimulating hormone (TSH), adrenocorticotrophic hormone (ACTH) and follicle-stimulating hormone (FSH). The posterior pituitary hormones are rarely affected.
3 *Hormone excess*: hormone-secreting adenomas may present with symptoms from the hormone, for example, Cushing's disease[3] from ACTH excess.

They are named according to their staining on light microscopy.

Chromophobe adenoma (80%)

This is the most common pituitary tumour, which, as it enlarges, compresses the optic chiasm, producing

---

[2] Theodore Schwann (1810–1882), German Physiologist, one of the first to establish the cellular nature of all tissues.

[3] Harvey Cushing (1869–1939), Professor of Surgery, Harvard Medical School, Boston, MA, USA. He was one of the founders of neurosurgery.

a bitemporal hemianopia. Half are non-secretory tumours, which gradually destroy the normally functioning pituitary, producing hypopituitarism with secondary hypogonadism, hypothyroidism and hypoadrenalism. In childhood, there is arrest of growth together with infantilism. Half produce prolactin, which causes infertility, amenorrhoea and galactorrhoea (discharge of milk from the nipple) in females. These tumours rarely extend to involve the hypothalamus, producing diabetes insipidus and obesity.

Eosinophil (acidophil) adenoma (15%)

These are slow-growing tumours, which secrete growth hormone. If they occur before puberty, which is unusual, they induce gigantism. After puberty, acromegaly results.

Basophil adenoma (5%)

These are small tumours that produce no pressure effects and may be associated with Cushing's syndrome (ACTH production, see Chapter 42).

Special investigations

- *MR imaging* demonstrates the pituitary fossa, encroachment on the optic chiasm superiorly and laterally into the cavernous sinus.
- *Visual field mapping* looking for evidence of bitemporal hemianopia.
- *Hormone assessment*, with basal assays of each pituitary hormone and change in hormone concentrations after stress created by insulin-induced hypoglycaemia. For microadenomas (less than 1 cm diameter) that are frequently not seen on MRI, there may be the need to sample the inferior petrous sinus for differences in hormone secretion to determine the site of ectopic hormone secretion.

Treatment

Pituitary tumours that are producing pressure symptoms on the optic chiasm are treated by removal through a trans-sphenoidal (or occasionally transcranial) route. Endoscopic approaches now allow extracapsular removal. Radiotherapy is reserved for subtotal resections. Prolactin-secreting tumours (prolactinomas) usually respond to treatment with a dopamine agonist (e.g. cabergoline) to suppress prolactin secretion and reduce tumour size.

Craniopharyngioma

Craniopharyngioma is a benign but locally invasive tumour, usually cystic, which arises in the remnant of the craniopharyngeal duct (the precursor of the anterior pituitary). It presents in childhood or early adult life, and lies above and/or within the sella turcica.

The tumour produces hypopituitarism, raised intracranial pressure and optic chiasmal involvement. Craniopharyngiomas may be very difficult to remove completely because of their close relationship to the hypothalamus, so treatment often involves subtotal removal with postoperative radiotherapy.

Secondary tumours

These account for about 30% of intracranial tumours seen on a neurosurgical unit but are more common on the general wards. Common primary tumours are those of the lung, breast, kidney and melanoma, with the last occasionally presenting with intracranial haemorrhage.

Intracranial abscess

Aetiology

Intracranial abscesses may be intracerebral, subdural or extradural. There are three common causes for them:

1 *Penetrating wound* of the skull usually with a staphylococcal secondary infection. Such wounds usually cause extradural abscesses.
2 *Direct spread* – the cause in 75% of cases:
  a an infected middle ear or mastoid; initially causes a subdural abscess that subsequently spreads to either the temporal lobe or cerebellum;
  b an infected frontal or ethmoid sinus, spreading to the frontal lobe.
3 *Blood-borne spread*. A septic embolus, especially from a focus of infection in a lung such as bronchiectasis or lung abscess, or occasionally from the systemic circulation in the presence of congenital cyanotic heart disease in which there is a right-to-left shunt. Such abscesses commonly occur in the middle cerebral artery territory.

Clinical features

The clinical features are those of:

- the underlying cause (e.g. chronic mastoiditis);
- evidence of the development of an intracerebral space-occupying lesion (raised intracranial pressure);
- localizing features (e.g. epilepsy or a focal neurological defect);
- toxaemia, fever, meningism and a leucocytosis, particularly if there is rapidly spreading cerebral infection. Often, the abscess is walled off by a relatively thick capsule so that the general manifestations of infection (fever and toxaemia) are not evident.

Special investigations

- *Blood tests* looking for systemic infection (increased white cell count and increased CRP) can be normal in 60% of patients.
- *Chest X-ray* may show a primary focus in the lung.
- *CT and MR imaging* provide accurate diagnosis and localization of the abscess, typically appearing as a ring-enhancing lesion with extensive oedema; sinus views may reveal the source. Differentiating abscesses from cystic brain tumours may be difficult, but on diffusion-weighted MRI, the viscous contents of abscesses will show restricted diffusion.

Treatment

In the first instance, the abscess is aspirated through a burr-hole by means of a brain needle. Intravenous antibiotics are given at high dose depending on the antimicrobial sensitivities of organisms grown from the pus. Serial CT scans are used to follow the resolution of the abscess. The aspirations may need to be repeated. Occasionally, the abscess fails to respond to aspiration and its capsule must be excised.

Epilepsy develops in one-third of patients and requires anticonvulsant therapy.

Intracranial vascular lesions

Intracranial vascular lesions may present as either subarachnoid or intracerebral haemorrhage, or a combination of the two. Subarachnoid haemorrhage (SAH) is commonly caused by rupture of an aneurysm of a cerebral artery or due to trauma. Rarer causes include bleeds from tumours or arteriovenous malformations. In up to 15% of cases no cause can be found.

Intracerebral haemorrhage is commonly due to the following:

- *Hypertensive bleeds* – due to rupture of microaneurysms (Charcot–Bouchard aneurysms[4]). They commonly affect the basal ganglia, thalamus and cerebellum.
- *Amyloid angiopathy* – frequently leads to lobar haemorrhage.
- *Arteriovenous malformations.*
- *Capillary haemangioma* (cavernomas) – cluster of abnormal capillaries. Often produce small haemorrhages and can be associated with epilepsy.
- *Tumours* – glioblastomas and oligodendrogliomas are the most common primary tumours to present with haemorrhage. Metastases from melanoma or renal tumours are the most common metastatic tumours. Occasionally, haematoma can obscure an underlying tumour – it is, therefore, important to arrange for repeat imaging once the haemorrhage has resolved.

Intracranial aneurysms

Pathology

Intracranial (berry) aneurysms are primary aneurysms of the cerebral arteries. They are saccular, generally arise near the bifurcation of an artery, and are probably due to aplasia or hypoplasia of the tunica media. Eighty-five percent occur in the anterior half of the circle of Willis,[5] with equal distribution between the anterior communicating artery, internal carotid artery and middle cerebral artery (Figure 16.1). Internal carotid artery aneurysms occur at its terminal bifurcation, origin of the posterior communicating artery and

[4] Jean-Martin Charcot (1825–1893), Neurologist and Anatomist, Hôpital Salpêtrière, Paris, France. One of the fathers of neurology, Charcot was also the first to describe multiple sclerosis, amongst other conditions. Charles-Jospeh Bouchard (1837–1915), Pathologist, Paris. Described the aneurysms while a student of Charcot at Salpêtrière. Bouchard also described the nodes characteristic of osteoarthritis of the proximal interphalangeal joints.

[5] Thomas Willis (1621–1675), Physician and Anatomist, first in Oxford and then in London.

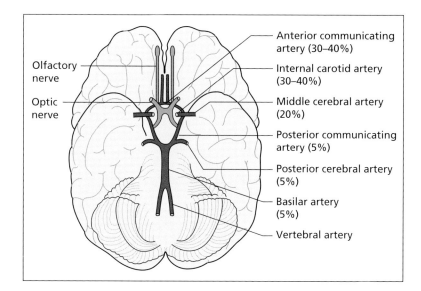

Olfactory nerve

Optic nerve

Anterior communicating artery (30–40%)

Internal carotid artery (30–40%)

Middle cerebral artery (20%)

Posterior communicating artery (5%)

Posterior cerebral artery (5%)

Basilar artery (5%)

Vertebral artery

Figure 16.1 The common sites of intracranial aneurysms.

occasionally in the cavernous sinus or at the origin of the ophthalmic artery. Fifteen percent occur on the basilar or vertebral arteries. About 20% are multiple. Men and women are equally affected, and the aneurysms may be familial. They are associated with hypertension and cigarette smoking, and also occasionally with polycystic kidney disease, coarctation of the aorta and collagen disorders such as Ehlers–Danlos syndrome.[6] They are rarely due to arteriosclerosis, trauma or infection (mycotic aneurysms).

Clinical features

These can be divided into two groups.

1 *Subarachnoid haemorrhage:* bleeding into the CSF from a ruptured intracranial aneurysm is the most common cause of spontaneous subarachnoid haemorrhage. Between 6% and 8% of all strokes are due to SAH. Rupture most commonly occurs at times of stress or exercise, and presents with the following:
   a severe headache of sudden onset ('as if I was hit across the back of my head');
   b vomiting;
   c photophobia;
   d irritability;

e neck stiffness and a positive Kernig's sign[7] (flexion of the hip with extension of the leg causes pain when meningeal irritation is present);
f impairment of consciousness;
g focal neurological signs or generalized seizures.

Prior to the haemorrhage, there is often a history of severe headache within the previous 2 weeks, an event that might be due to a small bleed. Aneurysm rupture may also cause intracerebral or subdural bleeding with neurological signs depending on the site of the haematoma. Most cases occur after the age of 40 years, when increasing atheromatous degenerative changes in the arteries and hypertension are probably precipitating factors. The clinical diagnosis is confirmed by CT, or if CT is negative, lumbar puncture will reveal xanthochromia – yellow-stained CSF.

2 *Pressure symptoms due to the aneurysm:* especially third-nerve palsy from an aneurysm of the posterior communicating artery.

Haemorrhage from a ruptured aneurysm is serious and one-quarter of patients die without recovering consciousness. Further deterioration results from the intense spasm that follows several days after the haemorrhage and from further bleeding. About 50%

---

[6] Edvard Lauritz Ehlers (1863–1937), Professor of Clinical Dermatology, Copenhagen, Denmark. Henri-Alexandre Danlos (1844–1912), dermatologist, Paris, France.

[7] Vladimir Kernig (1840–1917), German Physician and Neurologist, St Petersburg, Russia.

will bleed again within 6 weeks of the initial haemor-rhage, and the mortality of such bleeds is high.

Treatment

If the patient is in coma or has significant neurological deficit, but does not have hydrocephalus or a signifi-cant intracerebral bleed, conservative management is adopted. This involves flat bed rest, adequate fluid, sodium replacement and analgesia, and nimodipine to reduce the risk of development of delayed cerebral ischaemia from vasospasm.

If the patient recovers from the initial bleed, cere-bral angiography is performed to locate the site of the aneurysm. If the aneurysm is demonstrated, treat-ment comprises either:

- *endovascular approaches using platinum coils to thrombose the aneurysm.* These are now consid-ered first-line treatment, and are preferred to sur-gical clipping in patients with posterior circulation aneurysms (because of the difficult surgical approach) and those with significant co-morbidity; or
- *craniotomy with the direct application of a clip across the base of the aneurysm.* Clipping is also associated with a low incidence of recanalization and hence rebleeding. The results of clipping are good in 80% of patients, with a 2–8% mortality.

About 15% of the angiograms are negative and prob-ably indicate that thrombosis has taken place in a microaneurysm. Such patients are treated conserva-tively, and the prognosis is good.

Arteriovenous malformations

Developmental vascular malformations may occur in any part of the CNS, particularly over the surface of the cerebral hemispheres in the distribution of the middle cerebral artery. They comprise a tangle of abnormal vessels, ranging from telangiectasia to cavernous and venous malformations often with arte-riovenous fistulas.

They may produce focal epilepsy, headaches or slowly progressive paralysis, and 50% present with subarachnoid or intracerebral bleeding. The suba-rachnoid haemorrhage is less catastrophic than in rupture of an aneurysm but accounts for about 10% of all cases of spontaneous subarachnoid bleeding. Half of the cases have a bruit, which may be heard over the eye, skull vault or carotid arteries in the neck. Exact

diagnosis and localization are made by cerebral angiography.

The haemorrhage rate is around 4% per year. Accessible malformations in non-eloquent parts of the brain (i.e. those not involved in speech produc-tion) might be treated by surgery, although stereotac-tic radiosurgery (known as the gamma knife) is now employed for many patients with a nidus under 3 cm in diameter. The aim of radiosurgery is to induce endarteritis obliterans in the nidus of the lesion. This may take many months to achieve during which the patient is not protected. Both surgery and stereotactic radiosurgery may be facilitated by prior embolization.

Sturge–Weber syndrome[8] is an association between a port-wine stain localized to one or more segments of the cutaneous distribution of the trigeminal nerve and a corresponding extensive venous angioma (which may cause contralateral focal fits).

Hydrocephalus

The circulation of cerebrospinal fluid

CSF is produced by the choroid plexuses of the lateral, third and fourth ventricles (Figure 16.2). It escapes from the fourth ventricle through the median fora-men of Magendie[9] and the lateral foramina of Luschka[10] into the cerebral subarachnoid space. About 80% of the fluid is reabsorbed via the cranial arachnoid villi. The remaining 20% of the CSF is absorbed by the spinal arachnoid villi or escapes along the nerve sheaths into the lymphatics.

Obstruction along the CSF pathway produces a rise in pressure and dilation within the system proximal to the block. Hydrocephalus may be classified according to whether the block occurs within the ventricular system or outside it.

---

[8] William Allen Sturge (1850–1919), Physician, Royal Free Hospital, London, UK. Frederick Parkes Weber (1863–1962), Physician, London, UK, with a life-long interest in rare diseases.

[9] François Magendie (1783–1855), Physiologist and Professor of Medicine, Collège de France, Paris, France.

[10] Hubert von Lushka (1820–1875), Professor of Anatomy, Tubingen, Germany.

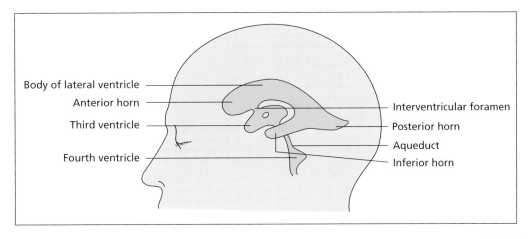

Figure 16.2 The ventricular system. Reproduced from Ellis H, Mahadevan V (2019) *Clinical Anatomy*, 14th edn. Oxford: Wiley-Blackwell.

Non-communicating or obstructive hydrocephalus

CSF cannot escape from within the brain to the basal cisterns. This may be due to congenital narrowing of the aqueduct of Sylvius[11] or the Chiari malformation,[12] which is a congenital downward protrusion of the cerebellum into the foramen magnum (with consequent occlusion of the foramina of the fourth ventricle) frequently associated with spina bifida. It may also be acquired as a result of cerebral abscess or tumour, either within or adjacent to a ventricle.

Communicating hydrocephalus

CSF can escape from within the brain, but absorption via the villi is prevented as a result of the obliteration of subarachnoid channels. It may be congenital, as a result of failure of development of the arachnoid villi, or it may be secondary to meningitis or bleeding into the subarachnoid space (e.g. head injury, aneurysm rupture, arteriovenous malformation).

[11] Franciscus Sylvius (1614–1672), Professor of Medicine, Leiden, The Netherlands.

[12] Hans Chiari (1851–1916), Viennese Pathologist, successively Professor at Strasbourg, France, and Prague, Czech Republic; he also described the syndrome of hepatic venous outflow obstruction.

Clinical features

Clinically, hydrocephalus may be divided into two important groups. The first is the acquired variety, which presents with features of raised intracranial pressure described at the beginning of this chapter. The second comprises patients with congenital hydrocephalus, who show the characteristic picture of enlargement of the skull (comparison should be made with the size of an infant's skull of the same age obtained from standard charts) over which the scalp is stretched with dilated cutaneous veins. The fontanelles are enlarged and tense, and fail to close at the normal times. Typical of this condition is the downward displacement of the eyes ('sun setting'), and there may be an associated squint and nystagmus. Papilloedema is not present in these cases. There may be late epilepsy, and mental impairment may be considerable when there is extensive thinning of the cerebral cortex. There may be associated congenital deformities, especially spina bifida.

In some infants with congenital hydrocephalus, natural arrest occurs, presumably as a result of recanalization of the subarachnoid spaces. In the remainder, there is steady progression with inevitable mental deterioration and high mortality unless adequate treatment is instituted.

Special investigations

- *CT or MR scans* confirm ventricular enlargement and can identify causes of obstruction.

- *Cranial ultrasound* through the fontanelle is useful in children.
- *Dynamic CSF studies* allow monitoring of CSF pressures over time as well as the measurement of the resistance to CSF outflow.

Treatment

The goal of treatment is to divert the CSF around the blockage by means of a shunt. For non-communicating (obstructive) hydrocephalus, direct removal of the occluding mass lesion is desirable.

Decompression of the hydrocephalus can be achieved by diverting the CSF into the peritoneum (ventriculoperitoneal shunt) or right atrium via the internal jugular vein (ventriculoatrial shunt). The shunts comprise silicone catheters with a regulator valve mechanism in the middle to permit CSF flow at a certain ventricular pressure without overdrainage of the CSF.

In non-communicating (obstructive) hydrocephalus, an artificial outlet may be created through the floor of the third ventricle into the basal cisterns (endoscopic third ventriculostomy).

Normal pressure hydrocephalus

In elderly patients, there is a form of chronic hydrocephalus that is associated with normal CSF pressures but disordered CSF dynamics. This normal pressure hydrocephalus is characterized by a triad of gait disturbance, dementia and urinary problems. It is important as it is a treatable cause of dementia.

Additional resources

17

Head injury

Stephen Price

Learning objectives

✓ To know the common causes of coma.

✓ To be able to recognize the severity of a head injury and understand the principles of management.

Head injury is a major cause of death in children and young adults. Many survivors of head injury are catastrophically disabled. Recognizing a severe head injury and administering prompt and appropriate care is important for all medical practitioners who, if not receiving patients with such injuries under their care, may nevertheless be bystanders witnessing such an injury. If presented with a patient in 'coma' (see Box 17.1) other causes of unresponsiveness should be considered.

Head injuries are generally classified as closed (concussional) or open (penetrating).

Types of injury

Injuries are usefully classified according to the structures involved (scalp, skull and underlying brain) together with the mechanism of the injury, be it penetrating or blunt, and whether an acceleration/deceleration and/or a rotational brain injury occurred. In reality, isolated injuries are uncommon, and patients more typically experience blunt injury fracturing the skull in which acceleration/deceleration of the brain also occurs.

Ellis and Calne's Lecture Notes in General Surgery, Fourteenth Edition.
Edited by Christopher Watson and Justin Davies.
© 2023 John Wiley & Sons Ltd. Published 2023 by John Wiley & Sons Ltd.
Companion website: www.wiley.com/go/Watson/GeneralSurgery14

Scalp injuries

Most scalp injuries are simple penetrating injuries, which are readily managed by debridement and suture. When the skull is also penetrated, the brain may be lacerated. However, if the injury occurred when the head was stationary, in the absence of acceleration and deceleration, consciousness may not be lost and neither the patient nor the doctor may appreciate the true extent of the injury.

Skull injuries

Injuries to the skull are a result of crushing or some other severe force. The skull fractures along its weakest plane, which varies according to the position of the injuring force. Typically, this is a linear fracture of the skull vault, but may extend into the skull base. A simple crush injury to a stationary head may leave the scalp intact and not disturb consciousness in the absence of acceleration and deceleration forces, although the subsequent skull X-ray may show extensive fractures.

A skull fracture is most important as an indicator of the force of the injury, and the risk of intracranial haemorrhage. There are several other facets of a skull fracture that are important to note (see Box 17.2).

Fractures involving paranasal air sinuses: cerebrospinal fluid rhinorrhoea

Fractures extending through any of the paranasal air sinuses (frontal, ethmoid or sphenoid) communicate

Fractures of the petrous temporal bone: CSF otorrhoea or rhinorrhoea

Fractures through the petrous temporal bone may result in CSF otorrhoea, as CSF passes through into the external auditory meatus either directly or via the mastoid air cells or middle ear in the presence of a ruptured tympanic membrane. If the tympanic membrane is intact, CSF rhinorrhoea occurs via the Eustachian tube. Involvement of the inner ear will result in deafness and is frequently associated with a lower motor neuron facial nerve palsy. Spontaneous resolution of the leak is usual.

Fractures through the temporal bone: middle meningeal vessels

A fracture through the temporal bone may disrupt the middle meningeal artery and/or vein as they traverse the bone, and result in an extradural haemorrhage, which may not manifest immediately (see later in this chapter).

Depressed fractures

A localized blow drives a fragment of bone below the level of the surrounding skull vault. Such fractures are often compound, as the overlying scalp is torn.

with the outside and are, therefore, compound (open) fractures, as the overlying dura is usually breached. This external communication may manifest as a runny nose (rhinorrhoea), the clear cerebrospinal fluid (CSF) being rich in glucose and low in mucin content (and positive for beta trace protein), compared with the normal nasal secretion, which contains no sugar and is rich in mucin. Such a connection may also be indicated by intracranial air (aerocele) or fluid in one of the sinuses on a computed tomography (CT) scan. Anosmia may occur if the fracture crosses the cribriform plate. Such patients are at risk of meningitis. Some CSF leaks heal spontaneously, particularly those involving the temporal bone, but a persistent leak will require craniotomy and dural repair or endonasal repair. Vaccination against *Pneumococcus* is recommended where there is any suggestion of a CSF leak.

[1]William Henry Battle (1855–1936), Surgeon, St Thomas's Hospital, London, UK.

The depressed bone may be left if it is not deeply depressed (less than the skull thickness) and not otherwise troublesome. Indications for elevation include the debridement of a contaminated wound, depression greater than the bone thickness, associated intracranial haematoma or epileptic focus.

Orbital haematoma

Fractures of the anterior and middle cranial fossae are very frequently associated with orbital haematoma; blood tracks forward into the orbital tissues, into the eyelids and behind the conjunctiva. It may be difficult to differentiate this from a 'black eye', which is a superficial haematoma of the eyelid and surrounding soft tissues produced by direct injury.

An orbital haematoma is suggested by the following features:

- *Subconjunctival haemorrhage*, the posterior limit of which cannot be seen.
- *Absence of grazing of the surrounding skin.*
- *Confined to the margin of the orbit* (owing to its fascial attachments), whereas a black eye frequently extends onto the surrounding cheek.
- *Mild exophthalmos and a degree of ophthalmoplegia.*
- *Bilateral haematoma.*

There may also be some confusion in making a diagnosis between a subconjunctival and conjunctival haemorrhage. The subconjunctival haemorrhage extends from the orbit, forwards and deep to the conjunctiva; there is, therefore, no posterior limit to the haemorrhage. A conjunctival haemorrhage results from a direct blow on the eye and produces a small haematoma clearly delimited on the conjunctiva itself.

Brain injuries

Brain injury can be divided into primary and secondary injuries.

Primary brain injuries are the direct result of trauma, and may have several components which, apart from direct penetrating injuries, are the result of the brain being relatively mobile within the skull and it being violently forced into sudden acceleration and deceleration. These result in both diffuse and local effects.

Secondary brain injuries occur after the initial event and are the result of hypoxia, hypercapnia, hypotension (ischaemia), intracranial haemorrhage or meningitis. These are the main causes of in-hospital mortality after head injury.

Diffuse brain injury

Diffuse neuronal injury occurs as a result of shearing movements, the worst being rotational shearing, as occurs when a blow is delivered off centre. The result is axon damage and rupture of the small vessels, particularly serious in the brain stem. A severe rotational shearing force may be transmitted down along the axis of the brain, and such forces shearing through the brain stem are usually fatal.

Localized brain injury

Local brain damage occurs as the brain impacts against the skull.

Coup and contre-coup (Figure 17.1)

The direct impact of the brain on the skull at the site of injury and the contre-coup injury as it rebounds against the opposite wall of the skull result in oedema and bruising at the sites of impact. Common sites of impaction are the frontal lobes in the anterior fossa and temporal lobes within the middle fossa, with contre-coup to the occipital lobes.

Laceration within the skull

The brain may impinge on sharp bony edges within the skull, such as the sphenoid ridge, and sustain a laceration.

Cerebral perfusion

Understanding the mechanisms underlying the regulation of cerebral perfusion, and how these may be affected in trauma, is important in the management of patients with a head injury. The main regulatory factors are described below.

Systemic arterial pressure

Cerebral perfusion is normally autoregulated by the vasoactive cerebral arterioles to maintain constant cerebral blood flow over a wide range of systemic blood pressures. If systemic arterial pressure falls, cerebral vasodilation occurs to compensate; a further fall may

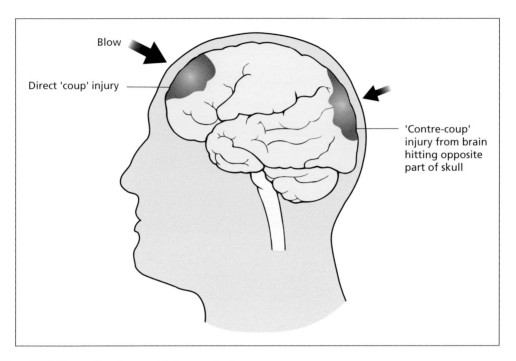

Blow

Direct 'coup' injury

'Contre-coup' injury from brain hitting opposite part of skull

Figure 17.1 Coup and contre-coup injuries – mechanism.

exceed the arterioles' ability to compensate, and cerebral ischaemia occurs. The arterioles are also sensitive to the presence of vasoactive mediators, the most important being pH, and its proxy, Pco$_2$. An increase in arterial Pco$_2$ (hypercapnia) causes cerebral vasodilation, and in the presence of oedema may further raise intracranial pressure and result in exacerbation of the brain injury, one of the causative factors in secondary brain injury. Intensive care management aims to avoid hypercapnia. Reduction of the Pco$_2$ can lead to vasoconstriction and hence more ischaemia. As a result, hyperventilation, once employed to reduce Pco$_2$, is now rarely used and only with suitable monitoring.

Intracranial pressure

Since the skull is a closed compartment, a rise in intracranial pressure (ICP) will reduce the cerebral perfusion pressure.

Cerebral perfusion pressure = MAP − ICP

where MAP is the mean arterial blood pressure. Initial increases in ICP (i.e. due to an expanding haematoma) are compensated by reduction of CSF volumes within the cranial cavity. Once the compensatory mechanisms are overcome then small changes in volume

will lead to very large increases in ICP. A rise in ICP coupled with hypotension in trauma victims with head injuries reduces cerebral blood flow, and the resultant ischaemia increases ICP further as well as affecting the cardiorespiratory centres in the floor of the fourth ventricle, leading to reflex increase in systemic pressure and bradycardia – the Cushing reflex.[2] Hence, hypotension in head injury victims is seldom due to the head injury.

Management of the patient with a head injury

The management of a patient with a head injury can be divided into the following:

- Initial assessment.
- Immediate management.
- Delayed management.

[2]Harvey Cushing (1869–1939), Professor of Surgery, Harvard Medical School, Boston, MA, USA. He was one of the founders of neurosurgery.

In practice, the initial assessment and immediate management frequently overlap according to clinical priorities.

Initial assessment

The initial assessment is an active process and not just a period of history taking. However, the history is most important, in particular the account of a witness, as most victims of major head injuries are unable to give an accurate history.

History

Important points to note in the history are as follows.

- *The mechanism of the injury.* This may enable some prediction as to the likely injuries, both visible and within the cranium. The nature of the injurious force and its direction relative to the recipient are important.
- *The immediate condition of the injured person.* What was the patient like immediately after the injury? In particular, note the level of consciousness in terms of an accepted scale such as the Glasgow Coma Scale (see Box 17.3), as well as other vital signs (pulse, respiration, blood pressure), the size and reaction of the pupils and recorded limb movements (was the patient moving their arms and legs after the accident?).
- *Any change in the condition of the injured person.* As well as establishing the patient's condition when first seen after the injury, it is also important to establish whether the condition has changed at all. For example, if the patient was talking and moving all limbs and is now comatose, it suggests that an intracranial mass lesion such as an intracranial haemorrhage is developing.
- *The prior condition of the injured person.* As much history as possible about the injured person should be obtained from relatives and friends. Was the patient drunk at the time? Is the patient diabetic and so could the coma be hypoglycaemic? Does the patient have a glass eye or is he or she on treatment for chronic glaucoma to account for the absence of pupillary responses?
- *What other injuries has the person sustained?* Patients who are unstable due to severe chest or abdominal trauma need these managing first to prevent secondary brain injury.

Examination

Your examination should reassess the patient's conscious level to decide whether the condition has worsened or improved, and look for associated injuries, in particular major occult injuries such as a tension pneumothorax or fractured spine. In patients with major injuries, the priorities for examination are usually quoted in terms of the ABC of resuscitation, to which may be added an additional C.

- *Airway.* Is the airway clear without obstruction such as vomitus or blood? If the patient is not maintaining the airway, intubation with an endotracheal tube should be performed. Occasionally, this may not be possible and a tracheostomy may be required.
- *Breathing.* Is the patient breathing spontaneously or should ventilation be instituted? Avoiding hypercapnia is desirable to reduce ICP (see Chapter 16). An arterial blood sample for estimation of oxygen carriage should be taken as soon as convenient, and the patient should be monitored by pulse oximeter to ensure adequate haemoglobin oxygen saturation.
- *Circulation.* The patient's pulse and blood pressure should be taken and monitored. Raised ICP results in bradycardia and hypertension (Cushing reflex; see earlier in this chapter). Hypotension is rarely due to head injury and an alternative cause should be sought (a ruptured spleen, a haemothorax or a fractured pelvis, for example). Occasionally, extensive scalp bleeding may result in hypotension, as may a head injury in a child.
- *Cervical spine.* Every patient who sustains a head injury should be considered to have a cervical spine injury as well until proved otherwise by good-quality radiography or CT scan. The neck should, therefore, be immobilized in a hard collar.

Following the initial ABC, a full central nervous system (CNS) examination should be performed as well as complete examination of the chest, abdomen and limbs. Particular attention should be paid to the parts that are usually forgotten, including examining the back for evidence of trauma and integrity of the spine, and a rectal examination with particular attention to anal tone (or its absence in spinal injury) and the position of the prostate in the male (a ruptured urethra results in a displaced prostate).

Box 17.3 The Glasgow Coma Scale (GCS)

Eye opening

4 Spontaneously.

3 To speech/command.

2 To pain.

1 None.

Best verbal response

5 Orientated – knows who and where they are.

4 Confused conversation – disorientated; gives confused answers to questions.

3 Inappropriate words – random words; no conversation.

2 Incomprehensible sounds.

1 None.

Best motor response

6 Obeys commands.

5 Localizes pain.

4 Flexes to pain – flexion withdrawal of limb to painful stimulus.

3 Abnormal (decorticate) flexion – upper limb adducts, flexes and internally rotates so that it lies across chest; lower limbs extend (Figure 17.2).

2 Extends to pain (decerebrate) – painful stimulus causes extension of all limbs.

1 None.

When assessing the GCS, it is very important that an adequate stimulus is applied.

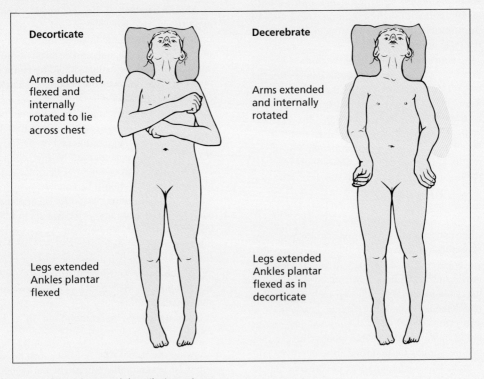

Decorticate

Arms adducted, flexed and internally rotated to lie across chest

Legs extended
Ankles plantar flexed

Decerebrate

Arms extended and internally rotated

Legs extended
Ankles plantar flexed as in decorticate

Figure 17.2 Decerebrate and decorticate postures.

The conscious level: the Glasgow Coma Scale

Vague terms such as comatose, semi-comatose, unconscious, stuporose and so on should be avoided. Instead, the conscious level is charted according to the patient's motor, verbal and eye-opening responses to stimuli; these are very much the reactions of a patient recovering from deep anaesthesia. The most commonly used scale is the Glasgow Coma Scale (GCS) (see Box 17.3), in which the responses within each group are allotted a score, the normal being 15. A mild head injury may score 13–15, a severe injury 8 or less.

Pupil size and responses

If a cerebral hemisphere is pressed upon by an enlarging blood clot, the third cranial nerve on that side becomes compressed by descent of the uncus over the edge of the tentorium cerebelli. Paralysis of the third nerve (which transmits parasympathetic pupilloconstrictor fibres) results in dilation of the corresponding pupil (owing to the intact unopposed sympathetic supply) and failure of the pupil to respond to light. An important sign of cerebral compression is, therefore, dilation and loss of light reaction of the pupil on the affected side although, occasionally, pupillary dilation will be a false localizing sign and will be on the side opposite the mass lesion. Because the optic nerve pathway is intact, a light shone into this unreacting pupil produces constriction in the opposite pupil (consensual reaction to light). As compression continues, the contralateral third nerve becomes compressed, and the opposite pupil in turn dilates and becomes fixed to light.

Bilateral fixed dilated pupils in a patient with head injury indicate very great cerebral compression from which the patient rarely recovers. Occasionally, local trauma to the nerves from extensive skull-base fractures may produce the same findings.

Pulse, respiration and blood pressure

With increasing ICP, the pulse slows and the blood pressure rises (Cushing reflex; see earlier in this chapter), the respirations become stertorious and eventually Cheyne–Stokes[3] in nature.

Special investigations

With respect to head injury, there are three immediate investigations that may be indicated.

1 *Skull X-ray* used to be the initial investigation but has been replaced owing to the ready availability of CT. It may have a role in children as part of a skeletal survey in suspected non-accidental injury.
2 *CT scan* should be performed on all patients with significant head injuries (see Box 17.4) as indicated by impaired conscious level (GCS <15), history of penetrating injury or suspected fracture, signs of a basal skull fracture (e.g. CSF rhinorrhoea or otor-

---

> **Box 17.4 Indications for CT scan**
>
> - Impaired conscious level, GCS <13 on initial assessment or GCS <15 at 2 hours after the injury.
> - Suspected open or depressed skull fracture or suspected penetrating injury.
> - Basal fracture of skull (possibly indicated by cerebrospinal fluid rhinorrhoea or otorrhoea, periorbital haematoma – Battle's sign).
> - Focal neurological signs, fits or any other neurological symptoms.
> - Deteriorating conscious level.
> - More than one episode of vomiting.
> - Amnesia for 30 min before impact.
> - Coagulopathy/anticoagulation in patients with a history of significant trauma or impaired consciousness.

rhoea, bilateral orbital haematoma [Battle's sign]), post-traumatic seizure, focal neurological deficit or recurrent (>1) vomiting or amnesia for more than 30 min prior to impact. Other indications include a history of loss of consciousness or amnesia and a history of significant trauma, coagulopathy (e.g. patient on anticoagulation), or age over 65 years. The resulting images may then be viewed locally or transmitted to a regional neurosurgical centre for specialist opinion.

3 *Cervical spine X-ray* is necessary in all unconscious patients following head injury, unless included in the CT scan. Other indications include neck pain and/or tenderness with a history of possible neck trauma, or where exclusion of neck trauma is necessary prior to intubation for other surgery.

Immediate management

Admission to hospital (see Box 17.5), CT scanning (see Box 17.4) and neurosurgical referral should all be considered. Consultation with a neurosurgeon is indicated for persistent coma (GCS ≤8), persistent unexplained confusion lasting more than 4 hours, deterioration in GCS and progressive focal neurological signs as well as those in whom neurosurgery is indicated (see later in this chapter). Transfer should only occur after initial resuscitation and stabilization of the patient.

The immediate management of complicated cases will include correcting any problems identified in the

---

[3] John Cheyne (1777–1836), an Edinburgh-trained Physician who migrated to Ireland. William Stokes (1804–1878), Physician, Meath Hospital, Dublin, Ireland.

initial assessment, such as draining a pneumothorax, instituting ventilation if the patient is unable to maintain the airway or to breathe, and performing a laparotomy and/or orthopaedic procedures when appropriate.

Following the initial brain injury, further deterioration may be due to the following factors:

- Increasing cerebral oedema as the brain swells consequent upon the damage it sustained.
- Intracranial haemorrhage – extradural, subdural or intracerebral.
- Hypoxia, due to impaired ventilation or ischaemia.
- Infection, secondary to compound fractures including fractures involving the paranasal sinuses or petrous temporal bone.
- Hydrocephalus, either communicating or noncommunicating.

Delayed management

Management of minor head injuries

With respect to the head injury, there follows a period of observation, with attention paid to the following:

- Conscious level – according to the GCS.
- Vital signs – pulse, blood pressure, temperature, oxygen saturation.
- Pupil size and responses – dilation of a pupil, loss of response to light or asymmetry are late signs of increasing ICP; ICP monitoring – done with a catheter placed within the ventricles, which will help direct treatment and facilitate drainage of intracranial fluid to lower pressure.

Management of severe head injuries

With severe head injuries the aim of management is to prevent secondary injury. This is done by:

- Maintaining blood pressure – patients need accurate fluid balance and may need inotropic support.
- Maintaining adequate oxygenation and avoidance of hypercapnia.
- Avoidance of hyperthermia.
- Monitoring ICP.

Managing high intracranial pressure

In an unconscious, ventilated patient, it is important to monitor ICP.

Intraparenchymal probes are commonly used for this. A high ICP can be treated as follows.

- *Paralyse and sedate the patient*: this prevents the patient 'fighting' with the ventilator and having increases in intrathoracic pressure. Most sedatives used (e.g. propofol) reduce cerebral metabolic activity, thus reducing the demand for blood to the brain. In extreme cases with uncontrolled ICP, attempts to cause 'electrical silence' of the brain with barbiturates can be considered.
- *Reduce venous congestion*: this is done by nursing in a slight head-up position and ensuring ties for endotracheal tubes do not compress the neck.
- *Ensuring adequate blood pressure*: falls in blood pressure lead to vasodilation in areas of the brain that are autoregulating. Reversing even slight falls in blood pressure can have a profound improvement in ICP.

- *Cooling*: moderate cooling of patients can help ICP control. More intensive cooling can have its own problems and there is little evidence that it is neuroprotective.
- *Osmotic diuretics*: mannitol is commonly used to reduce ICP. The exact mechanism is not fully understood but it is thought to draw water from normal brain and improve the viscosity and hence flow of blood. Being a relatively large molecule, it crosses areas of damaged blood–brain barrier and can accumulate, causing a rebound increase in ICP. As a result, it is used before a definitive treatment to 'buy time', such as transferring a patient for surgery.
- *Avoiding hyponatraemia*: low serum sodium levels can lead to further oedema. Hypertonic saline can be used to increase the serum sodium and act as an osmotic diuretic with fewer problems with rebound increases in ICP.
- *Drainage of CSF*: this is done most commonly from the ventricular CSF (using an external ventricular drain) or occasionally with lumbar drainage, providing there are no contraindications.
- *Evacuation of haematomas*: these can develop over time and may need evacuating. This is discussed in more detail later.
- *Decompressive craniectomy*: if the ICP is uncontrollable, then one consideration is to remove part of the skull and open the dura to allow the brain to swell. This will require later reconstruction of the skull. The RESCUEicp clinical trial showed decompression reduces mortality but this may be at the expense of leaving those survivors in a vegetative or severely disabled state.

Nursing care of the unconscious patient

The airway

The most important single factor in the care of the deeply unconscious patient who has lost the cough reflex, whatever the cause, is maintenance of the airway. The patient is transported and nursed in the recovery position, that is, on one side with the body tilted head downwards, which allows the tongue to fall forward and bronchial secretions or vomit to drain from the mouth rather than be inhaled. Suction may be required to remove excessive secretions or vomit from the pharynx.

An endotracheal tube will be necessary if the airway is not satisfactory and, if after some days it is still difficult to maintain an adequate airway, tracheostomy may be required.

Restlessness

Opiates, particularly morphine, are generally contraindicated, as they will depress respiration and disguise the level of consciousness and will also produce constricted pupils, which may mask a valuable physical sign. Paracetamol, benzodiazepines or codeine preparations may be necessary but often all that is required is to protect the patient from self-injury by judicious restraint and padding.

A cause of restlessness may be a distended bladder; if the retention is relieved, the patient may then calm down.

In most cases where it is not possible to assess the patient properly due to restlessness, it is often best to anaesthetize the patient and ventilate them to assess them properly (especially with imaging).

Feeding

Many patients with head injury died in the past owing to dehydration and starvation. Orogastric feeding is instituted if the patient remains unable to swallow. A nasogastric tube is contraindicated in patients with craniofacial injuries because of the danger of intracranial penetration.

Skin care

A deeply unconscious patient is susceptible to bed sores. Careful nursing care and the use of an intermittently inflatable mattress are required for their prevention.

Sphincters

The unconscious patient may be incontinent, and the resultant excoriation of the skin makes the patient still more susceptible to pressure sores. The use of a penile sheath on the penis or an indwelling catheter in female patients will help in the nursing care. Retention of urine may require catheter relief.

Indications for surgery in head injuries

Early

- The excision and suture of scalp lacerations.
- Surgical toilet of a compound fracture.
- Cerebral decompression and evacuation of the haematoma for intracranial bleeding.

Delayed

- Repair of a dural tear with CSF rhinorrhoea.
- Late repair of skull defects.
- Late plastic surgery for deforming facial injuries.

Traumatic intracranial bleeding

Classification

Haemorrhage within the skull following injury may be classified as follows.

1 Extradural.
2 Subdural:
   a Acute.
   b Chronic.
3 Subarachnoid.
4 Intracerebral.
5 Intraventricular.

Extradural haemorrhage

This is sometimes wrongly named 'middle meningeal haemorrhage'. It may indeed arise from a tear of the middle meningeal artery, but an extradural collection of blood may also develop from a laceration of one of the other meningeal vessels, from the torn sagittal sinus or as a result of oozing from the diploë, bone and stripped dura mater on each side of any associated fracture (Figure 17.3a). As the dura mater is more adherent to the skull in older patients, extradural haematomas are very uncommon in the elderly.

Clinical features

The classic story is of a relatively minor head injury producing temporary concussion, recovery ('the lucid period') then, some hours later, the development of headache and progressively deeper coma due to cerebral compression by the extradural clot. This picture may give rise to the tragedies of the drunk who is put into the cells for the night and is found dead in the morning, or the cricketer who goes home to bed after being mildly concussed by a cricket ball and dies during the evening. It is important to note that this classic picture is not as common as is thought. Often, there is no lucid period; the patient progressively passes into deeper coma from the time of the initial injury.

The physical signs are those of rapidly increasing ICP, which have already been discussed (see Chapter 16). In addition, there are certain localizing signs that may help the surgeon. These are as follows.

- *The pupils*: a good neurosurgical aphorism is 'explore the side of the dilated pupil' (see earlier in

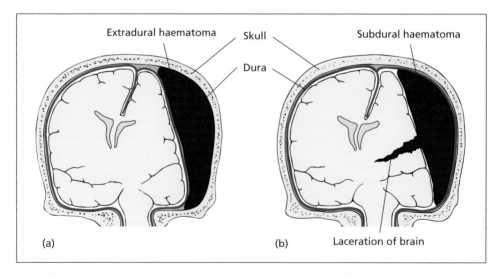

Figure 17.3 (a) Extradural haematoma and (b) acute subdural haematoma. The latter is usually associated with a severe brain injury.

this chapter). In 10% of patients, the dilated pupil will be a false localizing sign.

- *Hemiparesis or hemiplegia* (common) or focal fits (uncommon) usually indicate contralateral compression. This, however, can be a false localizing sign – compression of the contralateral cerebral peduncle on the tentorial hiatus can cause a contralateral weakness.
- A boggy *scalp haematoma* usually overlies the extradural clot.

Special investigations

CT scan is diagnostic and allows accurate localization of the position and size of the clot.

Treatment

An extradural haemorrhage is one of the few surgical emergencies where minutes really can matter. If a neurosurgeon is available, a bone flap will be turned over the clot. The major bleeding point on the dura is controlled either with diathermy or silver clips or by under-running. Bleeding from the bone edges is plugged by means of bone wax.

Subdural haematoma

Acute subdural haematoma (Figure 17.3b)

This results from bleeding into the subdural space from lacerated brain or torn vessels. It is usually part of a severe head injury. The patient is frequently in deep coma from the moment of injury but the condition deteriorates still further.

Treatment

Release of the subdural clot through a craniotomy may give some improvement in the neurological state, but the outcome may be poor because of the severity of the underlying brain trauma.

Chronic subdural haematoma or hygroma

This follows a trivial (often forgotten) injury, usually in an elderly patient, sustained weeks or months before. There is a small tear in a cerebral vein as it traverses the subdural space. Whenever the patient coughs, strains or bends over, a little blood extravasates. The resulting haematoma becomes encapsulated; as the clot breaks down, smaller molecules are formed with a rise in the osmotic pressure within the haematoma. Consequent absorption of tissue fluid produces gradual enlargement of the local collection,

which may comprise liquid blood, clot or clear yellow fluid (hygroma).

Clinical features

Clinical features are those of a developing intracranial mass lesion. There is mental deterioration, headaches, vomiting and drowsiness, which progresses to coma. Moderate papilloedema is seen in about half the cases. The condition is indeed often confused with an intracerebral tumour but contrast enhanced CT imaging will demonstrate the outline of the clot.

Treatment

Treatment comprises the evacuation of the clot or fluid collection through burr-holes. The addition of a subdural drain has been shown to reduce the rate of re-accumulation.

Subarachnoid haemorrhage

Clinical features

Blood in the CSF is incidental to most severe head injuries and gives the clinical picture of meningeal irritability with headache, neck stiffness and a positive Kernig's sign.[4] There may be a mild pyrexia.

Treatment

Analgesia and bed rest are required until the severe headache has subsided; rapid rehabilitation follows.

Intracerebral haemorrhage

Scattered small haemorrhages throughout the brain substance are a common postmortem finding in severe head injuries and may be demonstrated at CT scanning in extensive cerebral injury. At other times, a clot may develop within the brain substance, often in the frontal or temporal lobes. If it is exerting a mass effect and the ICP is high, the haematoma is evacuated and the injured lobe may have to be removed.

Intraventricular haemorrhage

Haemorrhage into a ventricle may occur from tearing of the choroid plexus at the time of injury or rupture of an intracerebral clot into the ventricle. It occurs particularly in childhood and is usually part of an overwhelming head injury.

[4]Vladimir Kernig (1840–1917), Neurologist, St Petersburg, Russia. He described neck stiffness in meningitis, which at the time was commonly tuberculous in origin.

Other complications

Meningitis

Infection of the meninges may complicate a fracture of the skull that is compound, either directly to the exterior or via a dural tear into the nasal or aural cavities (see earlier in this chapter). Immunization against *Pneumococcus* is recommended where there is evidence of a CSF leak.

Confirmation of the diagnosis of meningitis is the only positive indication for performing a lumbar puncture on a patient with a head injury.

Treatment

The treatment of established meningitis is antibiotic therapy. Infection via the nasal route is probably due to *Pneumococcus*; here, penicillin should be the first drug of choice. For infection complicating a compound fracture, or in patients with long inpatient stays or previous antibiotic exposure, *Staphylococcus aureus* or Gram-negative bacilli may be responsible and a broad-spectrum antibiotic which can cross the blood–brain barrier is indicated. The antibiotic may have to be changed when the sensitivity of the organism obtained on lumbar puncture becomes known.

Hyperpyrexia

The temperature of a patient with severe brain-stem injury may soar to 40 °C (105 °F) or more as a result of injury to the heat-regulating centre. This is a serious complication and must be treated vigorously by means of cooling blankets.

Late complications

Postconcussional syndrome

Persistent headache, dizziness and poor concentration are common following even minor head injuries and may take many months to resolve. Anxiety following a head injury is not uncommon. Unless reassured and rapidly rehabilitated, the patient who has had concussion is easily led to believe that the brain has been damaged and not fit to lead a normal life again.

Neurological deficits

These are common following traumatic brain injury and will often require extensive periods of neuro-rehabilitation. Cognitive and behavioural changes are very common and are often the most distressing for relatives. Input from neuropsychology is important.

Amnesia

Some idea of the severity of the injury is given by the period of amnesia, both the retrograde amnesia up to the time of the accident and the post-traumatic amnesia following injury. Interestingly, the retrograde amnesia is always considerably shorter than the post-traumatic amnesia. If the period of amnesia amounts to a few minutes or hours, the ultimate prognosis is good; amnesia of several days or even weeks indicates a severe injury and poor prognosis for return of full mental function.

Epilepsy

Persistent epilepsy may complicate penetrating compound wounds with resultant cortical scarring. In such cases, anticonvulsant therapy, such as phenytoin, is given for at least 6 months following injury. Established post-traumatic epilepsy is treated medically by means of anticonvulsants. Occasionally, success may follow excision of a cortical scar.

Post-traumatic hypopituitarism

Damage to the pituitary is common due to shearing of the hypophyseal vessels and stalk. Partial or complete hypopituitarism occurs in 33–50% of patients and can occur in all severities of injury. It manifests in a number of ways including fatigue, myopathy, cognitive difficulties, depression, behavioural changes or adrenal crises. Early identification and prompt endocrine referral are important.

Brain death

The medical and nursing care of patients with severe brain damage due to trauma, haemorrhage or intracranial tumour is now so good that the doctors and nurses are often faced with the sad case of a patient whose brain is completely and irreversibly destroyed, but whose heart and circulation are intact, provided the lungs are mechanically ventilated. This state of affairs may persist for some weeks with severe distress to the patient's relatives and the ward staff.

The diagnosis of brain death depends on the demonstration of permanent and irreversible destruction of brain-stem function. The tests must be performed by two people with experience in the diagnosis of brain-stem death and should be performed together on two occasions. *All brain-stem reflexes should be absent*. The following should first be excluded before tests for brain-stem death can be performed:

- Hypothermia.
- Intoxication.
- Sedative drugs – particularly any barbiturate drugs that are used to reduce cerebral metabolism. As they are distributed in fat, it can take many hours for the levels to drop below therapeutic levels.
- Neuromuscular blocking drugs.
- Severe electrolyte and acid–base abnormalities.

In addition, there must be a clearly identified cause of death, which is usually obvious in the presence of head injury but may be less clear in other circumstances.

The specific features of brain-stem death are as follows.

- The patient is in a coma and on a ventilator.
- The pupils are dilated and do not respond to direct or consensual light.
- There is no corneal reflex.
- Vestibulo-ocular (doll's eye) reflexes are absent, such that when the head is passively turned, the eyes remained fixed relative to the head.
- Caloric reflexes are absent. These are tested by slow injection of 20 mL of ice-cold water into each external auditory meatus in turn, clear access to

the tympanic membrane having been established by direct inspection. If no eye movement occurs during or after the test, it is considered positive.

- No motor responses within the cranial nerve distribution can be elicited by adequate stimulation of any somatic area.
- There is no gag reflex response to bronchial stimulation by a suction catheter passed down the trachea.
- No respiratory movements occur when the patient is disconnected from the mechanical ventilator for long enough to ensure that the arterial $P\text{co}_2$ rises above the threshold for stimulating respiration, that is, the $P\text{co}_2$ must be above 6.65 kPa (50 mmHg).

If this situation persists over a period of observation and is confirmed by a second practitioner, death can be certified. The period of observation depends upon the age of the patient (child or adult) and the cause of the coma.

The decision to stop mechanical ventilation rests on the above factors. Once this decision has been made, the possibility of the patient becoming an organ donor for transplantation should be considered. This should be discussed fully and sympathetically with available relatives so that their informed consent is obtained for the removal of organs.

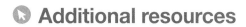 # Additional resources

18

The spine

Rodney J. C. Laing

Learning objectives

✓ To be familiar with the types of spinal injury, associated clinical signs and appropriate management.

✓ To understand the age-related (degenerative) spinal disorders, associated symptoms and treatment options.

Spina bifida (Figure 18.1)

The neural tube develops by an infolding of the neural ectoderm to become the spinal cord. The surrounding meninges and vertebral column derive from mesodermal tissue. Failure of embryonic fusion may result in various anomalies, collectively described as dysraphism.

- *Spina bifida occulta*: bony and soft tissue developmental anomalies, meninges and nervous tissue normal. Incidence less than 10% of the population.
- *Meningocele*: a cystic protrusion of the meninges through a posterior vertebral defect.
- *Myelomeningocele*: neural tissue (the cord or spinal roots) protrudes into, and may be adherent to, the meningeal sac.
- *Myelocele*: failure of fusion of the neural tube; an open spinal plate is flush with the skin and occupies the defect as a red, granular area with cerebrospinal fluid (CSF) leaking from its centre. Folic acid supplements in food and antenatal screening with ultrasound have resulted in a significant decline of spinal dysraphism. Worldwide the incidence of neural tube defects has reduced to between 0.2 and 6%.

Clinical features

These defects are usually in the lumbosacral area, although any part of the spine may be involved. There may be an associated overlying lipoma, tuft of hair or skin anomaly. When nervous tissue is involved, there may be associated weakness, sensory disturbances in the limbs and loss of normal bladder and bowel control.

Hydrocephalus nearly always co-exists with open neural tube defects probably as a consequence of the descent of the cerebellar tonsils below the foramen magnum with consequent obstruction of the CSF pathway (*Arnold–Chiari malformation*[1]).

In some dysraphic conditions, the spinal cord may be tethered to the dura by a fibrous band and, as the child grows, weakness and sensory loss in the legs may occur leading to deformity of the feet and disturbance of bladder and bowel control (tethered cord syndrome).

Treatment

Dietary supplementation with folic acid before and in the first trimester of pregnancy reduces the occurrence of neural tube defects. In many countries, like

Ellis and Calne's Lecture Notes in General Surgery, Fourteenth Edition. Edited by Christopher Watson and Justin Davies.
© 2023 John Wiley & Sons Ltd. Published 2023 by John Wiley & Sons Ltd.
Companion website: www.wiley.com/go/Watson/GeneralSurgery14

[1] Julius Arnold (1835–1915), Professor of Pathology, Heidelberg, Germany. Hans Chiari (1851–1916), Viennese Pathologist, successively Professor at Strasbourg, France, and Prague, Czech Republic.

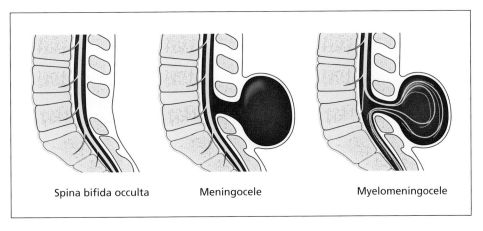

Spina bifida occulta   Meningocele   Myelomeningocele

Figure 18.1 Spina bifida.

the UK, folic acid has been added to certain foods in an effort to ensure that adequate dietary supplementation is achieved.

Minor degrees of dysraphism do not require any intervention. If a dermal sinus is communicating with the dura, there is a risk of infection and surgical excision/closure is needed. Skin-covered lesions may require cosmetic surgery. All cases with an exposed neural plate should be repaired as soon as possible to prevent meningitis and reduce the risk of hydrocephalus. Associated hydrocephalus needs to be monitored by measuring head circumference and interval ultrasound scanning to measure ventricular size. Not all children require CSF diversion and for those that do the options are a ventriculo-peritoneal shunt, endoscopic third ventriculostomy and/or choroid plexus cauterization. Surgery to improve bladder function and to correct orthopaedic limb problems arising as a result of muscle imbalance or weakness may be required as the child grows.

Spinal injuries

Spinal injuries have two components – bony/ligamentous injury and neurological injury – both of which may occur in patients following spinal trauma.

The bony-ligamentous injury

The bony injury may comprise either a disco-ligamentous injury, a fracture or a combination of both which may result in a fracture dislocation. The most important consideration is the stability of the fracture. A stable fracture is one that is unlikely to undergo further displacement causing neurological damage or deformity or both. An unstable fracture may undergo further displacement with the risk of further neurological injury.

Initial management

The normal trauma principles apply and protocols should be followed (see Chapter 9). Assessment and protection of the airway, breathing and circulation take precedence. The vast majority of injuries will not displace further when a patient is lying horizontal on their back or side. When moving position, patients should be log rolled for comfort as well as to reduce any rotational forces on the injured spine. The assessment of stability is fundamental to the subsequent management of the patient. It depends upon the integrity of the structures that make up the normal spinal column, namely the vertebrae, intervertebral discs and ligaments. In making an assessment, the concept of the three-column spine is useful (Figure 18.2).

The three columns are made up as follows.

- *The anterior column* comprises the anterior longitudinal ligament, anterior parts of the vertebral body, disc and annulus fibrosus.
- *The middle column* comprises the posterior parts of the vertebral body, disc and annulus fibrosus, and the posterior longitudinal ligament.

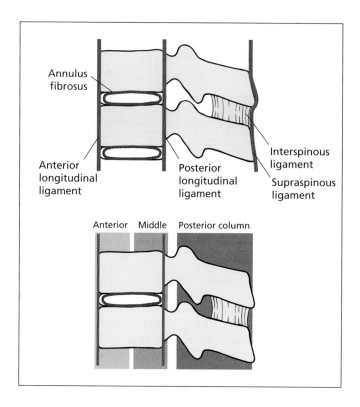

Figure 18.2 The three-column spine concept.

- *The posterior column* comprises the facet joints, the posterior arch and the intervening ligament complex, itself comprising supraspinous ligaments, interspinous ligaments and ligamentum flavum.

Disruption of two or all of these columns indicates a greater risk of spinal instability. Disruption of a single column, such as in a compression fracture affecting the anterior half of the vertebral body, is a stable injury without any risk of further displacement or neurological damage. The vast majority of spinal fractures will heal with conservative management. Contemporary trauma principles apply to the spine and in selected cases internal fixation allows patients to be mobilized early and be discharged from hospital sooner thus avoiding complications associated with prolonged immobilization.

Types of fracture

Most fractures are caused by hyperextension or hyperflexion, often combined with compression or distraction. The results of these forces may be subdivided into five levels in the spine.

1 *Upper cervical spine (C1, C2).* In the upper cervical spine, flexion/extension injuries may result in fracture of the dens (odontoid process) at its base, atlantoaxial dislocation or fracture of the atlas (Jefferson's fracture[2]) or axis (hangman's fracture). The spinal canal is wide in the upper cervical region and spinal cord damage is uncommon although in severe high velocity injuries fatal damage to the cord may occur.

2 *Lower cervical spine (C3–C7).*
   a *Hyperflexion injuries* may result in anterior dislocation of facet joints, disco-ligamentous injury and vertebral body fracture, all with consequent narrowing of the spinal canal and potential neurological injury. Either one or both facet joints may be involved. The spinal

[2] Sir Geoffrey Jefferson (1886–1961), Professor of Neurosurgery, Manchester, UK.

canal has a smaller cross-sectional area than in other regions and so the incidence of spinal cord injury is much higher and may result in incomplete or complete injuries.

   b *Hyperextension* may result in rupture of the anterior longitudinal ligament and disc with backward displacement of the vertebral body narrowing the spinal canal and contusing the cord, before normal alignment is restored.

   c *Compression, combined with flexion*, may result in a wedge-shaped fracture of the vertebral body. Severe compression injuries may result in a burst fracture with a fragment protruding backwards into the spinal canal.

3 *Thoracic.* The thoracic spine is relatively stable owing to the splinting afforded by the rib cage and sternum. Pathological fractures in patients with osteoporosis, metastatic cancer or myeloma are more common in this region.

4 *Thoracolumbar.* The thoracolumbar junction is susceptible to injuries caused by flexion, rotation and compression. Such injuries may follow a fall from a height landing on the feet or the buttocks, or forward flexion of the spine in a decelerating road traffic accident, or a heavy weight falling on the shoulders.

5 *Lumbar.*

   a *Compression* injuries may cause wedge-shaped fractures where the body of the vertebra collapses asymmetrically.

   b *Burst fractures* with comminution of the vertebral body and disruption of the anterior and middle columns may occur following axial compression and may result in a potentially unstable fracture, sometimes with nerve root or cauda equina damage if bone fragments encroach into the canal. Such fractures may be associated with damage to the intervertebral disc.

In practice, the most common fractures are those in the cervical and thoracolumbar regions.

Clinical features

There is the typical history of injury followed by localized pain, bruising, tenderness and occasionally obvious deformity. Careful neurological examination Box 18.1 should be recorded on an American Spinal Injury Association (ASIA) chart.

It is essential to rule out a spinal fracture in head-injured unconscious patients and once haemodynamically stable and with appropriate protection of the airway a full-body computed tomography (CT) scan to include the head and whole spine should be undertaken.

Special investigations

- *Spine X-ray.* There are very few indications for spinal X-rays. In certain circumstances, dynamic (flexion/extension) views may be indicated but only after cross-sectional imaging with CT/magnetic resonance (MR).
- *Computed tomography (CT)* is the primary radiological investigation to assess injury to the vertebral column.
- *Magnetic resonance imaging (MRI).* All patients with neurological symptoms or signs need an MRI scan to assess injury to the spinal cord, intervertebral discs and ligaments. Short T1 inversion recovery MRI sequences (fat supressed T2) are particularly sensitive to the presence of ligamentous injury.

The neurological injury

Mechanism of cord injury

Cord compression

The cord may be compressed by bone, intervertebral disc or haematoma. It is particularly common when a previous abnormality exists, such as spinal canal narrowing most often seen in the context of cervical spondylosis. Bilateral facet joint dislocation, in which the spinal cord is compressed in a compromised canal at the level of the dislocation, is often associated with incomplete or complete spinal cord injury.

Direct injury

Open injuries, or shards of fractured bone may penetrate the neural canal and injure the spinal cord.

Ischaemia

A vascular insult to the spinal cord may result in neurological deficit, which may be exacerbated by cord oedema. The blood supply to the cord is from the anterior spinal artery and paired posterior spinal arteries. Ischaemia may result from an associated aortic injury such as a dissection.

Box 18.1 Examining neurological injury

The examination of spinal injuries requires a full neurological examination with recording of sensation, power and reflexes. The components of sensation include light touch, vibration and joint position sense (dorsal columns), and temperature and pain (spinothalamic tract). Abnormalities should be noted in relation to both dermatome and, in the case of peripheral nerve injuries, innervation.

Motor responses should be examined in relation to spinal level.

Movement	Muscle responsible	Innervation
Arm abduction	Deltoid	C5, 6
Elbow flexion	Biceps	C5, 6
Wrist extension	Forearm extensors	C6, 7
Elbow extension	Triceps	C7, 8
Finger abduction	Intrinsic muscles of hand	T1
Hip flexion	Iliopsoas	L2, 3
Knee extension	Quadriceps femoris	L3, 4
Foot dorsiflexion	Tibialis anterior, extensor hallucis longus, extensor digitorum longus	L4, 5
Knee flexion	Hamstrings	L5, S1
Hallux extension	Extensor hallucis longus	L5
Foot plantarflexion	Gastrocnemius, soleus, tibialis posterior, flexor hallucis longus, flexor digitorum longus	S1, 2
Anal tone	Anal sphincter	S2, 3, 4

Motor responses should be graded according to the Medical Research Council (MRC) scale:

0 Total paralysis
1 Flicker of movement
2 Active movement with gravity eliminated
3 Normal movement against gravity but not against additional resistance
4 Movement against both gravity and resistance, but less than normal
5 Normal power

The reflexes are innervated as follows:

Biceps	C5, 6
Triceps	C7, 8
Knee	L3, 4
Ankle	S1, 2

- *Plantar reflex.* Extension is abnormal and indicates an upper motor neurone lesion (brain or spinal cord).

Two other reflexes are useful in the assessment of patients with spinal cord injuries, the presence of which suggests an incomplete cord lesion:

- *Bulbocavernosus reflex.* Contraction of the anal sphincter in response to pinching of the penile shaft.
- *Anal reflex.* Contraction of the anus in response to stroking of the perianal skin.

Types of neurological injury

Spinal contusion

Functional continuity is not lost, paralysis below the level of injury is incomplete and recovery may start within a few hours. Full return of function is possible.

Complete spinal cord injury

Loss of all neurological function below the level of the injury is irrecoverable, as the axons within the cord have no power of regeneration. There is an initial period of spinal shock with complete flaccid paralysis, loss of tendon reflexes, atonicity of the bladder (which becomes distended), faecal retention and priapism. This phase may last for a few days. The cord below the level of injury then recovers reflex function, and the paralysis becomes associated with increased muscle tone (spasticity) and with muscle spasms. The plantar responses become extensor, and the bladder and bowel may begin to empty spontaneously (Box 18.2).

> **Box 18.2 Components of neurological injury**
>
> The neurological injury following spinal cord damage can be divided into three components.
>
> **Sensory loss**
> Somatic and visceral sensations are lost below the level of injury. Hyperaesthesia may be present at the level of injury.
>
> **Motor loss**
> Spinal cord injuries result in an upper motor neurone spastic paralysis with increased reflexes. Cauda equina injuries, being injuries of nerve roots, produce a lower motor neurone paralysis characterized by reduced tone and loss of reflexes.
>
> **Autonomic loss**
> Loss of sympathetic outflow results in hypotension as a result of loss of vasomotor tone. Thermoregulation, which also depends on vasomotor activity, is also impaired. Sphincter control is also autonomic. With injuries above the level of the sacral outflow, the spinal reflex arc triggering micturition remains intact so the bladder can empty automatically. Injuries below this level interrupt the reflex and an atonic bladder results.

Cauda equina injury

This may complicate fractures below the conus, which is usually at the lower border of the first lumbar vertebra. There is saddle anaesthesia (over the buttocks, anus and perineum), weakness of the lower leg muscles, absent ankle reflexes and painless urinary retention. The cauda equina are peripheral nerve fibres and possess some regenerative potential provided the continuity of the nerve root is not lost. Recovery is rarely complete if compression is prolonged.

Combined cord and cauda equina injury

As many spinal injuries take place at the thoracolumbar junction, there can be a combination of spinal cord and nerve root injury. For example, a fracture dislocation at the T12/L1 junction may injure the cord at the first sacral segment but clinical examination may reveal paralysis being due to damage to the spinal roots as they pass the site of the fracture dislocation (Figure 18.3). In this instance, the roots may recover with return of knee and hip movement, although the sacral paralysis will be permanent.

Cord injury syndromes

Although other patterns of injury may occur, the three most common syndromes of cord injury are as follows.

Anterior cord syndrome

Injury to the anterior part of the spinal cord as a result of hyperflexion or occlusion of the anterior spinal artery causes paralysis below the injury (involvement of the pyramidal tracts) with loss of pain and temperature sensation (involvement of the anterior spinothalamic tracts) but preserved touch, movement and vibration sense (posterior column involvement).

Central cord syndrome

Occurs following ischaemia or trauma e.g. a hyperextension injury in the cervical spine in the elderly. Sensory and motor fibres for the legs are situated more peripherally in the cord than those for the arms, so central cord swelling results in greater neurological impairment in the arms than the legs. In the arms, there is a mixture of upper and lower motor neurone damage while in the legs the weakness is predominantly upper motor neurone (spastic paralysis).

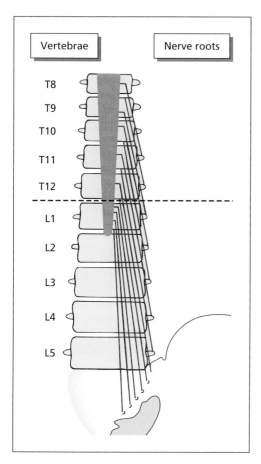

Figure 18.3 The relationship of the spinal cord and nerve roots to the vertebrae. Because of the disparity between the two, a fracture dislocation at the thoracolumbar junction, shown here by the dotted line may injure the sacral segments of the spinal cord together with injury to the lumbar nerve roots.

Brown-Séquard syndrome[3]

A unilateral penetrating injury of the spinal cord may cause loss of power on the affected side (ipsilateral pyramidal tract), loss of joint position and vibration sense (ipsilateral dorsal column) and loss of pain and temperature sensation on the opposite side to the

[3] Charles Edward Brown-Séquard (1817–1894), born in Mauritius, trained in Paris. Neurologist at the National Hospital for Nervous Diseases, London, and later Professor of Medicine at Harvard, Boston, MA, USA, and then the Collège de France in Paris, France.

lesion (the spinothalamic tract). Such an injury is often partial, and rarely occurs after a closed injury.

Treatment of spinal injuries

The treatment of spinal injuries depends on whether or not there has been neurological injury, and also upon the stability of the fracture.

Immediate management

Spinal injury should be suspected in anyone following severe trauma or who is unconscious following trauma. In addition, any patient with sensory or motor symptoms following minor trauma should be treated as having had a spinal injury until proved otherwise. Protection of the airway is paramount. Before such a patient is moved, neck movements should be minimized with a collar and the patient carefully moved onto a properly designed stretcher for transfer. Provided a patient is lying down, they will not come to further harm. Patients should not lie on hard surfaces for prolonged periods as their skin integrity may be compromised.

Airway management and circulatory support are the immediate considerations. The principles are the same as those following head injury. In addition, following spinal cord injury, loss of sympathetic tone may lead to vasodilation and hypotension, on top of any blood loss that may result from trauma, and so replacing circulating volume is important to prevent ischaemia.

Treatment with no neurological injury

Stable fractures of the spine are treated by a short initial period of bed rest, to allow the associated soft tissue injury to subside and pain to become manageable. Patients should be out of bed as soon as possible with support from physiotherapists.

Potentially unstable fractures require more active intervention in order to minimize the small risk of secondary neurological injury and to reduce deformity. A fracture/dislocation with cord compression and incomplete neurological injury is an indication for urgent operative reduction and fixation.

Unstable cervical fractures should be managed by open reduction and internal fixation when facilities are available. Closed reduction and traction are no longer in widespread use in developed countries. A Halo vest remains a good method of immobilizing the cervical spine when internal fixation is either not possible or not available.

Thoracolumbar burst fractures are often treated by operative reduction and internal fixation to relieve pain, allow early mobilization and reduce the risk of deformity.

Treatment of paraplegia or tetraplegia

The patient is transported in a neutral position to a spinal or neurosurgical centre, the spine being supported by suitably arranged pillows and the patient being moved from side to side to relieve pressure on the skin. The distended bladder should be catheterized under full aseptic precautions to prevent infection.

The following are the main principles of treatment.

- *Management of a complete spinal cord injury.* A complete injury is one where there is no motor or sensory function below the level of the injury. There will be no neurological recovery and there is no indication for emergency intervention.
- *Management of an incomplete spinal cord injury.* If the injury is incomplete and there is evidence of spinal cord compression then decompression and internal fixation should be organized as soon as feasible but only when the patient is stable.
- *Management of the spinal column injury.* Open reduction and internal fixation of the fracture as soon as the patient is haemodynamically stable (i.e. urgent not emergency surgery) allows early mobilization and reduces the risk of complications associated with prolonged bed rest.
- *Care of the skin.* Pressure sores may develop very quickly in the first weeks because of the combination of anaesthesia and immobilization. Two-hourly turning and meticulous skin care are required.
- *The bladder.* In the initial phase of complete bladder paralysis, acute urinary retention is common and continuous catheter drainage by means of a urethral catheter is necessary. The vast majority of patients will need permanent urinary diversion usually with a suprapubic catheter, intermittent self-catheterization or an indwelling urethral catheter.
- *The bowels.* Acute spinal injury results in paralytic ileus. Following recovery of motility, constipation is common and is best managed by regular enemas.

Faecal impaction must be avoided and the rectum emptied by digital evacuation.

- *Venous thromboembolism prophylaxis.* Patients with paralysis of the legs following spinal cord injury are at risk of venous thrombosis and pulmonary emboli. Prophylaxis with subcutaneous low molecular weight heparin should be instituted and continued as long as necessary.
- *Rehabilitation.* Active development of muscles with an intact or partial innervation by expert physiotherapy can restore mobility in many patients with significant neurological injury. Patients have complex rehabilitation and enablement needs, which are best delivered in dedicated spinal cord injury centres.

Age-related (degenerative) spinal disorders

Age-related spinal disorders arise from changes in the intervertebral joints and intervertebral discs. Axial spinal pain is multifactorial and poorly characterized. Occasionally, age-related changes result in compression of the neural structures. These are the spinal cord (myelopathy), nerve roots (radiculopathy) and cauda equina (neurogenic claudication or cauda equina syndrome).

Clinical presentations associated with age-related changes

- *Back or neck (axial) pain* may be associated with age-related changes but there is a very poor correlation between radiological findings and symptoms in patients with non-specific low back or neck pain. Some patients develop an abnormal curvature of the spine (scoliosis) which may be associated with pain.
- *Radiculopathy*, causing pain and lower motor neurone symptoms, arises from compression of nerve roots either in the spinal canal or as they exit through the intervertebral foramina. Compression may be due to disc prolapse, facet joint hypertrophy, ligamentous thickening or osteophytes.
- *Degenerative cervical myelopathy* causes upper motor neurone symptoms and results from compression of the spinal cord. It can be caused by

prolapse of an intervertebral disc, ligamentous and facet joint hypertrophy and osteophytes encroaching into the spinal canal. Myelopathy occurs more frequently in patients with congenital narrowing of the spinal canal.

- *Neurogenic claudication* may arise as a result of lumbar canal stenosis. Symptoms overlap with those resulting from peripheral vascular disease. There is usually bilateral leg pain with sensory disturbance that is worse when standing or walking and relieved promptly by sitting down. Walking distance may be reduced to less than 100 m before the patient has to sit or bend forwards to relieve their symptoms. In contrast, symptoms of claudication from vascular disease are often unilateral, worse when walking uphill and relieved by standing.

Prolapsed intervertebral disc

Disc herniation (prolapse) comprises a protrusion of disc material posteriorly into the spinal canal. Disc prolapse is common and can be triggered by minor events but is often associated with bending, lifting and twisting. The most common levels in the lumbar spine are between L4/L5 and L5/S1. Cervical disc protrusions are most common at C5/C6 and C6/C7. Disc prolapses occur more frequently in younger patients and neurological symptoms in older patients are more often associated with age-related changes in the spine.

Lumbar disc herniation

Clinical features

The onset of symptoms is often with low back pain and patients often report a specific time of onset following straining or heavy lifting. The majority of patients complain of leg pain (sciatica) radiating from the buttock down the back of the thigh and knee and down the lateral side of the leg to the foot. There may be paraesthesiae or altered sensation in the foot. This pain is made worse by coughing, sneezing or straining (all of which raise intrathecal pressure) or by straight leg raising (which stretches the inflamed nerve root across the disc prolapse). Sometimes there may be motor weakness affecting dorsiflexion (L5) or plantar flexion (S1). A central lumbar disc prolapse, if large enough, can fill the

spinal canal causing compression of the cauda equina with bilateral leg pain and disturbance of bladder, bowel and sexual function (cauda equina syndrome).

Examination may reveal flattening of the normal lumbar lordosis, lateral curvature of the spine and reduced spinal movements. The para-spinal muscles are in spasm and straight leg raising is limited and painful. There may be weakness of the ankle and sensory loss on the medial side of the dorsum of the foot and the great toe (L5) which suggests an L4/L5 disc lesion. Sensory loss on the lateral side of the foot (S1) and loss of the ankle reflex may occur in L5/S1 disc lesions.

Special investigations

- *Magnetic resonance imaging (MRI) of the spine* will reveal vertebral fractures (common in elderly osteoporotic spines), bone marrow changes (in metastatic disease) and compression of the neural structures in the spinal canal or neural foramina.
- *Computed tomography (CT)* is the primary modality for imaging patients following trauma.
- *Inflammatory markers including C-reactive protein (CRP) are normally raised in spinal infection.* Haematological and biochemical screening can be helpful in detecting otherwise unsuspected malignancy.

Differential diagnosis

This includes other causes of radicular pain including lateral recess and lumbar canal stenosis, spondylolisthesis (ventral subluxation), spinal tumours and rarely lesions affecting the sacral plexus such as tumours of the prostate or rectum. Intermittent claudication can usually be differentiated by careful history, examination and a Doppler probe. An abdominal aortic aneurysm may occasionally cause low back pain.

Treatment

Severe acute pain is treated with analgesia including anti-inflammatories and an initial period of rest. As soon as the patient is more comfortable, gentle mobilization should start. Without treatment, most lumbar disc prolapses will heal and the symptoms they cause will resolve spontaneously. Most people get better without any medical intervention and after three months seventy per cent of people will have had significant reduction in their leg pain. An epidural or nerve root block may provide relief of symptoms during this period. A spinal injection cannot cure the underlying pressure on the nerve, which is the cause of the pain, but may provide significant pain relief while waiting for the disc prolapse to heal. Operative treatment of the prolapsed disc is indicated if conservative measures fail, if repeated attacks occur or if the symptoms severely impair an individual's quality of life. If bladder sphincter disturbance occurs and an MRI scan reveals a large central disc prolapse filling the spinal canal with loss of CSF signal from the dural sac, then surgical decompression with excision of the prolapsed disc fragment must be performed without avoidable delay.

Spinal stenosis

The cross-sectional area of the spinal canal follows a normal distribution in the population. Patients with congenital narrowing are more likely to develop symptoms of spinal stenosis as the normal age-related changes become superimposed on the pre-existing narrowing. These changes include thickening of the ligamentum flavum, over growth of the facet joints and changes in vertebral body alignment (spondylolisthesis). Symptomatic lumbar canal stenosis only occurs with significant reduction in the cross-sectional area to less than 20% of normal and most frequently occurs at L4/5 and L3/4.

The clinical features overlap with intermittent vascular claudication (see Chapter 12), but in spinal claudication the patient presents with pain, numbness and weakness in the legs brought on by standing or walking, and, in contrast to vascular claudication, it is not relieved by standing still but by sitting down or bending forwards. Neurological examination of the legs is usually normal.

The diagnosis is confirmed by MRI (or CT if patients are unable to have an MRI) which shows a reduction of the cross-sectional area of the lumbar spinal canal. Once stenosis is severe and symptomatic, decompression surgery will provide effective relief of symptoms. Minimally invasive techniques allow adequate decompression, minimize operative morbidity and allow early mobilization and discharge from hospital.

Cervical spondylosis

Cervical spondylosis refers to age-related (degenerative) changes that occur in the neck, with similar pathological processes to those that occur in the lumbar spine. In the cervical spine, these changes can be associated with spinal cord compression (myelopathy) and nerve root compression (radiculopathy).

Clinical features

Non-specific neck pain is common. Radicular symptoms include severe pain radiating into the arm accompanied by sensory disturbance in a specific dermatome. Patients with myelopathy often present with numb, clumsy hands, impaired balance and difficulty walking. Occasionally, patients notice a change in bladder function, most often urinary frequency and urgency. Examination of the arms can reveal a mixture of lower and upper motor neurone signs. In cervical myelopathy, examination of the legs will reveal upper motor neurone findings with increased tone, leg weakness (especially hip flexion), brisk reflexes and extensor plantars.

Differential diagnosis

The differential diagnosis of cervical myelopathy includes spinal tumour, multiple sclerosis and motor neurone disease. When arm pain alone is present, the differential diagnosis includes a cervical rib, carpal tunnel syndrome and angina pectoris.

Treatment

Radiculopathy usually settles with conservative treatment, including early rest and anti-inflammatory medication with gentle physiotherapy once the pain begins to settle. The natural history and indications for surgery are the same for a prolapsed cervical disc as for a lumbar disc prolapse.

Spinal infection

An abscess in the extradural (epidural) spinal compartment can either be blood-borne infection as part of a *Staphylococcus aureus* septicaemia or is often associated with spondylodiscitis (osteomyelitis) of the spine. Diagnosis is often delayed due to an insidious presentation in patients with other comorbidities.

Clinical features

Clinical features are progressive local pain, fever, malaise and anorexia, and in rare cases, rapidly progressive paraplegia. The white blood cell count may be raised, CRP and erythrocyte sedimentation rate (ESR) are elevated and the diagnosis is confirmed with contrast enhanced MRI.

Treatment

If there is an abscess in the spinal canal, then urgent treatment is required to drain any pus usually via a posterior or postero-lateral approach. In patients with spinal infection, the causative organism should be identified with repeated blood cultures and CT-guided aspiration/biopsy. Prolonged intravenous antibiotic therapy is started, preferably guided by the results of culture and sensitivities. The involvement of infectious diseases specialists is needed to guide antibiotic therapy. Patients with profound neurological deficits can make a worthwhile recovery but delay in diagnosis and treatment carries with it the risk of permanent cord damage.

Spinal tumours

Spinal tumours are conveniently classified, from both the pathological and clinical points of view, into those which occur outside the dura (extradural), those inside the dura but outside the spinal cord (intradural, extramedullary) and those occurring within the substance of the spinal cord (intramedullary).

The tumours most commonly encountered are the following.

1 *Extradural.*
   a Metastatic spinal tumours – are by far the most common spinal tumour and are usually found in the vertebral body. The primary is most commonly the breast, kidney or prostate.
   b Primary vertebral bony tumours – (e.g. osteoclastoma, chondrosarcoma, Ewing's tumour and osteosarcoma.).
   c Haematological malignancies – Lymphoma including Hodgkin's disease and myeloma.

2 *Intradural extramedullary.*
   a Meningioma.
   b Schwannoma.
3 *Intramedullary* (rare).
   a Astrocytoma.
   b Ependymoma.
   c Haemangioblastoma which can be sporadic or be found in patients with von Hippel-Lindau disease[4].

Clinical features

The three groups of spinal tumours listed above each tend to have a fairly distinctive clinical picture.

- *Metastatic tumours.* Commonly there is a pre-existing diagnosis of cancer. There can be weeks or even months of back pain and sometimes radicular pain. Progressive cord compression leading to postural pain and paraplegia can occur.
- *The intradural extramedullary tumours* are usually slow growing and benign. As the tumour increases in size, cord compression takes place with neurological symptoms resulting in weakness with a sensory level at or below the site of the tumour. Neurological examination reveals upper motor neurone signs with increased tendon reflexes and extensor plantar responses. Urinary symptoms are typically urgency and frequency.

  Cauda equina tumours cause lower motor neurone signs with weakness, which may be radicular, diminished reflexes and impairment of bladder and bowel control.
- *The intramedullary tumours* may be accompanied by axial pain and followed by a slow and delayed onset of motor weakness below the lesion. There may be a suspended (normal above and below the lesion) dissociated sensory loss, with loss of pain and temperature (spinothalamic tract) but preservation of vibration and position sense (dorsal column) initially which may be lost later on in the progress of the disease.

---

[4] Eugen von Hippel (1867–1939), Professor of Ophthalmology, Göttingen, Germany, described haemangiomas in the eye; Arvid Lindau (1892–1958), Pathologist, Lund, Sweden, described haemangioblastomas in the brain and spinal cord of affected individuals.

Differential diagnosis

Spinal tumours are relatively uncommon and most occur in patients over 60 years who are being investigated for gait disturbance. In this group, the main differential diagnosis is of age-related disorders such as degenerative cervical myelopathy and thoracic disc prolapse. In younger patients, inflammatory lesions such as multiple sclerosis may present with spinal cord lesions but careful history taking often distinguishes these pathologies.

Special investigations

- *MRI with contrast enhancement* is the definitive investigation and provides precise localization of the level of the tumour and its relationship to the spinal cord and other structures.
- *CT myelography* may rarely be necessary in patients who are unable to have an MRI scan.
- *X-rays of the spine* are no longer indicated in the investigation of patients with spinal pain/symptoms.

Treatment

Many intradural tumours can be safely removed using modern microsurgical techniques. Localization of the correct spinal level is fundamental and is achieved with intraoperative X-rays and cross-referencing the MRI scan to these intraoperative films. Wherever possible, the tumour is completely excised and this can normally be achieved in meningiomas, schwannomas, ependymomas and haemangioblastomas. In meningiomas, careful consideration needs to be given to excising the dural origin, which reduces the risk of recurrence but increases morbidity associated with a postoperative CSF leak.

In metastatic tumours, radiotherapy and chemotherapy are the mainstay of treatment in the majority of patients. Surgery has a role in highly selected patients with a good prognosis and postural pain.

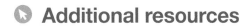 **Additional resources**

Case 36: A spinal abnormality in a newborn child
Case 37: Back injury

19

Peripheral nerve injuries

Ian Grant

Learning objectives

✓ To know the different types of acute and chronic peripheral nerve injuries and their prognosis.

✓ To be able to recognize the pattern of symptoms and signs associated with injury to the major peripheral nerves in the upper and lower limbs.

The central nervous system is protected by the bones of the skull and spine. The peripheral nervous system is vulnerable to acute and chronic injury as a consequence of compression, traction and division. The potential for a peripheral nerve to recover from injury is dependent upon the extent of the injury, and the proximity of the injury to the target organ.

Classification

Acute peripheral nerve injuries

Acute peripheral nerve injuries are commonly the result of laceration, traction (stretching) or compression (crush) injuries. There are three types of injury.

1 *Neurapraxia.* This is the mildest and most transient peripheral nerve injury. It is associated with localized loss of the myelin around the axons of the injured nerve (demyelination). As a consequence, the amplitude and velocity of electrical conduction is greatly diminished causing temporary weakness or numbness which resolves in most patients within 4–6 weeks.

2 *Axonotmesis.* This is injury to the axon and myelin sheath without disruption of the continuity of its perineural sheath. The axons distal to the lesion degenerate (Wallerian degeneration[1]) leaving the endoneurium (the connective tissue around the axons) as a scaffold. Axons and Schwann cells migrate from the proximal injured nerve at approximately 1 mm/day; therefore, the time to recovery depends upon the distance between the injury and end organ. The rate of recovery can be followed by tapping the path of the injured nerve and at suitable intervals mapping the point of maximal tenderness which represents the leading point of the advancing regenerating axons (The Hoffmann-Tinel sign).

3 *Neurotmesis.* This is the physical division of a peripheral nerve. Regeneration will only occur if the fascicles of the proximal and distal ends of the nerve are in close intimacy (or are sutured together). In the absence of treatment, most divided nerves will produce a tender lump called a neuroma.

A peripheral nerve contains a large number of individual fibres, so it is quite possible in a nerve injury for some fibres to suffer from a mixture of neurapraxia, axonotmesis and neurotmesis.

Ellis and Calne's Lecture Notes in General Surgery, Fourteenth Edition.
Edited by Christopher Watson and Justin Davies.
© 2023 John Wiley & Sons Ltd. Published 2023 by John Wiley & Sons Ltd.
Companion website: www.wiley.com/go/Watson/GeneralSurgery14

[1] Augustus Waller (1816–1870), a General Practitioner in London, UK, for 10 years before working as a Physiologist in Bonn, Germany, Paris, France and Birmingham, UK.

Chronic peripheral nerve injuries

Chronic peripheral nerve injuries are commonly the result of compression or traction over a period of 6 weeks or more. This can be a consequence of entrapment below a ligament (e.g. carpal tunnel syndrome), or pressure from a prominent bone or soft tissue structure (e.g. the median nerve neuropathy occasionally seen after malunion of a distal radial fracture), or persistent traction (e.g. the ulna nerve neuropathy seen in throwing athletes as a consequence of repetitive elbow flexion).

Patients initially report episodic symptoms such as tingling, pain, weakness and numbness. This is thought to be caused by cycles of demyelination and remyelination of the injured nerve. If the cause is left untreated, the symptoms are likely to worsen and become continuous, and eventually the disability becomes irreversible.

Patients with systemic conditions affecting the peripheral nerve system (such as insulin dependent diabetes) or with inherited neuropathies that affect the ability to produce myelin (such as Charcot-Marie-Tooth disease) are more vulnerable to chronic peripheral nerve injuries.

Special investigations

Electrophysiological studies assess the speed and amplitude of electrical conduction through a peripheral nerve (*nerve conduction studies)* and the electrical activity with the target muscle (*electromyography*, *EMG*). This can help localize the site of injury in a symptomatic patient.

For an acute injury with a peripheral nerve thought to be 'in-continuity', it can help distinguish between neurapraxia and axonotmesis. For a nerve that cannot be readily explored or imaged, it can help distinguish between axonotmesis and neurotmesis.

Neurapraxia and axonotmesis

Those joints whose muscles have been paralysed are splinted in the position of function to avoid contractures. They are put through passive movements several times a day so that, when recovery of the nerve lesion occurs, the joints will be fully mobile.

Neurotmesis

Best outcomes are achieved with early repair (ideally within 4 days of injury) of the divided nerve using an operating microscope. The proximal and distal ends of the nerve are sequentially resected until healthy fascicles are visible before repair is started. The fascicles of the proximal and distal nerve ends are aligned and the epineurium approximated using fine sutures.

If a tension-free anastomosis is not possible, a nerve graft may be required. This can be a section of a less valuable nerve such as the sural nerve. Smaller nerve gaps of <1 cm can be bridged with a conduit such as a section of vein or a commercial product. Generally, the recovery of sensibility after nerve repair is, at best, partial, and the muscle strength is reduced.

Nerve transfers

When a nerve is acutely injured proximally, the denervated target muscle will maintain the potential for recovery for about one year. If the nerve does not reach the target muscle within this period, the muscle atrophies, motor end plates disappear and any capacity for regeneration is lost. Patients with proximal nerve injuries can benefit from a nerve transfer in which a branch of an un-injured adjacent nerve is anastomosed distally to the nerve fascicles heading towards the target muscle. For example, in a patient with a proximal ulnar nerve injury in the upper arm, the anterior interosseous branch of the median nerve can be anastomosed to the side of the motor fascicle of the ulnar nerve at the wrist. This gives early recovery of the intrinsic muscles of the hand which are supplied by the ulnar nerve (which would otherwise atrophy due to the prolonged wait of over a year for the regenerating axons of the injured ulnar nerve to reach the hand).

Tendon transfers

If restoration of nerve function cannot be achieved after injury or where the prognosis for recovery is poor, tendon transfers may allow the patient to perform movements that would otherwise be impossible. For example, wrist drop after a radial nerve lesion may be treated by transposing the pronator teres muscle (supplied by the median nerve) onto the dorsum of the wrist and connecting the tendon to the paralysed wrist extensor tendons.

It is beyond the scope of this chapter to discuss lesions of all the individual nerves, but a few important peripheral nerve injuries will be mentioned.

Brachial plexus injuries

Upper trunk lesions (Erb's paralysis[2])

An acute injury of the upper trunk of the brachial plexus occurs when the patient's head is forced away from the shoulder, for example in a fall from a motor cycle. It may also occur as an obstetric injury. Injury to the upper trunk of the brachial plexus, or the C5 and C6 nerve roots, results in paralysis of the biceps, brachialis, brachioradialis, supinator, supraspinatus, infraspinatus and deltoid. The limb will assume the 'waiter's tip' position, being internally rotated with the forearm pronated (owing to the loss of the powerful supinating action of biceps). The arm hangs vertically (deltoid paralysis) and the elbow cannot be flexed (biceps and brachialis). There will be an area of impaired sensation over the outer side of the upper arm. Patients should be referred for assessment at a specialist centre.

Patients that have sustained neurapraxia or axonotmesis have the potential for recovery. Patients that have sustained neurotmesis can potentially benefit from exploration of the injury and repair of the divided nerves (usually with nerve grafts). In more severe injuries in which the nerve roots are avulsed, there is no potential for nerve repair. These patients are dependent upon improvements achieved by nerve and tendon transfers.

T1 injury (Klumpke's paralysis[3])

This can be caused by acute forced abduction of the shoulder for example when falling from a height and reaching out to grasp and to attempt to prevent the fall, or from an obstetric injury in a child delivered in a breech position. Chronic injuries can be caused by compression from structures in the neck such as a

[2] Wilhelm Erb (1840–1921), Professor of Neurology, Heidelberg, Germany.

[3] Auguste Dejerine-Klumpke (1859–1927), Neurologist, Paris, France.

cervical rib. The small muscles of the hand are wasted and there is loss of sensation on the inner side of the forearm. There may also be Horner's syndrome owing to associated damage of sympathetic fibres passing to the inferior cervical ganglion (see later in this chapter).

Radial nerve injuries (Figure 19.1a)

The radial nerve is most commonly acutely injured by a fracture of the humerus involving the spiral groove where the nerve is closely applied to the posterior aspect of the midshaft of the bone. The nerve supply to the triceps comes off the radial nerve before it enters the spiral groove, and the lesions distal to that point will not affect extension of the elbow. The patient will be unable to actively extend their wrist (sometimes called wrist drop) because of paralysis of the wrist extensors. If the nerve is divided or is crushed as the consequence of a iatrogenic injury from surgery to the fracture, the patient is best served by urgent exploration and nerve repair. Acute traction injuries associated with an absence of any loss of nerve continuity usually recover spontaneously.

Median nerve injuries (Figure 19.1b)

The median nerve may be acutely injured in fractures around the elbow joint (such as a supracondylar fracture of the distal humerus) or laceration of the forearm or wrist. In proximal injuries above the elbow, the pronators of the forearm and flexors of the wrist and fingers will be involved, with the exception of the flexor carpi ulnaris and the medial half of the flexor digitorum profundus, which are supplied by the ulnar nerve and which produce ulnar deviation of the wrist. Whether the injury is in the forearm or wrist, there will be paralysis of the abductor pollicis muscle at the base of the thumb, resulting in significant disability as the patient is unable to lift their thumb to allow it to oppose to the other digits. The associated sensory loss is significant, as humans generally explore the world with the combination of the thumb, index and middle fingers. This pattern of numbness makes it difficult for fine movements such as those required to fasten buttons.

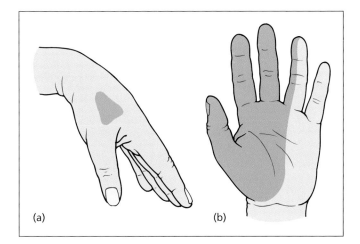

Figure 19.1 (a) Radial nerve injury: wrist drop, together with anaesthesia of a small area of the dorsal aspect of the hand at the base of the thumb and index finger. (b) Median nerve injury: thenar eminence paralysis with anaesthesia of the palmar aspect of the radial three and a half digits and corresponding palm.

Median nerve compression at the wrist (carpal tunnel syndrome)

The median nerve can be compressed as it passes through the carpal tunnel (formed by the flexor retinaculum stretching from the hook of the hamate and pisiform medially to the trapezium and scaphoid laterally). This results in a chronic compression neuropathy of the median nerve. Symptoms include tingling, diminished sensibility and weakness in the hand as well as pain in the hand and forearm. In the early and mild stage of carpal tunnel syndrome, the symptoms are episodic and worse at night (patients are often woken from sleep).

In the later and more severe stage, the symptoms are continuous. The thenar muscle area of the hand can become wasted. Women are affected four times more commonly than men, and there is an association with systemic conditions including obesity and diabetes, and also with pregnancy. In most patients, the diagnosis can be made from review of the history, and the severity confirmed by examination. Patients with mild carpal tunnel syndrome may benefit from weight loss, use of a splint across the wrist at night, and injection of steroids into the carpal tunnel. Severe carpal tunnel syndrome is effectively treated by surgery to divide the flexor retinaculum at the wrist.

Ulnar nerve injuries (Figure 19.2)

The ulnar nerve is acutely injured by fractures around the elbow joint, penetrating injuries to the upper inner arm and by lacerations of the forearm and the wrist. Chronic compression of the nerve occurs at the

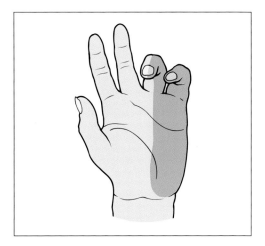

Figure 19.2 Ulnar nerve injury: *main en griffe* with anaesthesia of the ulnar one and a half digits and ulnar border of the hand on both palmar and dorsal aspects.

elbow (in the cubital tunnel) and less commonly at the wrist (Guyon's canal[4]).

The ulnar nerve supplies all the intrinsic muscles of the hand apart from the three muscles of the thenar eminence (abductor pollicis brevis, opponens pollicis and flexor pollicis brevis) and the two radial lumbricals, all of which are supplied by the median nerve. The affected intrinsic muscles are the adductor pollicis, the muscles of the hypothenar eminence, the ulnar two lumbricals and the interossei, which are the abductors and adductors of the fingers and which also extend the interphalangeal joints. In the forearm, the ulnar nerve supplies flexor carpi ulnaris and the medial half of flexor digitorum profundus.

The function of the ulnar nerve can be reliably assessed by testing the patient's capacity to adduct the thumb (using adductor pollicis) towards the index finger (Froment's test[5]).

Damage to the ulnar nerve produces the 'claw hand deformity' or *main en griffe*. This posture results from the unopposed action of the long flexors and extensors of the fingers. The paralysed intrinsic muscles of the hand are normally responsible for flexion of the metacarpophalangeal joints of the fingers. These joints are, therefore, extended in an ulnar nerve palsy. The flexor profundus and sublimis, flex the distal and middle phalanges at the interphalangeal joints, and these joints are held in a flexed posture. The patient is unable to make a normal grip around an object and instead flexes the interphalangeal joints pushing an object down the palm.

If the nerve is injured at the elbow, flexor digitorum profundus to the fourth and fifth finger is paralysed so that, rather anomalously, the clawing of these fingers is less intense than in injuries at the wrist. Paralysis of flexor carpi ulnaris produces a tendency to radial deviation at the wrist. In late cases, wasting of the intrinsic muscles is readily evident on inspecting the dorsum of the hand and the web space between the thumb and index finger. Sensory loss occurs over the dorsal and palmar aspects of the ulnar one and a half digits and the ulnar border of the hand on both palmar and dorsal aspects.

If the ulnar nerve is divided at the level of the wrist, the sensory loss is confined to the palmar surface, as the dorsal branch of the ulnar nerve, supplying the dorsal aspects of the ulnar one and a half fingers, is given off 5 cm proximal to the wrist and thus escapes injury.

Division of the ulnar nerve leaves a surprisingly efficient hand. The long flexors enable a good grip to be achieved; the thumb, apart from the loss of adductor pollicis, is intact, and the important sensation over the palm of the hand is largely maintained. Indeed, it may be difficult to be certain clinically that the nerve is injured. A reliable test is loss of the ability to abduct and adduct the fingers with the hand laid flat, palm downwards, on a table. This eliminates the trick movements of adduction and abduction of the fingers occurring as part of their flexion and extension, respectively.

Ulnar nerve compression at the elbow (cubital tunnel syndrome)

The ulnar nerve may be compressed as it passes through the cubital tunnel between the two heads of flexor carpi ulnaris and behind the medial epicondyle and medial collateral ligament of the elbow. In many patients, this is an idiopathic condition, but it can be caused by persistent elbow flexion, localized swelling, and fractures or arthritis of the elbow. Compression results in weakness in the hand and paraesthesia (numbness and tingling) in the ring and little fingers (and the ulnar border of the patient's hand). In patients with compression of the ulnar nerve at the wrist in Guyon's canal, the pattern of numbness is confined to the patient's fingers. Symptoms are worse at night.

Nerve conduction studies can confirm the diagnosis and its severity. Conservative treatment with elbow splints, and avoiding flexing or resting on the elbows may help. Surgery, when appropriate, involves division of the roof of the cubital tunnel at the elbow.

---

[4] Jean Casimir Félix Guyon (1831–1920), Professor of Surgical Pathology and Genitourinary Surgery, University of Paris. He described the canal at the start of his surgical training in 1861.

[5] Jules Fromont (1878–1946) described the sign while working with Babinski and examining wounded soldiers in World War 1 at Hôpital Pitié Salpêtrière in Paris.

Differential diagnosis of flexion deformities of the fingers

Ulnar nerve lesion

This has been described above; there is hyperextension of the metacarpophalangeal joints and clawing of the hand, with sensory loss along the ulnar border of the hand and ulnar one and a half fingers.

Dupuytren's contracture[6]

This is a common condition in the elderly, usually male, subject in whom there is fibrosis of the palmar aponeurosis. This produces a flexion deformity of the fingers at the metacarpophalangeal and proximal interphalangeal joints, usually starting at the ring finger and spreading to the little finger and sometimes the middle finger. As the aponeurosis extends distally only to the base of the middle phalanx, the distal interphalangeal joint escapes. The contracture is often bilateral and may occasionally affect the plantar fascia of the foot.

Volkmann's contracture[7] due to ischaemic fibrosis of flexors of the fingers

The fingers will be curled up in the hand with metacarpophalangeal and interphalangeal joint flexion. This deformity can to some extent be relieved by flexion of the wrist when the shortened tendons are no longer so taut and the fingers can be partially extended.

Congenital contracture

This usually affects the little finger and produces very little, if any, disability. The proximal interphalangeal joint is typically affected, the condition is usually bilateral and, by definition, it dates from birth.

[6] Baron Guillaume Dupuytren (1777–1835), Surgeon, Hôtel Dieu, Paris, France.

[7] Richard von Volkmann (1830–1889), Professor of Surgery, Halle, Germany.

Mallet finger

This follows trauma (common in cricketers) with flexion deformity of the distal interphalangeal joint due to avulsion of the extensor tendon insertion to the base of the distal phalanx.

Trauma

Scar formation following burns, injury or surgery to the fingers or the palm may produce gross flexion deformities wherever a scar crosses a joint line.

Sciatic nerve injuries

This nerve may be injured in penetrating injuries or torn in posterior dislocation of the hip associated with fracture of the posterior lip of the acetabulum, to which the nerve is closely related. Injury is followed by paralysis of the hamstrings and all the muscles of the leg and foot; there is loss of all movement below the knee joint with foot drop deformity. Sensory loss is complete below the knee, except for an area extending along the medial side of the leg over the medial malleolus to the base of the hallux, which is innervated by the saphenous branch of the femoral nerve, the longest cutaneous nerve in the body.

Common peroneal nerve injuries

The common peroneal nerve is in a particularly vulnerable subcutaneous position as it winds around the neck of the fibula. It may be injured at this site by direct trauma or compression, such as the pressure of a tight plaster cast, or in severe adduction injuries to the knee. It is the most common peripheral nerve injury in the lower limb and the majority of cases result from iatrogenic causes. Damage is followed by foot drop (due to paralysis of the ankle and foot extensors) and inversion of the foot (due to paralysis of the peroneal muscles with unopposed action of the foot flexors and inverters). There is anaesthesia over the anterior surface of the leg and foot. The medial side of the foot, innervated by the saphenous branch of the femoral nerve, and the lateral side of the foot, supplied by the sural branch of the tibial nerve, both escape.

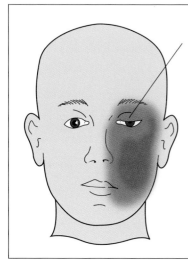

Ptosis: drooping upper eyelid
Enophthalmos: apparent, not real
Meiosis: small pupil

Dry skin and flushing on side of lesion (sudomotor and vasoconstrictor denervation)
Ipsilateral hand often also involved

Figure 19.3 Horner's syndrome.

Lateral cutaneous nerve of the thigh compression: meralgia paraesthetica

The lateral cutaneous nerve of the thigh (L2, 3) may be trapped as it emerges beneath the inguinal ligament, a finger's breadth medial to the anterior superior iliac spine. It commonly occurs in overweight middle-aged men and in athletes undergoing physical training. Symptoms comprise painful paraesthesiae over the anterolateral aspect of the thigh, worse on standing and relieved on sitting (hip flexion). Sensation in the distribution of the nerve is diminished.

Cervical sympathetic nerve injuries: Horner's syndrome[8]

If the T1 contribution to the cervical sympathetic chain is damaged, the result is known as Horner's syndrome (Figure 19.3), in which there are the following characteristics.

- *Meiosis*: paralysis of the dilator pupillae, resulting in constriction of the pupil.
- *Ptosis:* paralysis of the sympathetic muscle fibres transmitted via the oculomotor nerve to the levator palpebrae superioris results in drooping of the upper eyelid.
- *Anhidrosis*: loss of sweating on the affected side of the face and neck.
- *Enophthalmos*: the eye appears sunken within the orbit, an illusion due to the ptosis.

Horner's syndrome may follow operations on, or injuries to, the neck in which the cervical sympathetic trunk is damaged, malignant invasion from lymph nodes or adjacent tumour or spinal cord lesions at the T1 segment (e.g. syringomyelia).

Additional resources

Case 38: A lacerated wrist
Case 39: A hand deformity
Case 40: A deformed finger
Case 41: A boy with a droopy eyelid

---

[8] Johann Horner (1831–1886), Professor of Ophthalmology, Zurich, Switzerland.

The oral cavity

Kanwalraj Moar

Learning objectives

✓ To understand the embryology and anatomy of the oral cavity and lips.
✓ To know the common features of acquired and congenital diseases of the oral cavity and lips.

It is a useful exercise (and a favourite examination topic) to consider what can be learned by examining a specific anatomical site, such as the fingers, nails or eyes, in making a clinical diagnosis. The mouth and tongue can be conveniently used to illustrate how best to deal with this subject, which can be considered under three headings.

1 *Information about local disease.* Tumours of the mouth and tongue and congenital anomalies are diagnosed by local examination.
2 *Local manifestations of disease elsewhere.*
   - *Crohn's disease*: oral ulceration, cobble stoning, gingival hyperplasia, fissuring of lips, perioral erythema and angular cheilitis. Symptoms may precede gastrointestinal disease.
   - *Pernicious anaemia*: smooth tongue.
   - *Agranulocytosis/leukopaenia*: ulcerated mouth with no inflammatory halo.
   - *Leukaemia*: oral ulceration, petechiae, gingival haemorrhage and swelling, loose teeth.
   - *Addison's disease*[1]: brown pigmentation of gingiva and areas of trauma.

- *Peutz–Jeghers syndrome*[2] : perioral pigmentation.
- *Vitamin C deficiency*: swollen bleeding gums and loosened teeth.
- *Hypoglossal nerve palsy:* hemihypertrophy of the tongue.
- *Human immunodeficiency virus (HIV)*: many oral manifestations including candidiasis, hairy leukoplakia, gingivitis, acute necrotizing ulcerative gingivitis (ANUG), Kaposi's Sarcoma, atypical ulceration.
- *Sjogren's Syndrome*: xerostomia leading to caries, candidiasis, dry mucosa and lobulated tongue. Patient symptoms include disturbed taste, speech and swallow and enlarged major salivary glands.
- *Hereditary haemorrhagic telangiectasia*: telangiectasia on lips and intraoral mucosa.

3 *Information given about the general condition and habits of the patient.* Examples include the dry tongue of dehydration, the brown dry tongue of uraemia and the coated tongue with foetor oris of acute appendicitis.

[1] Thomas Addison (1773–1860), Physician, Guy's Hospital, London, UK.

Ellis and Calne's Lecture Notes in General Surgery, Fourteenth Edition. Edited by Christopher Watson and Justin Davies.
© 2023 John Wiley & Sons Ltd. Published 2023 by John Wiley & Sons Ltd.
Companion website: www.wiley.com/go/Watson/GeneralSurgery14

[2] Johannes Peutz (1886–1957), Physician, the Hague, the Netherlands. Harold Jeghers (1940–1990), Professor of Medicine, Georgetown University School of Medicine, Washington, DC, and Tufts University Medical School, Boston, MA, USA.

The oral cavity

The oral cavity (see Figure 20.1) is an integral part of the orofacial skeleton and is a unique combination of hard and soft tissues. It is the cephalic limit of the oro-digestive tract and forms the junction between the external and internal aspects of the body. The external boundary is the vermillion of the lips ante-riorly and buccal mucosa of the cheeks laterally. It extends posterior and inferior where it adjoins the oropharynx, at the anterior pillars of the fauces. Posteriorly, the oropharynx comprises the soft pal-ate, tonsillar fossae, tongue base and posterior and lateral walls inferiorly to the epiglottis. The distinc-tion between oral cavity and oropharynx is of par-ticular importance when treating cancers of the head and neck.

The oral cavity is divided into several regions by the dental alveolus and teeth into the oral vestibule between teeth and cheeks, and the oral cavity proper internally. The hard and soft palate form the superior margin or ceiling. The lower border is lim-ited by oral mucosal membrane overlying the mylo-hyoid muscle and formed from the floor of mouth and tongue.

Embryology

The embryology of the face, oral cavity and lips is complex, but is important in understanding the pathology in this region. The various structures within the orofacial region are derived from the four primary germ layers and summarized as follows:

- *Ectoderm*: enamel of teeth, adjacent oral epithe-lium, tastebuds and major salivary glands.
- *Mesoderm*: muscle of tongue, cementum and peri-odontal ligament of teeth.
- *Endoderm*: minor salivary glands and pharyngeal pouch derivatives.
- *Neural crest*: underlying skeleton, cartilages and musculature, the inner layers of the tooth – dentine and pulp.

Oral facial development is recognizable from 14 days post-conception (see Figure 20.2) with the formation of a prechordal plate in the bilaminar germ disc. This will contribute to the oropharyngeal membrane; a junction of ectoderm and endoderm with no inter-vening mesoderm (mimicked by the cloacal mem-brane of the hindgut) that will separate the primitive oral cavity from the forming pharynx.

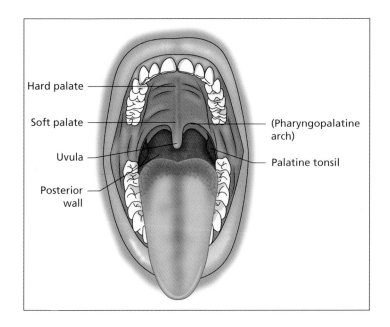

Hard palate

Soft palate

Uvula

Posterior wall

(Pharyngopalatine arch)

Palatine tonsil

Figure 20.1 The oral cavity and oropharynx viewed from the front.

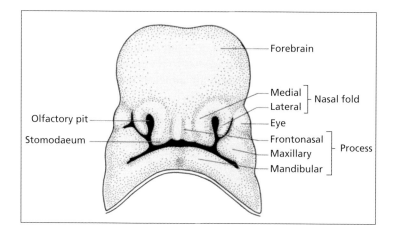

Figure 20.2 The ventral aspect of a foetal head showing the three prominences – frontonasal, maxillary and mandibular – from which the face, nose and jaw are derived.

Facial prominences

The face forms from the three embryological prominences (frontonasal, paired maxillary and paired mandibular) surrounding a central stomodeum (a depression with will go on to become the mouth). The frontonasal prominence will develop the nasal and optic placodes from ectodermal thickenings that will form forehead, nose and upper lip.

The upper lip is a fusion of the nasal and maxillary prominences, separating mouth from nose. The medial nasal prominence also forms the tip of nose and 'primary' palate or premaxilla. Midline fusion of the paired mandibular prominences forms the lower lip and jaw, with the commissures of the oral aperture formed by lateral fusion of the maxillary and mandibular prominences. Failure of fusion at any of the sites can give rise to the more common cleft lip or less frequent facial clefts.

The separation of nasal from oral cavity occurs with formation of the palate from horizontal extensions of the frontonasal and maxillary prominences to form the primary palate and two lateral palatal shelves. These will fuse horizontally in a Y shape, with the nasal septum superiorly, to form the hard and soft palate at 6–8 weeks. Mesenchyme migrates into the posterior third, which remains unossified, to form the musculature of the velum.

Development of the tongue

The anterior two-thirds of the tongue develops from the fusion of two lateral lingual swellings of first branchial arch origin. The posterior part of the tongue develops from median swellings of second, third and fourth branchial arch, with the central junction of first arch and second arch swellings being the foramen caecum. The innervation of the tongue reflects its branchial arch origin. The body of the tongue receives sensory supply from the lingual nerve (V), special taste sensation from chorda tympani (VII) and motor innervation from the hypoglossal (XII). The palatoglossus muscle and the root of the tongue are innervated by a plexus of glossopharyngeal (IX) and vagus (X) nerves.

Embryology of teeth

Teeth are unique in their structure and development and derive from their own dedicated epithelium known as 'odontogenic' epithelium.

Teeth develop initially within the alveolar crypt of the jaw and uniquely erupt from their bony envelopment into the oral cavity. Buds for permanent teeth form on the lingual side of the deciduous teeth during embryological development. They remain dormant until around the sixth year of life, when they push through the underside of the deciduous teeth. The roots of the deciduous teeth undergo osteoclasis and reabsorption.

Congenital disease of the oral cavity and lips

Cleft lip and palate

Cleft lip and palate is second only to talipes as the most common congenital deformity with a UK incidence of approximately 1:800 live births, although there is significant worldwide variation being more common in Chinese and less common in people of African-Caribbean descent. Many of these children will have additional congenital malformations with the musculoskeletal, circulatory and digestive systems most commonly affected.

Aetiology

Cleft lip and palate can be caused by a single gene defect in which case it is associated with a syndrome. It more commonly arises due to the interaction of several genes (polygenic) with associated environmental factors (epigenetic), such as smoking, alcohol usage, folate deficiency, obesity and medications including steroids and anticonvulsants. This results in sporadic cases and unpredictable inheritance.

Manifestations

Cleft deformities may involve the lip (44%), the palate (23%), or a combination of the two with either a single cleft lip (22%) or bilateral cleft lip (11%). It may be complete, incomplete, microform (lip) or submucous (palate), and may extend beyond the lip as a facial cleft.

Embryology and anatomy

Cleft pathologies are an example of what happens when embryological development is disrupted. The deformities can be understood by understanding the embryology of the developing face and oral cavity.

Cleft lip

The lip is formed from the conjunction of the nasal and maxillary processes. Fusion begins as the tripoint junction of the premaxilla (from the nasal process) and the secondary palatal shelves (from the maxillary processes), which later becomes the incisive foramen. In the lip, fusion travels from posterior to anterior in a V shape, fusing anterior palate, alveolus and lip from nasal sill to vermillion. The earlier the failure of fusion the more significant and complete the cleft.

Cleft lip is the result of failure of fusion resulting in discontinuity of the skin, muscle (orbicularis oris and nasalis) and mucosa. This can be continuous, through the nasal floor, with a discontinuity in the anterior maxilla and alveolus. Although the nose is intact, there is a characteristic nasal deformity due to adverse

muscle activity resulting in asymmetry (flat and wide nostril on cleft side) and internal obstruction of the ipsilateral nasal passage due to a bowed and deviated septum.

Diagnosis can be as early as 12 weeks postconception by ultrasound scan or at birth. If there is no palate involvement, a baby should be able to suckle and feed normally, but this is dependent on the severity of the lip deformity and ability to form a lip seal.

Cleft palate

The palate is formed from the fusion of the secondary palatal shelves with the premaxilla anterior and the vomer superior. Fusion progresses from the future incisive foramen anteriorly in a posterior direction towards the uvula.

Cleft palate is a result of failure of fusion in the midline between the shelves of the secondary palate and the vomer. It can be a complete cleft of hard and soft palate or incomplete. When the hard palate is involved, there may be bilateral or unilateral failure of fusion of the palatal shelves with the vomer. On occasion, there will be continuity of the oral/nasal mucosa but failure of fusion of the underlying bone or musculature resulting in a submucous cleft palate which is often diagnosed later in life. A submucous cleft is typified by bifid uvula, notching of the posterior border of hard palate, and a central sagittal lucid zone in the soft palate.

Diagnosis of cleft palate is usually made at birth either by direct observation and palpation of the palate or following failure to feed and associated nasal regurgitation; occasionally, it is identified on antenatal ultrasound scan. The difficulty in feeding is because of the inability to form a seal between mouth and nose, so the baby cannot suck. Patients may also suffer from recurrent otitis media due to tensor palatine dysfunction resulting in reduced hearing with an associated impact on speech development.

Management of clefts

Cleft lip and palate is ideally treated in specialist centres by a multidisciplinary team typically comprising cleft surgeons (maxillofacial, plastic and ENT), cleft nurse specialist, speech and language therapist, psychologist, paediatric dentist, orthodontist and audiologist. While advice on how to feed the baby is crucial, the ultimate treatment is surgical, the aim being to return the anatomy to as normal form and function as possible. This is done in three stages.

1 *Cleft lip and anterior palate repair (age 3–6 months).* Repair by 6 months will allow parents to form a bond with their child and improves lip function including speech, as babble starts from around this time.
2 *Cleft palate repair (age 9–12 months).* At least 3 months following lip repair. Exact timing depends on the width of the cleft and any underlying medical conditions. There is a trade-off between repairing the palatal apparatus in time to facilitate normal speech to develop and the potentially negative impact of surgery on the growing maxilla.
3 *Alveolar bone graft (age 8–10 years).* A cleft of the lip will often involve a discontinuity of the bone in the underlying anterior maxilla and through the alveolus. This will have an impact on the ability of teeth, particularly the adult canines, to erupt and so a bone graft may be considered.

Other craniofacial clefts

Intrauterine failure of fusion in other areas of the face can result in other craniofacial clefts. These are rare and complex clefts involving underlying bone and organs with the severity dictated by the anatomical position and extent. They may be associated with ocular defects and communications between the cranial and oral cavity.

Acquired disease of the oral cavity and lips

Dental disease

Anatomy

The human body has two sets of teeth:

Deciduous (milk) teeth

These 20 teeth erupt after birth, and are exfoliated by age 13 to be replaced by the permanent dentition. They comprise eight incisors, four canines, eight molars. Notation is by quadrant and capital letter starting at the midline.

Permanent teeth

These start to erupt from 6 years of age, usually completed by the late teens. There are 32 adult teeth,

made up of 8 incisors, 4 canines, 8 premolars and 12 molars. Notation is by quadrant and number starting at the midline.

The nerve supply of each tooth lies within the rich neurovascular complex of the pulp, which is protected by layers of hard tissue (dentine and enamel). It is responsible for the proprioception of the dentition and for the sensation of *odontalgia* – commonly known as toothache.

Dental caries

This is the most common disease of the oral cavity and poses a major health burden. It can affect both the permanent and deciduous dentition and is the most common indication for a general anaesthetic in the paediatric population.

Pathogenesis

Dental caries is bacteria-mediated breakdown of the hard tissues of the teeth. Bacteria, usually *Streptococcus mutans* found in plaque, will break down dietary sugars to produce acid. These acids dissolve the mineral content of the hard tissues, resulting in caries. The caries will progress through the layers of the tooth causing cavities and eventually pulp death.

Clinical features

Presence of plaque, dark discolouration of teeth, cavities, pain in response to eating, drinking and temperature changes, and unprovoked toothache. Risk factors include poor oral hygiene, high sugar diet, dry mouth secondary to medications, autoimmune disease and radiotherapy.

Special investigations

- *Dental radiography*: the scanning dental/orthopantomogram (OPG) is used for a broad assessment but if caries is suspected an intraoral dental radiograph should be used to assess the extent of the disease.
- *Pulp test*: sensitivity to hot, cold or electricity may be used to assess if the pulp of the tooth is alive.

Differential diagnosis

Includes erosion, abrasion, enamel hypoplasia, amelogenesis imperfecta, dentinogenesis imperfecta, fluoride/tetracycline staining.

Treatment

Removal of caries and dental restoration, extraction of affected tooth. Future prevention by improvement in oral hygiene.

Dental abscess

Pathogenesis

A dental abscess is a mixed bacterial infection (*bacteroides, streptococci*) that can develop subsequent to caries (necrotic pulp), but also with periodontal disease and unerupted wisdom teeth (pericoronitis). Although the majority of abscesses are self-limiting and localized, they can progress to life-threatening *Ludwig's angina*[3], where large submandibular swelling can threaten to occlude the airway.

Clinical features

Initially:

- Pain on biting onto a tooth.
- Bad taste in mouth.
- Visible discharging sinus through gingiva (gums).

Subsequently:

- Buccal, palatal or lingual swelling adjacent to tooth.
- Extraoral swelling in submandibular region or cheek.
- Difficulty opening mouth (trismus) or swallowing.

Symptoms may progress to an airway, sight and/or life-threatening emergency if spread to the fascial spaces within head and neck, as indicated by extreme trismus, drooling and stridor (*Ludwig's angina*). Signs of systemic infection including pyrexia, tachycardia and raised white cell count. This will require urgent incision and drainage under general anaesthetic.

Special investigations

- *Dental radiography,* usually OPG to identify causative tooth.
- *Computed tomography (CT) or ultrasound scan* of large swellings to identify position and extent of abscess.

Differential diagnosis

Infected cyst of sebaceous, dermoid, or branchial origin, or an oral cancer or other skin infection (e.g. actinomycosis).

Treatment

Depending on the extent of the abscess, this may range from removal of dental pulp and root canal treatment, to removal of tooth and drainage of any associated abscess via tooth socket, intraoral incision or extraoral incision together with broad spectrum antibiotics.

Cysts and tumours of dental origin
Odontogenic tumours

These are not common and usually benign in nature.

- *Odontomes: hamartomas* of odontogenic tissue, which may contain dental tissues or odontomas.
- *Ameloblastoma:* derived from ameloblasts (epithelial cells which produce enamel for the developing tooth). It can be locally invasive in nature but can rarely undergo malignant transformation; it rarely metastasizes. Usually multilocular and commonly found at the angle of the mandible. Any age may be affected, but the majority present in the second and third decades with equal sex distribution.

Treatment of both conditions is surgical resection.

Odontogenic cysts:

Present as asymptomatic radiolucencies on radiographs.

- *Dentigerous cyst:* occurs around the crown of unerupted teeth.
- *Radicular (apical periodontal) cyst:* occurs in association with root apex of non-vital teeth.
- *Keratocysts or keratinizing odontogenic tumours* are potentially aggressive cysts that can act as a locally invasive tumour and will mimic other cysts. High chance of recurrence with resection due to presence of daughter/ satellite cysts. Multiple cysts and basal cell carcinomas characterize the autosomal dominant Gorlin-Goltz syndrome[4].

[3] Wilhelm Frederick von Ludwig (1790–1865). A prisoner of war in the Napoleonic wars, he later practised in Stuttgart and was personal Physician to King Wilhlem I.

[4] Robert J Gorlin (1923–2006), Pathologist, University of Minnesota School of Dentistry. Robert W Goltz (1923–2014), Dermatologist at the same institution, and co-author of the 1960 paper describing the syndrome.

Non-malignant disease of oral mucosa and oral cavity

Lesions of the cutaneous lip

The lip is at the junction of the skin and mucosa, which makes it prone to disease processes from both. Lesions here can be usefully divided into infective and non-infective lesions.

Infective lesions

Herpes labialis (cold sore)

This is a secondary reactivation of a previous herpes simplex virus (HSV) infection, latent in the trigeminal ganglia. Initially an itching and burning sensation, a crop of vesicles will develop into a confluent crusting ulcer before resolving. Maybe precipitated by trauma, sunlight, menstruation, underlying physiological stress and immunosuppression. Treatment usually symptomatic but infection may be curtailed by early and regular application of a topical antiviral such as aciclovir or famciclovir. Should be differentiated from other infective causes such as varicella zoster or impetigo and malignancy including basal or squamous cell carcinoma.

Herpes zoster (shingles)

This is a secondary reactivation of previous varicella zoster infection. It presents as a dull ache or mimics toothache, followed by the classical presentation of an itchy or painful rash following the trigeminal dermatomes. It can progress to mouth ulcers.

It is usually triggered by underlying physiological stress or immunosuppression. A positive *Hutchinson's sign*[5] (rash of the tip of nose) is important as it indicates nasociliary nerve involvement, a prelude to herpes zoster ophthalmicus. This can result in reduced vision, eye pain and photophobia, with a potential for severe eye damage and blindness. Treatment is with an antiviral (usually aciclovir).

[5] Sir Jonathan Hutchinson (1828–1913); Surgeon, London. He described many signs, including Hutchinson's freckle (a premalignant melanoma) and the pegged teeth of congenital syphilis.

Impetigo contagiosa

This *Staphylococcus aureus* or *Streptococcus pyogenes* infection causes papules on the skin, which progress to erythematous vesicles then pustules with golden crusts. It is highly infectious and spread by contact. It rarely has systemic symptoms. Usually found in young children especially those suffering from underlying malnutrition. The diagnosis is confirmed on culture, but should be differentiated from other vesiculo-bullous lesions such as HSV. Treatment is with topical antibacterial creams or oral flucloxacillin if systemic symptoms.

Angular stomatitis (angular cheilitis)

Inflammatory condition of the corners of the mouth, usually due to infection with *Candida albicans* but bacterial species such as *Staphylococcus aureus* and/ or *Streptococcus* may also be present. Other causes include underlying iron or vitamin B deficiency, immunocompromise and overhang of the upper lip resulting in deep furrows. Seen most commonly in the elderly edentulous patient. Clinical features include sore erythematous fissures at the oral commissure with concomitant mucosal leucoplakia.

Treatment is of the underlying cause and topical antifungals. New dentures may be needed to reduce any associated denture-induced stomatitis and increase lower face height.

Non-infective lesions

Erythema multiforme

Immune-mediated hypersensitivity reaction to drugs such as NSAIDs, carbamazepine, phenytoin and penicillins. It may also be triggered by HSV infection, UV light, pregnancy, malignancy and chemicals. The cause cannot always be identified.

Symptoms can range from mild to life-threatening. It can affect skin, mucosa or both. There is circumoral crusting with serosanguinous exudate. In its minor form, it will affect only one site. Treatment is withdrawal of any identified triggering factors and supportive with analgesia and rehydration. Steroids and antivirals may also be required, depending on aetiology.

In its major form, *Stevens-Johnson's Syndrome*, it can cause significant systemic illness and affect multiple sites including eyes and genitals and will require admission for parenteral steroids or other immunosuppressants and supportive therapy including intravenous rehydration and nutrition.

Other oral lesions

Several other non-infective oral lesions may be identified which are associated with either genetic or inflammatory conditions:

- *Peutz-Jeghers[2] circumoral pigmentation*: autosomal dominant condition associated with intestinal hamartomatous polyps which may cause obstruction due to intussusception.
- *Hereditary haemorrhagic telangiectasia (Osler-Weber-Rendu syndrome[6])*: associated with intestinal telangiectasia and associated gastrointestinal bleeding.
- *Lichen planus*: white striae, atrophic, erosive, can affect multiple intra- and extraoral sites.
- *Lip swelling*: may be symptomatic of allergic angioedema, hereditary angioedema, orofacial granulomatosis (Crohn's disease or sarcoidosis).

Lesions of the oral mucosa including lip mucosa

Lesions within the mouth are related to the oral mucosa and underlying connective tissue and glands. Many will also have cutaneous/extraoral manifestations as already described.

Infective oral ulceration

Primary herpes simplex (gingivostomatitis)

Oral lesions usually due to HSV1 and carried by 60% of the population. Transmitted by direct contact or bodily fluids with incubation period of 3–7 days. Infection is usually subclinical. Presents with painful punched out

ulceration at gingival margins and multiple vesiculobullous ulcers of the oral mucosa which can become confluent. Systemic symptoms of infection include malaise, fever, lymphadenopathy and anorexia. Diagnosis is usually clinical. Treatment is supportive; analgesia, bed rest, fluids, antipyrexials, analgesia, antiviral agents if immunosuppressed or early diagnosis.

Other infective causes may need to be excluded, as should *erythema multiforme and leukaemia*. Herpes simplex may recur as cold sores.

Herpangina

Multiple small vesicular ulcers (2–4 mm) secondary to coxsackie type A infection. Commonest in children under 4 and spread by the faeco-oral route; it can be epidemic in nature. Most cases are mild and can present with associated fever and malaise. Treatment is supportive as the infection is self-limiting.

Primary varicella (chickenpox)

Oral lesions may precede skin presentations and mimic primary HSV on the mucosa but without gingival lesions. Long incubation of 14–21 days with prodromal symptoms of malaise, pharyngitis and rhinitis. Treatment is mainly supportive or antivirals where immunocompromised or ocular involvement. May recur as shingles.

Other infective causes of oral ulceration include hand foot and mouth disease, Epstein Barr virus, syphilis, tuberculosis and measles.

Non-infective oral ulceration

Oral ulceration is disruption in the continuity of the oral epithelium leading to exposure of the underlying connective tissue.

Ulcers of local aetiology

These are usually solitary and solo in nature, and are related to localized trauma including biting habits, sharp teeth or dental restorations, burns including irradiation, ill-fitting dentures. Other causes of ulceration should be excluded, in particular malignancy. Treatment is symptomatic and removal of causative agent if chronic.

Recurrent aphthous stomatitis (aphthae)

This is a common cause of oral ulceration often with no clear causative agent. Predisposing factors include

---

[6] Sir William Osler (1849–1919), Professor of Medicine, successively at McGill University, Montreal, Canada; Johns Hopkins University, Baltimore, MD, USA; and the University of Oxford. Henri Rendu (1844–1902), Physician, Necker Hospital, Paris, France. Frederick Parkes Weber (1863–1962), a London Physician with an interest in rare disorders. The disease was actually first described by Henry Sutton in 1864.

haematinic deficiency, phase of menstrual cycle, food allergies and stress.

Investigations: check underlying medical history for systemic disorders. Blood tests for haematinics and autoantibodies. Consider biopsy if no evidence of resolution to exclude other causes and malignancy.

Treatment: Treat any underlying conditions. Treat symptoms with chlorhexidine or benzydamine mouthwash. May require topical corticosteroids (mouthwash, pellets) including eclomethasone or oral prednisolone.

Behçet's syndrome[7]

Autoimmune vasculitis characterized by recurrent oral ulcers, genital ulcers, uveitis and arthritis. Treatment includes topical/ intralesional steroids, and immunosuppression.

Drug reactions

Oral mucosal ulceration can occur secondary to medications, such as the immunosuppressants everolimus and sirolimus. Pathogenesis can be due to focal irritation, allergic hypersensitivity or cytotoxicity. Common drugs implicated include NSAIDs and nicorandil.

Pemphigus vulgaris

This vesiculobullous autoimmune disease produces circulating autoantibodies to epithelial desmosomes (sticky areas on the surface of keratinocytes near the bottom of the epidermis) resulting in intraepithelial clefting. Clinical presentation includes fragile bullae/ erosions of mucosa preceding skin lesions. Lateral sheer pressure on skin may cause epithelial separation (positive Nikolsky sign[8]).

Investigations: Biopsy will show intraepithelial vesicles, and immune deposits on direct immunofluorescence. Plasma anti-desmosomal antibodies (Dsg1 and Dsg3) will be raised and correlate to disease activity.

Differential diagnosis includes mucous membrane pemphigoid. Treatment is with immunosuppression

including steroids, immune sparing drugs and other medications such as dapsone or monoclonal antibodies such as rituximab.

Mucous membrane pemphigoid

Most common of all the vesiculobullous lesions, presenting in the older populations. Subepithelial clefting is caused by anti-basement membrane autoantibodies, resulting in thick walled bullae that are less likely to rupture, but will scar. In addition to oral manifestations, it may affect genital, nasal, oesophageal, laryngeal tissues and skin. Biopsy will show subepithelial clefting and linear IgG and C3 deposits at the basement membrane. Treatment is similar to that for pemphigus and includes immunosuppression with steroids and other systemic therapies.

Other autoimmune disease resulting in oral ulceration includes Epidermolysis Bullosa, Systemic Lupus Erythematosus.

Potential malignant disorders of the mouth

Lichen planus

A relatively common immune-mediated condition of the stratified squamous epithelium affecting mouth, skin and genitalia. 2% of the population are affected by oral lichen planus. When in response to a drug it is described as a lichenoid reaction.

Clinical features

Often bilateral white striae or erosions of oral mucosa. May be asymptomatic or painful and sore if atrophic or ulcerated. Extra oral manifestations include violet papules on flexor surfaces, vertical ridges of nails, alopecia, lesions on genitalia.

Special investigations

Biopsy of non-ulcerated lesion, blood tests (full blood count and haematinics). Erosive and atrophic areas are at small risk of malignant change.

Treatment

Treatment is only necessary if symptomatic. Topical steroids such as hydrocortisone or betamethasone

---

[7] Hulusi Behçet (1889–1948), Professor of Dermatology, Istanbul, Turkey.

[8] Pyotr Vasilyewich Nikolsky (1858–1940), Professor of Dermatology, University of Warsaw. The sign differentiates intra-epidermal blisters from subdermal blisters.

lozenges, spray or inhaler with escalation to intralesional or oral steroids. Occasionally further immunosuppression is necessary.

Candidiasis

Candida albicans is a commensal organism in the oral cavity but can become a source of infection if there is a change in the local environment (denture wear, xerostomia) or underlying immune status of the patient (steroids, diabetes). Malnutrition, smoking, and broad spectrum antibiotics can also predispose to infection.

Clinical features

There are three common types of *candida* infection:

- *Pseudomembranous:* Acute (thrush) or chronic. Creamy white plaques or deposits that can be wiped away leaving erythematous areas.
- *Erythematous:* smooth red mucosa of tongue, hard palate and buccal mucosa.
- *Hyperplastic:* Leukoplastic lesions are considered at high risk of malignant transformation to squamous cell carcinoma.

Special investigations

Mucosal swabs should confirm the infection. Diabetes should always be excluded as a cause. Concerning lesions should be biopsied.

Treatment

Topical (e.g. nystatin) or systemic (e.g. fluconazole) antifungal medication. Oral and denture hygiene should be improved and underlying risk factors eliminated.

Leukoplakia

Leukoplakia is the diagnosis of exclusion for a white patch or plaque on the oral mucosa that cannot be characterized clinically or pathologically as any other lesion. It is found in 3% of adults, usually middle aged or elderly and presents as a thickened white area of mucosa that cannot be removed on wiping. It can be found at any site within the oral cavity. Leukoplakia affecting the lateral border of tongue and floor of mouth are considered high risk for malignant transformation. Chronic irritation including the 5 S's (smoking, spices, sharp tooth, syphilis and alcohol (spirits)) are aetiological factors.

Heterogenous lesions, they can variably be white, erythematous or speckled, with a flat or exophytic cross-section. This is reflected in the variable histology; atrophic epithelium, hyperplasia without hyperkeratosis, dysplasia of varying degrees (none, mild, moderate, severe), or even carcinoma.

Biopsy is recommended if an irregular appearance or evidence of erythroplakia and will guide treatment. Risk factors should be modified and consideration given to long-term follow-up including photography. Severely dysplastic lesions should be removed in their entirety and mandate close follow-up.

Other white patches

Include trauma such as cheek biting, keratosis (frictional, smokers, other tobacco related, sublingual), hairy leukoplakia. Malignancy should be excluded.

Intraoral pigmented lesions

Haemangioma

These lesions represent a congenital vascular malformation or tumour that presents and grows rapidly after birth, which later stabilizes and then gradually regresses. Treatment is conservative unless these is impact on functional development such as vision or there is significant bleeding. Active management includes intralesional steroid, interferon, laser or surgery.

Other benign causes of intraoral pigmentation include drug induced, amalgam tattoo, racial pigmentation, purpura and naevi.

Intraoral lumps

The majority of intraoral lumps are benign in nature and related to trauma.

Mucocele

Described as mucous retention cysts, these are extremely common. They are considered secondary to trauma to a minor salivary gland within the submucosa, such as the lower labial mucosa, and may go through a cycle of recurrent swelling and discharge. They appear as a blue domed, well-defined swelling just underlying the mucosa and may transilluminate if large enough. Some will resolve spontaneously but treatment is surgical excision under local anaesthetic.

Ranula

A ranula, from the Latin for frog, is a mucous extravasation cyst in the floor of the mouth commonly related to the sublingual gland. It is usually a large, blue, translucent swelling. Although many are managed conservatively, definitive treatment requires removal of the ipsilateral sublingual gland, rather than direct excision or marsupialization of the cyst.

Trauma-induced hyperplasia

Chronic irritation from a denture flange or dental restoration, rather than causing ulceration, can induce hyperplasia of the affected mucosa. This may be seen as a painless lump or leaf underlying the flange of a denture (*denture granuloma*) particularly in the lower labial sulcus. Definitive diagnosis is by excision biopsy, and recurrence prevented by reducing the denture flange or source of irritation.

Fibroepithelial polyp

These are trauma/ irritation induced pedunculated or sessile overgrowths of epithelial or submucosal tissue and are found throughout the oral cavity. It is described as an *epulis* when found presenting on the gingiva. They may bleed or become ulcerated if acutely traumatized so mimicking a soft tissue tumour. Definitive diagnosis and treatment is by excision biopsy under local anaesthetic.

Malignant disease of the cutaneous lip

Malignant disease of the cutaneous lip is treated as per the protocols for other cutaneous cancers of the face. Basal cell carcinoma and squamous cell carcinoma are seen most commonly. These are discussed in Chapter 11.

Surgical excision of lesions of the lip

Cutaneous lesions of the lip should be excised with sufficient margin to ensure full clearance. This can range from a superficial excision to full thickness resection of skin, muscle and mucosa or distinct anatomical areas such as the philtrum or commissure. Up to one-third of the lip can be removed using a wedge excision and reconstructed with primary closure. For larger resections, local or free flaps may be needed.

Malignant disease of oral mucosa and oral cavity

Malignant disease of the head and neck is the 7th most commonly occurring cancer in the UK. It is more common in men and with a median age at diagnosis of 60. Cancer in patients under 45 is often associated with an oncogenic virus. Head and neck cancer is a diverse group. Arising from the structures within the oral cavity and oropharynx, over 90% are squamous cell carcinoma. The cancer can arise *de novo*, in a previous premalignant lesion, such as leucoplakia, erythroplakia, chronic hyperplastic candidiasis, lichen planus, and oral submucous fibrosis. Other tumours can include those of the minor salivary glands such as adenocarcinoma and mucoepidermoid carcinoma.

Squamous cell carcinoma of the oral cavity

Predisposing factors

Tobacco usage and increased alcohol consumption are considered the primary causative factors. Betel nut chewing increases the risk, and in India 40% of all cancers are oropharyngeal.

Oncogenic viruses such as human papilloma virus (HPV), especially types 16 and 18, and the Epstein Barr[9] virus are independent risk factors for oropharyngeal cancer.

---

[9] Michael Anthony Epstein (b. 1921), Professor of Pathology, University of Bristol, Bristol, UK. Yvonne Barr (1932–2016), Virologist and research assistant of Epstein when both were at the Middlesex Hospital, London, UK.

Clinical features

Many oral cancers are diagnosed incidentally after examination by a dentist or primary care physician. Symptoms can include a painless ulcer, sore throat, difficulty swallowing or sensation of a foreign body, pain (either local to the tumour or distant including toothache and earache), a lump in the neck or local mass, and weight loss.

On clinical examination it may appear as an indurated ulcer, an exophytic mass or an area of erythroplakia. There may also be evidence of a cranial nerve lesion such as loss of sensation (trigeminal nerve), a facial palsy (facial nerve), deviation of the tongue (hypoglossal nerve) or voice changes (glossopharyngeal nerve).

Common sites for SCC in the oral cavity include the lateral border of tongue, floor of mouth and buccal mucosa. If a lesion is suspected examination should include full assessment of the oral cavity, endoscopic examination of the nasopharynx, oropharynx and larynx, and examination of the neck for palpable masses and lymph nodes.

Diagnosis

This requires histological examination of tissue by direct biopsy of a visible lesion or fine needle aspiration of a suspected mass or node. Open biopsy of a neck lump is avoided. If previous biopsies are inconclusive and in absence of an identifiable primary lesion, a planned resection of the lymph nodes of the neck will be completed to aid diagnosis and avoid metastatic spread.

Special investigations

- *Plain radiography* (OPG) is helpful in assessment for dental health.
- *Cross-sectional imaging* of the site of tumour to assess local invasion, and neck and chest to exclude metastases. *Magnetic resonance imaging (MRI)* is preferred to CT for its increased accuracy in assessing depth and volume of tumours and neck disease, and is superior in demonstrating the presence of perineural invasion in salivary gland tumours.

Prognostic features

As with most squamous cell cancers, features suggesting aggressive disease include poor differentiation, perineural invasion, lymphatic invasion, lymph node metastases and extracapsular spread. The presence of HPV should also be assessed.

Treatment

Treatment aims to eradicate disease, minimizing morbidity and effecting the highest possible cure rates. The three modalities of treatment are surgery, radiotherapy and chemotherapy, and these may be used in isolation or combination depending on the primary site, histological appearance and stage.

Surgery

A surgical approach is used to remove the tumour, control disease in the neck and reconstruct the site to reduce post-treatment morbidity.

- *Primary site* – access to many tumours of the oral cavity are via a transoral approach, but as tumours increase in size or are more posterior, access may be necessary via a lip split and mandibulotomy, the neck or transfacial. The size and location of the tumour will determine the need for reconstruction beyond primary closure or healing by secondary intention.
- *The neck*: Block dissection of the lymph nodes of the neck may be done as a staging or therapeutic procedure. Alternatively, sentinel node sampling of the neck may be done if no abnormal neck nodes are identified on imaging.

A patient may require tracheostomy to support the airway through the surgical period, and potentially long term.

Other cancers of the oral cavity

Tumours of minor salivary glands

See chapter 21.

Tumours of the jaw

Tumours of the jaw are of extremely wide pathological variety because they may arise from the bone of the jaw itself, from the tissues over the surface of the jaw or, in the case of the maxilla, from the mucosa lining the maxillary antrum.

Tumours adjacent to the oral cavity

Nasopharyngeal tumours

These lie in the nasopharynx, posterior and superior to the soft palate. They may present with epistaxis and congestion or neck lump, and should be differentiated from nasal polyps and rhinitis. They are linked with Epstein- Barr virus infection and diets rich in cured fish or meat, so are common in south-east Asia and China. Treatment is with a combination of surgery and radiotherapy.

Oropharyngeal tumours

These are tumours that lie posterior and inferior to the oral cavity and in general are managed in the same way, as they are usually mucosal squamous carcinomas. They are also associated with HPV.

Tongue base and tonsillar tumours may be treated with primary chemoradiotherapy.

Tonsil tumours

Usually a squamous carcinoma, more common in males over the age of 50 and strongly associated with HPV infection. Differential diagnosis includes lymphoma, small cell carcinoma and secondary deposits of Merkel cell carcinoma, renal cell carcinoma and small cell lung cancer. Patients may complain of sore throat, unilateral otalgia, sensation of foreign body or difficulty opening their mouth. They may also present with enlarged cervical lymph nodes. Treatment depends on size and location.

Antral tumours

Most commonly squamous carcinomas arising from the mucous membrane of the maxillary antrum, and treated with surgery. Other tumours include adenocarcinoma, adenoid cystic carcinoma and lymphoma.

Clinical features

Symptoms and signs are late in manifesting themselves as the tumour can expand into the antrum before becoming clinically obvious. Its clinical presentation depends on the pattern of spread.

- *Medial extension:* Blockage of the ostium of the maxillary antrum with consequent infection of the sinus, or with nasal obstruction and epistaxis.
- *Lateral extension:* Swelling of the face, which often has an inflammatory appearance and may well be mistaken for an acute infection.
- *Superior extension:* Orbital invasion with proptosis, diplopia and lacrimation due to blockage of the tear duct. Anaesthesia of the cheek may result

from invasion of the maxillary branch of the trigeminal nerve.
- *Inferior extension:* Bulging and ulceration into the palate. Dental pain and tooth mobility.

Metastases to the upper jugular lymph nodes occur at a relatively late stage.

Special investigations

- *Orthopantomogram* may show local bony destruction, involvement of teeth and opacity of maxillary sinus.
- *Nasal endoscopy* may visualize the tumour if it is invading the medial wall of the maxilla, and may permit biopsy under direct vision.
- *CT and MR imaging* are invaluable in defining the extent of tumour spread, including orbital soft tissue involvement.

Treatment

Treatment is usually surgical resection followed by radiotherapy. The patient may require orbital exenteration depending on extent of ocular involvement and the need for follow-up radiotherapy. Reconstruction includes free tissue transfer, obturation or implant-retained prosthesis.

Reconstructive surgery in head and neck cancer

The head, face and neck is a complex structure that is a conduit for communication, eating and breathing. It is also the social interface for most people so adequate cosmesis is vital.

The defect size and site will determine the reconstruction, as will the required tissue and health of the patient. Reconstruction should be immediate, as simple as possible, with low morbidity and not impact on the ability to resect the tumour.

Reconstructive ladder

A hierarchy of surgical options is as follows:

- *Healing by secondary intention*: used following laser resection of superficial lesions. Not suitable in conventional resection due to scarring.
- *Primary closure*: for small defects, where there is minimal distortion of adjacent tissues. No donor site morbidity.

- *Graft*: mucosa, split or full thickness skin, bone, cartilage, vascular or nerve as determined by the defect. Sometimes used in conjunction with other reconstructive techniques such as flaps.
- *Flaps:*
  - *Local* – donor tissue is transferred into an adjacent small defect and benefits from being of similar tissue and retaining its vascular supply. Examples include the nasolabial flap.
  - *Regional and distant flaps* – the donor site is distant from the defect but the flap is transferred while maintaining its blood supply. The temporalis flap is considered local to the head and neck whereas flaps such as pectoralis major myocutaneous flap or the deltopectoral flap are distant. These flaps are useful when other techniques have failed or free tissue transfer is considered inappropriate due to associated patient morbidity.
  - *Free tissue transfer* – the donor site is separate from the defect. The flap is raised with its associated vascular pedicle and detached before being anastomosed to vessels in the neck. Although technically challenging and complex this surgery allows transfer of tissue without restriction and in larger volumes. These flaps can be soft tissue, bony or a combination. Three commonly used flaps are:
    - *Radial forearm flap* – usually skin only but can be composite.
    - *Fibula flap* – comprised bone +/- muscle and skin. Used following mandibular or maxillary resection.
    - *Anterolateral thigh flap* – large skin and muscle flap.

Complications of surgery

Head and neck cancer surgery with resection includes specific risks of:

- Airway compromise due to swelling and problems with the tracheostomy.

- Collection of fluids:
  - Seroma.
  - Saliva collections.
  - Chylous leak.
- Wound dehiscence and breakdown resulting in oro-cutaneous fistula.
- Nerve injuries – facial nerve (marginal mandibular branch), phrenic nerve, vagus (recurrent laryngeal), accessory nerve, sympathetic chain.
- Failure of reconstruction, especially loss of blood supply to free tissue flaps.

Adjunctive therapy for oral SCC

Radiotherapy: Many patients with oral cavity SCC will require adjunctive radiotherapy to the site of the tumour and the neck depending on disease size and spread, and the success of the resection. Usually, it is delivered by external beam over a number of sessions, and although it is useful for disease control it is associated with high levels of morbidity.

Morbidity includes mucositis, skin erythema and ulceration, loss of taste, impaired nutrition and weight loss, dry mouth with associated dental disease, lymphoedema, fibrosis and osteoradionecrosis.

Chemotherapy: This is used less frequently as the role remains controversial. It is used as a primary therapy in tumours of the tonsil, tongue base and nasopharynx.

⊗ Additional resources

Case 42: A lump on the lip
Case 43: A white plaque on the tongue
Case 44: A baby with two congenital deformities

21

The salivary glands

Brian Fish

Learning objective

✓ To know the common benign and malignant conditions of the salivary glands and their treatment.

The salivary glands comprise three paired major glands – the parotid, submandibular and sublingual – together with numerous minor salivary glands scattered throughout the oral mucosa and in the posterior third of the tongue, cheeks and palate. The parotid gland secretes serous saliva, in contrast to the mucus product of the sublingual glands. The submandibular saliva is seromucus, and represents 70% of the total saliva produced by the major glands. The minor glands can either be serous or mucous and produce 10% of total saliva volume.

The parotid and submandibular glands drain into the mouth via long ducts, the parotid (Stensen's[1]) duct opening adjacent to the second upper molar tooth, while the submandibular (Wharton's[2]) duct opens on the floor of the mouth through a papilla at the base of the frenulum of the tongue. Their orifices are easily visible in your own mouth and saliva will be seen to flow if you press on the glands themselves. The sublingual gland's mucus secretion drains by a series of very short ducts into the floor of the mouth.

The two principal surgical conditions of the salivary glands are inflammation, with or without calculus, and neoplasm. The nature of the glandular cells determines the saliva's composition, explaining the different incidence of these conditions in each of the salivary glands.

Inflammation

Aetiology

- *Infection (viral or bacterial)* usually affects the parotid, rarely the submandibular gland.
- *Chronic recurrent sialadenitis*, usually occurs in the parotid.
- *Sjogren's syndrome*, involving all the salivary and the lacrimal glands.
- *Calculus*, usually affecting the submandibular gland.

Viral infections

The commonest viral infection to affect the salivary glands is mumps but human immunodeficiency virus (HIV) and hepatitis C should also be considered.

Mumps

A viral infection (incubation period 17–21 days), which is common in children and affects the parotid glands; it

---

[1] Niels Stensen (1638–1686), Professor of Anatomy, University of Copenhagen, Denmark. Gave up his Chair in 1669 to become a bishop.

[2] Thomas Wharton (1614–1673), Physician, St Thomas's Hospital, London, UK.

Ellis and Calne's Lecture Notes in General Surgery, Fourteenth Edition. Edited by Christopher Watson and Justin Davies. © 2023 John Wiley & Sons Ltd. Published 2023 by John Wiley & Sons Ltd. Companion website: www.wiley.com/go/Watson/GeneralSurgery14

is usually bilateral. Rarely, the submandibular or sublingual glands may also be involved. Most children are now immunized against mumps before starting school.

Mumps may present to the surgeon in the following ways.

- *Acute parotitis:* usual in childhood but may occasionally occur as a painful parotid swelling in an adult (Boxes 21.1 and 21.2).
- *Mumps orchitis:* usually presents in adolescents or young adults, and rare before puberty. Pain and swelling in the testicle occur 7–10 days after the onset of the parotitis and may lead to testicular atrophy. If bilateral orchitis occurs, there may be sterility or eunuchoidism. Very rarely, the orchitis occurs without prodromal parotitis.
- *Pancreatitis, mastitis, thyroiditis or oophoritis* are also rarely caused by mumps.

Acute bacterial parotitis

Reduction of salivary flow is an important prerequisite for ascending infection of the parotid gland via its duct. Aetiological factors include dental sepsis, dehydration, prolonged presence of a nasogastric tube and poor oral hygiene. This complication may occur in any severe debilitating illness and in uraemia. The infection is usually streptococcal (*Streptococcus viridans*) or staphylococcal (*Staphylococcus aureus*). It used to be common after major abdominal surgery but is less so now due to the use of antibiotics.

Clinical features

Clinically, there is swelling and intense pain in one or both parotid glands, which are hard, enlarged and tender, often with associated trismus. There may be a purulent discharge from the duct. Abscess formation occasionally occurs.

Treatment

Prophylaxis is important with adequate hydration and elimination of the above aetiological factors. In the established case, the patient must be kept fully hydrated and the flow of saliva encouraged by sucking citrus sweets or chewing gum. Parenteral antibiotic therapy is commenced. Occasionally, surgical drainage is required.

Chronic recurrent parotid sialadenitis

Repeated episodes of pain and swelling in one or both parotids are not uncommon and are caused by a combination of obstruction and infection of the gland. There may be an associated dilation of the duct system and alveoli of the gland, termed 'sialectasia' (which resembles bronchiectasis in the lung), associated with a stricture of the duct or a stone. These changes are best demonstrated by performing a *sialogram*.

Treatment

An associated stricture is treated by dilation, and if stones are present these must be removed. Massage of the gland several times a day, and the use of sialogogues (such as 'acid drops'), encourage drainage. Sialoendoscopy can be used to help with diagnosis and treatment of stenoses and stones. Occasionally, in severe and refractory cases, excision of the gland with preservation of the facial nerve is required.

Sjögren's syndrome

Sjögren's syndrome[3] is an autoimmune disease characterized by periductal lymphocytes in multiple organs. The salivary glands are affected in approximately 40% of cases and one in six patients will progress to lymphoma. It is associated with dry eyes (xerophthalmia), leading to conjunctivokeratitis, and dry mouth (xerostomia). If there is no connective tissue component, it is described as primary and if there is a connective tissue disorder, usually rheumatoid arthritis, it is secondary.

Calculi

Stone formation is common in the submandibular gland and its duct, rare in the parotid and rarer still in the sublingual. The different composition of the saliva from each gland probably explains this difference. Stasis of the more viscid secretion of the submandibular gland in its long duct, changes in composition of the saliva, trauma to the duct, infection, and stricture may predispose to stone formation. Calcium phosphate is the predominant salt of the calculi and the majority are radio-opaque particularly in the submandibular gland or duct.

[3] Henrik Sjogren (1899–1986) a Swedish Ophthalmologist.

Clinical features

There is painful swelling of the affected gland, aggravated by food (classically, by sucking a lemon), and there may be an unpleasant taste in the mouth due to the purulent discharge. On examination, the obstructed gland is enlarged and tender. The orifice of the submandibular duct, visible in the floor of the mouth, is red and swollen and the calculus may be visible or palpable on bimanual examination of the duct. Gentle pressure on the gland may produce a purulent exudate from the orifice of the duct.

Special investigations

- *X-rays* invariably confirm the presence of the stone.
- A *sialogram*, in which contrast material is injected into the duct, may be necessary if no stone is visible. This may reveal stenosis of the ostium of the duct, which mimics the symptoms of a stone, or sialectasis.
- *Sialoendoscopy*.

Treatment

If the stone lies within the submandibular duct, it can be removed from within the mouth, with the duct being marsupialized at the site of extraction. It can also be removed via sialoendoscopy. If one or more stones are impacted in the gland substance, excision of the whole gland is required.

Salivary tumours

There are over 35 variants of salivary gland tumours and a simplified classification is shown below. A good approximation is that 80% of all salivary gland tumours are in the parotid, 80% of parotid tumours are benign and 80% of the benign parotid tumours are pleomorphic adenomas. One in three tumours arising in the submandibular gland and one in two arising in the minor salivary glands are malignant.

Benign

- Pleomorphic adenoma (mixed salivary tumour).
- Adenolymphoma (Warthin's tumour).

Malignant

- *Primary:* carcinoma – adenoid cystic, acinic, mucoepidermoid, carcinoma ex-pleomorphic adenoma.
- *Secondary:* secondarily involved intraparotid lymph nodes, usually from primary skin squamous cell carcinomas.

Pleomorphic adenoma

These account for 70–80% of all salivary gland neoplasms with 80% appearing in the parotid gland. Mean age of presentation is 46 years although any age may be affected. Sex distribution is roughly equal.

Pathology

Macroscopic appearance

The tumour is lobulated and lies within a capsule of varying thickness. In minor salivary gland sites, the capsule may be completely absent. The outer surface is bosselated with finger like processes extending into and occasionally through the capsule.

Microscopic appearance

Epithelial and modified myoepithelial elements intermingle most commonly with tissue of mucoid, myxoid or chondroid appearance hence the synonym of 'mixed tumour.'

Clinical features

The patient presents with a slow-growing swelling anywhere within the parotid gland, but usually in the lower pole and in the region of the angle of the jaw. The lump is well-defined, usually firm or hard but sometimes cystic in consistency. It is usually placed in the superficial part of the gland but may occasionally be in its deep lobe in the parapharyngeal space and indeed may project into the pharynx. The facial nerve is never involved, except by frankly malignant tumours. Its integrity should be confirmed.

Surgical considerations

Complete surgical excision is the treatment of choice as, although pleomorphic adenoma is a benign tumour, there is a risk of recurrence and malignant transformation. Because of the variability of the capsule and protuberances through it, excision with a cuff of normal salivary gland tissue is recommended to reduce the chance of recurrence.

Removal of the tumour with an appropriate part of the superficial part of the gland (superficial parotidectomy) is adequate treatment for the majority of tumours. If the tumour involves the deep lobe, a total conservative parotidectomy may be required with removal of all or nearly all of the parotid tissue with preservation of the facial nerve.

Prognosis

Providing the tumour is completely excised, the prognosis is excellent but inadequate surgery is followed by a recurrence in a high percentage of cases.

Adenolymphoma

Adenolymphoma (Warthin's tumour[4]) accounts for about 10% of parotid tumours and 10% present bilaterally. Adenolymphomas usually occur in men over the age of 50 years, and there is a strong association with cigarette smoking.

Macroscopically, the tumour is soft and cystic. Microscopically, it consists of columnar cells forming papillary fringes, which project into cystic spaces and are supported by a lymphoid stroma. These tumours probably arise from ectopic salivary duct epithelium within intra- or para-parotid lymph nodes. Presence of the lymphoid tissue may lead to confusion with lymphoproliferative disorders. Prognosis is excellent after local removal.

Carcinoma

Clinical features

There is a significant correlation between tumour stage and survival. Sex distribution is equal, and the patients are usually over the age of 50 years. All ages, however, can be affected with mucoepidermoid tumours being the commonest salivary neoplasm in children. The tumour is hard and infiltrating. Clinically, malignancy should be suspected if there is rapid growth, pain and

---

[4] Aldred Scott Warthin (1866–1931), Professor of Pathology, University of Michigan, Ann Arbor, MI, USA.

involvement of the facial nerve and regional lymph nodes. Eventually, surrounding tissues are infiltrated and the overlying skin becomes ulcerated.

Adenoid cystic, acinic and mucoepidermoid carcinomas are the commonest primary salivary gland malignancies. Growth rates may be variable as is spread to regional lymph nodes. Adenoid cystic tumours tend to spread along nerve sheaths and acinic and mucoepidermoid tumours are more likely to spread to cervical lymph nodes. All may metastasize distantly.

Treatment

Treatment of these tumours is primarily surgical if there has been no distant spread. Wide local excision with clear surgical margins is preferred with or without an associated neck dissection to remove the cervical lymph nodes. Preservation of the facial nerve in parotid tumours may be possible if it is not involved preoperatively. However, it may need to be sacrificed if involved or to achieve adequate clearance. Postoperative radiotherapy may be considered in some cases.

Additional resources

Case 45: A painful submandibular swelling
Case 46: A lump over the angle of the jaw

22

The oesophagus

Peter Safranek

Learning objectives

✓ To know the common causes of dysphagia.

✓ To know the presentation and management of oesophageal perforation.

✓ To know the presentation and management of oesophageal carcinoma.

Dysphagia

Dysphagia is difficulty in swallowing. The causes may be local or general. The local causes of obstruction of any tube in the body can be subdivided into those in the lumen, those in the wall and those outside the wall.

Local causes

In the lumen

- Foreign body.

In the wall

- Congenital atresia.
- Inflammatory stricture, secondary to reflux oesophagitis.
- Caustic stricture.
- Achalasia.
- Eosinophilic oesophagitis causing dysmotility and/or stricture.
- Plummer–Vinson syndrome with oesophageal web.
- Pharyngeal pouch.
- Epiphrenic diverticulum.

- Schatzki's ring.[1]
- Tumour of oesophagus or cardia.
- Systemic sclerosis (scleroderma).

Outside the wall

- Pressure of enlarged lymph nodes (secondary cancer or lymphoma).
- Thoracic aortic aneurysm.
- Bronchial carcinoma.
- Retrosternal goitre.
- Hiatus hernia.

General causes

- Myasthenia gravis.
- Bulbar palsy.
- Bulbar poliomyelitis.
- Diphtheria.
- Hysteria.

Investigations

History

The subjective site of obstruction is not always exact; the patient often merely points vaguely to behind the sternum. The diagnosis may be given by a history of

Ellis and Calne's Lecture Notes in General Surgery, Fourteenth Edition.
Edited by Christopher Watson and Justin Davies.
© 2023 John Wiley & Sons Ltd. Published 2023 by John Wiley & Sons Ltd.
Companion website: www.wiley.com/go/Watson/GeneralSurgery14

[1] Richard Schatzki (1901–1992), Radiologist, Boston, MA, USA. Described a circumferential ring of mucosal tissue in the distal oesophagus.

swallowed caustic in the past. A previous story of reflux oesophagitis may suggest peptic stricture. Patients with achalasia tend to be younger and the history may be longer.

Malignant stricture has a short history, occurs usually in older people and tends to be associated with significant weight loss.

Examination

Often this is negative, but search is made for clinical evidence of Plummer–Vinson syndrome (a smooth tongue, anaemia and koilonychia; see later in this chapter), secondary nodes from a carcinoma of the oesophagus which may be felt in the neck and supraclavicular fossae, and the upper abdomen is carefully palpated, as a carcinoma of the cardia is also a common cause of dysphagia in older patients.

Special investigations

- *Fibreoptic endoscopy* enables biopsies to be taken to confirm malignancy, and permits therapeutic dilation of benign strictures and palliative stenting of incurable malignant obstruction.
- *Barium swallow*, with cine-radiography, may demonstrate the characteristic appearances of a cervical web, extrinsic compression and the dilated oesophagus of achalasia (Figure 22.1).

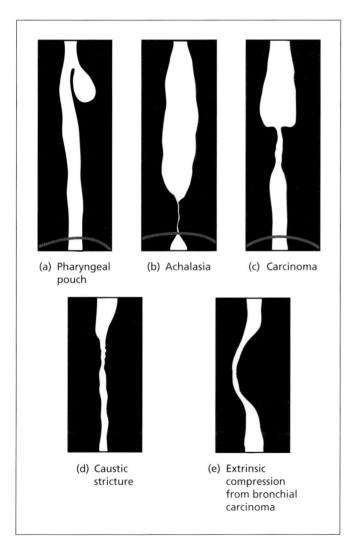

(a) Pharyngeal pouch

(b) Achalasia

(c) Carcinoma

(d) Caustic stricture

(e) Extrinsic compression from bronchial carcinoma

Figure 22.1 (a–e) Barium swallow appearances of common causes of dysphagia.

Endoscopy is the primary investigation but they are complementary and a barium swallow may add useful information.

Swallowed foreign bodies

Foreign bodies are swallowed either accidentally, usually by children, or deliberately by those with psychiatric illness, and prison inmates. Button batteries, which can generate sodium hydroxide when in contact with body fluids, are a particular hazard in children, since they can stick in the oesophagus and cause caustic ulceration and perforation or haemorrhage.

Obstruction of the oropharynx and tracheal opening by a large portion of meat can rapidly become fatal. A sharp blow just below the xiphoid, Heimlich's manoeuvre,[2] causing a sudden rise in intra-abdominal pressure, may dislodge the plug and save the patient's life.

Unless they are sharp or irregular, amazingly large foreign bodies will pass into the stomach. If a smooth object such as a bolus of food impacts in the oesophagus, one must suspect the presence of a stricture or dysmotility such as that caused by eosinophilic oesophagitis. Occasionally, a carcinoma of the oesophagus presents with acute dysphagia when a morsel of food lodges above it. Absolute dysphagia, with failure to swallow even saliva, is then characteristic and needs urgent treatment.

The presenting feature is painful dysphagia. The danger depends on the nature of the foreign body. Perforation may occur with resultant mediastinitis; rarely, perforation of the aorta occurs with fatal haematemesis. The diagnosis is usually made with a computed tomography (CT) scan often with the addition of oral contrast medium if perforation is suspected.

Treatment

Endoscopic removal is indicated when the foreign body is stuck in the oesophagus. With advances in flexible endoscopy, surgery for removal of foreign bodies is seldom necessary in the absence of perforation. The great majority of foreign bodies, once they have passed into the stomach, proceed uneventfully along the gastrointestinal tract and are passed per

rectum. Occasionally, a sharp foreign body penetrates the wall of the bowel (there is a particular tendency for it to lodge in, and pierce, a Meckel's diverticulum; see Chapter 25).

The treatment of a foreign body that has passed the cardia is initially conservative. The patient is watched and serial X-rays can be taken to observe the object's progress if it is radio-opaque. Operation is performed if a sharp object fails to progress or if abdominal pain or tenderness develop.

If the foreign body is potentially toxic when ingested, emetics or laxatives may be indicated.

Perforations of the oesophagus

Classification

From within

- Swallowed foreign body – may occur anywhere in the oesophagus.
- Rupture at rigid oesophagoscopy – usually at the level of cricopharyngeus or above a stricture.
- Rupture during dilation or biopsy – usually at the lower end of the oesophagus and especially likely in the presence of oesophageal disease (carcinoma or stricture).
- Rupture during oesophageal echocardiography – again usually at the lower end, often in the presence of a hitherto unknown stricture or pharyngeal pouch.
- Rupture during endoscopic retrograde cholangiopancreatography (ERCP) - the side viewing endoscope inadvertently enters an undiagnosed pharyngeal pouch which is thin and perforates easily.

From without

- Perforating wounds (rare).

Spontaneous

- Lower thoracic oesophagus (Boerhaave's syndrome[3]).

---

[2] Henry J. Heimlich (1920–2016), Thoracic Surgeon, Xavier University, Cincinnati, OH, USA.

[3] Hermann Boerhaave (1668–1738), Physician, Leiden, the Netherlands. Diagnosed spontaneous rupture of the oesophagus at postmortem on the Grand Admiral of the Dutch Fleet.

Clinical features

After instrumentation, perforation is suspected if the patient complains of pain in the neck, chest or upper abdomen, together with dysphagia and pyrexia. Diagnosis is certain if subcutaneous emphysema is felt in the supraclavicular area.

Spontaneous rupture of the oesophagus occurs rarely and is associated with vomiting after a large meal (Boerhaave's syndrome) where perforation occurs when luminal pressure is increased and cricopharyngeus fails to relax. There is severe pain in the chest, the dorsal region of the spine or the upper abdomen (acute mediastinitis). The patient shows signs of sepsis (fever/tachycardia/raised inflammatory markers). The abdomen may be rigid if perforation extends below the diaphragm. Surgical emphysema (subcutaneous crepitation) can be palpable in the neck owing to gas escaping into the mediastinum.

Special investigations

- *Chest X-ray* shows gas in the neck and mediastinum and there may be fluid and gas in the pleural cavity.
- *Thoraco-abdominal computed tomography (CT)*, combined with oral gastrografin (a water-soluble contrast medium), will confirm the perforation and define its position.

Treatment

Cervical perforation is managed conservatively with parenteral antibiotics, nil by mouth and intravenous fluids. Abscess formation in the superior mediastinum requires drainage via a thoracoscopic or radiological approach.

Thoracic rupture is treated by immediate surgical repair (with or without a T-tube). A perforated carcinoma may potentially be resected. The prognosis from spontaneous rupture is inversely related to the time to surgery, and after 12 hours can be very poor with rapid progression from systemic sepsis to multi-organ failure.

A novel therapy which has gained popularity in the treatment of both iatrogenic and spontaneous oesophageal perforation is Endoluminal Vacuum Therapy. This involves endoscopic placement of a vacuum device through the perforation to control any leak, collapse the mediastinal or pleural cavity and promote healing. This can be used successfully in patients who would not survive the major surgery that conventional treatment entails.

Caustic stricture of the oesophagus

This follows accidental or suicidal ingestion of strong acids or alkalis (particularly, caustic soda and ammonia). It occurs more commonly in children.

In the acute phase, there are associated burns of the mouth and pharynx. The mid- and lower oesophagus are usually affected, as these are the sites of temporary hold-up of the caustic material where the oesophagus is crossed by the aortic arch and at the cardiac sphincter.

Treatment

In the acute phase, treatment aims to neutralize the cause, so alkali ingestion may be neutralized with vinegar and acid ingestion with bicarbonate of soda. The damaged oesophagus is rested by instituting feeding via a gastrostomy or jejunostomy, nil being given by mouth. Systemic steroids are given to reduce scar formation. If a stricture develops, gentle balloon dilation is commenced after 3 or 4 weeks. An established, impassable stricture is treated by resection and reconstruction with either stomach (if this remains healthy) or a colonic conduit if not.

Achalasia of the cardia

This is a neuromuscular condition of the oesophagus where there is failure of both peristalsis and relaxation of the lower oesophageal sphincter, resulting in progressive dilation and tortuosity. The pathological process involves loss of inhibitory ganglion cells from the wall of the oesophagus. It is thought that the cause of the neurone loss may relate to a viral infection or autoimmune response to infection in susceptible individuals. The condition is indistinguishable from Chagas' disease,[4] which occurs in South America secondary to

[4] Carlos Chagas (1879–1934), Professor of Tropical Medicine, Rio de Janeiro, Brazil.

Trypanosoma cruzi infection. The parasite destroys the intermuscular ganglion cells of the oesophagus.

Clinical features

Achalasia may occur at any age but particularly in the third decade. The ratio of women to men is 3:2.

There is progressive dysphagia (particularly to fluids) over months to years, sometimes associated with a spasm-like chest pain. Regurgitation of fluids from the dilated oesophagus may cause an aspiration pneumonia. The failure of clearance of fluid and food can sometimes lead to symptoms which can be mistaken for reflux in the early stages. Occasionally, malignant change occurs in the oesophagus.

Special investigations

- *Chest X-ray* may reveal the dilated oesophagus as a mediastinal mass, with an air–fluid level, and pneumonitis from aspiration of oesophageal contents. (Note that there are three other 'pseudotumours': scoliosis, tuberculous paravertebral abscess and thoracic aortic aneurysm, all of which may simulate a mediastinal tumour on a chest X-ray.)
- *Barium swallow* shows gross dilation and tortuosity of the oesophagus leading to an unrelaxing narrowed segment at the lower end (said to resemble a bird's beak) (see Figure 22.1).
- *Endoscopy* demonstrates a dilated and tortuous oesophagus containing food and fluid residue despite a period of fasting.
- *Oesophageal high resolution manometry* is the gold standard investigation and shows failure of peristalsis with impaired lower oesophageal sphincter relaxation.

Treatment

Good relief of symptoms is obtained by Heller's operation,[5] which is a cardiomyotomy dividing the muscle of the lower end of the oesophagus and the upper stomach down to the mucosa in a similar manner to Ramstedt's operation (see Chapter 23) for congenital pyloric hypertrophy. This procedure can be performed laparoscopically, thus reducing morbidity. It is often combined with an anterior fundoplication which reduces the risk of postoperative reflux.

The same effect may be achieved by forcible dilation of the oesophagogastric junction by means of an endoscopic balloon that is inflated under fluoroscopic (X-ray) control. Although this avoids an operation, there is a risk of rupture of the oesophagus. A temporary non-invasive approach involves endoscopic injection of botulinum toxin (Botox) to paralyse the lower oesophageal sphincter. This can be useful for frail patients unsuitable for surgery or as a temporary means of relieving symptoms.

There is a new endoscopic therapy, per-oral endoscopic myotomy (POEM) which is gaining some popularity. In this technique, the myotomy is performed from the oesophageal lumen using an endoscope.

Plummer–Vinson syndrome[6]

A syndrome actually described by Paterson and Kelly before Plummer and Vinson, and which sometimes rejoices in all four names, comprising dysphagia and iron deficiency anaemia (with its associated smooth tongue and koilonychia – spoon-shaped nails) usually in middle-aged or elderly women.

The dysphagia is associated with hyperkeratinization of the oesophagus and often with the formation of a web in the upper part of the oesophagus. The condition is premalignant and is associated with the development of a carcinoma in the cricopharyngeal region.

Treatment

The dysphagia responds to treatment with iron, although the web may require endoscopic dilatation.

Oesophageal diverticula

The only common diverticulum of the oesophagus is the pharyngeal pouch.

---

[5] Ernst Heller (1877–1964), Surgeon, Leipzig, Germany.

[6] Henry S. Plummer (1874–1937) and Porter Paisley Vinson (1890–1959), Physicians, Mayo Clinic, Rochester, MN, USA. Donald Ross Paterson (1863–1939), ENT Surgeon, Royal Infirmary, Cardiff, UK. Adam Brown-Kelly (1865–1914), ENT Surgeon, Victoria Infirmary, Glasgow, UK.

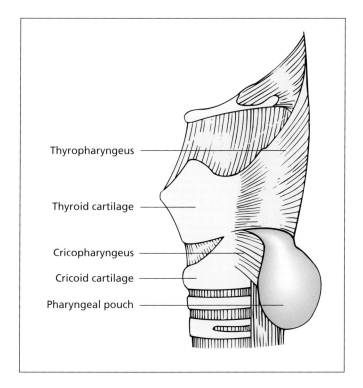

Figure 22.2 A pharyngeal pouch emerging between the two components of the inferior constrictor muscle.

Labels on figure:
- Thyropharyngeus
- Thyroid cartilage
- Cricopharyngeus
- Cricoid cartilage
- Pharyngeal pouch

Other oesophageal diverticula

Other oesophageal diverticula are very rare.

- *Traction diverticula* may occur in association with fixation to tuberculous nodes or to pleural adhesions.
- *Pulsion or epiphrenic diverticula* may be associated with cardiospasm and occur at the lower end of the oesophagus.
- *Congenital diverticula* are occasionally found. These are usually X-ray findings only, although they may occasionally produce dysphagia.

Pharyngeal pouch

This is a mucosal protrusion between the two parts of the inferior pharyngeal constrictor – the thyropharyngeus and cricopharyngeus (Figure 22.2). The weak area between these portions of the muscle is situated posteriorly (Killian's dehiscence[7]). The pouch is believed to

[7] Gustav Killian (1860–1921), Professor of Otorhinolaryngology, Freiburg and Berlin, Germany.

originate above the cricopharyngeus muscle which is in spasm; it develops first posteriorly but cannot then expand in this direction and protrudes to one or the other side, usually the left. As the pouch enlarges, it displaces the oesophagus laterally. It is an example of a pulsion diverticulum, forming as a result of increased intraluminal pressure.

Clinical features

It occurs more often in men and usually in the elderly. There is dysphagia, regurgitation of the food that has collected in the pouch, and often a palpable swelling in the neck, which gurgles. Food retained in the pouch leads to a foetor, and late regurgitation may lead to aspiration pneumonia and lung abscess. Diagnosis is confirmed by a barium swallow.

Treatment

Traditional surgery involved a cervical incision with excision of the pouch combined with a posterior myotomy of the cricopharyngeus. More commonly now, the pouch can be treated by division of the wall between pouch and oesophagus using an endoscopic stapling device (endoscopic diverticulotomy), leaving the pouch *in situ* and avoiding the risk of fistula formation and leaks associated with the open operation.

Reflux oesophagitis

This is produced by the reflux of peptic juice through the incompetent cardiac sphincter into the lower oesophagus, resulting in ulceration and inflammation and eventually in stricture formation. The exact mechanism of the cardio-oesophageal sphincter is not understood; it is sufficient to prevent regurgitation into the oesophagus when standing on one's head or in forced inspiration, when there is a pressure difference of some 80 mmHg between the intragastric and intraoesophageal pressure, yet it can relax readily to allow vomiting or belching to occur. The mechanism is probably a complex affair comprising the following:

- Positive intra-abdominal pressure acting on the lower (intra-abdominal) oesophagus, maintaining a high-pressure zone at the cardia.
- Physiological muscle sphincter at the lower end of the oesophagus.
- Valve-like effect of the obliquity of the oesophago-gastric angle.
- Pinch-cock effect on the lower oesophagus of the diaphragmatic sling when the diaphragm contracts in full inspiration.
- Plug-like action of the mucosal folds at the cardia.

The diaphragm is an important but not essential part of the cardiac sphincter mechanism, as sliding hiatus hernias are not necessarily accompanied by regurgitation. Similarly, free regurgitation occurs in some subjects with a normal oesophageal hiatus, presumably because of some defect in the function of the physiological sphincter.

Reflux oesophagitis may also occur in association with the following:

- Repeated vomiting, especially in the presence of a duodenal ulcer with high acid content of gastric juice.
- Long-standing nasogastric intubation.
- Resections of the cardia with gastro-oesophageal anastomosis.
- Most commonly, in association with hiatal hernia and a weak lower oesophageal sphincter.

Special investigations

- *Endoscopy* demonstrates the presence of oesophagitis and hiatus hernia, and facilitates biopsy to exclude carcinoma, or the presence of Barrett's metaplasia or dysplasia.
- *Twenty-four-hour oesophageal pH and Impedance studies*: a probe in the oesophagus will demonstrate reflux of gastric acid, intestinal fluid and gas and their temporal relation to symptoms.
- *Barium swallow*: this will demonstrate the outline of a hernia and the presence of any associated stricture. Tilting the patient head down will demonstrate reflux, but does not necessarily confirm that the symptoms are due to reflux.

Differential diagnosis

The pain of oesophagitis may be confused with cholecystitis, peptic ulcer or angina pectoris; indeed, these conditions often co-exist.

The obstructive symptoms of an associated stricture must be differentiated from carcinoma of the oesophagus or of the cardia.

Treatment

Medical treatment comprises weight loss, stopping smoking and dietary manipulation. Regurgitation is discouraged by avoiding stooping or lying and by sleeping propped up in bed. Alginate antacids (e.g. Gaviscon) taken after meals neutralize the acidity as well as lining the oesophagus. The mainstay of medical treatment is proton pump inhibitors (e.g. omeprazole), which directly block acid production. H_2-receptor antagonist drugs (e.g. cimetidine) are less effective. Prokinetic drugs to increase gastric emptying, such as metoclopramide, are occasionally used. Many patients with mild symptoms obtain relief of their symptoms with medical treatment.

Laparoscopic surgery for reflux is undertaken when medical treatment fails, if there is significant volume reflux, or if medical therapy cannot be tolerated due to side effects. It usually consists of repair of any hiatal hernia combined with a complete (360 degree, Nissen[8]), or partial (270 degree, Toupet[9]) fundoplication which

---

[8] Rudolph Nissen (1896–1981), Professor of Surgery, Berlin, Turkey, USA and Switzerland.

[9] André Toupet (1915–2015) Surgeon, St Cloud Hospital Paris, France.

sutures the gastric fundus around the lower oesophagus.

In the presence of *stricture*, continuous acid reduction treatment with a proton pump inhibitor and endoscopic balloon dilation will provide effective treatment in most cases. Anti-reflux surgery in younger patients combined with preoperative endoscopic dilation is also an effective treatment. It is very rare for non-caustic strictures to require surgical resection.

Tumours of the oesophagus

Classification

Benign

- Leiomyoma.

Malignant

- Primary:
  - Carcinoma.
  - Leiomyosarcoma.
- Secondary: direct invasion from lung or stomach.

Carcinoma

Postcricoid carcinoma usually occurs in women and is associated with the Plummer–Vinson syndrome (see earlier in this chapter). The remaining oesophageal tumours occur more often in men, usually elderly men. The most common site has changed in recent years, with distal tumours becoming more common than tumours of the mid-third, and upper oesophageal tumours being least common.

Tobacco is a risk factor for oesophageal carcinoma, with squamous carcinoma also being linked to alcohol, long-standing achalasia and coeliac disease. Adenocarcinoma may occur in association with Barrett's oesophagus as a consequence of metaplastic change and subsequent dysplasia in the lower oesophagus or at the gastro-oesophageal junction; it is also associated with obesity.

Carcinoma of the oesophagus is a relatively common tumour in the UK (18 per 100 000 incidence), but is 20 times more common in China, and twice as common in France. The incidence is rising in the Western world. The overall prognosis is about 20% survival at 5 years. This is mainly a reflection of the advanced stage at presentation.

Pathology

The tumour commences as a nodule, which then develops into an ulcer, a papillomatous mass or an annular constriction.

Microscopically, the majority are now adenocarcinomas arising at the lower end of the oesophagus, either in Barrett's oesophagus or as a result of extension into the oesophagus by a tumour developing in the cardia of the stomach. Tumours of the upper two-thirds are usually squamous carcinomas.

Spread

- *Local*: into the mediastinal structures – the trachea, aorta, mediastinal pleura, diaphragm and lung. Also peritoneal in subdiaphragmatic tumours.
- *Lymphatic*: to para-oesophageal, tracheobronchial, supraclavicular and subdiaphragmatic nodes.
- *Bloodstream*: to liver and lungs (relatively late).

Clinical features

Carcinoma of the oesophagus may present because of the following:

- *Local symptoms* – dysphagia, haematemesis.
- *Secondary deposits* – enlarged neck nodes, occasionally jaundice and/or hepatomegaly.
- *General manifestations of malignant disease* – loss of weight, anorexia, anaemia.

Dysphagia in an elderly male with a short history is almost invariably due to carcinoma of the oesophagus or the upper end of the stomach. Progression is from dysphagia for solids to dysphagia for liquids. Hoarseness and a bovine cough suggest invasion of the left recurrent laryngeal nerve by an upper oesophageal tumour, or malignant nodes in the aorto-pulmonary window.

Special investigations

The purpose of these investigations is to confirm the diagnosis and to assess extent (stage) of disease.

- *Endoscopy* enables the tumour to be inspected and a biopsy taken. This may be combined with endo-luminal ultrasound to evaluate local invasion.
- *Endoscopic ultrasound* enables assessment of the tumour's depth of invasion and detection of local and lymphatic spread; it also facilitates fine needle aspiration of lymph nodes to facilitate preoperative staging.
- *CT scan* of the thorax and abdomen to assess the primary growth, local invasion and secondary spread to the liver, lungs and lymph nodes.
- *Positron emission tomography (PET)*, in conjunction with CT, is also used to stage oesophageal carcinoma and is more sensitive for metastatic disease.
- *Laparoscopy* is used to exclude peritoneal metastatic disease in tumours extending below the diaphragm.

Differential diagnosis

Other causes of dysphagia (see list at the beginning of this chapter).

Treatment

The treatment aim is to cure the cancer when possible, and if not to palliate the symptoms including dysphagia.

Curative resection

When cure is possible, resection is undertaken following a course of chemotherapy and/or radiotherapy which have been shown to significantly increase survival in large randomized trials. The tumour is removed and the oesophagus is usually reconstructed by mobilizing the stomach up into the chest, with anastomosis to residual oesophagus in the thorax or the neck. With multimodal therapies and radical surgery in specialist centres, the long-term survival following oesophagectomy continues to improve with 3 year survival around 57% in the latest national audit.

Palliation

- *Intubation* with a stent may relieve dysphagia if the tumour is inoperable.
- *Radiotherapy*, either external beam or intraluminal, is useful for squamous tumours.
- *Chemotherapy*, particularly with a platinum-based regimen, has shown increasing promise.

- *Immunotherapy* has recently shown benefit with programmed death ligand (PDL) inhibitors in advanced disease.

The average expectation of life has improved with high-quality palliative treatments and relief of dysphagia is achievable in most cases but few patients with advanced metastatic disease survive more than a year.

Barrett's oesophagus[10] and adenocarcinoma

This is an increasingly common condition with an estimated prevalence of about 2% of adults in the UK. The normal oesophagus is lined by stratified squamous epithelium. In patients with long-standing reflux of duodenogastric contents, the lower oesophageal epithelium undergoes metaplasia to an intestinal-type columnar epithelium. Continued inflammation may lead to dysplasia and subsequently to malignant change. Carcinomas in such cases are adenocarcinomas, and most occur in the lower third of the oesophagus or at the gastro-oesophageal junction. They are most common in male smokers, with a long history (over 10 years) of Barrett's metaplasia and frequent symptoms (more than three times a week) of gastro-oesophageal reflux.

Barrett's metaplasia of the oesophagus is premalignant, and such patients should undergo regular endoscopic surveillance, with biopsies to look for dysplasia. When dysplasia becomes high grade, there is a high chance of progression to invasive cancer. Therefore, endoscopic treatment in the form of radiofrequency ablation and/or endoscopic resections of small areas or lesions should be undertaken. Early adenocarcinoma in Barrett's which does not invade the submucosa has a high chance of being cured with endoscopic resection. Surgical resection is recommended if there is significant invasion of submucosa or lymphovascular invasion which would increase the risk of lymph node involvement. Persistent low-grade dysplasia is increasingly being considered for endoscopic therapy.

---

[10] Norman Barrett (1903–1979), Thoracic Surgeon, St Thomas's Hospital, London, UK.

The risk of malignant change in someone with Barrett's oesophagus is approximately 0.5% per patient per year. The important thing is to diagnose those patients who often have a significant history of reflux, so they can undergo surveillance. This allows any dysplasia to be identified early when it can be cured by endoscopic therapy.

Additional resources

23

The stomach and duodenum

Stavros Gourgiotis

Learning objectives

✓ To have knowledge of gastric tumours (benign and malignant), gastroparesis and pyloric stenosis; pathology, symptoms, diagnosis and indications for surgical management.

✓ To have knowledge of peptic ulceration and its aetiology and complications and how treatment has changed with recognition of *Helicobacter pylori*.

✓ To have knowledge of gastric volvulus and its treatment options.

Congenital hypertrophic pyloric stenosis

Aetiology

The aetiology of pyloric stenosis in infants is unknown, but it includes genetic and environmental factors. Although a specific gene has not been identified, it has long been recognized to have a familial tendency; 80% of cases occur in male infants; 50% are first born; and the condition often occurs in siblings including a six-fold increased incidence in monozygotic compared to dizygotic twins. There is also an association with the administration of macrolide antibiotics (e.g. erythromycin) to the mother in late pregnancy or to the infant in the first 2 weeks of life.

Ellis and Calne's Lecture Notes in General Surgery, Fourteenth Edition.
Edited by Christopher Watson and Justin Davies.
© 2023 John Wiley & Sons Ltd. Published 2023 by John Wiley & Sons Ltd.
Companion website: www.wiley.com/go/Watson/GeneralSurgery14

The mechanism of pyloric stenosis may relate to an abnormality of the ganglion cells of the myenteric plexus, or failure of the pyloric sphincter to relax due to disturbance in nitric oxide neurotransmission resulting in intense work hypertrophy of the adjacent circular pyloric muscle.

Clinical features

The child usually presents at three to eight weeks of age, although symptoms may be present, rarely, at or soon after birth. It is extremely uncommon for a previously healthy infant to develop this condition after 12 weeks.

The presenting symptom is projectile vomiting. The vomit never contains bile and the child takes food avidly immediately after vomiting, that is, the infant is always hungry. There is failure to gain weight and, as a result of dehydration, the baby is constipated (the stools resembling the faecal pellets of a rabbit).

The infant may be dehydrated and visible peristalsis of the dilated stomach may be seen in the

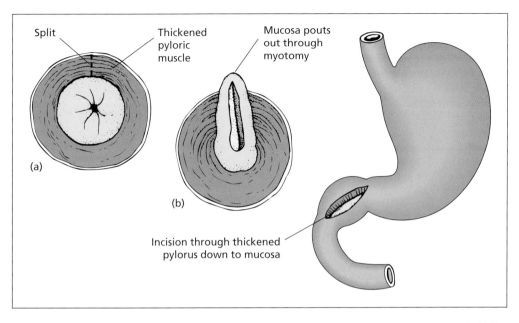

Split | Thickened pyloric muscle | Mucosa pouts out through myotomy

(a)

(b)

Incision through thickened pylorus down to mucosa

Figure 23.1 Ramstedt's pyloromyotomy. The thickened muscle at the pylorus is split down to the mucosa. (a, b) The pathology and the operative procedure in transverse section.

epigastrium. Ninety-five per cent of infants have a palpable pyloric mass, which is felt as a firm 'bobbin' in the right upper abdomen, especially after vomiting a feed.

Differential diagnosis

- *Enteritis*: diarrhoea accompanies this.
- *Neonatal intestinal obstruction* from duodenal atresia, volvulus neonatorum or intestinal atresia: symptoms commence within a day or two of birth and the vomit contains bile.
- *Intracranial birth injury*.
- *Overfeeding*: here there are no other features to suggest pyloric stenosis apart from vomiting.

If the clinical features are characteristic and a pyloric mass is palpable, no further investigations are necessary.

- *Ultrasound scan* demonstrates the thickened and elongated pylorus and large stomach.
- *Abdominal X-ray* reveals a dilated stomach with minimal gas in the bowel, in contrast to dilated loops of small bowel in intestinal obstruction.
- *Barium meal* reveals the pyloric obstruction with characteristic shouldering of the pyloric antrum

due to the impression made on it by the hypertrophied pyloric muscle. Neither plain X-ray or barium study are usually necessary.

Management

This is anomalous in that the more seriously ill the child, the less urgent is the operation. With prolonged vomiting, the infant becomes dehydrated with a hypochloraemic metabolic alkalosis. In such cases, a day or two must be spent with gastric decompression and fluid replacement (saline with added potassium chloride). Children with minimal electrolyte abnormalities can undergo surgery soon after admission.

Surgical treatment (*Ramstedt's pyloromyotomy*)[1]

A longitudinal incision is made through the hypertrophied muscle of the pylorus down to mucosa and the cut edges are separated (Figure 23.1). This is now commonly performed laparoscopically, and is one of

[1]Conrad Ramstedt (1867–1963), Surgeon, Munster, Germany. The procedure was first described by Sir Harold Stiles (1863–1946) in Edinburgh earlier in the same year, 1912.

the most common procedures in children. The infant is given glucose water 3 hours after the operation and this is followed by 3-hourly milk feeds, which are steadily increased in amount. Results are excellent and the mortality is extremely low. Complication rates vary between 4 and 12%.

Duodenal atresia

Duodenal atresia is a congenital intestinal obstruction that can cause bilious or non-bilious vomiting within the first 24 to 48 hours of neonatal life. The diagnosis is suggested *in utero* by the presence of polyhydramnios. It is one of the most common causes of foetal bowel obstruction.

Aetiology

Duodenal atresia is caused by obstruction of the duodenum, usually distal to the ampulla of Vater in the second part of the duodenum. During the eighth to the tenth week of embryological development, errors of duodenal re-canalization are the main cause of duodenal atresia. In duodenal atresia, there is complete obstruction of the duodenal lumen, in contrast to duodenal stenosis where there is narrowing, resulting in an incomplete obstruction of the duodenum lumen.

Epidemiology

Duodenal atresia occurs in 1 in 5 000 to 10 000 live births and is often associated with other anomalies, including trisomy 21 (Down syndrome) and cardiac malformations. Around a third of children with duodenal atresia have trisomy 21. There is a 3% prevalence of congenital duodenal atresia among patients with Down syndrome. Duodenal atresia is associated with annular pancreas, and other bowel atresias, including jejunal atresia, ileal atresia and rectal atresia.

Differential diagnosis

- *Oesophageal atresia*: there is choking rather than vomiting.
- *Pyloric stenosis*: bile is absent from the vomit, there is a palpable pyloric mass, and onset is later.

- *Congenital intestinal obstruction*: there is abdominal distension and X-rays show multiple distended loops of bowel with fluid levels.

In cases of duodenal atresia, the abdominal X-ray is diagnostic and shows distension of the stomach and proximal duodenum with absence of gas throughout the rest of the bowel (the 'double bubble' sign).

Treatment

Duodenojejunostomy or gastrojejunostomy is performed after rehydration and gastric aspiration.

Peptic ulcer

Peptic ulcer is ulceration of the upper gastrointestinal (GI) tract and accounts for about half of all episodes of upper GI tract bleeding in the UK. This includes gastric ulcers and duodenal ulcers. *Helicobacter pylori* is associated with ~70% of gastric ulcers and 90% of duodenal ulcers. However, only 20% of people with *H. pylori* will develop a peptic ulcer. Although the overall incidence of peptic ulcer appears to be decreasing, rates of bleeding from ulcers remain the same.

Pathology

The pathogenesis of peptic ulcer involves a disturbance in the balance between the secretion of acid and pepsin by the stomach on the one hand and the mucosal barrier (a thick layer of mucus) on the other. The normal stomach mucosa is adapted to contain the acid produced by the parietal (oxyntic) cells. Where the mucosal defence is compromised, or non-existent, the acid causes mucosal ulceration. Ulcers also occur where acid attacks mucosa not specialized to deal with it. Hence, typical sites for peptic ulcers are the oesophagus (reflux oesophagitis), stomach, first part of duodenum, at the stoma of a gastrojejunal anastomosis or adjacent to a Meckel's diverticulum[2] when ectopic parietal cells are present.

[2]Johann Frederick Meckel (1781–1833), Professor of Anatomy and Surgery, Halle, Germany. His grandfather and father were both Professors of Anatomy.

Historical background

The vast majority of peptic ulcers are caused by infection with *H. pylori*. Until the publication of the link between this organism and ulcers in 1983, the majority of peptic ulcers were thought to be due to overactivity of the gastric parietal cells. The stimuli to parietal cell function are neural (via the vagus nerve) and humoral (gastrin and histamine). Earlier treatments were, therefore, directed at reducing acid secretion by surgical denervation of the stomach (vagotomy) or removal of the parietal cells (partial gastrectomy). More recently, pharmacological control has been possible with histamine H2-receptor antagonists (e.g. cimetidine) and proton pump inhibitors (e.g. omeprazole). With hindsight, we now realize that none of these treatments dealt with the most important cause of the peptic ulceration, *H. pylori*.

Helicobacter pylori

Helicobacter pylori (previously called *Campylobacter pyloridis*) is a spiral-shaped, Gram-negative, motile rod that is able to penetrate the viscid mucus layer lining the stomach. Its potent urease activity splits any urea in the vicinity, producing ammonia and thus neutralizing the pH in the local milieu surrounding the organism. Many *H. pylori* strains also produce cytotoxins that possess protease and phospholipase activity, allowing them to attack and damage mucosal membranes. This direct damage, together with the resultant inflammation, impairs the gastric mucosal barrier and allows further damage by gastric acid. Non-cytotoxin-producing strains explain asymptomatic carriage of the organism.

Patients with duodenal ulcer have impaired bicarbonate secretion in the proximal duodenum in the face of influx of gastric acid. This impaired response is reversed by the eradication of *H. pylori*. The mechanism by which *H. pylori* hampers duodenal bicarbonate secretion is not understood. One proposed mechanism is that nitric oxide synthase activity in the duodenum interferes with bicarbonate secretion.

Evidence identifying *H. pylori* as a causative agent in peptic ulceration includes the following observations:

- Ingestion of *H. pylori* results in chronic gastritis (as demonstrated by Barry Marshall, who with

Robin Warren[3], identified the relationship between infection with the organism and peptic ulceration, and proved it by inoculating himself).
- Animal inoculation with *H. pylori* mimics human gastritis.
- Antimicrobial treatment that eradicates *H. pylori* also eliminates gastritis.
- *H. pylori* can be identified in almost all patients with duodenal ulcers, and most patients with gastric ulcers.

Zollinger–Ellison syndrome[4]

This is a syndrome in which a non-insulin-secreting islet cell tumour of the pancreas produces a potent gastrin-like hormone (see Chapter 34). It is an uncommon cause of peptic ulceration. In this syndrome, the ulcers are often multiple, and ulceration may be more widespread within the small bowel.

Other factors in the aetiology of peptic ulceration

A number of other factors decrease the effectiveness of the mucosal defences against gastric juice. In particular, non-steroidal anti-inflammatory drugs (NSAIDs) inhibit the production of protective prostaglandins in the mucosa. Steroids also predispose to ulceration, as do smoking and stress, which are thought to have an effect on both acid secretion and mucosal defences.

The acute peptic ulcer

This may be single or multiple (multiple erosions), may occur without apparent cause or may be associated with ingestion of alcohol or NSAIDs (aspirin is a common culprit), steroid therapy, acute stress, a major

[3]Barry Marshall (b. 1951), Gastroenterologist, Royal Perth Hospital, Australia. J. Robin Warren (b. 1937), Pathologist, Royal Perth Hospital, Australia. Won the Nobel Prize for their observation in 2005. Spiral-shaped organisms were identified in stomach biopsies in 1875, and their relation to gastritis suggested in 1899 by Walery Jaworski, a Polish Physician; the observation was largely overlooked until the work of Marshall and Warren in 1982.

[4]Robert Milton Zollinger (1903–1992), Professor of Surgery, Ohio State University, Columbus, Ohio; Edwin Homer Ellison (1918–1970), Associate Professor at the same institution.

operation, head injury (Cushing's ulcer[5]) or severe burns (Curling's ulcer[6]). It may present with sudden pain, haemorrhage or perforation. A proportion of acute ulcers probably go on to become chronic.

The chronic peptic ulcer

At least 80% of peptic ulcers occur in the duodenum. *Duodenal ulcers* may occur at any age, but especially in the thirties to forties; about 80% occur in men. Women are relatively immune to duodenal ulceration before menopause and especially during pregnancy.

    Gastric ulcers occur predominantly in men, but the sex preponderance is less marked - about 3:1 for men to women. Any age may be affected, but especially the forties to fifties (i.e. a decade later than the peak for duodenal ulceration).

Clinical features

Physical signs in the uncomplicated case are absent or confined to epigastric tenderness. Clinical diagnosis depends on a careful history.

    The pain is typically epigastric, occurs in attacks that last for days or weeks and is interspersed with periods of relief. Pain that radiates into the back suggests a posterior penetrating ulcer. Peptic ulcer pain may come on immediately after a meal but more typically commences about 2 hrs after, so that the patient says it precedes a meal ('hunger pain'). Characteristically, it wakes the patient in the early morning, so much so that the patient may adopt the habit of taking a glass of milk or an alkali preparation to bed.

    It is a myth to say that one can differentiate between a gastric and a duodenal ulcer merely on the time relationship of the pain. The pain is aggravated by spicy foods and relieved by milk and alkalis, although the relief is lost in deep and penetrating ulcers. There may be associated heartburn, nausea and vomiting.

[5] Harvey Cushing (1869–1939), Professor of Surgery, Harvard Medical School, Boston, Massachusetts.

[6] Thomas Blizzard Curling (1811–1888), Surgeon, the London Hospital, London.

The patient may lose weight because of the pain produced by food but often may gain weight because of the high intake of milk.

Special investigations

- *Fibreoptic endoscopy*: enables the oesophagus, stomach and duodenum to be examined. The ulcer can be identified and, particularly in the case of a gastric lesion, biopsy material obtained to enable differentiation between a benign and malignant ulcer.
- *H. pylori detection*:
  - *Endoscopic biopsy*. Histological examination will confirm the presence of the organism and identify mucosal damage. A urease test, in which a biopsy sample is placed in a solution of urea together with a pH indicator, is highly specific and sensitive for the organism. *H. pylori* splits urea, releasing ammonia, which changes the pH of the solution.
  - *^{13}C-labelled urea breath test*. The patient ingests a solution containing ^{13}C-labelled urea (non-radioactive). The urease from the organism cleaves the urea load and bicarbonate (HCO_3^-) is released into the blood and expired as $^{13}CO_2$. Measurement of labelled CO_2 in breath samples taken before and after ingestion of the urea solution confirms the diagnosis, and serial tests can be used to confirm eradication of the organism.
  - *Serological testing*. Infection with *H. pylori* results in generation of antibodies, which may be detected. Antibody titre falls slowly after eradication.

Treatment

Treatment of a peptic ulcer is medical in the first instance; surgery is indicated when complications occur. The complications are perforation, stenosis, haemorrhage and, in the case of gastric ulcer, malignant change. They are considered in detail later in this chapter.

Principles of medical treatment

The main principles of treatment are to eradicate *H. pylori* and to reduce and neutralize (using alkalis and milk) acid secretion. Failure to eradicate *H. pylori* by giving antacid therapy alone results in high relapse rates.

- *H. pylori eradication.* A 2-week course of antimicrobial therapy combined with acid reduction therapy will eradicate *H. pylori*. Acid reduction is usually afforded by a proton pump inhibitor (e.g. omeprazole, lansoprazole) and the antimicrobial therapy is based on either clarithromycin or amoxicillin, together with metronidazole. The combination of two antibiotics is recommended because of the high incidence of antibiotic resistance. Such protocols will eradicate *H. pylori* in over 90% of patients.
- *Acid reduction.* Acid reduction with a proton pump inhibitor (or less commonly a H_2-receptor blocker such as cimetidine) alone results in the majority of ulcers healing within 1–2 months; the ulcers will recur if *H. pylori* has not been eradicated.

Significant gastric acid stimulants such as alcohol should be avoided. Rest, avoidance of smoking and dealing with underlying anxiety states are helpful. Aspirin and other NSAIDs should be avoided wherever possible.

Principles of surgical treatment

Surgical treatment is now reserved for those patients in whom complications of ulceration occur. In the emergency situation, minimal surgery is practised with the confidence that medical cure of the underlying disease may be effected. The most common indications for emergency surgery are bleeding or perforation.

Gastric ulcers

Gastric ulcers are treated by removing the ulcer together with the gastrin-secreting zone of the antrum. Traditionally, this was done by the Billroth I gastrectomy[7] (Figure 23.2), but is now more commonly achieved by an antrectomy combined with a Roux-en-Y gastroenterostomy, the latter to limit bile reflux.

Duodenal ulcers

Duodenal ulcers will heal providing the high acid production of the stomach is abolished. This can be effected by removing the bulk of the acid-secreting area of the stomach (the body and the lesser curve), and re-establishing gastric drainage via a Roux-en-Y gastroenterostomy. The traditional procedures involved a partial (Pólya) gastrectomy[8] with closure of the duodenum and a gastrojejunostomy, or division of the vagus nerves. As total vagotomy interferes with the mechanism of gastric emptying, this operation must be accompanied by a drainage procedure, either gastrojejunostomy or pyloroplasty. If the branches of the vagus nerve that supply the pyloric sphincter (the nerves of Latarjet[9]) are left intact, the remaining vagal fibres can be divided without the necessity of gastric drainage (highly selective vagotomy), but nevertheless the goal of reduction in the vagal phase of acid secretion is achieved.

Post-gastrectomy syndromes

Even though about 85% of patients are well following Pólya partial gastrectomy for peptic ulcer, a large number of unpleasant sequelae may occur. These may be classified into the following.

- *Small stomach syndrome*: a feeling of fullness after a moderate-sized meal.
- *Bilious vomiting* due to emptying of the afferent loop of a Pólya gastrectomy into the stomach remnant.
- *Anaemia* due usually to iron deficiency (HCl is required for adequate iron absorption) or, occasionally, vitamin B_{12} deficiency owing to loss of intrinsic factor with extensive gastric resection.
- *Dumping*: comprises attacks of fainting, vertigo and sweating after food, rather like a hypoglycaemic attack. This is probably an osmotic effect due to gastric contents of high osmolarity passing rapidly into the jejunum, absorbing fluid into the gut lumen and producing a temporary reduction in circulating blood volume.

---

[7]Theodor Billroth (1829–1894), Professor of Surgery, Vienna, Austria. He performed the first successful gastrectomy for cancer at the pyloric end of the stomach in 1881.

[8]Eugen Alexander Pólya (1876–1944), Surgeon, St Stephen's Hospital, Budapest, Hungary.

[9]André Latarjet (1876–1947), Professor of Anatomy, Lyon, France.

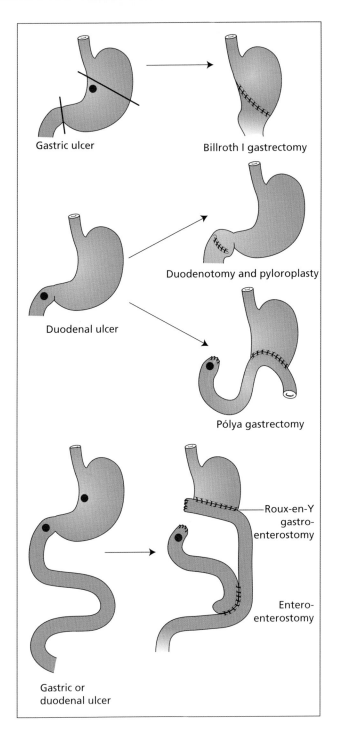

Gastric ulcer

Billroth I gastrectomy

Duodenal ulcer

Duodenotomy and pyloroplasty

Pólya gastrectomy

Gastric or duodenal ulcer

Roux-en-Y gastro-enterostomy

Entero-enterostomy

Figure 23.2 The principal operations once commonly performed for peptic ulcer. Surgery is still indicated in the presence of haemorrhage from an ulcer, and usually comprises a partial gastrectomy with drainage into a Roux-en-Y loop of jejunum. The more traditional procedures are also shown here: for a gastric ulcer, a Billroth I gastrectomy with gastroduodenal anastomosis was performed; for a duodenal ulcer, a simple longitudinal duodenotomy, closed as a pyloroplasty, with under-running of the bleeding vessel, was performed, combined with acid suppression with a proton pump inhibitor (instead of the traditional vagotomy); a Pólya gastrectomy[8] with under-running of the vessel was an alternative. Eradication of *Helicobacter pylori* should be undertaken when necessary. For gastric cancer, a gastrectomy with Roux-en-Y drainage is now preferred.

- *Steatorrhoea*: in the presence of a long afferent loop, food passing into the jejunum traverses the bowel without mixing adequately with pancreatic and biliary secretions. Calcium deficiency and osteomalacia may occur.
- *Stomal ulceration* complicates about 2% of gastrectomies for duodenal ulcer; it is extremely rare after resection for gastric ulcer. It may be due to inadequate removal of the acid-secreting area of the stomach or, rarely, because of the Zollinger–Ellison syndrome. A stomal ulcer, like any other peptic ulcer, may perforate, stenose, invade surrounding structures or bleed. It is treated by either vagotomy or higher gastric resection.

Post-vagotomy syndromes

The following sequelae may occur after truncal vagotomy.

- *Steatorrhoea and diarrhoea*: frequently transient or episodic, they may be severe and persistent in about 2% of patients. The incidence is reduced in patients subjected to highly selective vagotomy without drainage.
- *Stomal ulceration* may occur if vagotomy is incomplete.

Complications of peptic ulceration

Peptic ulcer at any site may undergo the following complications:

- *Perforation* either into the peritoneal cavity or into adjacent structures, for example the pancreas, liver or colon.
- *Stenosis*.
- *Haemorrhage*.
- *Chronicity* due to formation of fibrous tissue in the ulcer base.
- *Malignant change*, which does not occur in duodenal ulcers but may rarely take place in a gastric ulcer; a long history does not necessarily mean that the ulcer was not malignant *de novo*. Both benign gastric ulcer and gastric carcinoma are common conditions and there may merely be a

chance association between the two. Around 1% of all gastric carcinomas arise in a gastric ulcer.

Perforated peptic ulcer

Pathology

Perforation of a peptic ulcer is a relatively common and important emergency, and the incidence of peptic ulcer perforation is decreasing due to early diagnosis and effective medical management. Male preponderance, once very high, is now about 2:1. Until recently, perforation occurred particularly in young adults, but now the shift is towards the older age groups, especially in patients who are on either steroids or NSAIDs.

Clinical features

A previous history of peptic ulceration is obtained in about half the cases, although this may be forgotten by the patient in agony. Typically, the pain is of sudden onset and of extreme severity; the patient can often recall the exact moment of the onset of the pain. Subphrenic irritation may be indicated by referred pain to one or both shoulders, usually the right. The pain is aggravated by movement and the patient lies rigidly still. There is nausea, but only occasionally vomiting. Sometimes, there is accompanying haematemesis or melaena.

Examination reveals a patient in severe pain, cold and sweating with rapid, shallow respirations. In the early stages (hours), there may be no clinical evidence of true shock: the pulse is steady and the blood pressure normal; the temperature is either normal or a little depressed. The abdomen is rigid and silent, although in some instances an occasional bowel sound may be heard. Liver dullness is diminished in about half the cases owing to escape of gas into the peritoneal cavity. Rectal examination may reveal pelvic tenderness.

In the delayed case, after 12 hours or more, the features of generalized peritonitis with paralytic ileus become manifest; the abdomen is distended, effortless vomiting occurs and the patient is in septic shock.

Special investigations

- *Chest X-ray*, with the patient erect, shows free gas below the diaphragm in over 70% of cases.
- *Computed tomography (CT) scan* is more sensitive in the detection of free intraperitoneal gas, and can exclude common differential diagnoses such as pancreatitis when doubt exists.

Differential diagnosis

The four conditions with which perforated ulcer is most commonly confused are:

- Perforated appendicitis.
- Acute cholecystitis.
- Acute pancreatitis.
- Myocardial infarction.

Treatment

Indications for surgery

- *Generalized peritonitis* and typically, but not always, free gas under the diaphragm on erect chest X-ray (CXR).
- *Failed conservative management* in selected patients. Conservative management can be chosen in patients with a confirmed diagnosis of peptic perforation who are haemodynamically stable and have no, or localized, signs of peritonitis.

Preoperative management

A nasogastric (NG) tube is passed to empty the stomach and diminish further leakage. This is an essential pre-anaesthetic measure. Opiate analgesia is given to relieve pain and intravenous fluid resuscitation is started. Antibiotics are given to contend with the peritoneal infection, and an intravenous proton pump inhibitor commenced. Most surgeons are in favour of immediate operative repair of the perforation.

Operative management

Perforations usually occur on the anterior wall of the first part of the duodenum. Surgery involves suturing an omental plug to seal the perforation, together with lavage of the peritoneal cavity (Figure 23.3). In addition, a gastric ulcer is biopsied at all four quadrants to exclude malignancy; an

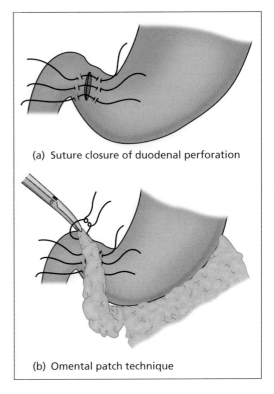

(a) Suture closure of duodenal perforation

(b) Omental patch technique

Figure 23.3 Techniques to close a perforated ulcer.

obviously malignant gastric ulcer is removed by partial gastrectomy.

Laparoscopic closure of the peptic ulcer should be considered in all cases. Advantages of laparoscopic surgery include similar results as open surgery with the additional advantage of decreased postoperative pain, hospital stay, wound infections and incisional hernia. However, the procedure can be technically more challenging and time-consuming.

Prognosis

The mortality for perforated peptic ulcer lies between 5% and 10%. Most deaths are in patients incorrectly diagnosed, with consequent delay in correct treatment, or in those who are too ill for operation. The subjects who die are typically either over the age of 70 years or reach hospital 12 hours or more after the time of perforation or are shocked on admission. The long-term prognosis following perforation depends on whether or not the ulcer is chronic, and whether a treatable cause, such as *H. pylori* or NSAIDs, is present.

Pyloric stenosis

This is an inaccurate term when applied to duodenal ulceration, as the obstruction is in the first part of the duodenum.

Pathology

At first, fibrotic scarring is compensated by dilation and hypertrophy of the stomach muscle. Eventually, failure of compensation occurs, much like the failure of a hypertrophied ventricle of the heart with valvular stenosis.

Clinical features

During the phase of compensation, there is nothing in the history to suggest stenosis. Once failure occurs, there is characteristic profuse vomiting, which is free from bile. The vomitus may contain food eaten days previously and appears and smells faeculent. Because of copious vomiting, there is associated loss of weight, constipation (because of dehydration) and weakness because of electrolyte disturbance.

On examination, the patient may appear dehydrated and wasted. Progressive dilation and hypertrophy of the stomach occurs. At first, a gastric splash (*succussion splash*) can be elicited by shaking the patient's abdomen several hours after a meal. As the stomach enlarges, visible peristalsis can also be seen, passing from left to right across the upper abdomen. Finally, the grossly dilated, hypertrophied stomach, full of stale food and fluid, can actually be palpated.

Gastric aspiration normally yields a morning resting juice of over 100 mL. In advanced cases of pyloric stenosis, it may amount to several litres of foul-smelling gastric contents.

Special investigations

- *Gastroscopy* following decompression of the stomach with a nasogastric tube will identify the cause in most cases.
- *CT scan* will provide further anatomical information about the diagnosis and its aetiology.
- *Arterial blood gases and electrolyte estimation* may show a hypochloraemic alkalosis, with hypokalaemia and uraemia.

Biochemical disturbances

Pyloric obstruction with copious vomiting results in not only dehydration from fluid loss but also alkalosis due to loss of hydrogen ions from the stomach. The alkalotic tendency is compensated by the renal excretion of sodium bicarbonate, which may keep the blood pH within normal limits. During this phase, the dehydration results in diminished volume and increased concentration of urine, the chloride content of which is first diminished and then disappears and the pH of which is alkaline. If vomiting continues, a large sodium deficit becomes manifest. This loss of sodium is partly accounted for by loss in the vomitus but it is mainly the result of urinary excretion consequent upon the bicarbonate lost in the urine as sodium bicarbonate. As the body's sodium reserves become depleted, hydrogen and potassium ions are substituted for sodium as the cations that are excreted with the bicarbonate. This results in the paradox that the patient with advanced alkalosis now excretes an acid urine.

The blood urea rises, partly because of dehydration and partly because of renal impairment secondary to the electrolyte disturbances. Eventually, the patient may develop tetany as a result of a shift of the ionized, weakly alkaline calcium phosphate to its unionized state, in attempted compensation for the alkalosis. The concentration of calcium ions in the plasma, therefore, falls, although the total calcium concentration is not affected.

The metabolic disturbances may be summarized as follows:

- The patient is dehydrated and the haematocrit level is raised.
- The urine is scanty, concentrated, initially alkaline, but later acid; the chloride content of the urine is reduced or absent.
- Serum chloride, sodium and potassium are lowered and the plasma bicarbonate and urea are raised.

Differential diagnosis

- Carcinoma of the pylorus.

Other causes of pyloric obstruction are unusual in the adult:

- Scarring associated with a benign gastric ulcer near the pylorus.

- Carcinoma of the head of the pancreas infiltrating the duodenum and pylorus.
- Chronic pancreatitis.
- Invasion of the pylorus by malignant nodes.

The differential diagnosis from a pyloric carcinoma cannot always be established until endoscopy and biopsy, or even laparotomy, but a reasonable attempt can be made on the following points.

- *Length of history:* a history of several years of characteristic peptic ulcer pain is in favour of benign ulcer. Cancer usually has a history of only months and indeed may be painless.
- *Gross dilation of the stomach favours a benign lesion*, as it may take several years for this to develop.
- *The presence of a mass at the pylorus indicates malignant disease*, although, rarely, a palpable inflammatory mass in association with a large duodenal ulcer can be detected.

Treatment

The treatment of established pyloric obstruction is invariably surgical. Before operation, dehydration and electrolyte depletion are corrected by intravenous replacement of saline together with potassium. Daily gastric lavage is performed to remove the debris from the stomach. In addition, this often restores function to the stomach and allows fluid absorption to take place by mouth. Vitamin C is given, as the patient with a chronic duodenal ulcer is often deficient in ascorbic acid. This may be a direct effect of *H. pylori* or it may be the result of a diet low in fruit and vegetables.

Surgical correction is carried out after a few days of preoperative preparation. Surgery usually involves an antrectomy with a Roux-en-Y gastroenterostomy.

Gastrointestinal haemorrhage

Management

The management of patients presenting with haematemesis and/or melaena is threefold:

1 Assessment and resuscitation of the patient.
2 Diagnosis of the source of the bleeding.
3 Treatment and control of the source of bleeding.

Assessment of the patient

An initial appraisal of the patient's airway and breathing is undertaken; oxygen is administered when necessary. Indicators of severe blood loss are the features of shock, namely pallor, cold, clammy and peripherally shut down, with a tachycardia and a systolic blood pressure below 100 mmHg. It should be remembered that patients on β-blockers tend not to become tachycardic, and if the patient is known to have hypertension a systolic pressure well above 100 mmHg does not rule out shock.

The presence of shock is an indication for immediate fluid replacement with normal saline or compound sodium lactate (Hartmann's) solution; at the same time, blood should be taken for cross-matching. Additional evidence of significant bleeding is a marked difference between lying and standing blood pressure (postural hypotension) and a low central venous pressure. Every patient presenting with GI haemorrhage should have blood taken for grouping and cross-matching.

Once resuscitation is under way, a further history should be taken to establish the possible aetiology of the bleeding.

Aetiology

In considering the aetiology of the bleeding, both general and local causes should be borne in mind (see Box 23.1).

General bleeding diatheses seldom cause bleeding by themselves, they alter the course of bleeding from a local lesion. About 55% of patients in the UK with upper GI bleeding of an acute form have a peptic ulcer or erosion of the stomach or duodenum. About 5% of patients have oesophageal varices, and the remainder are accounted for by the other causes listed above.

Bleeding peptic ulcer

Overview

Gastrointestinal bleeding is the most common complication associated with peptic ulcer disease. Vomiting of fresh blood, or haematemesis, indicates that bleeding originates from a site

Box 23.1 Cause of gastrointestinal haemorrhage

Local causes

1 Oesophagus:
   a Reflux oesophagitis (associated with hiatus hernia).
   b Oesophageal varices (associated with portal hypertension, see Chapter 32).
   c Peptic ulcer.
   d Tumours (benign and malignant).

2 Stomach:
   a Gastric ulcer.
   b Acute erosions (small ulcers <5 mm; associated with aspirin, other NSAIDs and corticosteroids).
   c Gastritis (generalized inflammation, appearing as red dots through the endoscope).
   d Mallory–Weiss[10] syndrome (see later in this chapter).
   e Vascular malformation (e.g. Dieulafoy lesion[11]).
   f Tumours (benign and malignant).

3 Duodenum:
   a Duodenitis.
   b Duodenal ulcer.
   c Erosion of the duodenum by a pancreatic tumour.
   d Aortoduodenal fistula, usually in patients with previous aortic graft.

4 Small intestine:
   a Tumours.
   b Meckel's diverticulum.
   c Angiodysplasia.
   d Aortoenteric fistula.

5 Large bowel:
   a Tumours (benign and malignant, commonly adenocarcinomas).
   b Diverticular disease.
   c Angiodysplasia.
   d Colitis (ulcerative colitis, ischaemic colitis and infective colitis).

General causes

   a Haemophilia.
   b Leukaemia.
   c Anticoagulant therapy.
   d Thrombocytopenia.

[10]George Kenneth Mallory (1900–1986), Professor of Pathology, Boston University, Boston, MA, USA. Soma Weiss (1898–1942), Professor of Medicine, Harvard University, Boston, MA, USA.
[11]Paul Georges Dieulafoy (1839–1911), Physician, Paris. The lesion is a submucosal artery running abnormally close to the mucosa, typically occurring in the gastric fundus near the oesophagogastric junction and a cause of recurrent bleeding.

proximal to the duodenal-jejunal flexure (ligament of Treitz[12]).

A history of fresh haematemesis usually implies a significant bleed and the patients may go into haemodynamic instability due to hypovolaemia. 'Coffee ground' vomiting, usually arising from altered black blood, often indicates that active bleeding may have ceased.

Melaena is the passage of black tarry stool. It occurs when haemoglobin in the gut is converted to haematin by bacterial degradation. As little as 200 mL of bleeding inside the digestive tract can produce melaena. Although melaena generally denotes bleeding proximal to the duodenal-jejunal flexure, bleeding from small bowel or proximal colon may also cause it, especially when colonic transit is slow.

Haematochezia, passage of pure red blood or blood mixed with the stool, generally occurs when bleeding comes from the lower GI tract. It can also present due to massive upper GI bleeding. When a substantial amount of blood is lost into the GI lumen, tachycardia and hypotension develop. The haemoglobin concentration at this stage may not reflect the actual amount of blood loss before haemodilution sets in. A close monitoring of vital signs and estimation of volume of vomitus offer a better prognostic indicator of the severity of the illness.

Management (Table 23.1)

Bleeding from a peptic ulcer can be life-threatening. Urgent endoscopy is performed to identify the site and cause of bleeding, and also to institute appropriate therapeutic intervention. Early endoscopy within 24 hours of admission has been shown to reduce blood transfusion and length of hospital stay. Bleeding vessels may be managed by endoscopic clipping or adrenaline injection and most, but not all, bleeding can be controlled in this way. Urgent interventional radiology with embolization of the bleeding vessel or surgical intervention may occasionally be required.

Indications for surgery

- Failure of endoscopic control.
- Rebleeding after successful endoscopic therapy.

[12]Václav Treitz (1819–1872). Professor of Pathological Anatomy, Prague.

Table 23.1 Summary of Recommendations for gastroduodenal ulcer disease

Clinical problem	Operative risk	Recommended approach
Perforated duodenal ulcer	Low or high	Laparoscopic or open repair with omental or falciform patch. Postoperative management with evaluation for H. pylori infection, acid suppression therapy, management of risk factors (NSAIDs, alcohol, tobacco).
Perforated gastric ulcer	Low	Open or laparoscopic excision of ulcer and closure. Gastric resection if obviously malignant ulcer.
Perforated gastric ulcer	High	Open or laparoscopic excision of ulcer and closure. Postoperative management as above.
Bleeding duodenal or gastric ulcer refractory to endoscopic management	Low	Open exploration, biopsy of gastric ulcer with suture ligation of all branches of arteries feeding the ulcer bed. Consider truncal vagotomy and pyloroplasty or highly selective vagotomy (if appropriately experienced) or gastric wall closure and postoperative management.
Bleeding duodenal or gastric ulcer refractory to endoscopic management	High	Angioembolization with open surgery and suture ligation of bleeding vessel if this fails.
Gastric outlet obstruction refractory to endoscopic dilation	Low	Gastric resection and reconstruction with postoperative therapy.
Refractory gastroduodenal ulcer disease positive for gastrinoma or other hypersecretory state	Low	Resection of gastrinoma.
Refractory gastroduodenal ulcer disease	High	Truncal vagotomy with antrectomy and reconstruction if medical therapies fail.

- Elderly and unfit patients may not tolerate bleeding – consider early surgery.
- Patients with ongoing blood transfusion requirements.

In some patients, particularly those unfit for major surgery, radiological embolization of the gastroduodenal artery may be preferred to surgery for duodenal ulcer haemorrhage.

Gastroparesis

Gastroparesis is a motility disorder defined by the manifestations of chronic upper GI symptoms and prolonged gastric emptying in the absence of mechanical obstruction. It affects predominantly females with an incidence of 14–25 in 100 000.

Symptoms

Symptoms can be mild to severe, tend to be intermittent and include: early satiety (fullness), nausea, vomiting that may lead to dehydration, loss of appetite, weight loss, malnutrition, bloating, abdominal pain or discomfort, gastroesophageal reflux disease (GORD) and unpredictable blood sugars in people with diabetes.

Causes

Gastroparesis may be without obvious cause (idiopathic), or the result of problems with nerves and muscles controlling the emptying of the stomach. Other causes include: poorly controlled diabetes, bariatric surgery, gastrectomy, medication such as opioids, scleroderma, Parkinson's disease and amyloidosis.

Special investigations

- *Barium X-ray.*
- *Gastric emptying scan using scintigraphy:* food containing a very small amount of a radioactive substance is ingested with a subsequent scan.
- *Endoscopy* to exclude any intrinsic or extrinsic cause.
- *Capsule endoscopy.*

Treatment

There is no cure for gastroparesis. Symptoms can be reduced/resolved with dietary changes such as eating small and frequent meals, eating soft and liquid foods that are easier to digest, chewing food well before swallowing, drinking non-fizzy liquids with meals and avoiding or reducing certain foods such as high-fibre and foods high in fat.

Other treatments include:

- *Gastroelectrical stimulation (GES):* surgical implantation of a battery-operated device, to deliver electrical impulses to stimulate the muscles involved in controlling the passage of food through the stomach (often inappropriately referred to as a 'gastric pacemaker').
- *Botulinum toxin* injected endoscopically into the pyloric sphincter offers temporary relief, and may need repeating.
- *Transpyloric stenting,* but effectiveness limited by risk of stent migration.
- *Laparoscopic or endoscopic pyloromyotomy and gastrectomy.*
- *Symptomatic control* with antiemetics and antibiotics.
- *Alternative feeding methods:* nasojejunal tube or jejunostomy feeding, or parenteral nutrition.
- A gastric bypass procedure (gastroenterostomy or gastrojejunostomy) may benefit some patients, releasing gas and relieving bloating.

The latest guidelines from the European Society of Gastrointestinal Endoscopy recommend against the use of botulinum toxin injection, balloon dilations, and transpyloric stenting in unselected patients with gastroparesis, while a gastrectomy is seldom currently performed due to the appearance of minimally invasive procedures, including different modalities of pyloromyotomy and GES. The optimum intervention option for gastroparesis remains elusive.

Gastric volvulus

Gastric volvulus is a rare condition whereby the stomach rotates more than 180°, creating a closed-loop obstruction that can result in strangulation. It can manifest either as an acute abdominal emergency or as a chronic intermittent problem.

Classification of gastric volvulus

The most frequently used classification system of gastric volvulus relates to the axis around which the stomach rotates and includes the following three types:

- *Organoaxial:* the stomach rotates around an axis that connects the gastro-oesophageal junction (GOJ) and the pylorus. The antrum rotates in the opposite direction to the fundus of the stomach. This is the most common type of gastric volvulus, occurring in approximately 59% of cases and it is usually associated with diaphragmatic defects.
- *Mesenteroaxial:* the mesenteroaxial axis bisects the lesser and greater curvatures. The antrum rotates anteriorly and superiorly so that the posterior surface of the stomach comes to lie anteriorly. The rotation is usually incomplete and occurs intermittently. Vascular compromise is uncommon. This aetiology accounts for approximately 29% of cases of gastric volvulus.
- *Combined:* is a rare form in which the stomach twists both mesenteroaxially and organoaxially. This type of gastric volvulus makes up the remainder of cases and is usually observed in patients with chronic volvulus.

In aetiologic terms, gastric volvulus can be classified as either:

- *Type 1 (idiopathic):* makes up two-thirds of cases and is presumably due to abnormal laxity of the gastrosplenic, gastroduodenal, gastrophrenic and gastrohepatic ligaments. This allows approximation of the cardia and pylorus when the stomach is full, predisposing to volvulus.
- *Type 2 (congenital or acquired):* is found in one-third of patients and is usually associated with congenital or acquired abnormalities that result in abnormal mobility of the stomach.

Epidemiology

Males and females are equally affected. About 10–20% of cases occur in children, usually before the age of one year, but cases have been reported in children as old as 15 years.

Symptoms

The presenting symptoms depend on the degree of twisting and the rapidity of onset. The classic Borchardt triad of features comprises:

- Severe epigastric pain.
- Retching without vomiting.
- Inability to pass a NG tube.

Acute gastric volvulus

The Borchardt triad is diagnostic of acute volvulus and reportedly occurs in 70% of cases. Other symptoms are: hiccups, sudden onset of severe epigastric or left-upper-quadrant pain, sharp chest pain radiating to the left side of the neck, shoulder, arms and back, progressive distention and non-productive retching follow the pain, while some patients present with hematemesis secondary to mucosal ischaemia and sloughing.

Chronic gastric volvulus

Intermittent epigastric pain and abdominal fullness after meals, early satiety, dyspnoea, chest discomfort and dysphagia are the most common symptoms.

Complications

Strangulation and necrosis are the most feared complications of gastric volvulus; they can be life-threatening and occur most commonly with organoaxial gastric volvulus (5–28% of cases). Gastric perforation occurs secondary to ischaemia and necrosis and can result in sepsis and cardiovascular collapse; it can also complicate endoscopic reduction.

Special investigations

- *Chest X-ray:* a retrocardiac gas-filled viscus may be seen in cases of intrathoracic stomach, which confirms the diagnosis.
- *Abdominal X-ray:* reveals a massively distended viscus in the upper abdomen.

- *CT scan* is the imaging modality of choice, outlining the anatomy.
- *Upper GI endoscopy* may be helpful in the diagnosis of gastric volvulus.
- *Contrast studies* are less commonly performed now.
- *Other investigations* may be necessary to exclude the differential diagnoses, which include gallstones, hiatus hernia, myocardial infarction and peptic ulcer.

Management

In general, treatment of an acute gastric volvulus involves emergency surgical repair. In patients who are not surgical candidates, endoscopic reduction may be attempted and may allow adequate resuscitation and medical optimization before definitive surgical repair. Chronic gastric volvulus may be treated on a non-emergency basis.

Gastric tumours

Classification

Benign

1 *Epithelial*: adenoma:
   a Single.
   b Multiple (gastric polyposis).
2 *Connective tissue*: gastrointestinal stromal tumour.
3 *Vascular*: haemangioma.

Malignant

1 *Primary*:
   a Adenocarcinoma.
   b Gastrointestinal stromal tumour.
   c Lymphoma.
2 *Secondary*: invasion from adjacent tumours (pancreas or colon).

Epidemiology

Benign tumours of the stomach are uncommon, with an incidence of 0.4% in autopsy series and 3–5% in upper endoscopic series, most of them performed for unrelated reasons. Polyps account for 3.1% of all gastric tumours and their frequency increases to almost 90% of benign gastric tumours. Age and sex distribution depend on the type of tumour. There is no difference in distribution by race.

Many benign gastric tumours are found incidentally on gastroscopy. Small tumours are usually asymptomatic, but larger tumours can ulcerate and cause occult bleeding and anaemia. Large antral tumours cause intermittent gastric outlet obstruction, as manifested by nausea, vomiting and early satiety. If ulcerated, these tumours may cause epigastric pain similar to that caused by a peptic ulcer.

Gastric polyps

Gastric polyps are usually found incidentally during endoscopy. According to the cell of origin, polyps can be epithelial (fundic gland polyp, hyperplastic polyp, adenomatous polyp), neuroendocrine, lympho-histiocytic (xanthelasma, lymphoid hyperplasia), mesenchymal (gastrointestinal stromal tumour, neural or vascular tumours) or mixed. They can be sporadic or occur as part of a syndrome.

- *Fundic gland polyps* are the most common type of gastric polyps and were originally described in patients with familial adenomatous polyposis (FAP). The incidence of fundic gland polyps is low in patients with *Helicobacter pylori* infection and relatively high in patients taking proton pump inhibitors. While low-grade dysplasia is frequent in FAP patients with fundic gland polyps, dysplasia is rare in sporadic cases.
- *Hyperplastic polyps* are composed of epithelial and stromal components and are most frequently found in the antrum of patients with inflamed or atrophic gastric mucosa, and represent around 14% of gastric polyps. Removal of the underlying cause, such as *H. pylori* infection, results in regression of the hyperplastic polyps in 70% of patients. Hyperplastic polyps should be regarded as surrogate markers of cancer risk and synchronous or metachronous gastric carcinomas have been reported in up to 6% of cases.
- *Adenomatous polyps* are subdivided into classic intestinal-type adenomas and non-intestinal-type adenomas. Adenomatous polyps are precursors of gastric adenocarcinomas with the risk of adenocarcinoma increasing with increasing size; 50% of adenomatous polyps > 2 cm harbour malignancy.

- *Polyposis syndromes.* Hamartomatous polyps in the stomach have been found in patients with Peutz-Jeghers syndrome, juvenile polyposis, Cronkhite-Canada syndrome and Cowden disease. All patients with these polyposis syndromes have an increased risk of developing gastric carcinoma, which appears to be highest in patients with Peutz-Jeghers syndrome, at 30%.

Symptoms

The majority of patients are asymptomatic. Occasionally, polyps bleed, presenting as haematemesis or melaena. Rarely, large pedunculated polyps can obstruct the pylorus, leading to nausea, abdominal distension and vomiting.

Special investigation

Upper GI endoscopy is indicated to elicit the cause. Histological assessment of all polyps is essential because early gastric cancers can look insignificant.

Treatment

Removal or resection of adenomatous polyps is essential. Otherwise, treatment is related to symptoms and may include a polypectomy (polyp removal). Polyps smaller than 2 cm are easily snared endoscopically and removed. Larger polyps or sessile polyps are best removed operatively to obtain a clear margin and complete removal. Occasionally, staged piecemeal endoscopic removal can be performed in patients with severe comorbidities.

Wide, local or segmental resection of the stomach may be performed for multiple polyps, depending on their histology and location. Gastrectomy is justified in patients with diffuse involvement of the stomach by polyps, which can make detection of a synchronous focus of cancer difficult.

Gastrointestinal stromal tumours

Gastrointestinal stromal tumours (GISTs) are soft-tissue sarcomas of mesenchymal origin that arise in the gastrointestinal tract; they are rare, representing <3% of all gut tumours and 5% of all soft-tissue sarcomas.

Pathology

GISTs were previously thought to arise from the muscular layer or from nerve cells in the gut wall; in fact, they are now believed to arise from the interstitial cells of Cajal[13] (ICCs), the pacemaker cells of the gastrointestinal tract. ICCs are part of the autonomic nervous system and when the tumour has the appearance of neural tissue it is often called a gastrointestinal autonomic nervous tumour (GANT). Other tumours may have an appearance more like smooth muscle cells; hence, they were previously thought to be leiomyomas.

GISTs may be malignant or benign, and, although they may occur anywhere in the gastrointestinal tract, they are most common in the stomach, but not infrequent in the rest of the small intestine. They appear as small tumours within the muscular wall or larger tumours growing out from the bowel wall. Large tumours may outstrip their blood supply and become partly cystic; sometimes, the cyst communicates with the bowel lumen. GISTs typically present with either intestinal bleeding or obstruction; some are found during investigation of non-specific abdominal pain.

Aetiology

The aetiology of GISTs is unclear, but they are associated with type 1 neurofibromatosis in some cases. Typically, patients are over 40 years and there is no sex difference in incidence. The pathogenesis is a spontaneous mutation in the *c-kit* gene, which codes for a transmembrane receptor (*c-kit*/CD117) for a growth factor called stem cell factor. The *c-kit* mutation results in a continuous signal for cell growth which is mediated via a tyrosine kinase in the intracellular domain of the molecule. Some GISTs arise from mutations in platelet-derived growth factor receptor α (PDGFA); occasional cases demonstrate an inherited predisposition.

Clinical features

The symptoms of GISTs are non-specific and depend on the size and location of the lesion. Small GISTs (2 cm or less) are usually asymptomatic and are

[13]Santiago Ramóny Cajal (1852–1934), Histologist and Professor, successively in Valencia, Barcelona and Madrid, Spain. Awarded the Nobel Prize in 1906 with Golgi for studies of the neurone.

detected during investigations or surgical procedures for unrelated disease. The vast majority of these are of low-risk for malignancy. The most common symptom is gastrointestinal bleeding which is present in around half of patients. Patients with larger tumours may experience abdominal discomfort or develop a palpable mass. GISTs are often clinically silent until they reach a large size, bleed or rupture. Most duodenal GISTs occur in the second part of the duodenum where they can cause obstructive symptoms or infiltrate into the pancreas.

Special investigations

- *Endoscopy* usually detects the tumour, which appears as a submucosal polyp and which often has an ulcerated surface.
- *CT scan* may also identify the presence of a tumour.
- *Endoscopic ultrasound (EUS)* can be used to confirm the nature of the polyp and demonstrates clearly the origin of the polyp from the muscular layer of the stomach wall.
- *Positron emission tomography (PET)* is used both for detection and for staging of the tumours.

Once a tumour is found, diagnosis is by biopsy. Owing to the polyp's submucosal origin, mucosal biopsies are frequently non-diagnostic and confirmation of the diagnosis relies on EUS appearances with or without EUS-guided biopsy. Percutaneous biopsies are undertaken in the presence of metastases, but not undertaken otherwise to avoid the risk of seeding tumour cells along the biopsy track. The presence of c-kit protein (CD117) on the cell surface is almost diagnostic. Most small GISTs (< 5 cm) have a low mitotic rate and behave like benign tumours; larger GISTs (> 5 cm) have a more malignant phenotype and require adjuvant chemotherapy.

Treatment

- *Surgical*: complete resection by wide excision is the treatment of choice, and is often possible laparoscopically.
- *Endoscopic resection* may be possible and effective for smaller (≤ 4.0 cm) GISTs originating from the muscularis propria.
- *Chemotherapy: m*olecular targeted chemotherapy with imatinib mesilate (Glivec), an inhibitor of the *c-kit* tyrosine kinase, is very effective. It can be

given either prior to surgery, to shrink a large tumour in order to make it operable, or postoperatively to treat metastases or when complete resection was not possible.

Gastric lymphoma

Primary gastric lymphoma is rare, accounting for about 5% of gastric tumours, but one of the commonest sites for 'extra-nodal' lymphoma. It is twice as common in men as in women and median age at diagnosis is 60–65 years, except in patients with human immunodeficiency virus (HIV), who develop the disease earlier. It often presents with the same non-specific signs of dyspepsia and vague epigastric discomfort. Surgery, therefore, has a limited role in the modern management of gastric lymphoma; it is used for resection of locoregional disease if medical treatment fails or in the emergency setting for bleeding or perforation.

Gastroenteropancreatic neuroendocrine tumours (GEP-NETs)

Gastroenteropancreatic neuroendocrine tumours (GEP-NETs) are classified into intestinal neuroendocrine tumours (previously termed 'carcinoids'), accounting for about two-thirds, and pancreatic endocrine tumours, accounting for the remaining one-third. Gastric NETs make up just under 2% of all gastric neoplasms and are often discovered incidentally during upper GI endoscopy. Alternatively, they may present with bleeding (iron deficiency anaemia or frank GI blood loss), abdominal pain or dyspepsia. Rarely, they present late with metastatic disease and symptoms from the release of bioactive substances.

Gastric carcinoma

It is the fifth most common carcinoma in the world, although not as common in the UK where the incidence is falling. It is twice as common in men as in women, with the highest geographical incidence in

Eastern Asia (42 per 100 000, compared to 10 per 100 000 in the UK). Approximately, 75% of all gastric carcinoma is diagnosed in Asia. Gastric carcinoma is the third leading cause of cancer death in both sexes worldwide, responsible for 10% of all cancer deaths.

Gastric cancer develops through a well-established precancerous cascade: from atrophic gastritis (AG) to gastrointestinal metaplasia, low-grade dysplasia, high-grade dysplasia and eventually carcinoma, with the likelihood of progression increasing as this cascade advances.

Aetiology and risk factors

The risk factors for gastric cancer can be classified into three groups:

1 *Predisposing conditions*
   - Pernicious anaemia and AG, conditions where achlorhydria is present.
   - Previous gastric resection (two- to threefold increased incidence).
   - Chronic peptic ulcer (believed to give rise to 1% of gastric cancer cases).
2 *Environmental factors*
   - *H. pylori* infection. Seropositive patients (indicating past or present infection) have a six-to nine-fold increased risk of gastric cancer. However, fewer than 1% of those infected with *H. pylori* will go on to develop gastric cancer.
   - *Epstein-Barr virus (EBV)* infection: it has been estimated that 10% of gastric carcinomas are associated with EBV.
   - Low socioeconomic status.
   - Smoking.
   - Nationality: gastric cancer is much more common in Japan, although recent work suggests that much of this excess is related to *H. pylori*. The incidence declines in Japanese immigrants to America.
3 *Genetic factors*
   - Blood group A.
   - Hereditary non-polyposis colon cancer syndrome, associated with an increased incidence of gastric as well as colon and other cancers.

Pathology
Macroscopic pathology

One-third diffusely involve the stomach; one-quarter arise in the pyloric region; and the remainder are distributed fairly evenly throughout the rest of the stomach.

There are three macroscopic appearances:

- A *malignant ulcer* with raised, everted edges.
- A *polypoid tumour* proliferating into the stomach lumen.
- *Linitis plastica* (the *'leather-bottle stomach'*) caused by submucosal infiltration of tumour with marked fibrous reaction. This produces a small, thickened, contracted stomach without, or with only superficial, ulceration; hence, occult bleeding is rare in this group.

Microscopic appearances

These tumours are all adenocarcinomas with varying degrees of differentiation. Linitis plastica consists of anaplastic cells arranged in clumps with surrounding fibrosis.

Malignant change in a benign ulcer is suggested when a chronic ulcer, with characteristic complete destruction of the whole muscle coat and its replacement by fibrous tissue and chronic inflammatory cells, has a carcinoma developing in its edge.

Early and advanced gastric carcinoma

Early gastric carcinoma is defined as adenocarcinoma limited to the mucosa or submucosa with or without regional lymph node metastases. The term 'early' does not refer to the size or age of the lesion. Gastric carcinoma infiltrating into the muscularis propria and beyond is defined as 'advanced'.

Spread

- *Local.* Spread is often well beyond the naked-eye limits of the tumour, and the oesophagus or the first part of the duodenum may be infiltrated. Adjacent organs (pancreas, abdominal wall, liver, transverse mesocolon and transverse colon) may be directly invaded. A gastrocolic fistula may develop.
- *Lymphatic.* Lymph nodes along the lesser and greater curves are commonly involved. Lymph drainage from the cardiac end of the stomach may invade the mediastinal nodes and thence the

supraclavicular nodes of Virchow[14] on the left side (Troisier's sign[15]). At the pyloric end, involvement of the subpyloric and hepatic nodes may occur.
- *Bloodstream.* Dissemination occurs via the portal vein to the liver and thence occasionally to the lungs and the skeletal system.
- *Transcoelomic spread.* May produce peritoneal seedlings, ascites and bilateral Krukenberg[16] tumours owing to implantation in both ovaries.

Clinical features

Symptoms may be produced by the local effects of the tumour, by secondary deposits or by the general features of malignant disease.

Local symptoms

These are epigastric pain and discomfort, pain radiating into the back (suggesting pancreatic involvement), vomiting, especially with a pyloric or antral tumour producing pyloric obstruction (see earlier in this chapter) and dysphagia in tumours of the cardia. The patient may also report a feeling of fullness after eating little (early satiety). Occasionally, carcinoma of the stomach may present with perforation or haemorrhage (melaena and/or haematemesis).

Symptoms from secondaries (metastases)

The patient may first report with jaundice owing to liver involvement or abdominal distension with ascites.

General features

Anorexia (an extremely common presenting symptom), loss of weight and anaemia.

Examination may reveal features corresponding to these three headings. Local examination may reveal a mass in the upper abdomen. A search for secondaries may show enlargement of the liver with or without jaundice, ascites, enlarged, hard left supraclavicular

[14]Rudolf Ludwig Karl Virchow (1821–1902), Professor of Pathology in Würzburg and later Berlin, Germany.

[15]Charles Émile Troisier (1844–1919), Professor of Pathology, Paris, France.

[16]Friedrich Krukenberg (1871–1946), Pathologist, Halle, Germany. Described transcoelomic cancer spread, such as gastric cancer metastasizing to the ovaries.

nodes, or a palpable mass on pelvic examination due to secondary deposits in the pouch of Douglas or recto-vesical pouch. There may be obvious signs of loss of weight or anaemia.

Paraneoplastic syndromes

Haemolytic anaemia, membranous glomerulonephritis and chronic disseminated intravascular coagulation leading to vascular thrombosis (Trousseau's sign[17]) are occasionally seen.

Special investigations

- *Gastroscopy* enables direct inspection and multiple biopsies of any lesion.
- *CT scan* may show nodal and metastatic spread.
- *EUS* enables assessment of lymph node spread and local tumour infiltration into pancreas, diaphragmatic crura and liver.
- *Staging laparoscopy* allows assessment of the primary tumour, including its mobility and invasion into adjacent organs, and examination of the peritoneal cavity to exclude small metastases (peritoneal or liver) that are not detectable by CT scanning. If ascites is found, this can be sampled for cytology. The presence of even small metastases means the patient has incurable disease.

It is important to note that considerable pain relief may occur when a gastric carcinoma is treated with acid suppression (H2-antagonists or proton pump inhibitors), owing to diminution in the adjacent oedema, and may lead to a false diagnosis of benign ulcer.

Differential diagnosis

There are five common diseases that give a very similar clinical picture, of a patient with a slight lemon-yellow tinge, anaemia and loss of weight:

1 Carcinoma of the stomach.
2 Carcinoma of the caecum.
3 Carcinoma of the pancreas.
4 Pernicious anaemia.
5 Uraemia.

---

[17]Armand Trousseau (1801–1867), Physician, Hôpital Necker, Hôpital St Antoine and Hôpital Dieu, Paris. Noted this sign in himself as confirmation of his own gastric cancer. He also described carpopedal spasm in hypocalcaemic tetany.

They form an important quintet, and should always be considered together in terms of appropriate special investigations.

Endoscopic gastric cancer screening

Countries with a high prevalence of gastric cancer, such as Japan, have implemented systematic screening programs and demonstrated the benefit of early detection and endoscopic resection of precancerous gastric lesions and early gastric cancers, offering curative treatment with considerably less morbidity. Japanese guidelines suggest biennial or triennial endoscopic screening for those over the age of 50. This approach could prevent up to 63% of gastric cancer-related mortality.

In the UK, screening is recommended in patients with multiple risk factors for gastric cancer (male, smoker, pernicious anaemia, family history in first degree relative) due to the lower incidence in the population as a whole.

Treatment of gastric cancer

Endoscopic treatment

- *Endoscopic mucosal resection* is the removal of a mucosal lesion by resecting it from its deeper layers using a snare instrument. This method does not allow for lesions larger than 2 cm to be removed *en bloc*.
- *Endoscopic submucosal dissection* was developed for the local treatment of superficial early gastric cancer limited to the mucosal layer or with minimal invasion of the submucosal layer. The main goal of submucosal dissection is to retrieve the lesion *en bloc* for histopathological staging and to minimize the chance for local recurrence.

Gastrectomy

The three common types of gastrectomy for gastric cancer are:

1 *Total gastrectomy:* this involves removal of the whole stomach including the cardia (oesophagogastric junction) and the pylorus (Figure 23.4a). It is indicated for tumours arising at or invading the proximal stomach.

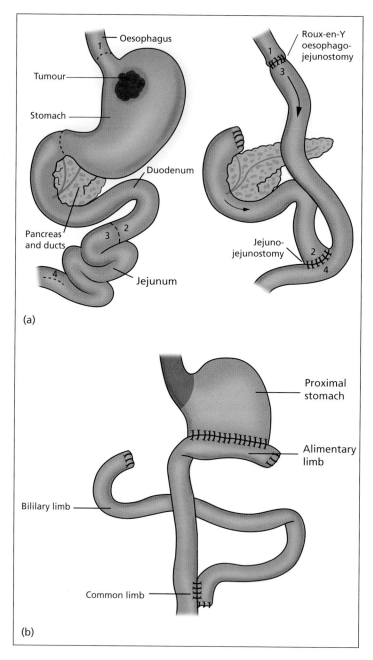

Figure 23.4 The upper panel (a) illustrates a total gastrectomy with a Roux-en-Y reconstruction. The lower panel (b) illustrates a subtotal gastrectomy with a Roux-en-Y reconstruction.

2 *Distal (subtotal) gastrectomy:* this involves removal of the stomach including the pylorus but preserving the cardia (Figure 23.4b). Two-thirds or more of the stomach is usually removed for gastric cancer.

3 *Proximal gastrectomy:* this involves removal of the stomach including the cardia but preserving the pylorus. It is indicated for proximal tumours with or without oesophageal invasion, where more than half of the distal stomach can be preserved.

Prognosis

This depends on the extent of spread and degree of differentiation of the tumour. Microscopic spread is often much further than apparent at operation, and lymph node spread has a poor prognosis. Early gastric carcinomas confined to the stomach wall and no more than two local lymph nodes (stage 1) have a 65% 5-year survival with resection. Invasion through the muscle wall but not into adjacent organs, or involvement of more than two perigastric lymph nodes (stage 2) reduces survival to 35%, whereas a more advanced local cancer with infiltration into surrounding tissues or more distant nodal involvement (stage 3) has a poorer survival rate. The presence of metastases (stage 4) is associated with death before 5 years.

Additional resources

Case 52: Vomiting in a baby
Case 53: A gastric ulcer
Case 54: A bloody vomit
Case 55. An acute abdominal emergency
Case 56: A serious gastric lesion
Case 57: A surgical specimen of stomach

24

The surgery of obesity

Christopher Pring

Learning objectives

✓ To recognize the link between obesity and health.

✓ To understand the evidence base with respect to treatment options for obesity.

✓ To understand the three main surgical procedures for treating obesity.

Bariatric surgery refers to the surgical treatment for obesity and its associated comorbidities. Bariatric derives from the ancient Greek word *baros*, meaning weight/pressure.

Given the effectiveness of bariatric surgery in treating metabolic diseases (type 2 diabetes, hypertension, dyslipidaemia), bariatric surgery is also referred to as '*metabolic surgery*'.

> **Box 24.1 Classification of obesity by body mass index**
>
> Body mass index (BMI) is a function of a person's weight and height – i.e.
>
> $$\frac{\textbf{weight in kg}}{\textbf{height in metres}^2} :$$
>
> <18.5 kg/m^2 = underweight
>
> 18.5–25 kg/m^2 = normal weight
>
> 25–30 kg/m^2 = overweight
>
> 30–35 kg/m^2 = class I obesity
>
> 35–40 kg/m^2 = class II obesity
>
> >40 kg/m^2 = class III obesity

Obesity

Prevalence

It is widely acknowledged that there is a worldwide obesity pandemic. Mean worldwide body mass index (BMI) has been steadily increasing since 1975 and current trends predict that 20% of the global population will be classified as having obesity by 2030 (Box 24.1). In the UK, 27% of the population is already classified as having obesity.

The estimated healthcare spend on obesity in 2014/15 was £6.1 billion, and this is projected to reach £9.7 billion by 2050, with an estimated societal cost of almost £50 billion.

Aetiology

Like all medical conditions, obesity is the cumulative outcome of genetic and environmental influences. There are very few genetically driven syndromes that cause obesity (e.g. Prader–Willi syndrome[1]) and only a handful of susceptibility genes have been identified (e.g. *MC4R, FTO*). The doubling of the prevalence

Ellis and Calne's Lecture Notes in General Surgery, Fourteenth Edition. Edited by Christopher Watson and Justin Davies.
© 2023 John Wiley & Sons Ltd. Published 2023 by John Wiley & Sons Ltd.
Companion website: www.wiley.com/go/Watson/GeneralSurgery14

[1] Andrea Prader (1919–2001) and Heinrich Willi (1900–1971), Paediatricians, Kinderspital, Zurich. The condition was first described by John Langdon Down of Down Syndrome description in 1887.

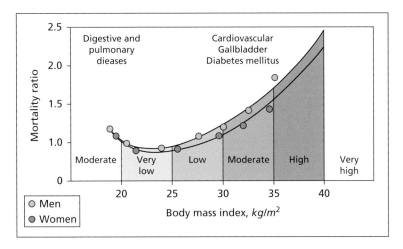

Figure 24.1 Relative risk of death from all causes according to body mass index.

of any condition in less than 40 years cannot be accounted for by a change in our genetic framework; the only explanation can be environmental factors.

A fundamental shift in the availability/consumption of various foodstuffs (energy dense, micronutrient-poor foods) and changes in our physical environment have created what is referred to as the 'obesogenic environment'.

Consequences of obesity

Health and body weight are intricately linked. This was established in a 1999 population study, clearly demonstrating that mortality risk increases as BMI increases (Figure 24.1). It is estimated that obesity reduces life expectancy by 8–10 years.

Obesity is associated with higher risks of type 2 diabetes, cardiovascular disease, osteoarthritis, and some cancers, among other conditions. Table 24.1 demonstrates this increased risk of disease states once a person's BMI > 30 kg/m².

Treatments for obesity

Conservative treatments

A common 'throw away comment' is that people who suffer with excess weight (and its associated comorbidities) need to eat less and move more. The epidemiology of obesity tells us that this paradigm is not working (worldwide prevalence continues to increase).

Table 24.1 Estimated increased risk for the obese of developing associated diseases

Disease	Relative risk (women)	Relative risk (men)
Type 2 diabetes	12.7	5.2
Hypertension	4.2	2.6
Heart attack	3.2	1.5
Colon cancer	2.7	3
Angina	1.8	1.8
Gall bladder disease	1.8	1.8
Ovarian cancer	1.7	
Osteoarthritis	1.4	1.9
Stroke	1.3	1.3

Robust scientific literature also demonstrates the challenge of successfully implementing conservative treatments. The highly regarded Look AHEAD study published in 2013 demonstrated that an intensive programme of eat less, move more, plus behavioural therapy did not result in sustained weight loss or improved cardiovascular morbidity and mortality. In fact after four years, 23% of participants weighed more than they did at the start and only 20% of participants had lost 10% of their body weight.

Medical treatments

For the pharmaceutical industry, developing a tablet that effectively controls weight is a huge prize. The research and development funds available for this quest are enormous. Our evolving understanding of the link between body weight and gut hormones has enabled the development of analogues that manipulate these gut hormones in order to support weight loss. Currently however, the European Medicines Agency has approved only three drug therapies (orlistat, bupropion/naltrexone and liraglutide). Nonetheless, recent studies indicate that liraglutide may offer reasonable efficacy.

Surgical treatment

Bariatric/metabolic surgery has evolved considerably since its inception in 1954 (the jejuno-ileal bypass) and subsequently the gastric bypass first performed by Mason in Iowa in 1966[2]. The advent of laparoscopic surgery in the early 1990s, alongside the publication of long-term surgical outcome data, have precipitated a paradigm shift in recognizing that surgery offers effective and low risk treatment for obesity and metabolic disease.

The Swedish Obese Subjects study published in 2007 demonstrated that people with class II obesity who underwent bariatric surgery had a 24% greater chance of being alive after 15 years compared to those who underwent standard non-surgical care. A 2021 meta-analysis has underscored the same finding, documenting that for people with type 2 diabetes who underwent bariatric surgery, life expectancy increased by 9.3 years compared to those with type 2 diabetes undergoing standard care. A further systematic review and meta-analysis observed that following bariatric surgery, the relative risk reductions for the development of type 2 diabetes, hypertension and dyslipidaemia were 61%, 64% and 77%, respectively.

The evidence base to support bariatric surgery is very strong. The National Institute for Health and Care Excellence (NICE) recognized this by publishing clinical guidance in 2014 (CG189). This supported treatment with bariatric surgery for people with class III obesity and for those with class II obesity who also have a metabolic disorder. Despite the overwhelming evidence that surgery offers effective treatment, as well as the recommendations of NICE CG189, fewer than 1% of those who are eligible for bariatric surgery in the UK actually receive it.

Mechanism of action

Essentially, all bariatric surgery works by reducing absorption of calories from the intestinal tract. Our understanding of the mechanisms by which this is achieved is evolving, and includes:

- Neuronal pathways.
- Hormonal changes.
- Alterations in the gut microbiome.
- Bile salt function.

The relative contributions of these mechanisms varies between the different procedures. The three main bariatric operations are gastric band, gastric bypass and gastric sleeve (Figure 24.2). There are other recognized bariatric procedures (biliopancreatic diversion; duodenal switch; one anastomosis gastric bypass) but these are beyond the scope of this chapter.

Gastric band

An adjustable band is placed around the proximal aspect of the stomach to create a small pouch above the band. The surgical complication rate for this procedure is so low that this is commonly performed as a day case procedure. There is no manipulation of gut anatomy and the band can be removed at any time (it is reversible).

Weight loss for this procedure is in the order of 16% total body weight. However, despite its simplicity, safety and effectiveness, its popularity has recently waned considerably due to the long-term risks of the band slipping, dysphagia, acid reflux and a high rate of reoperation.

Gastric bypass

The main body of the stomach and the duodenum/proximal small bowel are bypassed by stapling across the proximal stomach in order to create a small volume (20–30 mL) gastric pouch. The gastric pouch is reconnected to the gastrointestinal tract via a Roux[3]

---

[2] Edward Eatoon Mason (1920–2020), Surgeon, University of Iowa. Considered to be the father of bariatric surgery.

[3] César Roux (1857–1934), Professor of Surgery, Lausanne, Switzerland. His other claim to fame was for the first successful adrenalectomy for a phaeochromocytoma.

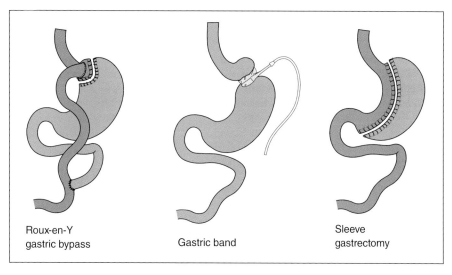

Roux-en-Y gastric bypass   Gastric band   Sleeve gastrectomy

Figure 24.2 The three common bariatric surgical procedures.

limb (sometimes called the alimentary limb) that is measured to approximately 60–120 cm long. The Roux limb is then reconnected to the bypassed duodenum/proximal small bowel (the biliopancreatic limb). Classically, this operation is described as a Roux-en-Y gastric bypass (the two prongs of the Y being the Roux limb and biliopancreatic limb; the stem of the Y being the common channel), similar to the operation performed for the treatment of peptic ulcer disease and distal gastric cancer.

Weight loss for this procedure is in the order of 31% total body weight and there is significant amelioration of the metabolic conditions (type 2 diabetes, hypertension, dyslipidaemia). Patients must take lifelong vitamin supplements.

Sleeve gastrectomy

Worldwide, sleeve gastrectomy is now the most popular bariatric procedure. Approximately 85% of the body of the stomach is resected to create a narrow stomach sleeve, but the duodenum/small bowel is left intact. Its simplicity, effectiveness and versatility (in terms of future operative procedures) are key to its popularity.

Weight loss for this procedure is in the order of 25% total body weight and there is significant amelioration of the metabolic conditions, although probably less so than for gastric bypass.

Complications of surgery (see Box 24.2)

Laparoscopic bariatric surgery is now recognized to be as safe as laparoscopic cholecystectomy, with postoperative length of stay around 1–2 days. Perioperative mortality is fewer than 1:1000 cases and surgical complications are in the order of 2–3% (bleeding, infection, staple line/anastomotic leak, ulceration at the gastric pouch anastomosis, gastro-oesophageal reflux).

In the long term, micronutrient deficiencies can occur, but these are mitigated against by adherence to daily multivitamin and mineral over-the-counter

---

Box 24.2 Complications of bariatric surgery

1 *Surgical complications.*
   a Staple line/anastomotic leaks.
   b Gastric ulceration.
   c Gastro-oesophageal reflux.
   d Gallstone formation.
   e Bolus intestinal obstruction.
   f Failure, with regain of weight.
2 *Nutritional deficiencies*
   a Vitamins: B12, folate, and the fat soluble vitamins A, D, E and K.
   b Chemical elements: calcium, copper, zinc and iron.

supplements. Weight regain and re-emergence of metabolic disease are also long-term risks, but again these are mitigated against by specialist input (particularly from the dietitian). Nonetheless, it is important to remember the evidence, that despite the risk of weight regain, people who undergo bariatric surgery have a survival advantage when compared to those who follow non-surgical treatments.

The decision as to which procedure is best suited to which patient is based upon multidisciplinary team assessment. The opinions, experience and support of bariatric physicians, dietitians, psychologists, anaesthetists and surgeons ensure that the right patients receive the right treatments. In the face of a continued obesity/metabolic epidemic, the application of bariatric surgery is now well-established and evolving quickly.

25

The small intestine

Justin Davies

Learning objectives

✓ To know the varying presentations of a Meckel's diverticulum.

✓ To have knowledge of Crohn's disease of the small intestine, in particular its varying presentations and treatment.

✓ To know the rare possibility of small bowel tumours, and how they may present.

Meckel's diverticulum

Meckel's diverticulum[1] is the remnant of the vitellointestinal duct of the embryo. It lies on the antimesenteric border of the ileum and, as an approximation, occurs in 2% of the population, arises approximately 60 cm (2 feet) from the caecum, and averages 5 cm (2 inches) in length.

Clinical features

Meckel's diverticulum may present in numerous ways.

- *A symptomless finding* at operation or autopsy.
- *Acute inflammation*, clinically similar to acute appendicitis.
- *Perforation by a foreign body*, presenting as peritonitis.

[1] Johann Frederick Meckel (1781–1833), Professor of Anatomy and Surgery, Halle, Germany. His grandfather and father were both Professors of Anatomy.

Ellis and Calne's Lecture Notes in General Surgery, Fourteenth Edition. Edited by Christopher Watson and Justin Davies.
© 2023 John Wiley & Sons Ltd. Published 2023 by John Wiley & Sons Ltd.
Companion website: www.wiley.com/go/Watson/GeneralSurgery14

- *Intussusception* (ileoileal), often gangrenous by the time the patient comes to operation.
- *Peptic ulceration* due to heterotopic gastric epithelium in the diverticulum, which bears HCl-secreting parietal cells. This particularly occurs in children and characteristically is the cause of melaena at about the age of 10 years. Rarely, the peptic ulceration perforates or gives rise to pain after eating. The diverticulum may also contain ectopic pancreatic tissue.
- *Patent vitellointestinal duct*, presenting as an umbilical fistula that discharges intestinal contents.
- *Raspberry tumour at the umbilicus* due to a persistent umbilical extremity of the duct.
- *Vitellointestinal band* stretching from the tip of the diverticulum to the umbilicus, which may obstruct a loop of small intestine or act as the apex of a small bowel volvulus.

Special investigations

Most diverticula are incidental findings. However, the following investigations may be indicated.

- *Computed tomography (CT)* scan may demonstrate the diverticulum, and given the increased access to CT scans in emergency presentations, the diagnosis may be increasingly made prior to surgery.

- *Technetium scan.* Radiolabelled technetium (^{99m}Tc) is taken up by gastric mucosa, and scintigraphy will outline the stomach and, in addition, the Meckel's diverticulum, usually near the right iliac fossa (RIF).
- *Barium follow-through or small bowel enema* may show the diverticulum arising from the antimesenteric border of the ileum, but these investigations are much less commonly performed nowadays.

Treatment involves surgical resection of the diverticulum if it is symptomatic.

Crohn's disease

Crohn's disease[2] is a non-specific inflammatory disease of the gastrointestinal tract, with diseased segments sandwiched between normal segments (i.e. it is discontinuous). Crohn and colleagues first described its occurrence in the ileum and termed it 'regional ileitis'. However, this description is inaccurate, as the disease may affect any part of the alimentary tract from the mouth to the anus. Crohn's disease may also affect the large bowel alone (see Chapter 27).

Aetiology

The aetiology of Crohn's disease likely has environmental (e.g. a triggering infection yet to be identified, smoking) and genetic (20% of patients have an affected relative) components. These aetiological factors remain poorly understood, and other factors such as stress and diet are more likely to trigger flares of the disease than be the initial cause. Recent work has pointed to a genetic mutation in the *NOD* gene family, among others. These genes are involved in the innate immune response to bacterial antigens within the gut. This observation may explain the success of dietary manipulation, such as the elemental diet (see later in this chapter). The presence of granulomas on histology previously led to suggestion of infection by a mycobacterium species, possibly *Mycobacterium avium* ssp. *paratuberculosis*. However, the success of immunosuppression in the control of Crohn's disease points to an autoimmune cause, although an initial infectious

 [2] Burrill Bernard Crohn (1884–1983), Gastroenterologist, Mount Sinai Hospital, New York, NY, USA. The disease was first described by Morgagni (1682–1771).

trigger (by an as-yet-unidentified causative organism) may turn out to be important. Acute ileitis can also be caused by bacteria such as *Yersinia enterocolitica*.

Pathology

Distribution

The small bowel is affected in two-thirds of cases, with the terminal ileum being the most common site, although the disease may affect any part of the gastrointestinal tract from the mouth to the anus. One-third of patients with ileal disease also have large bowel manifestations.

Macroscopic appearance

In the acute stage, the bowel is bright red and swollen; mucosal ulceration and intervening oedema result in a 'cobblestone' appearance of the mucosa. The wall of the intestine is greatly thickened, as is the adjacent mesentery, and the regional lymph nodes are enlarged. Mesenteric fat advances over the serosal surface in affected segments, known as 'fat wrapping' or 'creeping fat'. There may be skip areas of normal intestine between involved segments. Fistulas may occur into adjacent viscera, for example other loops of bowel, the bladder, uterus or vagina.

Microscopic appearance

There is fibrosis, lymphoedema and a chronic inflammatory infiltrate through the whole thickness of the bowel with non-caseating foci of epithelioid and giant cells. Ulceration is present, with characteristic fissuring ulcers extending deeply through the mucosa. These may extend through the bowel wall to form abscesses, or fistulas into adjacent viscera.

Clinical features

Crohn's disease occurs at any age, but is particularly common in young adults with a peak age of onset between 20 and 40 years of age. There is no sex difference. The typical clinical picture is a young adult with abdominal pain and diarrhoea, often with a palpable mass in the RIF. However, Crohn's disease may manifest clinically in several ways.

- *Acute Crohn's disease.* Crohn's disease may present like appendicitis with acute abdominal pain, usually in the RIF, and vomiting. Rarely, there is perforation of the bowel or acute haemorrhage.

Unlike appendicitis, the history is usually of several days or weeks, and investigation may reveal anaemia, or other features of Crohn's disease may be present. The typical features of Crohn's disease in the terminal ileum may be evident on CT scan, thus differentiating from appendicitis at presentation.

- *Intestinal obstruction.* Following inflammatory exacerbations, fibrosis of the intestinal wall occurs, leaving stenosed segments (strictures) that may result in intestinal obstruction. Obstruction may also follow an intraperitoneal abscess if this causes external compression of the bowel.
- *Fistula formation.* Fistulas may develop, penetrating adjacent loops of gut or the pelvic organs such as bladder, uterus or vagina or they may be perianal. External faecal fistulas may follow operative intervention.
- *Malabsorption.* Extensive involvement of the small bowel produces malabsorption with steatorrhoea and multiple vitamin deficiencies. It is exacerbated when bowel resections have already occurred.
- *Diarrhoea.* Diarrhoea may be due to inflammation and mucosal ulceration, colonic or rectal involvement, bacterial overgrowth in obstructed segments and malabsorption secondary to either disease or short bowel following previous surgery. Mucosal ulceration causes diarrhoea, with raised faecal calprotectin levels and often anaemia.
- *Perianal disease.* Ten per cent of patients with small bowel Crohn's disease also have perianal disease, including anal skin tags, fissures, fistulas and stenosis (see Chapter 28).

Special investigations

Crohn's disease is associated with anaemia, raised faecal calprotectin and occasionally steatorrhoea. Serum albumin is low, and inflammatory markers such as C-reactive protein (CRP) are a helpful index of disease activity. Additional investigations include the following.

- *CT or magnetic resonance enteroclysis* will demonstrate areas of active Crohn's disease, as well as areas of stricture and any pre-stenotic dilatation. It is also possible to demonstrate fistulas and to assess for any extraluminal disease. MRI has the advantage of no radiation exposure, but access to MRI scans is more limited and some individuals find the experience claustrophobic.
- *Small bowel enema,* or enteroclysis, in which contrast is instilled into the duodenum via a nasogastric tube and followed fluoroscopically as it passes through the bowel, is much less commonly employed now with advances in CT and MRI, but contrast injected via a likely fistula site on the abdominal wall (a fistulogram) can often help to delineate anatomy prior to surgery.
- *Technetium-labelled leucocyte (white cell) scan* is a sensitive way to show the extent of disease activity. Leucocytes are taken up in the inflamed segments, and also localize to abscesses. These are less commonly performed now due to increased access to CT and MRI scans.

Complications outside the gastrointestinal tract

In addition to those already mentioned, the following are associated with the disease.

- *Primary sclerosing cholangitis, arthritis, sacroiliitis, pyoderma gangrenosum, erythema nodosum, and uveitis* may occur, but are more common when the colon is also involved.
- *Renal calculi:* usually oxalate stones secondary to hyperoxaluria, which occurs as a consequence of steatorrhoea.
- *Gallstones* are more common in patients with ileal Crohn's disease, and in whom the ileum has been resected. This is due to the interruption of the enterohepatic bile salt circulation.

Treatment

Treatment is often medical initially, although surgery is appropriate in the management of complications and chronic disease. Surgery should always be carefully considered and planned because of the malabsorption that may follow extensive or multiple resections of the bowel or the production of blind loops of intestine.

Medical management

Initial management is often non-operative. Nutritional support may be required, and an elemental diet may be useful. Acute episodes are treated with steroids and immunosuppressants such as azathioprine; parenteral nutrition may be required.

Mild symptoms are treated with 5-aminosalicylate drugs such as mesalazine, and steroids may be required. Antibiotics, such as metronidazole, may also help.

Acute exacerbations and fistulating disease may be effectively treated with Infliximab and adalimumab, monoclonal antibodies to tumour necrosis factor alpha (TNF-α).

Increasing evidence now supports use of second and third line immunosuppressants/biologics but it is very important that decisions to escalate medical biologic therapy are made in a joint inflammatory bowel disease clinic setting that involves the patient, a gastroenterologist and a colorectal surgeon. These advanced agents include:

- *Ustekinumab*: a monoclonal antibody against the p40 protein subunit of interleukins IL-12 and IL-23.
- *Vedolizumab*: a monoclonal antibody against the α4β7 integrin preferentially expressed on gut-homing T lymphocytes.

Surgical management

If found at surgery in the acute stage, the condition should be left undisturbed since in a high proportion the acute phase may subside completely with medical therapy.

In the chronic stage of the disease, surgery is indicated for:

- Severe or recurrent obstructive symptoms.
- Symptomatic fistulas.
- When medical treatment either leads to complications or is not sufficient to allow the patient an adequate quality of life.

Recognizing that the disease is recurrent and that further resections may be required, surgery should be as conservative as possible. Either resection of the affected segment or a strictureplasty (widening of the narrowed segment, rather than removal) is performed; laparoscopic ('keyhole') surgery is increasingly used.

Prognosis

Recurrence of the disease after resection occurs in some 50% of cases within 10 years, and repeated operations may be required over time. Patients will often require ongoing medication after surgery in order to reduce the risk of recurrence. Stopping smoking is essential to lower this risk.

Tumours of the small intestine

One of the many mysteries of tumour formation is their rarity from beyond the pylorus to the ileocaecal valve.

Classification

Benign

- Adenoma.
- Gastrointestinal stromal tumour (see Chapter 23).
- Lipoma.
- Hamartoma (e.g. Peutz–Jeghers syndrome,[3] associated with circumoral pigmentation and multiple intestinal polyps).

Malignant

1 *Primary*:
   a Neuroendocrine tumour (previously known as 'carcinoid').
   b Adenocarcinoma.
   c Lymphoma.
   d Gastrointestinal stromal tumour (see Chapter 23).
2 *Secondary invasion* (e.g. from stomach, colon or bladder, or from a lymphoma).

Clinical features

Tumours of the small intestine may present with:

- Intestinal bleeding.
- Obstruction.
- Intussusception.
- Volvulus.
- Anaemia.

---

[3] Johannes Peutz (1886–1957), Physician, the Hague, the Netherlands. Harold Jeghers (1940–1990), Professor of Medicine, Georgetown University School of Medicine, Washington, DC, and Tufts University Medical School, Boston, MA, USA.

Neuroendocrine tumours

Neuroendocrine tumours (previously known as carcinoid tumours) are amine precursor uptake and decarboxylation (APUD) tumours, and share this property with cells of neural crest origin with which they were once confused. They belong to a group of neuroendocrine tumours called gastroenteropancreatic tumours; the other tumours in this group are pancreatic endocrine tumours such as gastrinomas and insulinomas. In 10% of cases, there is an association with the multiple endocrine neoplasia type 1 (MEN1) syndrome (see Chapter 38). Neuroendocrine tumours are most commonly found in the appendix, but may be found anywhere in the gastrointestinal tract and occasionally in the lung (10%). They commonly secrete 5-hydroxytryptamine (5-HT, also called serotonin), in addition to other hormones, but are rarely symptomatic until they have metastasized to the liver and are thus able to secrete their hormone directly into the systemic circulation, since the liver normally inactivates these hormones. This can lead to the symptoms of so-called 'carcinoid syndrome' (see later in this chapter).

Pathology

Macroscopic appearance

The tumour appears as a yellowish submucosal nodule. The overlying mucosa is at first intact but later ulcerates. Extension to the serosa leads to fibrosis and obstruction. Often, the tumour encircles the bowel at the time of diagnosis, and has infiltrated the mesenteric lymph nodes.

Microscopic appearance

The tumour is made up of Kulchitsky cells,[4] which take up silver stains and arise in the crypts of the intestinal mucosa.

The tumour is very slow growing, and usually presents after the fourth decade. Up to one-quarter are multiple. Neuroendocrine tumours of the appendix are relatively benign but 4% eventually metastasize. They may present early as appendicitis by obstructing

[4] Nikolai Kulchitsky (1865–1925), Professor of Histology, Kharkov, Russia. After the Russian Revolution he became Lecturer in Anatomy at University College, London, UK.

the appendix lumen, but most will be found incidentally when the removed appendix is examined under the microscope for histological diagnosis. Those arising in the ileum and large bowel may spread to the regional lymph nodes and the liver.

Clinical features

Neuroendocrine tumours present with local features related to the primary tumour or due to metastatic spread, including the so-called 'carcinoid syndrome' due to liver metastases and their endocrine products:

- Flushing (90%) with attacks of cyanosis and a chronic red-faced appearance, often precipitated by stress or ingestion of food or alcohol.
- Diarrhoea (70%), often profuse, with noisy borborygmi.
- Bronchospasm (15%).
- Abdominal pain (40%) owing to mesenteric fibrosis resulting in partial obstruction.

Abnormalities in the heart (pulmonary and tricuspid stenosis) are late manifestations; lung neuroendocrine tumours may cause stenosis of the left heart valves (mitral and aortic). Hepatomegaly and a palpable abdominal mass produced by the tumour and its secondaries may occasionally be present.

Special investigations

- *5-Hydroxyindole acetic acid (5-HIAA) urinary concentration.* 5-HT is broken down to 5-HIAA, which is excreted in the urine. A 24 h urine collection contains raised levels of 5-HIAA.
- *Chromogranin A serum concentration* is raised in patients with neuroendocrine tumours.
- *CT or ultrasound* of the liver to seek metastases. The primary tumour is often elusive, but CT may show mesenteric infiltration.
- *Radiolabelled octreotide scintigraphy* is a useful screening test for tumour and for detection of metastases; the octreotide binds to somatostatin receptors that are often expressed on the tumour.

Treatment

Resection of the tumour in early and symptomatic cases is the optimal treatment. Local metastases in the liver are also occasionally resectable. Palliation of more extensive tumour deposits can be achieved by embolizing the hepatic arterial supply via a catheter passed through the femoral artery. Cytotoxic therapy may induce worthwhile remission, but is not commonly used.

Symptoms may be controlled with octreotide, a somatostatin analogue that inhibits 5-HT release. Targeted radiotherapy, using radiolabelled octreotide, may have a place in treatment. Even if widespread deposits are present, the tumour is slow growing and the patient may survive for many years.

Additional resources

Case 62: An unusual case of severe rectal bleeding in a child

Case 63: An abdominal mass in a young man

Case 64: A striking facial appearance

26

The appendix

Ioanna G. Panagiotopoulou

Learning objective

✓ To learn the anatomical and histological features of the appendix.

✓ To appreciate the clinical presentation of acute appendicitis and its management.

✓ To be aware of rare appendiceal tumours.

The appendix (also known as the vermiform appendix) is considered a remnant in the human evolution process. Inflammation of the appendix is the most common abdominal surgical emergency. Acute appendicitis may present with a multitude of symptoms and signs, and has a wide differential diagnosis. Although the diagnosis of acute appendicitis is made largely on clinical grounds, relevant blood tests and imaging are important adjuncts of clinical practice. Finally, one needs to be aware of rare appendiceal tumours that may require referral and treatment, sometimes within specialist centres.

Embryology and anatomy

The appendix is a blind-ended, tubular, vermiform (worm-like) structure that arises from the posteromedial aspect of the caecal wall, and as such derives from midgut. During week 6 of gestation, the caecal diverticulum develops as the precursor of the appendix and the caecum. The caecum and appendix undergo medial rotation along with the midgut and descend in the right lower abdomen. The continued growth of the caecum even during childhood most

commonly rotates the appendix into a retrocaecal position (74% of cases). The appendix may assume several other different positions within the right lower abdominal cavity such as paracaecal/paracolic, subcaecal, pelvic and pre-/post-ileal, or may even adopt a position over the right upper abdomen in malrotation cases (Figure 26.1). The varying position of the appendix explains its varying presentations.

The appendix varies between 5 and 10 cm in length, with its base at the confluence of the three taenia coli of the caecum, which fuse to create the outer longitudinal muscular layer of the appendix. The mesentery of the appendix (mesoappendix) is triangular in shape and arises from the terminal ileal mesentery. It contains the appendiceal artery that originates from the ileocolic artery and passes posterior to the terminal ileum before it enters the mesoappendix. The appendicular artery is an end artery distal to the midpoint of the mesoappendix (Figure 26.2). Inflammation results in thrombosis of this end artery and this disruption of the blood supply leads to gangrene, and perforation.

Histology

Microscopically, the appendix consists of four layers: mucosa, submucosa, muscularis propria and serosa. The muscularis propria includes an outer longitudinal and an inner circular muscular layer. The submucosa contains blood vessels, nerves and lymphoid

Ellis and Calne's Lecture Notes in General Surgery, Fourteenth Edition.
Edited by Christopher Watson and Justin Davies.
© 2023 John Wiley & Sons Ltd. Published 2023 by John Wiley & Sons Ltd.
Companion website: www.wiley.com/go/Watson/GeneralSurgery14

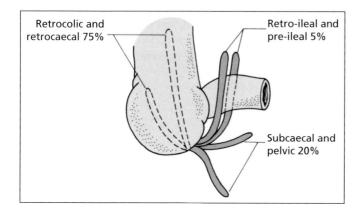

Figure 26.1 The positions in which the appendix may lie, together with their approximate incidence.

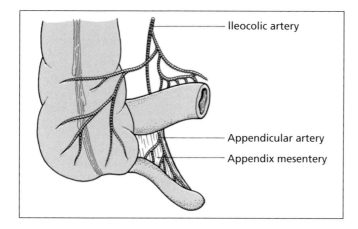

Figure 26.2 The blood supply of the appendix.

tissue. The lymphoid follicles seen within the appendix are not present at birth; they develop over the first 10 years of life and subsequently disappear. The mucosa of the appendix is similar to the colon. It contains tall columnar epithelial cells, mucin-secreting goblet cells and enteroendocrine or enterochromaffin cells that lie in the base of crypts.

Acute appendicitis

Acute appendicitis is the most common abdominal surgical emergency affecting around 10% of the population. Although it can occur at any age, it is uncommon in the very young, where the appendix has a wide mouth, and in the elderly where its lumen is obliterated; the peak incidence is in the third decade of life with a second peak in the seventh decade.

Aetiology and pathology

Various theories have been put forward to explain its occurrence.

a) Mechanical obstruction

Obstruction of the appendix lumen by faecoliths, or from enlargement of lymphoid aggregates or from tumours of the appendix or the caecum results in inflammation. Faecoliths, which are largely composed of fats (coprosterols), epithelial debris, calcium phosphates and vegetable fibres, form when there is slower stool transit time usually reflecting a low fibre intake. The mechanical hypothesis is thought to explain why there is a lower incidence of appendicitis in populations with a high fibre diet such as in Southern Africa.

Once obstruction of the appendix lumen occurs, the intraluminal pressure increases due to the ongoing inflammatory exudate production and mucus secretion. Lymphatic and venous drainage become impaired with the increased appendiceal intraluminal pressure resulting in oedema and mucosal ulceration. Bacterial translocation then sets on the already oedematous appendiceal wall leading to acute appendicitis. Inflammation of the appendix causes thrombosis of the appendicular artery, resulting in gangrenous appendicitis which then results in perforation and bacterial contamination of the peritoneal cavity.

b) Infection hypothesis

This is based on the finding of microbes in appendiceal specimens. Viruses (e.g. dengue, influenza, Epstein-Barr), bacteria (e.g. campylobacter, salmonella) and parasites (e.g. enterobius vermicularis) may proliferate in the appendix and invade the lamina propria leading to oedema of the appendix wall and luminal obstruction.

c) Hygiene

The hygiene hypothesis relates to improved hygiene and a change in childhood gastrointestinal infection and gut immune system interaction. This hypothesis has been considered due to the increase in the incidence of appendicitis in developing countries.

Clinical features

History

The clinical presentation of acute appendicitis varies widely among individuals.

- *Pain.* The classical presentation involves central peri-umbilical colicky pain that migrates to the right iliac fossa over 4–24 hours. The initial appendicular dilatation and inflammation result in poorly localized midgut pain experienced centrally around the umbilicus. Localization of the pain to the right iliac fossa (RIF) occurs when parietal peritoneal structures are involved in the inflammation, stimulating somatic nociceptors. Coughing and/or movement exacerbate the localized RIF pain.
- *Nausea and vomiting,* usually follow the onset of pain.

- *Anorexia* is almost universal.
- *Fever* and occasional diarrhoea or constipation.

Examination

- *Low-grade pyrexia,* around 37.5 °C, and flushed facies.
- *Foetor oris,* and coated tongue are usually present.
- *Motionless:* the patient lies still as movement exacerbates the pain.
- *Localized tenderness in the RIF,* with guarding and rebound tenderness.
- *Rebound tenderness* may be elicited with gentle percussion over the site of maximum tenderness or by asking the patient to cough. The finding of generalized peritonitis with the abdomen being diffusely tender and rigid would be a sign of uncontained appendiceal perforation.
- *Rectal examination* may reveal tenderness when the appendix is in the pelvic position with pus present in the rectovesical pouch or pouch of Douglas.

Further eponymous signs that could be consistent with the diagnosis of acute appendicitis are shown in Box 26.1.

Atypical presentation

The typical migratory RIF pain and associated tenderness probably occurs in 50% of patients presenting with acute appendicitis.

- *Retrocaecal appendix:* inflammation may result in right loin pain rather than RIF pain. Tenderness and guarding in the RIF are unlikely due to the caecum being present between the inflamed appendix and the anterior abdominal wall. The psoas sign may be present.
- *Pelvic appendix:* inflammation may result in suprapubic tenderness without RIF tenderness. Irritation of the rectum may result in diarrhoea, irritation of the bladder may cause frequency of micturition due to irritation of the bladder and spasm of the obturator internus muscle (obturator sign). Rectal examination may be painful as the inflamed pelvic peritoneum is irritated by the examining finger.
- *Obese patients* may not manifest guarding since the presence of an increased depth of

---

Box 26.1 Eponymous signs in acute appendicitis

Rovsing's sign[1]	Deep palpation over the left iliac fossa causing pain in the right iliac fossa, as the peritoneal contents are displaced irritating the inflamed parietal peritoneum on the right.
Psoas sign[2]	The patient lying with the right hip flexed due to spasm in the iliopsoas hip flexors against which the inflamed retrocaecal appendix lies. Pain may also be elicited by passive extension of the hip.
Obturator sign	Pain on flexion and internal rotation of the right hip joint, which stretches obturator internus against which the inflamed appendix lies.

---

subcutaneous fat may hamper efforts to elicit abdominal signs.

- *Pregnant women* with acute appendicitis in the second or third trimester of pregnancy are likely to show right upper quadrant tenderness rather than RIF tenderness in view of the appendix having been displaced cranially to the right upper quadrant by the gravid uterus.
- *Appendicitis in the elderly or in children* may not present with the typical localizing symptoms and signs in the RIF due to the poorly developed or atrophic omentum at those extremes of age. The surgeon should have a low threshold of clinical suspicion for atypical presentations of acute appendicitis in such cases.

Special investigations

Investigations are particularly useful in helping the surgeon diagnose or exclude acute appendicitis in patients presenting with RIF pain, since there is a wide differential diagnosis (see below).

- *Full blood count:* a neutrophilia is common. A microcytic anaemia would raise suspicion of a coincidental caecal cancer.
- *C-reactive protein (CRP)* is usually raised. Both CRP and WCC have good diagnostic accuracy for acute appendicitis but cannot exclude or confirm appendicitis. The diagnostic accuracy of WCC and CRP combined is higher for cases of perforated appendicitis, but 5% of cases have normal indices.

- *Urinalysis* looking for evidence of infection (pyelonephritis may mimic a retrocaecal appendix).
- *Pregnancy test* (β-human chorionic gonadotrophin [βHCG]) to rule out an ectopic pregnancy.
- *Ultrasound scan* may diagnose appendicitis, but its main role is in excluding gynaecological causes of pain.
- *CT scans* are accurate in diagnosing appendicitis, and in evaluating atypical presentations. They can also diagnose an appendix mass or abscess. Radiation exposure means it is less suited to the assessment of young adults or during pregnancy.
- *MR imaging (MRI):* valuable in the assessment of a pregnant patient where ultrasound is inconclusive and CT contraindicated. Appendicectomy during pregnancy is high risk for mother and foetus, as is untreated appendicitis, so an accurate preoperative diagnosis is essential.
- *Diagnostic laparoscopy* is an option for young females where there are more potential differential diagnoses in circumstances where appropriate imaging is not available, but carries a risk of bowel injury, infection and potential removal of a normal appendix. A detailed discussion is crucial to help the patient appreciate the available diagnostic modalities and their associated potential risks for shared decision-making.

Differential diagnosis of RIF pain

Nothing can be so easy, nor anything so difficult, as the diagnosis of acute appendicitis. The differential diagnosis of appendicitis includes most of the causes of acute abdominal pain. They should be considered systematically under the following headings:

- Other gastrointestinal causes of acute pain.
- The urogenital tract.

---

[1]Niels Thorkild Rovsing (1862–1927), Professor of Operative Surgery, University of Copenhagen, Denmark.
[2]The psoas sign is also known as Cope's sign, after Sir Vincent Zachary Cope (1881–1974), Surgeon, St Mary's Hospital, London.

- Gynaecological emergencies in female patients.
- The chest.
- The central nervous system.

Gastrointestinal disease

The following commonly simulate appendicitis.

- *Non-specific mesenteric adenitis*, particularly in young children, following upper respiratory tract infection. This may co-exist with appendicitis, so the diagnosis may be confirmed at the time of appendicectomy.
- *Meckel's diverticulitis*, often indistinguishable from appendicitis; the presence of an inflamed Meckel's diverticulum (see Chapter 25) should always be excluded if the appendix is normal at surgery.
- *Acute Crohn's ileitis* (see Chapter 25) affects young adults, usually with a long history of recurrent pain.
- *Non-Crohn's terminal ileitis* due to yersinia enterocolitica.
- *Intestinal obstruction*, with colicky pain and vomiting. Closed loop large bowel obstruction, where there is a distal obstruction and the ileocaecal valve is competent, results in the colon and caecum distending. Where there is impending caecal perforation there will be RIF pain and tenderness.
- *Gastroenteritis*, with diarrhoea and vomiting but more diffuse and less severe tenderness. Vomiting usually precedes any colic.
- *Acute colonic diverticulitis* usually affects the left colon but may give RIF pain if the sigmoid colon is sufficiently mobile, or if there is inflammation of a solitary caecal diverticulum lying in the RIF. The age group differs from the usually younger patient with appendicitis.
- *Caecal cancer* may present with a mass and a history of RIF discomfort/pain for a few weeks/months.
- *Perforated peptic ulcer*, normally a sudden onset pain. RIF pain may occur as fluid tracks down the right paracolic gutter.
- *Acute cholecystitis*, in which the initial colicky pain is foregut pain, experienced in the epigastrium. A distended, inflamed gallbladder may descend to the RIF.
- *Pancreatitis*, a central pain with central and sometimes RIF tenderness, diagnosed by a raised serum amylase concentration.

The urogenital tract

- *Testicular torsion* may occasionally present with periumbilical pain and vomiting. It is mandatory to examine the testes of all boys and young adults with abdominal pain, to exclude both torsion and maldescent (see Chapter 48).
- *Ureteric colic*. The urine must be tested for blood and pus cells in every case of acute abdominal pain. The patient with ureteric colic is usually restless and moving about, with pain radiating from loin to groin.
- *Acute pyelonephritis*. Typically associated with a history of dysuria, loin tenderness and a high fever (39 °C) with rigors. Note that an inflamed appendix adherent to the ureter or bladder may produce dysuria and microscopic haematuria or pyuria.

Gynaecological emergencies

The most common gynaecological pitfalls are acute salpingitis, ectopic pregnancy and ruptured cyst of the corpus luteum.

- *A ruptured or torted ovarian cyst* presents with sudden severe RIF pain radiating to the loin. An urgent pelvic ultrasound may reveal the diagnosis, or it may be confirmed at laparoscopy.
- *Pelvic inflammatory disease* is a range of diseases including acute salpingitis, endometritis and tubo-ovarian abscess. It is a more diffuse, bilateral, lower abdominal pain, usually accompanied by a vaginal discharge with a history of dyspareunia and dysmenorrhoea.
- *A ruptured ectopic pregnancy* may present with colicky RIF pain if the pregnancy is in the right fallopian tube, with peritonitis and shoulder tip pain when it ruptures due to free blood irritating the diaphragm. Diagnosis is suggested by a positive pregnancy test.

Neurological causes

The pain preceding the eruption of herpes zoster affecting the 11th and 12th dorsal segments, the irritation of these posterior nerve roots in spinal disease (invasive tumour or tuberculosis) and the lightning pains of tabes dorsalis all occasionally mimic appendicitis.

The chest

Basal pneumonia and pleurisy may give referred abdominal pain, which may be surprisingly difficult to differentiate, especially in children. Auscultation may reveal a rub, and chest X-ray may demonstrate pneumonia.

Management of acute appendicitis

When the patient is diagnosed with acute appendicitis, a broad-spectrum antibiotic, such as co-amoxiclav, should be commenced.

Appendicectomy

The mainstay of treatment of acute appendicitis is surgery and, therefore, appendicectomy should be offered to the patient. Appendicitis when perforated and complicated after delayed diagnosis leads to peritonitis, sepsis and ultimately death. Laparoscopic appendicectomy has become the surgical standard. Compared to the open technique, it is associated with less postoperative pain, faster recovery and lower incidence of wound infections and intra-abdominal abscesses.

Laparoscopic appendicectomy is particularly beneficial in obese patients and in young females. For the obese patient, laparoscopic surgery may provide much better views of the peritoneal cavity, in order to perform the procedure as well as washout of any collection of pus, compared with open surgery where the operation may be technically challenging or result in a larger wound (with the subsequent increased risk of wound infection) due to the obesity. For women, laparoscopy may also be diagnostic allowing examination of the ovaries and the pelvis in order to exclude other causes of RIF pain while avoiding the radiation risks of CT.

Conservative treatment

Conservative management with antibiotics may be considered in selected patients who present with uncomplicated acute appendicitis and an operative approach is best avoided or postponed, such as in the presence of severe comorbidities or active SARS-CoV-2 infection, where a general anaesthetic would pose a significant risk of death. Following this strategy, around a quarter of patients would need an appendicectomy within a year.

Appendiceal abscess

Some patients may present late having had ongoing pain in the RIF for 5–7 days. In these cases, the appendix may have perforated already forming a peri-appendiceal abscess walled off by omentum and/or small bowel. Cross-sectional imaging will confirm the diagnosis and assess the potential for percutaneous drainage of the abscess. Nutritional support may be needed with parenteral nutrition if the patient has ileus, and intravenous antibiotics are given following microbiology advice.

Radiological drainage is the best treatment to control infection. Surgery on the phlegmonous tissue is not generally indicated due to the risk of bowel injury resulting in enterocutaneous fistula or postoperative intra-abdominal sepsis, as well as the risk of more extensive surgery such as a limited right hemicolectomy because of the unhealthy inflamed appendix stump. If the appendix abscess is not amenable to radiological drainage and antibiotics do not work, surgery is the only option for drainage.

Appendix mass (Box 26.2)

An appendix mass may form when the omentum and adjacent viscera wall off the inflamed appendix and no abscess forms. The patient may be well

---

Box 26.2 A mass in the right iliac fossa (RIF)

The causes of a mass in the RIF are best thought of by considering the possible anatomical structures in this region.

- Appendix abscess or appendix mass.
- Carcinoma of caecum: differentiated from the above by usually an older age group, a longer history, often the presence of diarrhoea, anaemia with positive occult blood and finally the barium enema examination.
- Crohn's disease: always to be thought of when there is a local mass in a young patient with diarrhoea.
- A distended gallbladder, which may extend down as far as the RIF.
- Pelvic kidney (or renal transplant).
- Ovarian or tubal mass.
- Aneurysm of the common, internal or external iliac artery.
- Retroperitoneal tumour arising in the soft tissues or lymph nodes of the posterior abdominal wall or from the pelvis.
- Ileocaecal tuberculosis (rare in the UK, common in India).
- Psoas abscess – now rare.

systemically but may have tenderness in the RIF with a palpable mass. An appendix mass is also best managed conservatively with antibiotics as an operation poses similar risks to those described for an appendix abscess.

Interval appendicectomy

Following conservative management of an appendix abscess or mass, interval cross-sectional imaging will confirm resolution and exclude the presence of an underlying neoplasm. An interval colonoscopy may be undertaken to ensure the appendix orifice is visualized endoscopically and no underlying neoplasm or other pathology (e.g. Crohn's disease) is identified. Recurrent abdominal pain, the risk of recurrent appendicitis and the potential risk of an underlying appendix neoplasm (see below) warrant discussion of an elective interval laparoscopic appendicectomy.

Appendiceal neoplasms

Appendiceal neoplasms are not uncommon. There are four broad categories of invasive neoplasm that can potentially spread beyond the appendix:

- Neuroendocrine neoplasms (NEN).
- Mucinous neoplasms.
- Goblet cell adenocarcinomas.
- Non-mucinous adenocarcinomas.

There are also non-invasive lesions that, as in the colon, can be precursors of invasive tumours: sessile serrated lesion and adenoma.

Appendiceal neuroendocrine neoplasms

Appendiceal NENs (previously known as 'carcinoids') comprise between 30 and 80% of all appendiceal neoplasms and are found, usually incidentally, in around 1% of appendicectomy specimens. Rarely, appendiceal NENs with extensive local disease and/or distant metastases present with abdominal pain, bowel obstruction, a mass in the RIF or symptoms consistent with carcinoid syndrome.

NENs arise from the enterochromaffin (Kulchitsky) cells of the crypts of Lieberkuhn between villi. The histopathological diagnosis of appendiceal NENs includes immunohistochemical staining for synaptophysin and Chromogranin A. The Ki-67 index, based on the mitotic activity and appearance of the cells, is used to determine the proliferative capacity of the tumour and its overall grading as per the WHO classification. The Ki-67 index as well as the size of the appendiceal NEN, its localization within the appendix and the extent of vascular invasion and invasion into the mesoappendix determine the need for further surgery.

Treatment

For small <1 cm, well-differentiated tumours, appendicectomy alone may suffice whereas for larger or more aggressive tumours a right hemicolectomy is more appropriate in order to achieve cure.

Mucinous neoplasms of the appendix

Mucinous neoplasms of the appendix are the most frequent source of *pseudomyxoma peritonei*, a rare syndrome that is characterized by a slow and relentless accumulation of mucinous tumour in the peritoneal cavity. Mucinous appendiceal neoplasms with pushing-type invasion rather than infiltrative invasion are low-grade appendiceal mucinous neoplasms (LAMN) and high-grade appendiceal mucinous neoplasms (HAMN), whereas a mucinous adenocarcinoma of the appendix exhibits the ability of infiltrative invasion and is more likely to produce distant metastases. If there are signet ring cells in a mucinous adenocarcinoma, the prognosis is worse.

Mucinous neoplasms may be identified on cross-sectional imaging if the appendix appears dilated or diagnosed histologically after a patient presents with acute appendicitis and undergoes appendicectomy. LAMN are the most common, and an appendix containing LAMN is typically dilated with fibrotic or calcified walls containing intraluminal mucin. If a LAMN is removed intact with appendicectomy then no further surgery is required but subsequent follow-up to ensure no disease recurrence occurs. If pushing invasion leads to rupture then mucin can spread in the peritoneal cavity following the peritoneal fluid flow (pseudomyxoma peritonei, see below). In other words, although a LAMN has no infiltrative potential its rupture leads to disease spread anywhere in the peritoneal cavity that can act as a nidus for further disease development at that site.

Pseudomyxoma peritonei

Deposition of mucin in different parts of the peritoneal cavity alongside low-grade mucinous neoplastic cells leads to the formation of pseudomyxoma peritonei in a prolonged and indolent course.

Surgery for pseudomyxoma peritonei is performed in specialized centres and aims to clear all visible disease with peritonectomy, omentectomy, bilateral salpingo-oophorectomy, and bowel resection, followed by heated intraperitoneal chemotherapy (HIPEC) to clear any cancer cells that were not visible to the naked eye. Although patients with LAMN who had cytoreductive surgery and HIPEC have an 87% survival rate at 5 years, patients with appendiceal HAMN or mucinous adenocarcinoma have a more aggressive course of disease and poorer prognosis.

Goblet cell adenocarcinomas

Goblet cell adenocarcinomas are rare tumours and occur almost always in the appendix. Although goblet cell adenocarcinoma was previously termed 'goblet cell carcinoid', this is a misnomer as they are a type of adenocarcinoma.

Appendiceal adenocarcinoma

An appendiceal adenocarcinoma that is not mucinous is a form of adenocarcinoma resembling the colorectal type. Treatment is similar to colonic adenocarcinoma requiring a completion right hemicolectomy to ensure regional lymph node clearance after the diagnosis is made on an appendicectomy specimen. Despite right hemicolectomy conferring an improved survival advantage to appendicectomy alone, the overall prognosis of appendiceal adenocarcinoma is worse than that of colonic adenocarcinoma.

◗ Additional resources

Case 65: Acute abdomen in a medical student
Case 66: Yet another mass in the right iliac fossa

The colon

Justin Davies

Constipation and diarrhoea

Constipation and diarrhoea are two symptoms frequently attributable to diseases of the large bowel. There are, of course, many causes of these common complaints, owing not only to lesions of the large intestine but also to other parts of the gastrointestinal tract being affected or to general diseases. It is useful here to consider the more common causes of these two symptoms.

Constipation

1 *Organic obstruction due to a stricture*:
   a Carcinoma of the colon.
   b Diverticular disease.
   c Crohn's disease.
2 *Painful anal conditions*:
   a Anal fissure.
   b Prolapsed haemorrhoids (piles).

3 *Adynamic bowel*:
   a Hirschsprung's disease.[1]
   b Spinal cord injuries and disease.
   c Hypothyroidism/myxoedema.
   d Parkinson's disease.
4 *Drugs*:
   a Opiate analgesics.
   b Anticholinergics.
5 *Habit and diet*:
   a Dehydration.
   b Starvation.
   c Lack of fibre in diet.
   d Lack of exercise.

Diarrhoea

1 *Specific infections*:
   a Food poisoning (e.g. *Salmonella*).
   b Dysentery (amoebic and bacillary).
   c Cholera.
   d Viral enterocolitis.
2 *Inflammation or irritation of the intestine*:
   a Ulcerative colitis.
   b Tumours of the large bowel.

Ellis and Calne's Lecture Notes in General Surgery, Fourteenth Edition.
Edited by Christopher Watson and Justin Davies.
© 2023 John Wiley & Sons Ltd. Published 2023 by John Wiley & Sons Ltd.
Companion website: www.wiley.com/go/Watson/GeneralSurgery14

[1] Harald Hirschsprung (1830–1916), Professor of Paediatrics, Queen Louisa Hospital, Copenhagen, Denmark.

   c Diverticular disease.
   d Crohn's disease.
3 *Drugs*:
   a Antibiotics and antibiotic-induced colitis.
   b Erythromycin (stimulates the motilin receptor).
   c Laxatives.
   d Digoxin.
   e Orlistat (inhibits lipase and causes steatorrhoea).
4 *Loss of absorptive surface*:
   a Bowel resections and bypass surgery (short circuits).
   b Coeliac disease.
   c Idiopathic steatorrhoea.
5 *Pancreatic dysfunction*: steatorrhoea due to lipase deficiency.
6 *Post-gastrectomy and after bypass surgery for obesity (see Chapter 24)*.
7 *General diseases*:

   a Anxiety states.
   b Hyperthyroidism.
   c Uraemia.
   d Carcinoid syndrome (see Chapter 25).
   e Zollinger–Ellison syndrome (see Chapter 34).

Diverticular disease

Background (Table 27.1)

Diverticula of the colon consist of outpouchings of mucous membrane through the muscle wall of the bowel. Because they lack the normal muscle coats, they are examples of 'false' diverticula, in contrast to a Meckel's diverticulum of the small bowel, which is a true diverticulum. They lie alongside the taenia coli, often overlapped by the appendices epiploicae. Diverticula are found most commonly in the sigmoid colon, and in the Western world become increasingly rare in passing from the left to the right side of the colon. Right-sided diverticula are more commonly found in people from Asia. They are unusual before the age of 40 years, although becoming more common in younger people in recent years, but they are found in about 60% of 70-year-olds. The sex distribution is roughly equal.

Pathogenesis

The characteristic feature of diverticulosis (the presence of diverticula in the absence of any symptoms) is hypertrophy of the muscle of the sigmoid colon, with diverticula occurring at the sites of potential weakness in the bowel wall, corresponding to the points of entry of the supplying blood vessels to the bowel (Figure 27.1). Traditionally blamed on a low-fibre diet, evidence suggests a multifactorial cause of diverticulosis.

1 *Diet and lifestyle*: diverticula are less common in individuals with a high-quality diet (high in fruit, vegetables, whole grains, poultry and fish). Regular physical activity reduces the risk of diverticulitis.
2 *Structural abnormalities*: diverticula are common in patients with Marfan and Ehlers–Danlos syndromes, as well as polycystic kidney disease. This suggests a potential role for dysfunctional connective tissue.
3 *Abnormal motility and increased intraluminal pressure*: patients with diverticulosis may have abnormal motility, with chronic and excessive segmental contractions producing high intraluminal pressure. The dysmotility may also be related to an enteric neuropathy since a reduced number of pacemaker cells in the myenteric plexus has been observed.
4 *Genetics*: genes are thought to contribute to 40–50% risk of diverticulitis.
5 *Obesity* increases the risk of diverticulitis.

Table 27.1 Diverticulum terminology

True diverticulum	An outpouching covered by all the layers of the bowel wall (e.g. Meckel's diverticulum, jejunal diverticulum).
False diverticulum	Lacking the normal muscle coat of the bowel (e.g. colonic diverticula).
Diverticula	Plural of diverticulum.
Diverticulosis	The presence of (usually, colonic) diverticula without symptoms.
Diverticular disease	Diverticula that cause symptoms, usually due to inflammation.
Diverticulitis	Inflammation of a diverticulum.

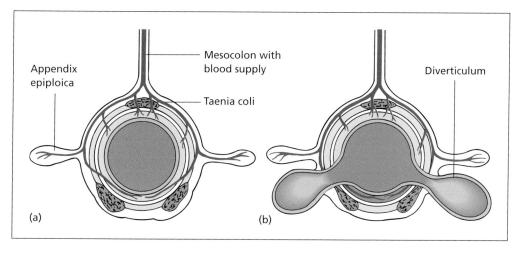

Figure 27.1 The relationship of diverticula of the colon to the taenia coli and to the penetrating blood vessels. (a) Normal colon. (b) Colon with diverticula. Both shown in transverse section.

6 *Non-steroidal anti-inflammatory drugs*: regular use increases the risk of diverticulitis.
7 *Immunosuppression:* patients who are immuno-suppressed are at higher risk of acute diverticulitis, complicated diverticulitis and mortality from diverticulitis.

Complications of diverticula

Diverticular disease may manifest in one of three ways.

1 *Diverticulitis, that may result in perforation into*:
   a The general peritoneal cavity, to cause peritonitis.
   b The pericolic tissues, with formation of a pericolic abscess.
   c Adjacent structures (e.g. bladder, small bowel, vagina), forming a fistula.
2 *Large bowel obstruction*, due to muscular hyper-trophy and inflammatory fibrosis leading to a stricture.
3 *Haemorrhage*, as a result of erosion of a vessel within the fundus of the diverticulum. The bleeding varies from acute and profuse to a chronic occult loss, and is more common in patients with hypertension, diabetes and those on NSAIDs.

Clinical features

Acute uncomplicated diverticulitis

This is characterized by an acute onset of low central abdominal pain, which shifts to the left iliac fossa (LIF) accompanied by fever, vomiting, local tenderness and guarding. A vague mass may be felt in the LIF and occasionally also on rectal examination.

Acute complicated diverticulitis

This is diverticular inflammation combined with obstruction, abscess, fistula or perforation. Perforation into the general peritoneal cavity produces the signs of general peritonitis. A pericolic abscess is comparable to an appendix abscess but on the left side: a tender mass accompanied by a swinging fever and leucocytosis.

Recurrent diverticulitis

This is diverticulitis that resolves completely but then abruptly returns.

Smouldering diverticulitis

This is an uncommon presentation that persists for weeks to months.
   Other presentations of diverticular disease include the following:

Profuse rectal bleeding

Bleeding from a diverticulum is the most likely cause of a sudden, profuse, bright red bleed in an elderly, often hypertensive patient.

Colovesical fistula

Diverticulitis may result in a fistula into the bladder with the passage of gas bubbles (pneumaturia) and faecal debris in the urine (faecaluria). Diverticulitis is the most common cause of a colovesical fistula, others being carcinoma of the colon, carcinoma of the bladder, Crohn's disease and trauma.

Ongoing chronic gastrointestinal symptoms

Ongoing abdominal pain is seen in around one in four patients 12 months after an acute episode of diverticulitis. This may be related to increased visceral hypersensitivity following inflammation.

Special investigations

- *Computed tomography (CT) scan* is the investigation of choice in the acute stage and can help exclude other causes of lower abdominal pain in difficult cases.
- *Endoscopy*: if the affected segment is low in the colon, there may be an oedematous block to the passage of the instrument beyond about 15 cm. Rigid sigmoidoscopes view only the rectum, and so do not visualize colonic diverticula. Flexible endoscopes are longer, and do allow full visualization of the sigmoid colon (flexible sigmoidoscopy) or the entire colon (colonoscopy).
- *CT colonography* demonstrates diverticula as globular outpouchings. Diverticular strictures may closely simulate an annular carcinoma. The length and density of the stricture can help with differentiation: diverticular wall thickening typically involves a long segment and is low density and smooth whereas carcinoma is higher density and involves a shorter segment. The presence of nodes in the adjacent fat (often the sigmoid mesentery) is also more common in carcinoma. A stricture identified on imaging will require direct visualization and biopsy at endoscopy in order to confirm the diagnosis.

Insufflation of gas required for endoscopy or colonography carries a risk of perforation of the inflamed, friable bowel if performed in the acute stage of diverticulitis, and if possible should be deferred until the acute inflammation has settled. Colonoscopy remains the gold standard and should be considered once an episode of acute diverticulitis has settled, as colorectal cancer is subsequently identified in 1% of those after uncomplicated and 7% of those after complicated acute diverticulitis.

Differential diagnosis

The important differential diagnosis is from neoplasm of the colon. It is impossible to be certain of this differentiation clinically or even on special investigations, unless a positive biopsy is obtained by endoscopy to definitively establish the diagnosis of carcinoma. Even at surgery, it may be difficult to be sure whether one is dealing with carcinoma or diverticular disease; indeed, these two common conditions may co-exist.

Treatment

Acute diverticulitis

When uncomplicated (i.e., no evidence of perforation, stricture or abscess), it is managed conservatively; the patient is usually placed on antibiotics (co-amoxiclav, or ciprofloxacin and metronidazole, are the combinations of choice). The great majority will settle on this regimen. There are some emerging data from randomized controlled trials that antibiotics may not be necessary in radiologically confirmed cases of acute uncomplicated sigmoid diverticulitis.

- *A pericolic abscess* is diagnosed by CT scan, and may be drained percutaneously if over 3 cm in size. Drainage may occasionally be complicated by formation of a faecal fistula. Once the sepsis is controlled, surgery with resection of the diseased segment should be considered but is not always necessary.
- *General peritonitis* from rupture of an acute diverticulitis is a dangerous condition. When peritonitis is the result of perforation of a diverticular abscess, laparoscopic lavage and drainage may suffice but is not commonly performed due to concerns that an underlying carcinoma may not be detected and that lavage alone may not be adequate to resolve the symptoms. Ideally, surgical resection is performed, either open or laparoscopic. A primary anastomosis, with or without a defunctioning loop ileostomy to divert the faecal stream until the anastomosis has healed, may be considered; the ileostomy is subsequently closed. Alternatively, an end colostomy is fashioned, usually as a Hartmann's procedure[2] (Figure 27.2). Full antibiotic therapy is given.

---

[2] Henri Hartmann (1860–1952), Professor of Surgery, Hôtel Dieu, Paris, France.

- *Acute obstruction* due to diverticulitis is often evident when a CT scan is performed in the emergency setting. It is important to determine whether or not the obstruction is caused by an adherent loop of small intestine, which is not uncommon. Surgical options are the same as for general peritonitis.

Chronic gastrointestinal symptoms

If the diagnosis is made with considerable certainty and symptoms are mild, this can be treated conservatively. The bowels are regulated by means of a regular stool softener. A high-roughage diet (fruit, vegetables,

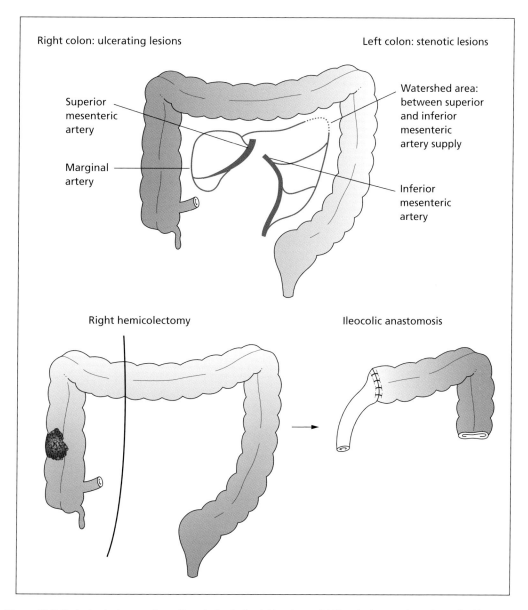

Figure 27.2 Typical colonic operations. For a lesion in the right colon, a right hemicolectomy is performed, with an ileocolic anastomosis. For a lesion in the left colon, a left hemicolectomy or sigmoid colectomy is performed, with anastomosis of the colon to the rectum; in an emergency situation, with unprepared bowel, a Hartmann's operation can be performed with the proximal bowel end exteriorized as a colostomy and the rectum oversewn. At a second stage, the continuity of the bowel can be restored by colorectal anastomosis.

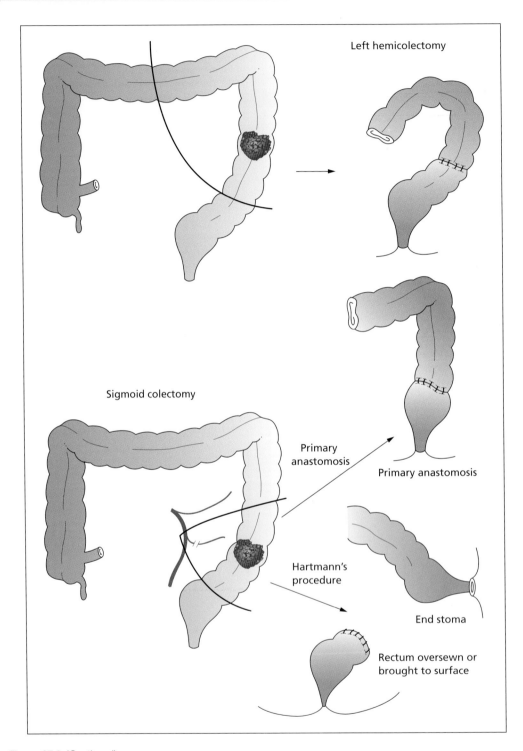

Left hemicolectomy

Sigmoid colectomy

Primary anastomosis

Primary anastomosis

Hartmann's procedure

End stoma

Rectum oversewn or brought to surface

Figure 27.2 (*Continued*)

wholemeal bread and bran) is often recommended, although in some patients with very sensitive colons and significant symptoms of pain, a lower fibre diet can often be helpful.

Colovesical fistula is treated by resection of the affected segment of the colon after disconnection from the bladder wall; a primary colorectal anastomosis is fashioned and the defect in the bladder repaired (although sometimes the bladder hole is so small that it will heal itself after a urinary catheter is left in place for a few days).

Angiodysplasia

This term is applied to one or multiple small (<5 mm) mucosal or submucosal vascular malformations, usually a dilated vein or sheaf of veins. Because they occur most commonly in the elderly, they are considered to be degenerative vascular anomalies. The caecum and ascending colon are the sites most usually involved, although they may be found anywhere in the small or large bowel.

Clinical features

They are usually asymptomatic, and were unknown before the advent of mesenteric angiography and colonoscopy. Their only clinical manifestation is bleeding, which may take the form of continuous chronic intestinal blood loss, presenting with anaemia, or recurrent acute dark or bright red rectal bleeding, which may occasionally be severe and life-threatening. Recurrent bleeding is common. They account for as much as 5% of such emergency cases.

Special investigations

- *Colonoscopy* is the investigation of choice, although it is often difficult to visualize the caecum acutely. The lesions appear as bright red 0.5–1 cm diameter submucosal lesions with small, dilated vessels visible on close inspection. They are not visible on CT colonography.
- *Mesenteric angiogram.* Actively bleeding angiodysplasias may be detected on angiography as contrast medium leaks into the bowel lumen.

Treatment

Blood transfusion is necessary if bleeding is severe. Colonoscopic electrocoagulation or argon plasma coagulation may be curative. Resection, usually a right hemicolectomy, is rarely required.

Colitis

Colitis, inflammation of the colon, presents with diarrhoea and often lower abdominal pain, with blood and mucus per rectum. The most common causes of colitis are:

1 *Inflammatory bowel disease*, including both ulcerative colitis and Crohn's colitis.
2 *Antibiotic-associated colitis*, for example pseudomembranous colitis due to *Clostridium difficile* (see Chapter 5).
3 *Infective colitis*, for example *Campylobacter* and amoebic colitis.
4 *Ischaemic colitis*, due to mesenteric ischaemia, occurring spontaneously (a poorly understood condition, as often the main supplying vasculature is patent on subsequent investigation), or following ligation of the inferior mesenteric artery in aortic surgery or its exclusion following placement of a covered aortic stent.

Ulcerative colitis

Ulcerative colitis is an inflammatory disease of the large bowel that involves the rectum and extends for a variable distance proximally in the colon. Women are more often affected than men, and it is found in any age from infancy to the elderly, but the maximum incidence is between the ages of 15 and 30 with a second peak between 50 and 70.

Aetiology

The aetiology of ulcerative colitis is unknown, although it appears to combine genetic factors, environmental stimuli and altered immune responses; it is one of the few diseases in which smoking appears to be protective.

1 *Genetic*:
   a First-degree relative affected in 10% of patients.
   b Monozygotic twins have a 10% concordance.

c Ashkenazi Jews have a five-fold higher risk than other groups.

d Association with human leucocyte antigen (HLA)-DRB1*0103.

2 *Environmental*:

a Incidence is higher in developed countries.

b Smoking is protective (half the incidence of non-smokers).

c Appendicectomy before the age of 20 appears protective.

d Previous episode of enteric infection (e.g. *Salmonella, Campylobacter*) doubles the risk of later ulcerative colitis.

3 *Immune response*:

a Epithelial barrier impaired.

b Dendritic cell numbers reduced.

c Exaggerated T-cell (Th2) response.

Pathology

The rectum and sigmoid colon are principally affected, but the whole colon may be involved. Initially, there is oedema of the mucosa, with contact bleeding and petechial haemorrhage, proceeding to ulceration; the ulcers are shallow and irregular. Oedematous islands of mucosa between the ulcers may form pseudopolyps. The wall of the colon is oedematous and fibrotic and, therefore, may become rigid with loss of its normal haustrations. The changes are confluent, with no unaffected 'skip lesions' as found in Crohn's disease. The inflamed colon does not generally become adherent to its neighbouring intra-abdominal viscera, as the inflammatory process in ulcerative colitis is not transmural (unlike in Crohn's disease).

Microscopically, the principal locus of the disease is mucosal; small abscesses form within the mucosal crypts ('crypt abscesses'). These abscesses break down into ulcers whose base is lined with granulation tissue. The walls of the colon are infiltrated with neutrophils; there is oedema and submucosal fibrosis. In the chronic, burnt-out disease, the mucosa is smooth and atrophic, and the bowel wall may be thinned.

Clinical features

Manifestations of ulcerative colitis may be fulminant, intermittent or chronic. The most common scenario is of diarrhoea, with urgency, frequency, blood and mucus. There may be accompanying cramp-like abdominal pains. Examination often reveals nothing but there may be mild tenderness in the LIF, and blood on the glove of the examining finger after rectal examination. The rectal mucosa may feel oedematous.

In severe attacks, there is fever, tachycardia, severe bleeding and risk of perforation. Anorexia and loss of weight occur in the acute episodes.

Special investigations

Investigations aim to make the diagnosis, differentiate it from Crohn's colitis, exclude complications and assess the proximal extent.

- *Sigmoidoscopy* reveals oedema of the mucosa with contact bleeding in the early mild cases, proceeding to granularity of the mucosa and then frank ulceration with pus and blood in the bowel lumen. Biopsy will provide histological confirmation of the diagnosis.
- *Colonoscopy* enables the whole of the large bowel to be inspected, the proximal extent of disease to be noted and biopsy material to be obtained. A full colonoscopy should not be performed in the acute phase due to increased risk of perforation.
- *CT scan* demonstrates typically left-sided mural thickening, which is symmetrical and continuous (compared with Crohn's disease which is asymmetrical with segmental involvement, although pancolitis can occur). Local perforations or abscesses may be identified, as may extracolonic manifestations, such as sacroiliitis and evidence of primary sclerosing cholangitis. The extent of colonic inflammation can also be assessed acutely by CT scan.
- *Barium enema* is very uncommonly used now. The classic picture of a smooth, narrow drainpipe colon due to oedema and fibrosis with loss of haustration is rarely seen nowadays.
- *Examination of the stools* reveals pus and blood visible to the naked eye or under the microscope; stool culture should be performed to exclude infections, including *Clostridium difficile*.

Differential diagnosis

Ulcerative colitis may be difficult to differentiate from other causes of diarrhoea (see earlier in this chapter), especially the dysenteries and carcinoma, or Crohn's colitis (Table 27.2). Differentiation from colonic Crohn's disease may be particularly difficult, even when the resected colon is examined by an expert

Table 27.2 Crohn's colitis and ulcerative colitis*

	Crohn's colitis	Ulcerative colitis
Clinical features	Perianal disease common, e.g. anal fissure and anal fistula.	Perianal disease rare, apart from *anal fissure*.
	Gross bleeding uncommon.	Often profuse haemorrhage.
	Small bowel may also be affected.	Small bowel not affected (although so-called 'backwash ileitis' may be seen).
Pathology		
Macroscopic differences	Any part of colon may be involved (skip lesions).	Disease extends proximally from rectum.
	Transmural involvement.	Mucosal involvement only.
	Fistulates into adjacent viscera.	No fistulas.
	Pseudopolyps less common.	Pseudopolyps of regenerating mucosa.
	Thickened bowel wall.	No thickening of bowel wall.
	Malignant change risk increases with length of time from diagnosis and extent of disease- surveillance required.	Malignant change risk increases with length of time from diagnosis and extent of disease – surveillance required.
Microscopic differences	Granulomas present.	No granulomas.

*Ten per cent of cases cannot be assigned clearly to one or other disease and are labelled as 'IBD-Unclassified'.

pathologist. Indeed, about 10% of cases have to be labelled as 'inflammatory bowel disease unclassified' (IBD-U). Colitis due to cytomegalovirus (CMV) should also be considered, especially in those who are immunosuppressed.

Complications

Local

- Toxic dilation, in which the colon dilates in a fulminant colitis, leading to perforation.
- Haemorrhage (acute, or chronic with progressive anaemia).
- Stricture.
- Malignant change (see later in this chapter).

General

- Weight loss and anaemia.
- Arthritis (including ankylosing spondylitis) and uveitis.
- Dermatological manifestations: pyoderma gangrenosum, erythema nodosum, other skin rashes and ulceration of the legs.
- Primary sclerosing cholangitis is associated with ulcerative colitis, as it is with Crohn's disease.

Malignant change

Patients with ulcerative colitis who have had chronic pancolitis (affecting the whole large bowel), particularly if the first attack was in childhood, have a higher risk of developing carcinoma of the colon than those without inflammatory bowel disease. Statistics indicate that 5–12% of patients with colitis of 20 years' duration will develop malignant change. Patients should, therefore, be offered surveillance colonoscopy in order to detect and treat the dysplasia that heralds malignant change.

Even in the absence of a pancolitis, patients with ulcerative colitis and Crohn's colitis are at greater risk of developing carcinoma of the large bowel than a normal individual. Moreover, the tumours occurring in patients with IBD are more likely to affect a younger age group, be poorly differentiated and be multiple compared with those arising in a sporadic nature. Often, the condition is diagnosed late, as both the patient and doctor may attribute the symptoms (bleeding, diarrhoea and pus) to the colitis.

Treatment

Initially this is medical in the uncomplicated case, but surgery is required when medical treatment fails or when complications arise.

Medical treatment

Corticosteroids given systemically, by rectal infusion or in combination, will often produce remission in an acute attack. Salicylates such as mesalazine are used to maintain a remission. In more severe cases, antibodies to tumour necrosis factor alpha, such as infliximab or adalimumab, or immunosuppressants such as azathioprine, ciclosporin or tacrolimus may be required. Increasing evidence now supports use of second and third line immunosuppressants/biologics, such as ustekinumab (a monoclonal antibody to the p40 subunit of interleukins 12 and 23) and vedolizumab (a monoclonal antibody to the α4β7-integrin expressed on gut-homing T-helper lymphocytes). It is very important that decisions to escalate medical biologic therapy are made in a joint inflammatory bowel disease clinic setting that involves the patient, a gastroenterologist and a colorectal surgeon.

Surgery

The indications for surgery are the following.

- *Fulminant disease* not responding to medical treatment (defined as the passage of more than six bloody motions per day, with fever, tachycardia and hypoalbuminaemia).
- *Chronic disease* not responding to medical treatment.
- *Malignancy or dysplasia that is not endoscopically resectable.*
- *Complications of colitis* already listed.

The initial procedure comprises removal of the colon (subtotal colectomy) with preservation of the rectal stump and formation of an end ileostomy. Subsequently, further surgery can be considered, once the patient has recovered from the acute episode. Options include:

a Removal of the rectum and anus with a permanent ileostomy.
b Removal of the rectum with restoration of intestinal continuity with an interposed pouch of ileum (ileoanal pouch, or Parks' pouch[3]).
c Formation of an ileorectal anastomosis in a small number of eligible patients, although this must be accompanied with an agreed plan for ongoing rectal surveillance for the presence of neoplasia and topical treatment to reduce inflammation in the rectum.

Most patients requiring urgent surgery for ulcerative colitis are either on corticosteroids or have recently received them. In these patients, surgical procedures must, therefore, be covered by an increased dosage of corticosteroids to compensate for presumed suppression of endogenous glucocorticoids, which can then be tailed off gradually in the postoperative period.

Crohn's colitis

Crohn's disease,[4] although most commonly found in the terminal ileum (see Chapter 25), may occur anywhere in the gastrointestinal tract from the mouth to the anus. It may be confined to the large bowel or there may be involvement of both the small and large intestine.

Clinical features

Colonic Crohn's disease closely mimics ulcerative colitis in its clinical manifestations. Unlike ulcerative colitis, the affected segment of colon may become adherent to adjacent structures with abscess formation and fistulation. Perianal involvement with abscesses, anal fissure(s) and multiple anal fistulas is also common and indeed may be the first manifestation of the disease.

Treatment

This is similar to that of Crohn's disease of the small intestine (see Chapter 25). Resection of involved large bowel may require segmental colectomy if there is limited disease involvement or total excision with a permanent ileostomy for extensive disease. Restorative proctocolectomy and ileoanal (Parks') pouch formation is only performed in very few cases of Crohn's disease affecting only the large bowel because of the immediate risks of sepsis and fistulation, and the chance of recurrence within the small bowel.

Tumours

Classification

Benign

- Adenomatous polyp.
- Papilloma.

[3] Sir Alan Parks (1920–1982), Colorectal Surgeon, St Mark's Hospital, London, UK.

[4] Burrill Bernard Crohn (1884–1983), Gastroenterologist, Mount Sinai Hospital, New York, USA.

- Lipoma.
- Neurofibroma.
- Haemangioma.

Malignant

1 *Primary*:
   a Carcinoma.
   b Lymphoma.
   c Neuroendocrine tumour (see Chapter 25).
2 *Secondary*: invasion from adjacent tumours, for example stomach, bladder, uterus and ovary.

Carcinoma

Carcinomas affecting the large bowel are common. They are the third most common cause of death from malignant disease in the UK, next in frequency to cancers of the lung and prostate in men, and lung and breast in women.

Colonic carcinoma may occur at any age. Women are affected slightly more often than men (although, interestingly, the incidence of rectal cancer is roughly equal in the two sexes). The sigmoid is the most common part of the colon affected, although the rectum accounts for one-third of all large bowel cancers. Five per cent of tumours of the large bowel are multiple (synchronous).

Predisposing factors

Increasing age, pre-existing adenomatous polyps, ulcerative and Crohn's colitis and a number of inherited colorectal cancer syndromes are risk factors for the development of carcinoma of the large bowel. Inherited syndromes such as familial adenomatous polyposis (FAP) and hereditary non-polyposis colon cancer (HNPCC) account for a small proportion of colorectal cancers, and potential carriers should be offered screening (see later in this chapter). Family history alone is sufficient to increase the risk, and it has been estimated that one first-degree relative having colon cancer aged over 45 years increases one's lifetime risk from 1 in 50 to 1 in 17; if the relative was diagnosed before 45, the lifetime risk increases to 1 in 10.

Familial adenomatous polyposis

This is a rare disease, but it is important because it invariably proceeds to colorectal carcinoma unless treated and accounts for 0.5% of all colon cancers. It has an autosomal dominant inheritance, and is associated with mutation in the FAP gene; 25% of cases are

spontaneous mutations. The polyps first appear in adolescence; symptoms of bleeding and diarrhoea commence about the age of 21 years and malignant change occurs between 20 and 40 years of age. Affected individuals usually have congenital hypertrophy of the retinal pigment epithelium (CHRPE) which is a useful, non-invasive screening test. Variants such as *Gardner's syndrome*[5] exist in which colonic polyps are associated with desmoid tumours and osteomas of the mandible and skull.

Treatment generally comprises a total colectomy with excision of the rectum, ideally before the age of 25. Options are to have a permanent ileostomy, or to consider restoration of intestinal continuity with an ileoanal (Parks') pouch. If the polyps are not profuse in the rectum, it is possible to resect the colon while leaving behind the rectum to which an ileorectal anastomosis is performed, and then carry out regular surveillance of the rectal stump via flexible sigmoidoscopy.

Hereditary non-polyposis colon cancer (HNPCC)

HNPCC accounts for less than 5% of colorectal cancers, and is also dominantly inherited. It results from mutations in a family of genes affecting DNA mismatch repair, which leads to genomic instability; 60% of cases are due to a mutation in the *MSH2* gene and 30% in the *MLH1* gene. Other implicated genes are *MSH6, PMS2, PMS1* and *MLH3*. Tumours tend to occur in the right colon, and arise before the age of 50. Occurrence of colon cancer in at least three family members spanning two generations, with one before the age of 45, strongly suggests this syndrome. It is also associated with tumours of the ovary, uterus, kidney, ureter, small bowel, stomach and skin.

Pathology

Macroscopically, the tumours can be classified into the following groups:

- Ulcerating.
- Papillomatous.
- Annular.
- Stricturing.

Microscopically, these are all adenocarcinomas.

---

[5] Eldon John Gardner (1909–1989), Geneticist, later Professor of Zoology, Utah State University, Logan, Utah.

Spread

- *Local*: encircling the wall of the bowel and invading the layers of the colon, eventually involving adjacent viscera (small intestine, stomach, duodenum, ureter, bladder, uterus, abdominal wall, etc.).
- *Lymphatic*: to the regional lymph nodes, eventually spreading via the thoracic duct, and may involve supraclavicular nodes in late cases.
- *Bloodstream*: to the liver via the portal vein, and also to the lungs.
- *Nerves:* perineural invasion is the process of neoplastic invasion of nerves.
- *Transcoelomic*: producing deposits of malignant nodules throughout the peritoneal cavity.

Staging

Historically, colorectal cancer was staged according to the classification of Dukes,[6] and depended upon the extent of transmural extension and lymph node spread (see Chapter 28), although the TNM staging system (see Chapter 7) is more commonly used nowadays. This leads to stages of disease from one to four according to how far the tumour has spread through the bowel wall (stages 1 and 2), to the draining lymph nodes (stage 3) or if there is metastatic (distant) spread (stage 4).

Clinical features

The manifestations of carcinoma of the colon can be divided, as with any tumour, into those produced by the tumour itself, those arising from the presence of secondaries (metastases), and the general effects of the tumour.

Local effects

1 *Change in bowel habit* is the most common symptom, usually with an increased frequency of looser stool (diarrhoea), or less frequently constipation. The diarrhoea may be accompanied by mucus (produced by the excessive secretion of mucus from the tumour) or bleeding, which may be bright, dark or occult, depending on the proximity of the tumour to the anus.

[6] Cuthbert Esquire Dukes (1890–1977), Pathologist, St Mark's Hospital, London, UK.

2 *Intestinal obstruction* due to a stricturing tumour, more commonly found in the left (sigmoid or descending) colon (see Chapter 30).
3 *Perforation* of the tumour, either into the general peritoneal cavity or locally with the formation of a pericolic abscess, or occasionally by fistulation into adjacent viscera, for example a gastrocolic fistula or colovesical fistula.

The effects of secondary deposits (metastases)

The patient may present with jaundice, hepatomegaly or abdominal distension due to ascites.

The general effects of malignant disease

Presenting features may be anaemia, anorexia or loss of weight.

Tumours of the left side of the colon, where the contained stool is solid, are typically stricturing tumours, so obstructive features predominate. In contrast, tumours of the right side tend to be proliferative and here the stools are semi-liquid, and, therefore, obstructive symptoms are relatively uncommon and the patient with a carcinoma of the caecum or ascending colon often presents with anaemia and loss of weight.

Examination

This should seek evidence of the following.

1 The presence of a mass palpable either per abdomen or per rectum.
2 Clinical evidence of intestinal obstruction.
3 Evidence of spread (hepatomegaly, ascites, jaundice or supraclavicular lymphadenopathy).
4 Clinical evidence of anaemia or loss of weight suggesting malignant disease.

Special investigations

- *Occult blood in the stool* is frequently present and should be tested for. This is now typically via a faecal immunochemical test (FIT).
- *Rigid or flexible sigmoidoscopy* in the outpatient setting will reveal tumours in the rectosigmoid region and allow positive evidence by biopsy to be obtained. Even if the tumour is not reached directly, the presence of blood or mucus coming

down from above is strongly suspicious of malignant disease, and warrants further investigation.

- *Colonoscopy*, enables the entire colon to be inspected and a biopsy to be obtained. This is the gold standard investigation.
- *CT colonography ('virtual colonoscopy')* has replaced barium enema as the investigation of choice if colonoscopy is not available or appropriate. It will usually reveal the tumour and associated stricture or filling defect ('apple-core' deformity), and can also detect associated liver metastases. It is important to remember that a negative CT scan does not definitely exclude the presence of a small tumour, particularly in the presence of extensive diverticulosis.
- *Staging CT scan* of the chest, abdomen and pelvis should be performed once the diagnosis has been confirmed, in order to assess the local extent of disease and whether there is any sign of metastatic disease.

Differential diagnosis

Diseases producing local symptoms

- Diverticular disease.
- Inflammatory bowel disease.
- Infective colitis and other causes of diarrhoea and constipation (see earlier in this chapter).

Treatment

Surgery

The principle of operative treatment is wide resection of the tumour together with its regional lymphatics and blood supply. In elective surgery, resection with restoration of intestinal continuity with a primary anastomosis can generally be achieved, with the risks of infection reduced with preoperative bowel preparation and oral antibiotics taken the day before. In cases of malignant large bowel obstruction, in which bowel preparation is contraindicated, the primary goal is to relieve obstruction. It may be possible to achieve primary resection with restoration of continuity at the same time, with or without a defunctioning stoma. The surgical alternatives are resection with a proximal end stoma (Hartmann's procedure, if the sigmoid colon is resected), or an initial defunctioning proximal stoma alone. If there is available expertise, an endoscopically placed colonic stent can be considered initially in order to relieve the obstruction, with a

view to a planned, elective surgical resection several weeks later.

Adjuvant therapy

Adjuvant chemotherapy with 5-fluorouracil (5-FU), in combination with folinic acid and oxaliplatin (FOLFOX) or with capecitabine and oxaliplatin (CAPOX), may reduce the risk of recurrent disease; for metastatic disease, oral therapy with capecitabine is the preferred choice. Biological therapy with monoclonal antibody therapy such as cetuximab and panitumumab (both against the epidermal growth factor receptor) or pembrolizumab (binds to the programmed cell death receptor 1, potentiating T-cell anti-tumour responses) may be considered as second line therapy for metastatic disease.

Follow-up

- *Cross-sectional CT imaging* is performed to detect local recurrence and the appearance of liver, lung and other metastases; metastatic spread to the liver in the absence of other disease may be treated by resection of the affected liver segment(s).
- *Surveillance colonoscopy* is undertaken at intervals to detect new tumours and local recurrence; having had one colorectal cancer is a risk factor for further ones.
- *Carcinoembryonic antigen (CEA)* blood test at intervals can highlight possible recurrence if the levels start to rise again after treatment.

The patient with incurable disease

Even if secondary spread is present and incurable, appropriate palliation is key. This may still be achieved by resection of the primary tumour, even if the primary is asymptomatic. If this is not possible or appropriate, the tumour may be stented to relieve obstruction. Where stenting is not possible, a palliative bypass or stoma may be considered. Systemic anti-cancer therapy, in particular chemotherapy, may help to alleviate symptoms. It is important to involve the palliative care team early in this process in order to provide a holistic and patient-centred approach to decision-making and symptom relief.

Prognosis

Stage 1 tumours (through the inner bowel lining of the bowel or into the muscle wall) are usually curable, with 91% 5-year survival. Five-year survival with stage 2 tumours (spread through to the outer muscle wall of the bowel), in which the disease is still confined to the bowel wall, is around 84%, and the presence of lymph node metastases in stage 3 disease gives a 65% 5-year survival. Metastatic disease (stage 4) has an overall 10% 5-year survival.

Colonic surgery (see Figure 27.2)

The different colonic resections are based on the blood supply to the colon coming from the superior mesenteric artery (midgut components, i.e. caecum, ascending colon and two-thirds of the transverse colon) and the inferior mesenteric artery (hindgut components, i.e. distal transverse colon, descending colon, sigmoid and rectum) together with a free vascular anastomosis between the principal arteries via the marginal artery (of Drummond[7]). Since survival from colonic cancer is, in the case of lymph node positive disease, at least in part dependent upon the adequacy of resection (adequately clearing the affected draining lymph nodes), surgery for cancer involves *en bloc* resection of the adjacent mesentery where lymphatic drainage occurs. This allows the best possible histopathological staging of the tumour, with adjuvant chemotherapy considered when tumour cells are present in the removed, draining lymph nodes or blood vessels. In practice, this means resecting as far down the principal artery as is possible and safe, since the lymphatic drainage runs alongside the arterial inflow. In non-cancer operations, more conservative surgical techniques may be employed.

Colostomy

When the bowel is brought to the surface and opened, it is termed a 'stoma' (from the Greek meaning mouth); in the case of the colon, such an opening is termed a 'colostomy'. Stomas may be permanent, for example when the distal bowel has been removed, or temporary, when there is a possibility of restoring continuity with more surgery at a future date.

---

[7] Sir David Drummond (1852–1932), Professor of Medicine, University of Durham, Durham, UK. He demonstrated the artery by tying off the right, middle, left colic and sigmoid arteries in cadavers and injecting contrast into the ileocolic artery and showing it flowed around to the rectum.

Indications for colostomy formation

The common indications for colostomy formation are:

- To divert faeces to allow healing of a more distal anastomosis or fistula.
- To decompress a dilated colon, as a prelude to resection of the obstructing lesion.
- Following removal of the distal colon and rectum in a patient who is either not fit enough to tolerate the effects of an anastomotic leak or whose anorectal function would lead to poor control/incontinence if bowel restoration is performed.
- Intractable faecal incontinence.

The ability of the patient to manage the colostomy needs to be borne in mind; in a patient with poor dexterity, such as following a stroke or secondary to severe Parkinson's disease, or with poor eyesight, creation of a stoma may be undesirable, even on a temporary basis.

Types of colostomy

Loop colostomy

The colon is brought to the surface and the antimesenteric border opened. A temporary rod or similar device may be used to stop the opened bowel loop from falling back inside, particularly if there is a thick abdominal wall. A loop colostomy is used temporarily to divert faeces and is more simple to reverse; more commonly, a loop ileostomy is preferred because of the better blood supply to the bowel facilitating subsequent closure.

End colostomy

An end colostomy is fashioned by dividing the colon and bringing the proximal end to the surface. It may be used as a definitive procedure in a patient undergoing total anorectal excision, or following perforated diverticular disease in which the diseased bowel is removed and gross faecal contamination makes performing a primary anastomosis to restore continuity undesirable. In the latter, the distal bowel may be closed off and left within the abdomen (a Hartmann's procedure if the sigmoid colon is removed and rectum closed off) or brought to the surface at a separate place as a mucus fistula.

Double-barrelled colostomy

A double-barrelled (Paul–Mikulicz[8]) colostomy comprises proximal and distal ends of colon brought out adjacent to each other, like a loop colostomy but with the intervening colon removed. This type of colostomy is not commonly used because the distal bowel is usually too short, but it is useful in the treatment of sigmoid volvulus, in which there is usually sufficient distal colon to allow a tension-free double-barrelled colostomy.

Complications of colostomy formation

- *Retraction*, in which the colon disappears down the hole out of which it was brought.
- *Stenosis*, in which the opening becomes smaller. This may be due to ischaemia or poor apposition of colonic mucosa with the skin edge.
- *Parastomal hernia*, in which peritoneal contents herniate through the abdominal wall defect made to accommodate the stoma.
- *Prolapse*, in which the colon prolapses out of the stoma.

In addition, there may be psychological issues to address, excess gas production with certain foods, and leakage with skin excoriation due to ill-fitting stoma appliances or poorly constructed stomas.

Stoma appliances: principles

Modern-day stoma appliances have made the management of stomas much more straightforward. The principal components are the collecting pouch, or bag, into which the faeces collect, and the adhesive flange, which adheres to the skin and keeps the pouch in position. The flange is cut to fit the stoma closely, and any exposed skin is covered with a barrier paste if needed. Colostomies contrast with ileostomies by the nature of the effluent. Ileostomy effluent is more liquid and irritant and may cause severe skin excoria-

[8] Frank Thomas Paul (1851–1941), Surgeon, Liverpool Royal Infirmary, Liverpool. Johann von Mikulicz-Radecki (1850–1905), Professor of Surgery, successively at Cracow, Konigsberg and Breslau, Poland.

tion. For this reason, an ileostomy is constructed with a prominent spout to keep the effluent off the skin, in contrast to a colostomy, which is constructed flush with the skin or preferably with a slight spout.

Siting a stoma

The optimal position of a stoma should be ascertained pre-operatively wherever possible. Typically, a colostomy is sited on the left, and an ileostomy on the right. The patient needs to be able to wear the appliance comfortably, so it should not be placed in an abdominal crease such that the appliance will not achieve a seal, or where a belt or waist band of a trouser or skirt usually sit. The stoma should be fully visible to the patient in its final position to enable them to empty it as required.

Management of a colostomy

In the first few weeks after performing a colostomy, the faecal discharge is often semi-liquid, but this gradually reverts to normal, solid stools. The colostomy appliances, which are waterproof, allow the patient to lead a normal life with little risk of leakage or unpleasant odour.

Although there is obviously no sphincteric control of the colostomy opening, many patients find that they pass a single stool a day. This can be helped by preparations such as Fybogel, which produce a bulky, formed stool. Patients may choose to reduce the amounts of vegetables or fruit eaten, which may produce diarrhoea and excessive flatus. Some patients undertake stoma irrigation in order to have more control over when the stoma produces its effluent.

 Additional resources

Case 67: A symptomless finding on a barium enema examination
Case 68: Ulcerative colitis
Case 69: A complication of long-standing ulcerative colitis
Case 70: An elderly woman with an abdominal mass
Case 71: A patient with bowel obstruction

28

The rectum and anal canal

Justin Davies

Learning objectives

✓ To know the causes and treatment of rectal bleeding.
✓ To know the presentation and management of benign and malignant anorectal conditions.

The distribution around the anal canal of various common conditions is shown in Figure 28.1.

Bright red rectal bleeding (Table 28.1)

The passage of bright red blood per anum is a common symptom, which the patient usually attributes to haemorrhoids, commonly known as 'piles'; indeed, haemorrhoids are by far the most common cause of rectal bleeding. It is important, however, to bear in mind a list of other possible causes of this symptom.

General causes

Bleeding diatheses (rare).

Local causes

- Haemorrhoids.
- Anal fissure.
- Tumours of the colon and rectum:
  - Benign.
  - Malignant.

Ellis and Calne's Lecture Notes in General Surgery, Fourteenth Edition.
Edited by Christopher Watson and Justin Davies.
© 2023 John Wiley & Sons Ltd. Published 2023 by John Wiley & Sons Ltd.
Companion website: www.wiley.com/go/Watson/GeneralSurgery14

- Diverticular disease.
- Ulcerative colitis.
- Infective colitis.
- Ischaemic colitis.
- Trauma.
- Angiodysplasia of the colon.
- Rarely, massive haemorrhage from higher up the alimentary canal – even a bleeding duodenal ulcer, may produce bright red blood per anum instead of the usual melaena, although such cases are commonly accompanied by haematemesis.

Haemorrhoids

Functional anatomy

Continence is mainly a function of the anal sphincters but also partly a consequence of the anal cushions. The anal cushions comprise highly vascular tissue lining the anal canal, with a rich blood supply from the rectal arteries, which anastomose with the draining veins both through capillaries and through direct arteriovenous shunts. The draining veins form saccules, commonly just below the dentate line, which then drain via the superior rectal vein. The venous saccules are supported by smooth muscle to form the cushions. Apposition of these subepithelial vascular cushions makes some contribution to continence of flatus and liquid.

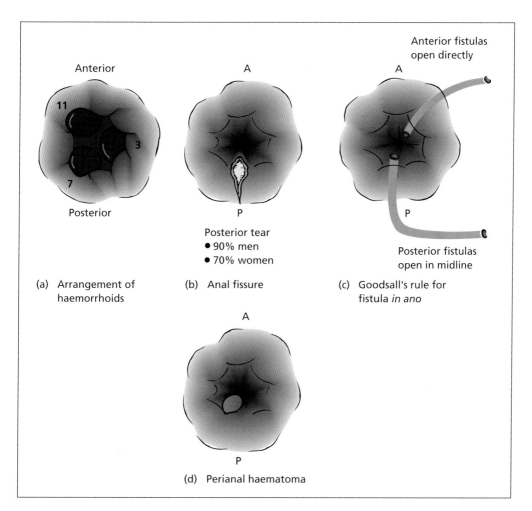

Anterior

A

A

11

3

7

Posterior

Posterior tear
● 90% men
● 70% women

Anterior fistulas
open directly

P

P

Posterior fistulas
open in midline

(a) Arrangement of
haemorrhoids

(b) Anal fissure

(c) Goodsall's rule for
fistula *in ano*

A

P

(d) Perianal haematoma

Figure 28.1 Distribution of different conditions around the anal canal.

Table 28.1 Rectal bleeding

	Blood	Pain
Haemorrhoids	Bright red blood on paper and in the toilet bowl. May prolapse.	Painless, unless prolapsed and/or thrombosed.
Fissure	Bright red blood on paper and outside of stool.	Painful; pain during and lasting long after passing stool.
Colon and rectal cancer	Blood often mixed in with stool, especially if proximal tumour.	Usually painless, unless distally placed in rectum or in anal canal, when causes tenesmus.
Diverticular disease	Large volume of blood in the pan.	Painless.
Ulcerative colitis	Blood and mucus mixed with loose, frequent stool.	Painless, unless co-existent fissure.

Classification

Haemorrhoids (or piles; the words are synonymous) may be classified according to their relationship to the anal orifice into internal, external and interoexternal. Internal haemorrhoids are congested vascular cushions with dilated venous components draining into the superior rectal veins. External haemorrhoids is a term that covers multiple different pathologies including perianal haematoma ('thrombosed external pile'), the 'sentinel pile' of anal fissure and anal skin tags. Strictly speaking, internal piles that prolapse should be termed 'interoexternal haemorrhoids', but this term is seldom used in clinical practice. In this chapter, the terms 'external' and 'interoexternal' haemorrhoids will not be used further.

Pathology

Internal haemorrhoids are abnormal anal cushions, usually congested as a result of straining at stool and/or pregnancy, and traumatized by the passage of hard stool. The anal cushions are particularly prominent in pregnancy owing to the venous congestion caused by the large gravid uterus and the laxity of the supporting tissues caused by the influence of progesterone. With the patient in the lithotomy position, the usual arrangement is that three major haemorrhoids occur at 3, 7 and 11 o'clock.

Grading haemorrhoids

- *First-degree haemorrhoids* are confined to the anal canal – they bleed but do not prolapse.
- *Second-degree haemorrhoids* prolapse on defaecation, then reduce spontaneously.
- *Third-degree haemorrhoids* prolapse outside the anal margin on defaecation; they need to be manually pushed back inside by the patient.
- *Fourth-degree haemorrhoids* remain prolapsed outside the anal margin at all times.

Predisposing factors

Most haemorrhoids are idiopathic, but they may be precipitated or aggravated by factors that produce congestion of the superior rectal veins. These include compression by any pelvic tumour (of which the most common is the pregnant uterus), lots of regular heavy lifting, chronic constipation and straining to pass a stool.

Occasionally, anorectal varices, similar in appearance to oesophageal varices, co-exist with haemorrhoids in patients with portal hypertension since the anorectal area is the site of a portosystemic anastomosis between the superior and inferior rectal veins (see Chapter 34).

Clinical features

Rectal bleeding is almost invariable; this is bright red and usually occurs at defaecation. In the case of first-degree haemorrhoids, this is the only symptom. Some haemorrhoids prolapse and may produce a mucus discharge and itching (pruritus ani). The prolapsed haemorrhoids may result in soiling.

Note that pain is not a feature of internal haemorrhoids except when these undergo thrombosis (see later in this chapter). When a patient complains of 'an attack of piles', it often means that some acute painful condition has developed at the anal margin. The most common and dramatic is strangulation of prolapsing haemorrhoids leading to thrombosis; apart from this, acute pain may be due to the following:

- Anal fissure.
- Perianal haematoma.
- Perianal or ischioanal abscess.
- Tumour of the anal margin.
- Proctalgia fugax: benign episodic, short-lived pain felt up inside the rectum.

Every patient presenting with a history suggestive of internal haemorrhoids should be considered for the following examinations:

1 *Examination of the abdomen* to exclude palpable lesions of the colon or aggravating factors for haemorrhoids, for example an enlarged liver or a pelvic mass, including the pregnant uterus.
2 *Rectal examination.* Internal haemorrhoids are not palpable but prolapsing haemorrhoids may be immediately obvious on inspection. The presence of prolapsing haemorrhoids does not exclude a lesion higher in the bowel. Rectal examination allows anal abscess, fissure and tumour to be excluded.
3 *Proctoscopy*, which will visualize the internal haemorrhoids.
4 *Sigmoidoscopy (rigid or flexible)* is performed to eliminate a lesion higher in the rectum – proctitis, polyp or carcinoma. Contrary to its name, the rigid sigmoidoscope does not afford a view of the

sigmoid colon, hence rigid sigmoidoscopy is more correctly termed 'rectoscopy'.

5 *Colonoscopy* is carried out when symptoms such as a change in bowel habit or blood mixed in with the faeces point to a more serious condition than internal haemorrhoids. Computed tomography (CT) colonography is carried out when colonoscopy is not readily available or appropriate.

Complications

- *Iron deficiency anaemia*: following severe or continued bleeding. This is uncommon, and a more serious cause of anaemia (colorectal or oesophagogastric cancer) should be considered in most cases.
- *Thrombosis*: this occurs when prolapsing haemorrhoids are gripped by the anal sphincter ('strangulated piles'). The venous return is occluded and thrombosis of the haemorrhoid occurs. The prolapsed haemorrhoids are swollen often to the size of large plums, purplish-black and tense, and are accompanied by considerable pain and distress. Suppuration or ulceration may occur. After 2–3 weeks, the thrombosed tissue become fibrosed, often with spontaneous cure. Haemorrhoidectomy can be considered acutely, especially if there is any concern for necrosis, but often surgery can be avoided in the acute phase and subsequent treatment options, including none, considered with the patient.

Treatment

Before commencing treatment, it is essential to exclude either any predisposing cause or an associated and more important lesion, such as carcinoma of the rectum.

Conservative management

Ideally, the patient should avoid straining at stool, and spending too long sat on the toilet. A bulk laxative, together with advice on an adequate fluid and fibre intake, are often required.

Sclerotherapy

This is suitable for some first-degree haemorrhoids; 2–3 mL of 5% phenol in almond oil is injected above each haemorrhoid as a sclerosing submucosal perivenous injection. (The phenol sterilizes the oil, which is the main sclerosant.) Because the injection is placed high in the anal canal/distal rectum above the dentate line, it is painless. One or more repeat injections may be required at intervals. This is now most commonly used in patients taking medication that predisposes to bleeding (e.g. warfarin, novel oral anticoagulants (NOACs)), as other interventions are likely to be contraindicated in this setting.

Suction banding

Application of a small rubber band to areas of protruding mucosa results in strangulation of the mucosa, which falls away after a few days. It can be successfully applied to first-, second- and third-degree haemorrhoids, but care must be taken to position the bands above the dentate line in order to avoid significant pain.

Surgery

Surgery is generally considered for recurrent third-degree and for fourth-degree haemorrhoids. There are several options that can be considered:

1 *Haemorrhoidectomy* involves excising the haemorrhoids after first ligating the vascular pedicle. This has the lowest recurrence rate of all operative interventions, but is very painful for a week or two afterwards.
2 *Haemorrhoidal artery ligation (HALO)* involves using a Doppler probe to identify the haemorrhoidal arteries which are then ligated above the dentate line. This may be combined with plication of the prolapsing mucosa if causing symptoms.
3 *Stapled haemorrhoidopexy* uses a circular stapling device to excise a band of mucous membrane above the dentate line. It also interrupts the blood supply to the haemorrhoids. This is less commonly considered now due to the very small risk of serious septic complications.

Thrombosed strangulated haemorrhoids

Conservative management is generally instituted for these. The patient may require several days of rest at home. Analgesia, often in combination with stool softeners, is given for the pain, which is also eased by local cold compresses. Often the thrombosed haemorrhoids fibrose completely with spontaneous cure. Acute haemorrhoidectomy can generally be avoided, unless there is a suggestion of tissue necrosis.

Specific complications of haemorrhoid surgery

Acute retention of urine

This is the result of acute anal discomfort postoperatively.

Postoperative haemorrhage

This may be reactionary, usually on the night of the operation, or secondary, on about the seventh or eighth day. The bleeding may not be apparent externally, as the source of haemorrhage may be above the anal sphincter, with the blood filling the large bowel with only a little escaping to the exterior.

General treatment comprises blood transfusion if haemorrhage is severe as evidenced by the general appearance of the patient and the presence of tachycardia and hypotension.

Local treatment is carried out under general anaesthetic in the operating theatre. The blood is washed out of the rectum with warm saline. Occasionally, in reactionary haemorrhage, a bleeding point is seen and can be suture-ligated. More often, there is a general oozing from the operation field and the anal canal requires packing with gauze and removal 24 hours later.

Anal stenosis

This only occurs when excessive amounts of mucosa and skin are excised at the time of a haemorrhoidectomy. It is important to leave a bridge of epithelium between each excised haemorrhoid.

Anal Incontinence

This is an uncommon complication of haemorrhoidectomy, and is generally incontinence of gas. Patient selection is paramount, with a history of previous anal surgery, significant obstetric history and pre-existing continence being carefully considered as part of the consent and shared decision-making process with the patient.

Perianal haematoma

This lesion, which is also sometimes incorrectly termed a 'thrombosed external pile', is produced by thrombosis within the subcutaneous tissue of the perianal skin. Unlike internal haemorrhoids, it is covered by squamous epithelium supplied by somatic nerves and is, therefore, initially very painful when it occurs. The onset is acute, often after straining at stool or after heavy lifting, with sudden pain and the appearance of a lump at the anal verge. Local examination shows a tense, smooth, dark-blue, cherry-sized lump at the anal margin.

Untreated, this perianal haematoma either subsides over a few days, eventually leaving a fibrous anal skin tag, or ruptures, discharging some clotted blood.

Treatment

In the acute phase, immediate relief is produced by evacuating the haematoma through a small incision, conveniently performed under local anaesthetic. This is generally most effective when performed within 24 hours of symptom onset. If the patient is seen when the haematoma is already discharging or becoming absorbed, hot baths may help symptoms and reassurance given that the symptoms will resolve over several weeks.

Anal fissure

An anal fissure is a tear in the anal canal, which most commonly follows the passage of a hard stool, but sometimes follows a prolonged bout of diarrhoea. The site is usually posterior in the midline (90% of men, 70% of women), occasionally anteriorly in the midline and rarely multiple. The posterior position of the majority of fissures has traditionally been explained by the anatomical arrangement of the external anal sphincter; its superficial fibres pass forward to the anal canal from the coccyx, leaving a relatively unsupported V posteriorly. However, mucosal tears are probably quite common and while most heal spontaneously, those occurring posteriorly (or anteriorly) are slow to heal because of the relatively poor blood supply to the anal mucosa in the midline. Anterior fissures in women may be associated with weakening of the pelvic floor following tears at childbirth. Multiple fissures may be a presenting feature of perianal Crohn's disease[1].

[1] Burrill Bernard Crohn (1884–1983), Gastroenterologist, Mount Sinai Hospital, New York, USA. The disease was first described by Morgagni (1682–1771).

Clinical features

Acute anal pain is characteristic. It is stinging in nature and lasts for a while after the passage of stool, sometimes several hours. Fissure is the most common cause of pain at the anal verge (see earlier in this chapter). There is often slight bleeding and, because of the pain, the patient is usually constipated. On examination, the anal sphincter is in spasm, and there may be a 'sentinel pile' protruding from the anus, which represents the torn tag of anal epithelium. The fissure can usually be seen by gently pulling open the anal verge. It may be impossible to do a rectal examination without anaesthetic; the fissure may then be evident as a tear in the anal canal.

Treatment

Early small acute anal fissures may heal spontaneously. A local anaesthetic ointment together with a stool softener may give relief. Application of 0.4% glyceryl trinitrate (GTN) or 2% diltiazem ointment relaxes the anal sphincter, allowing the torn epithelium to heal; these are indicated for chronic fissures, i.e. it has been present for at least six weeks.

Injection of botulinum A toxin into the anal sphincter to create a chemical sphincterotomy appears to be at least as effective as GTN or diltiazem ointment in facilitating fissure healing, works faster but with a small incidence of transient incontinence to gas afterwards. The effects are more sustained than topical creams, and last around 12 weeks.

Intractable cases usually respond to dividing the internal sphincter submucosally (lateral internal anal sphincterotomy) under general anaesthetic. It is important to take a detailed history of continence and to assess the anal tone prior to performing a sphincterotomy, as incontinence may result, particularly in patients who have suffered previous obstetric injury. Anal stretch, once a common treatment of fissures, has been abandoned because of the damage it caused to the sphincter with associated incontinence, and should no longer be performed.

A chronic recurring anal fissure may require excision and histological analysis to rule out malignancy.

Anorectal abscesses

Classification (Figure 28.2)

- *Perianal*: likely resulting from infection of a hair follicle, a sebaceous gland or perianal haematoma. These may be submucosal or subcutaneous.
- *Intersphincteric*: arising from between the internal and external anal sphincter muscles.
- *Ischioanal*: from infection of an anal gland leading from the anal canal into the submucosa and intersphincteric space, and then traversing the external

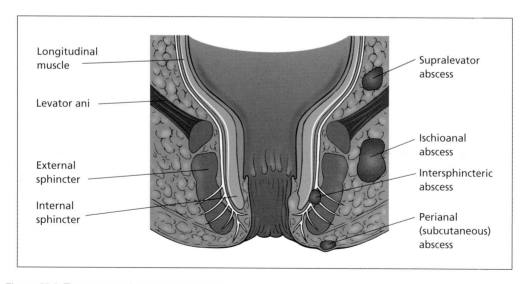

Figure 28.2 The anatomy of anorectal abscesses.

anal sphincter to spread to the ischioanal fossa. The abscess may occasionally form a track like a horseshoe behind the rectum to the opposite ischioanal fossa.

- *Supralevator*: most commonly due to downward extension from a pelvic source (e.g. diverticular abscess) although this is a rare finding.

Treatment

Early surgical drainage.

Anal fistula

Definitions

- A *fistula* is an abnormal communication between two epithelial surfaces, for example between a hollow viscus and the surface of the body or between two hollow viscera.
- A *sinus* is a granulating track leading from a source of infection to an epithelial surface.

Aetiology

The term 'anal fistula' or 'fistula in ano' is applied to fistulas in relation to the anal canal. The majority result from an initial abscess likely forming in one of the anal glands that pass from the intersphincteric space of the anal canal to open within its lumen. Anal fistulas are most commonly idiopathic, but they may also be associated with Crohn's disease and carcinoma of the anorectum (rarely, also, tuberculosis).

Anatomical classification (Figure 28.3)

Anal fistulas are classified according to their position and relation to the internal and external anal sphincters.

- Submucosal/subcutaneous.
- Intersphincteric.
- Transsphincteric.
- Suprasphincteric.
- Extrasphincteric.

Subcutaneous or submucosal fistulas are superficial tracks resulting from rupture, respectively, of subcutaneous and submucosal abscesses. They sometimes form from a partially healed anal fissure. Intersphincteric fistulas are examples of *low anal fistulas*, in which the track is below the dentate line; they constitute the majority of anal fistulas. Transsphincteric fistulas differ in their penetration through the external sphincter, and most are at a low level with the track passing through the subcutaneous part of the sphincter, although some may be classified as high if they traverse the majority of

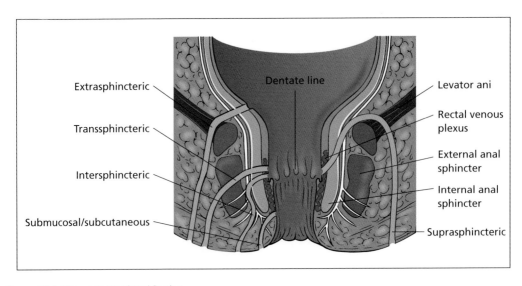

Figure 28.3 The anatomy of anal fistulas.

the external anal sphincter. Suprasphincteric fistulas pass via the intersphincteric space to open into the anus above the puborectalis and are *high anal fistulas*. Extrasphincteric fistulas, fortunately rare, extend through the levator ani to open above the anorectal junction, are a very challenging form of high anal fistula.

Fistulas with external openings posterior to the meridian in the lithotomy position usually open in the midline of the anus, whereas those with anterior external openings usually open directly into the anus – Goodsall's law[2] (see Figure 28.1); however, this rule is not absolute.

Clinical features

There is usually a story of an initial perianal abscess, which discharges or requires surgical drainage. Following this, there are recurrent episodes of perianal infection with persistent discharge of pus. Examination reveals the external opening of a fistula. The internal opening may be felt per rectum, but probing of the track is painful and should generally be deferred until the patient is under anaesthesia. Accurate assessment of the extent of the fistula track, in particular its relation to the anal sphincter, is crucial. Where doubt exists, and certainly when the fistula is recurrent, magnetic resonance imaging (MRI) can demonstrate the anatomy of a fistula very clearly, with endoanal ultrasound also useful.

Treatment

Superficial and low anal fistulas may be laid open and allowed to heal by secondary intention. When no sphincter needs to be divided, there is no loss of anal continence. If a few fibres of internal sphincter might need to be divided, then careful assessment of preoperative continence, prior anal surgery and an accurate obstetric history are required, along with a fully informed consent process as there will be a small risk of permanent flatus incontinence and staining of underwear. Careful clinical assessment, often augmented with information from the MRI scan, is, therefore, important in this shared decision-making process, and the final decision lies with the patient.

High fistulas (suprasphincteric and transsphincteric): sphincter-conserving procedures may be considered. These include injection with fibrin glue, placement of a bioprosthetic 'fistula plug' that is passed along the track or use of an 'over the scope' clip to close the internal opening. If these sphincter-preserving treatments fail, a long-term loose draining seton may be required, comprising a non-absorbable strong suture (e.g. Ethibond), passed through the track and left in place. The seton may need to be replaced every 5 years or so. Advancement flaps may be considered, but do have potential implications for continence, and an alternative approach is ligation of the intersphincteric tract (LIFT). Newer sphincter-preserving treatments include use of laser technology and also video-assisted fistula surgery, but longer-term outcome data are awaited.

Recurrent fistulas that are associated with Crohn's disease may respond to long-term antibiotics and additional medical treatment with an anti-tumour necrosis factor antibody such as infliximab, in addition to immunosuppressive therapy with azathioprine, in combination with drainage of any abscess and loose draining seton(s) placement. The role of stem cells in the treatment of Crohn's disease-related anal fistulas is the subject of ongoing research.

Stricture of the anal canal

Classification

- *Congenital*.
- *Iatrogenic*, particularly postoperative, after too radical excision of the skin and mucosa in haemorrhoidectomy.
- *Inflammatory*: lymphogranuloma inguinale (mostly female), Crohn's disease.
- *Post-radiotherapy*.
- *Malignant tumour*.

Treatment

Depends on the underlying pathology and may call for repeated dilation, plastic surgery reconstruction, defunctioning colostomy or, in the case of malignant disease, excision of the anorectum.

---

[2] David Goodsall (1843–1906), Surgeon, St Mark's Hospital, London, UK.

Prolapse of the rectum

This may be partial or complete.

- *Partial (mucosal) prolapse* is confined to the mucosa, which prolapses 2–5 cm from the anal verge. Palpation of the prolapse between the finger and thumb reveals that there is no muscular wall within it. It may occur in infants who are usually otherwise perfectly healthy. Treatment of these infants requires nothing more than reassurance of the parents that the condition is self-limiting. In adults, it usually accompanies prolapsing haemorrhoids or sphincter incompetence, and may present with pruritus ani and mucus discharge.
- *Full-thickness prolapse* involves all layers of the rectal wall. It most commonly occurs in elderly, multiparous women. Apart from the discomfort of the prolapse, there is associated incontinence owing to the stretching of the sphincter muscles and mucus discharge from the prolapsed mucosal surface.

Treatment

Treatment of mucosal prolapse in adults comprises excision of the redundant mucosa, or suction banding (see earlier in this chapter). In children, as already mentioned, self-cure without active treatment is the fortunate rule.

Repair of a full-thickness rectal prolapse may be performed by either a transabdominal or transperineal approach, the former being preferred in younger and fitter patients, the latter in more elderly and co-morbid patients.

Transabdominal rectopexy, whereby the mobilized rectum is secured to the presacral fascia, relies on the resultant brisk fibrous reaction to fix the rectum to the pelvic tissues. Mesh is less commonly used now to facilitate this apposition due to potential mesh-related complications such as erosion. The classic perineal approach was anal encirclement with a Thiersch wire,[3] in which a wire or nylon suture is passed around the anal orifice to narrow it and keep the prolapse reduced. This was complicated by obstruction and erosion of the wire and has largely fallen from favour. Today, a less traumatic approach involves excision of a sleeve of prolapsing rectal mucosa and pleating of the underlying muscle to form a doughnut-like ring (Delorme's procedure[4]), which holds the rectum in the pelvis rather as a ring pessary may control vaginal prolapse. An alternative is the Altemeier[5] perineal proctosigmoidectomy, in which a full-thickness resection of prolapsing rectum with coloanal anastomosis is performed.

Pruritus ani

There are four principal causes of pruritus ani.

1 *Local causes within the anus or rectum.* Any factor that causes moisture of the anal skin, for example poor anal hygiene, excessive sweating, leakage of mucus from haemorrhoids, proctitis, colitis, anal fistula, anorectal neoplasm or threadworms.
2 *Skin diseases*: psoriasis, scabies, pediculosis, fungal infections, such as *Candida albicans*.
3 *General diseases* associated with pruritus: diabetes mellitus, Hodgkin's disease, obstructive jaundice.
4 *Idiopathic:* Often the original cause has disappeared but the pruritus persists because of continued scratching and trauma of the anal region by the patient.

Treatment

Directed to the underlying cause. The idiopathic group often responds dramatically to attention to local hygiene, stopping the use of topical treatments and dietary changes.

Faecal incontinence

This is characterized by lack of anal control to flatus, liquid and/or solid stool, and is more common with increasing age. Other risk factors include vaginal delivery, prior anal surgery and cauda equina syndrome. The incontinence may be *urge* or *passive* in nature.

---

[3] Karl Thiersch (1822–1895), Professor of Surgery, Erlangen then Leipzig, Germany. He also devised the split skin graft.

[4] Edmond Delorme (1843–1929), Chief of Surgery in the French Army.

[5] William Arthur Altemeier (1910–1983), Professor of Surgery, Cincinnati, Ohio.

Treatment

This is most commonly non-operative, and includes measures to firm the stool and reduce gas production, such as a low fibre diet and regular loperamide, and measures to improve the strength and function of the sphincter complex (sphincter strengthening exercises and biofeedback therapy). In addition, use of suppositories, enemas and rectal irrigation can help to keep the rectum empty and reduce leakage; input from specialist nurse practitioners is valuable in this regard.

Surgery is uncommonly indicated, and only when non-operative measures have been exhausted and after discussion by a pelvic floor multidisciplinary team. Surgical approaches include external anal sphincter repair (anal sphincteroplasty), radiofrequency therapy and sacral nerve stimulation/neuromodulation. A colostomy is generally only considered when all other appropriate treatment options have not been successful.

Tumours

Pathology

Benign

- Adenoma.
- Papilloma.
- Lipoma.
- Endometrioma.

Malignant

1 *Primary*:
   A Adenocarcinoma.
   B Anal squamous cell carcinoma.
   C Melanoma.
   D Neuroendocrine tumour.
   E Lymphoma.
2 *Secondary*: invasion from prostate, uterus or pelvic peritoneal deposits.

Rectal polyps

Rectal polyps may be classified according to histology:

1 *Hyperplastic*: these are small, 2–3 mm, sessile lesions. Often multiple and always benign, this is an incidental finding on sigmoidoscopy.
2 *Adenomatous polyp*: there are three histological types of benign adenomatous polyp, all of which may undergo malignant change. Multiple polyps are present in familial adenomatous polyposis (see Chapter 27):
   a Tubular adenoma – usually small and rounded, the most common type of adenomatous polyp; the epithelium is arranged in tubular fashion.
   b Villous adenoma: appears like an anemone with many fronds growing from its base on the rectal wall. May grow very large, and produce large amounts of mucus. Greatest potential for malignant change, so should be completely removed.
   c Tubulovillous adenoma; histology that has an element of both.
3 *Hamartomatous*, for example the juvenile polyp; a developmental malformation which presents in children and adolescents and which looks like a cherry on a stalk. It is always benign, presents with bleeding and may prolapse during defaecation.
4 *Inflammatory (pseudopolyp)*: associated with colitis; is not a true polyp but is oedematous mucosa against a background of ulcerated, denuded bowel wall.

Diagnosis is by histological analysis after removal. Because of the propensity for malignant change of adenomatous polyps, particularly villous adenomas, these should always be excised in full to ensure that no area of malignant change is missed. Although very small polyps may be excised in the clinic, most polyps require endoscopic excision. Surgical excision may still be required for very large rectal polyps, and this can usually be performed via a minimally invasive, transanal approach.

Carcinoma of the rectum

Pathology

The sexes are equally affected. It occurs in any age group from the twenties onwards, but is particularly common in the age range of 50–70 years. There is a recent increase in the incidence of younger onset of rectal cancer, with the precise reasons remaining unclear. Carcinoma of the rectum accounts for approximately one-third of all tumours of the large intestine. Predisposing factors (as with carcinoma of the colon) are pre-existing adenomas, familial adenomatous polyposis and inflammatory bowel disease (both ulcerative and Crohn's colitis).

Macroscopic appearance

The tumours may be classified as follows:

- Papillomatous.
- Ulcerating (most common).
- Annular.
- Stenosing (more commonly at rectosigmoid junction).

Microscopic appearance

Rectal carcinomas are adenocarcinomas. At the anal verge and canal, anal squamous cell carcinoma may occur, but a malignant tumour protruding from the rectum through the anal canal is more likely to be an adenocarcinoma of the rectum invading the anal canal. True squamous cell carcinoma of the rectum is rare.

Spread

1 *Local*:
   a Circumferentially around the lumen of the bowel.
   b Invasion through the muscular wall.
   c Penetration into adjacent organs, for example prostate, bladder, vagina, uterus, sacrum, sacral plexus, ureters and lateral pelvic side wall.
2 *Lymphatic*: to regional lymph nodes along the inferior mesenteric vessels. At a later stage, there is invasion of the lateral pelvic side wall and external iliac lymph nodes and of the inguinal (groin) lymph nodes for very low tumours involving the anal canal and involvement of the supraclavicular nodes via the thoracic duct.
3 *Blood*: via the superior rectal venous plexus, thence via the portal vein to the liver and lungs.
4 *Nerves*: Perineural invasion is the process of neoplastic invasion of nerves.
5 *Transcoelomic*: seeding of the peritoneal cavity, which is more common in higher rectal cancers above the peritoneal reflection.

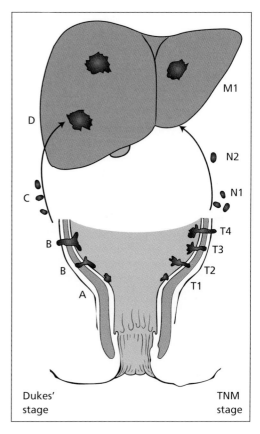

Figure 28.4 Staging of rectal cancer by modified Dukes' and TNM classifications. Dukes' A, confined to the bowel wall; B, penetrating the wall; C, involving regional lymph nodes; D, distant spread.

Staging

The extent of spread of rectal tumours was traditionally classified by Dukes[6] and later modified to include a stage for metastatic disease (Figure 28.4).

A The tumour is confined to the mucosa and submucosa.
B There is invasion of the muscle wall.
C The regional lymph nodes are involved.
D Distant spread has occurred, for example to the liver or invasion into the bladder.

[6] Cuthbert Esquire Dukes (1890–1977), Pathologist, St Mark's Hospital, London, UK.

More recently, colonic and rectal cancers have been staged using the TNM system (see Chapter 7), and a simplified version of this is shown below:

T1   The tumour is confined to submucosa.

T2   The tumour invades the muscle wall.

T3   The tumour invades through the muscle wall into the serosa or pericolic/perirectal tissue.

T4   The tumour invades other organs or has grown into the surface of the visceral peritoneum.

N0   No regional lymph node involvement.

N1   Tumour involves one to three lymph nodes in pericolic or perirectal tissue.

N2   Tumour involves more than three lymph nodes in pericolic or perirectal tissue.

M0   No distant metastasis.

M1   Distant metastasis.

This leads to stages of disease from one to four according to how far the tumour has spread through the bowel wall (stages 1 and 2), to the draining lymph nodes (stage 3) or if there is metastatic (distant) spread (stage 4).

Prognosis

Depends largely on the stage of progression of the tumour and its histological degree of differentiation (see Chapter 7). The more advanced its spread and the more poorly differentiated its cells, the worse the prognosis.

Clinical features

The patient may present with:

- Local disturbances owing to the presence of the tumour in the rectum.
- Manifestations of secondary deposits (metastases).
- The general effects of malignant disease.

Effects of secondary deposits and malignant disease are similar to those of carcinoma of the colon (see Chapter 27) with the addition that, rarely, carcinoma of the low rectum may spread to the inguinal lymph nodes as a late phenomenon. With carcinoma at the anal verge, this more commonly occurs.

Local symptoms

Local symptoms include bowel disturbance (constipation and/or diarrhoea occur in 80% of cases) and bleeding, which is almost invariable and is the presenting complaint in about 60% of patients. There may also be mucus discharge, rectal pain and tenesmus.

Examination

Abdominal palpation is often normal in early cases, but careful attention must be paid to the detection of hepatomegaly, ascites or abdominal distension. Other general features that may be detected in more advanced cases are enlarged supraclavicular nodes, enlarged inguinal nodes, hepatomegaly or jaundice. Rectal examination reveals the tumour in many cases.

Special investigations

- *Sigmoidoscopy* enables the great majority of tumours to be seen and a biopsy to be taken.
- *Colonoscopy* is indicated to rule out synchronous tumours (5% of tumours in the large bowel are multiple) or if there is ulcerative colitis or familial polyposis. CT colonography is indicated when colonoscopy is not readily available.
- *CT* of the chest, abdomen and pelvis is performed for staging in order to detect metastatic spread.
- *Magnetic resonance (MR) imaging* of the pelvis is necessary for preoperative staging of the tumour and for planning appropriate treatment, including preoperative radiotherapy and chemotherapy, as well as subsequent surgery.

Differential diagnosis of a rectal cancer

Differential diagnosis of a palpable malignant tumour in the rectum must be made from the following:

- Benign tumours.
- Carcinoma of the sigmoid colon prolapsing into the pouch of Douglas and felt through the rectal wall.
- Secondary deposits (metastases) in the pelvis.
- Ovarian or uterine tumours.
- Extension from carcinoma of the prostate or cervix.
- Endometriosis.
- Lymphogranuloma inguinale.
- The rare malignant tumours of the rectum (see earlier in this chapter).
- Faeces (these give the classic physical sign of indentation).

It may be possible to mistake the normal cervix for a palpable tumour, and note should be made of the presence of a ring pessary or tampon in the vagina, which are readily felt per rectum.

Treatment

Surgery

This may be performed by a traditional open approach (laparotomy), or by minimally invasive surgery (laparoscopic or robotic). The type of surgery performed generally depends upon the distance of the tumour from the dentate line, along with its local staging evident on MRI scan (Figure 28.5).

- *Upper third tumours* can be resected with restorative anastomosis between the colon and the lower rectum (anterior resection).
- *Lower third tumours*, less than 5 cm from the anal verge and adjacent to the dentate line, may require treatment by abdominoperineal excision of the rectum, with a permanent end colostomy. A low anastomosis can still be possible in carefully selected cases.
- *Mid-third rectal tumours* can usually be treated by low anterior resection, provided satisfactory distal clearance can be obtained. This can be a challenging procedure, given the constraints of a deep and narrow pelvis. A temporary covering loop ileostomy is often used in order to protect

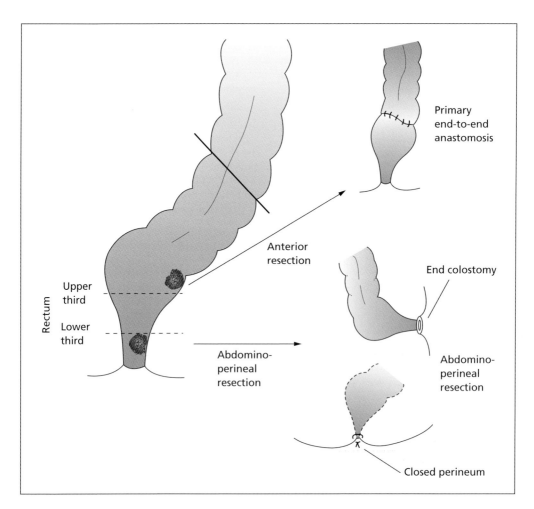

Figure 28.5 Surgical procedures for carcinoma of rectum.

the anastomosis, with subsequent closure of the stoma some months later.

Neoadjuvant therapy

Preoperative radiotherapy reduces the risk of local recurrence, and is commonly combined with chemotherapy (5-fluorouracil or capecitabine). Radiotherapy is typically delivered in the form of external beam, although brachytherapy (internal radiotherapy) may be delivered from a source placed in the rectum in some limited circumstances.

There is increasing evidence that some rectal cancers completely respond to chemoradiotherapy and are no longer clinically evident after this treatment (complete clinical response), potentially negating the need for subsequent surgical resection. National registries are assessing whether this will become an appropriate routine treatment option in the future.

Surveillance

After potentially curative treatment, ongoing surveillance will be advised, usually with annual CT scans and tumour marker (carcinoembryonic antigen – CEA) blood test to detect locally recurrent or metastatic disease, and colonoscopy at intervals to detect and remove further benign adenomas in order to prevent metachronous bowel cancer.

Palliative procedures

Even if there are metastases not amenable to potentially curative treatment, palliation may still be best achieved by excision of the primary tumour. A colostomy may be necessary for intestinal obstruction, but this does not relieve the bleeding, mucus discharge and sacral pain. In cases where surgery is not appropriate, radiotherapy is the palliative treatment option of choice for local symptoms such as bleeding, and palliative chemotherapy may be considered if there is incurable metastatic disease.

Anal cancer

Anal cancer is rare, affecting around 1 500 people a year in the UK. It is more common in women and the elderly, and its incidence is increasing. It is most commonly anal squamous cell carcinoma, and risk factors include:

- *Human papilloma virus*: around 90% of cases are linked to HPV infection, particular to the type 16 virus.
- *Genital warts and cervical cancer*, both conditions which share the HPV aetiology.
- *Immunosuppression*, whether for organ transplantation or as a consequence of disease (e.g. human immunodeficiency virus [HIV]).

Pathology

The anal canal is lined by squamous epithelium and anal carcinomas are usually squamous cell carcinomas and manifest as an ulcer near the anal verge. Rarely, adenocarcinoma, arising from the anal glands, basal cell carcinoma and melanoma may occur in this area.

Anal carcinomas spread to the inguinal lymph nodes as well as those within the pelvis; the anal canal should always be inspected in patients presenting with unexplained inguinal lymphadenopathy.

Clinical features

Anal cancers present with the passage of mucus or blood (similar to rectal cancer), anal pain, a lump at the anal verge and faecal incontinence. They are usually best examined under general anaesthetic when a biopsy can also be taken.

Special investigations

- *MRI imaging* to assess local invasion and *CT scan* to assess for distant spread.

Treatment

Abnormal anal lesions should be excised for histological analysis. High-grade squamous intraepithelial lesions (HSIL) and their low-grade equivalent (LSIL) may subsequently develop into malignancy and subsequent surveillance is required. These were previously known as anal intraepithelial neoplasia (AIN).

Anal squamous cell cancers less than 2 cm in size (T1) can be treated by local excision, preserving the anal sphincter. Larger tumours and those with confirmed or suspected lymph node involvement are treated by a combination of radiotherapy and chemotherapy. If chemoradiotherapy fails to control the disease, a salvage abdominoperineal resection is performed. Anal adenocarcinomas are treated in the same manner as rectal carcinomas.

Overall, about 70% of patients will be alive 5 years after diagnosis and treatment.

Additional resources

29

The acute abdomen

Constantinos Simillis

Learning objective

✓ To know the causes and assessment of the acute abdomen, and the general principles of treatment.

Aetiology

An acute abdomen refers to the rapid onset of severe abdominal pain requiring early diagnosis and treatment. There are many causes for an acute abdomen and the clinician should be able to consider all possible causes, investigate these accordingly, and provide the appropriate treatment urgently.

Diagnosis is difficult due to the numerous potential causes. The causes of an acute abdomen may usefully be considered in terms of the individual organs and their pathology (see Box 29.1)

Clinical assessment

A detailed history is invaluable in order to guide the clinician through the extensive list of differential diagnoses to the appropriate diagnosis and treatment. Meticulous physical examination is also important. For example, the location of abdominal tenderness may point towards the underlying diagnosis. Examination of the hernial orifices for incarcerated hernias and the scrotum for testicular torsion are particularly important areas that are often missed. Scars from previous surgical procedures may suggest postoperative complications or adhesions causing obstruction.

Ellis and Calne's Lecture Notes in General Surgery, Fourteenth Edition. Edited by Christopher Watson and Justin Davies.
© 2023 John Wiley & Sons Ltd. Published 2023 by John Wiley & Sons Ltd.
Companion website: www.wiley.com/go/Watson/GeneralSurgery14

The patient's temperature, heart rate, respiratory rate, oxygen saturation, blood pressure and urinary output are important to assess the extent of sepsis or shock, which may necessitate rapid escalation of treatment.

Special investigations

- *Full blood count:* to look for anaemia, leucocytosis, neutropenia, thrombocytosis and thrombocytopaenia.
- *Urea and electrolytes:* to identify acute kidney injury or electrolyte abnormalities. Knowledge of kidney function allows renal-dose adjustment of drugs and selection of appropriate antibiotics.
- *Liver function tests:* alanine transaminase (ALT) and aspartate transaminase (AST) as markers of hepatocellular injury, alkaline phosphatase (ALP) and bilirubin as a marker of biliary sepsis e.g. cholangitis, cholecystitis.
- *Serum amylase and lipase:* to identify acute pancreatitis.
- *C-reactive protein (CRP):* a marker of infection or inflammation.
- *Clotting screen:* to identify underlying bleeding risk, and important in anticoagulated patients in case of surgery.
- *Group and Save:* to identify the patient's blood group and save serum for future crossmatch, or crossmatch some blood immediately in readiness for emergency surgery.

Box 29.1 Causes of an acute abdomen

Oesophagus, stomach and duodenum

- Gastroesophageal reflux or heartburn.
- Gastritis or duodenitis.
- Peptic ulcer or peptic ulcer perforation.
- Perforated oesophagus.

Intestine

- Acute appendicitis.
- Bowel ischaemia.
- Diverticulitis with or without complications, e.g. perforation, abscess, obstruction.
- Meckel's diverticulitis.
- Inflammatory bowel disease e.g. Crohn's disease, ulcerative colitis.
- Small bowel obstruction e.g. due to adhesions, hernia.
- Large bowel obstruction e.g. due to neoplasm, sigmoid volvulus.
- Bowel volvulus e.g. sigmoid volvulus, caecal volvulus.
- Irritable bowel syndrome.
- Constipation.

Liver, biliary tree and pancreas

- Biliary colic.
- Cholecystitis.
- Cholangitis.
- Gallbladder perforation.
- Hepatitis.
- Liver abscess.
- Pancreatitis.

Abdominal wall hernia strangulation

- Groin hernia: inguinal and femoral.
- Other abdominal wall hernias e.g. umbilical, paraumbilical, incisional, epigastric, spigelian.

Gynaecological causes

- Ruptured ectopic pregnancy.
- Ovarian torsion.
- Ovarian cyst rupture.
- Pelvic inflammatory disease, e.g. salpingitis, tubo-ovarian abscess.
- Endometriosis.

Urological causes

- Ureteric colic.
- Pyelonephritis.
- Urinary tract infection.
- Testicular torsion.

Vascular causes

- Abdominal aortic aneurysm rupture.
- Other arterial aneurysm rupture, e.g. common and internal iliac arteries.

Trauma

- Organ injury e.g. splenic rupture, liver laceration, kidney injury.
- Haemoperitoneum.
- Penetrating or blunt injury.

Postoperative complications

- Iatrogenic injury e.g. bowel perforation, bowel ischaemia.
- Anastomotic leak.

Non-surgical causes

- Diabetic ketoacidosis.
- Myocardial infarction.
- Pulmonary embolism.
- Primary peritonitis or spontaneous bacterial peritonitis.
- Basal pneumonia.
- Adrenal crisis.
- Sickle cell crisis.
- Acute intermittent porphyria.
- Tuberculosis.

- *Arterial blood gas (ABG)* provides the lactate, pH, base excess, and some electrolyte concentrations quickly, as well as assessing oxygenation.
- *Glucose:* a marker of pancreatitis severity, of hepatocellular failure, and to identify diabetic ketoacidosis.

- *Urine dipstick:* leucocytes or nitrites may suggest urinary tract infection; blood may suggest renal colic; ketones may suggest malnutrition and dehydration or diabetic ketoacidosis; glucose in urine will suggest poorly controlled diabetes.

- *Pregnancy test*: β-human chorionic gonadotropin (β-HCG) to help diagnose ectopic pregnancy, and also to rule out pregnancy before exposure to X-rays.
- *Erect chest X-ray* may reveal free gas under the diaphragm in cases of a perforated abdominal viscus (seen in 70% of perforated peptic ulcers). It may also exclude pulmonary infection as a differential diagnosis.
- *Abdominal X-ray* may demonstrate small or large bowel dilation due to bowel obstruction; free intraperitoneal gas may also be noted if Rigler's sign[1] is present (the bowel wall is outlined by air both inside and outside). Plain X-rays are less commonly performed today in favour of a computed tomography scan.
- *Computed tomography (CT)*: the most important imaging tool because it provides rapid and accurate diagnostic information. CT is the most sensitive technique for detecting free intraperitoneal gas or free fluid and is valuable for determining the cause of the acute abdomen.
  - A *contrast enhanced CT scan* (done with intravenous contrast) is the technique of choice, but it can be done without contrast when investigating possible renal colic or if the patient is in renal failure.
  - *CT scan with oral contrast* may be requested in cases of bowel obstruction.
  - *CT angiogram* may be performed to assess the blood supply to the bowel or identify a bleeding point within the bowel.
- *Ultrasound scan* is the investigation of choice for suspected acute cholecystitis, biliary colic, or cholangitis. An ultrasound scan is often used to investigate acute abdomen in children to minimize exposure to ionizing radiation. In children, or patients with minimal central adiposity, ultrasound may identify the cause of the acute abdomen e.g. acute appendicitis.
- *Transvaginal ultrasound* may be useful when investigating pelvic pain in young female patients because it can visualize the gynaecological organs and assess for gynaecological pathology e.g. ovarian torsion, ovarian cyst, salpingitis, tubo-ovarian abscess.

- *Magnetic resonance imaging (MRI)* is useful as an alternative to CT where ionizing radiation exposure should be avoided, e.g. in children and pregnant patients.

Principles of treatment

In this section, only an outline of treatment is given, as specific causes of acute abdomen may require specific therapy, and these are dealt with in their appropriate chapters. The standard principles of resuscitation are followed, after an initial assessment of the patient's general condition.

1 *Oxygen therapy:* Oxygen is required if the patient is hypoxic based on their haemoglobin oxygen saturation or on ABG.
2 *Analgesia:* Relief of pain with opiates, such as intravenous morphine.
3 *Nil by mouth:* Patient should remain nil by mouth in case they require urgent surgery.
4 *Intravenous fluid and electrolyte replacement*: intravenous fluids or blood may be required in the presence of shock to correct hypovolaemia and improve organ perfusion (see chapter 8). This should lead to improved blood pressure, heart rate, and urine output.
5 *Antibiotic therapy* to treat the broad spectrum of bowel organisms, for example penicillin and gentamicin together with metronidazole, or co-amoxiclav; or in patients who have already been on antibiotic therapy the addition of an anti-candidal agent, such as fluconazole, is worthwhile.
   Cultures of blood, pus, urine and swabs of the peritoneal cavity should be taken to identify causative microorganisms and their microbiological sensitivities in order to guide antibiotic therapy in conjunction with the microbiology team.
6 *Inotropes:* If, despite intravenous fluid rehydration and antibiotics, the patient remains tachycardic, hypotensive and oliguric, then the patient may require inotropic support and intensive care management.
7 *Urinary catheter:* to monitor urine output as a measure of the patient's hydration and to monitor response to volume replacement.
8 *Nasogastric tube:* gastric aspiration by means of a nasogastric tube reduces the risk of inhalation of vomit (aspiration), prevents further abdominal distension and helps to ease symptoms of nausea

---

[1] Leo George Rigler (1896–1979); Professor of Radiology, serially at University of Minnesota and University of California Los Angeles.

and vomiting, hence it is used in bowel obstruction. It will also reduce the risk of aspiration at the time of induction of anaesthesia should surgery be necessary.

9 *Drainage:* Radiologically guided drainage is an option in order to drain any localized intraperitoneal collection of pus, thus avoiding the risks of surgery especially in high-risk patients. Surgery may still be an option if drainage fails, or sepsis recurs.

Non-surgical treatment

Conservative treatment is indicated, at least initially, when the infection has been localized, for example an appendix mass, or when the primary focus is irremovable, as in pancreatitis or postpartum infection. It may also be indicated when the patient is high risk for surgery or moribund.

Some causes of the acute abdomen may be treated without surgery, such as acute cholecystitis, urinary tract infection, pyelonephritis, pelvic inflammatory disease, uncomplicated diverticulitis and appendix mass. There are also circumstances when acute appendicitis can be managed non-operatively (see chapter 26).

Surgery

Surgery is indicated as the definitive treatment for many causes of the acute abdomen to manage the source of sepsis, for example the repair of a perforated ulcer, removal of a gangrenous and/or perforated appendix, resection of part of the colon for perforated diverticulitis or repair of a strangulated hernia.

Peritonitis

Aetiology

Peritonitis is localized or generalized inflammation of the peritoneum, caused by an infection or irritant entering the peritoneal cavity through one of four portals:

1 *From the exterior,* e.g. penetrating wound, peritoneal dialysis.
2 *From intra-abdominal viscera,* e.g. infected or perforated viscus.
3 *Via the blood stream,* e.g. as part of septicaemia (e.g. *Pneumococcus*, streptococcus, staphylococcus).
4 *Via the female genital tract,* e.g. acute salpingitis or puerperal infection.

Pathology

Peritonitis of bowel origin usually shows a mixed faecal flora (*Escherichia coli, Streptococcus faecalis, Pseudomonas, Klebsiella* and *Proteus*, together with the anaerobic *Clostridium* and *Bacteroides*). Gynaecological infections may be chlamydial, gonococcal or streptococcal. Blood-borne peritonitis may be streptococcal, pneumococcal, staphylococcal or tuberculous. In young girls, a rare gynaecological infection is due to *Pneumococcus*. Peritonitis is characterised by:

1 Widespread absorption of toxins from the large, inflamed surface.
2 The associated paralytic ileus with the following:
   a Loss of fluid.
   b Loss of electrolytes.
   c Loss of protein.
3 Gross abdominal distension with elevation of the diaphragm, which produces a susceptibility to lung collapse and pneumonia.

Clinical features

Peritonitis is usually secondary to a precipitating lesion, one of the causes of the acute abdomen listed above, which may have its own clinical features. For example, there may be features of peptic ulceration before the ulcer perforates to cause peritonitis.

Peritonitis is characterised by severe pain, exacerbated by movement such that the patient gains relief by lying still. Irritation of the parietal peritoneum on the underside of the diaphragm may produce referred pain to the shoulder tip which, like the diaphragm, is also innervated by the C3, 4, 5 nerve roots. There may be associated nausea and vomiting, and patients are usually pyrexial and tachycardic.

Examination elicits localized or generalised tenderness, depending on the extent and underlying cause of the peritonitis. The abdominal wall may be held rigidly or guarding may be present (increasing resistance to increasing depth of palpation), and rebound tenderness may be present. Rectal examination may show tenderness in the pouch of Douglas or pelvis, elicited by moving the examining finger anteriorly in the rectum; palpating posteriorly, against the sacrum, should not elicit pain as it does not stimulate peritoneum and is a useful 'control'.

The abdomen may become distended and tympanic. Depending on the underlying cause of peritonitis, other relevant signs or symptoms may also be present, for example, faeculent vomiting in bowel obstruction, or pain radiating to the back in pancreatitis.

Peritonitis is classified as primary, secondary or tertiary.

Primary peritonitis

In primary peritonitis, or *spontaneous bacterial peritonitis* (SBP), there is inflammation of the peritoneal surface without another intra-abdominal process or an identifiable anatomical derangement. It most commonly occurs in patients with hepatic cirrhosis and ascites, and less often in patients with ascites from other causes, such as heart failure and nephrotic syndrome. Such infections often precipitate hepatic decompensation in a patient with cirrhosis, resulting in encephalopathy, ascites and renal failure. The protein-rich ascitic fluid acts as a culture medium for organisms in these patients who often have a weakened immune response. Infection occurs when enteric organisms translocate across the intact bowel wall from the gut lumen into the ascites.

Bacteria may also gain access to the peritoneal fluid to cause primary peritonitis through different routes such as haematogenous or lymphatic dissemination, passing through the fallopian tubes from the vagina in women, through a peritoneal dialysis catheter or other iatrogenic sources of contamination. The majority of SBP cases are of monomicrobial origin. The commonest implicated pathogens are enteric gram-negative rods, such as *Escherichia coli* and *Klebsiella* species. A smaller number of cases are due to gram-positive organisms, such as *Streptococcus pneumoniae*. Primary peritonitis may be confirmed by a peritoneal tap rich in leucocytes and a positive bacterial culture. It is managed with antibiotics and organ support, without surgical intervention.

Secondary peritonitis

Secondary peritonitis is the most commonly encountered type of peritonitis in surgical patients and is defined as an infection or inflammation of the peritoneal cavity secondary to inflammation or infection from an abdominal viscus, such as appendicitis, diverticulitis, perforated bowel, pancreatitis, cholecystitis, bowel anastomotic leak, penetrating wound, bowel ischaemia and many others. The mainstay of treatment for secondary peritonitis is urgent surgery to achieve surgical control of the source of infection and reduction of the bacterial load, in conjunction with appropriate antibiotic therapy and organ support. There are cases of secondary peritonitis, however, not necessarily requiring urgent surgery, such as pancreatitis. Peritonitis of bowel origin usually shows mixed faecal flora (*Escherichia coli*, *Streptococcus faecalis*, *Pseudomonas*, *Klebsiella* and *Proteus*, together with the anaerobic *Clostridium* and *Bacteroides*).

Tertiary peritonitis

Tertiary peritonitis has been defined as a severe recurrent or persistent intra-abdominal infection 48 hours after apparently successful and adequate surgical source control of secondary peritonitis. For example, development of multiple intra-abdominal abscesses following an appendicectomy; or development of collections following the surgical management of perforated colonic diverticulitis.

After surgical treatment of secondary peritonitis, some patients develop persistent intra-abdominal infection which causes prolonged systemic inflammation leading to a high chance of severe sepsis or septic shock with multiorgan failure. There is a significant difference between the microbial flora in secondary and tertiary peritonitis, and the causal agents in tertiary peritonitis are mostly opportunistic and nosocomial facultative pathogenic bacteria and fungi (e.g. *enterococci*, *enterobacter*, and *candida*).

The development of multi-drug resistance has also been observed in microbes causing tertiary peritonitis due to use of broad-spectrum antibiotic therapy. Altered microbial flora, failure of the immune response, septic shock and progressive organ dysfunction lead to a high risk of mortality in tertiary peritonitis. Therefore, it is important to recognize tertiary peritonitis early in order to minimize complications and improve patient outcomes. Treatment involves appropriate antibiotics and antifungals, organ support, radiologically guided drainage of any source of intra-abdominal sepsis and reoperation if all other measures fail.

Special causes of peritonitis

Peritoneal dialysis peritonitis

Patients on peritoneal dialysis are prone to peritonitis either from organisms entering via the indwelling dialysis catheter (usually, skin flora such as *Staphylococcus* species) or from perforation of a viscus, in which case the flora are generally a mixture of faecal organisms. Diagnosis is made by the presence of abdominal pain and turbid dialysate. Single organisms are treated by intravenous and intraperitoneal antibiotics. Multiple organisms, particularly gut flora, suggest perforation and require surgery as well as antibiotics. Once infected, the peritoneal dialysis catheter may form a focus for sepsis, in which case it should be removed.

Pneumococcal peritonitis

This may be secondary to the septicaemia accompanying a pneumococcal lung infection, or can originate from an infected or colonized female genital tract. Clinically, there is peritonitis of sudden onset accompanied by septicaemia, and the white cell count is elevated. Peritoneal fluid is clear or turbid containing fibrin flakes without an obvious primary cause within the abdomen. The peritoneal fluid reveals characteristic gram-positive pneumococci arranged in chains and pairs. The condition responds to penicillin therapy.

Haemolytic streptococcal peritonitis

This may occur in children, secondary to streptococcal infection of the tonsils, otitis media, scarlet fever or erysipelas.

Staphylococcal peritonitis

Staphylococcal septicaemia may rarely cause staphylococcal peritonitis, which can be further complicated by intra-abdominal or perinephric abscess development.

Tuberculous peritonitis

Tuberculous peritonitis is a type of extrapulmonary tuberculosis affecting the peritoneum. It is frequently seen in the presence of other types of gastrointestinal tuberculosis. The majority of cases are due to the reactivation of dormant peritoneal tuberculous collections. It can also arise as a result of haematogenous spread from a primary active pulmonary focus or miliary tuberculosis. Less frequently, mycobacteria tuberculosis can enter the peritoneal cavity directly from the gastrointestinal tract (e.g. after a bowel perforation or transmurally from infected small intestine). There have also been cases of lymphatic spread (e.g. through mesenteric lymph nodes). In some female patients, spread has been noted via the genital tract (e.g. from primary tuberculous salpingitis).

Risk factors for tuberculous peritonitis include patients who are immunosuppressed, either iatrogenic (e.g. in peritoneal dialysis, chemotherapy or steroid therapy), or by disease (e.g. human immunodeficiency virus infection, liver cirrhosis). Lifestyle risk factors include alcoholism and intravenous drug abuse.

Tuberculous peritonitis is commonly classified into three types: wet, fixed fibrotic and dry plastic. The commonest type (>90% of cases) is the wet, or ascitic type, and it usually results from the haematogenous spread from a primary lung infection or through reactivation of latent tuberculous peritoneal lesions. As the name suggests, the wet type is characterized by large amount of either free or loculated viscous fluid. The fixed fibrotic type is characterized by large mesenteric and omental masses leading to fixed bowel loops with loculated ascites. The dry plastic type is the least common type and is characterized by caseous mesenteric lymphadenopathy, thickened omentum and fibrous adhesions.

Clinical features of tuberculous peritonitis include abdominal distension, night sweats, fevers, abdominal pain and weight loss. Treatment comprises of anti-tuberculous chemotherapy. Surgery may be required for complications including bowel perforation, intestinal obstruction secondary to adhesions, fistulae or abscesses.

Biliary peritonitis

Biliary peritonitis is caused by perforation of the gallbladder, bile duct or upper gastrointestinal tract. This may occur as a result of the following:

- *Traumatic rupture* of the gallbladder or biliary ducts.
- *Iatrogenic injury* after invasive procedures such as liver biopsy, percutaneous cholangiography or endoscopic retrograde cholangiopancreatography (ERCP).

- *Leakage from the liver, the gallbladder or its ducts after* a biliary tract operation, for example iatrogenic biliary injury during laparoscopic cholecystectomy.
- *Perforation of an acutely inflamed gallbladder* or transudation of the bile through a gangrenous but non-perforated gallbladder.
- *Non-traumatic perforation of the bile duct* where the extrahepatic duct or intrahepatic duct is perforated spontaneously without traumatic or iatrogenic injury.
- *Spontaneous perforation of the gallbladder*, associated with infections, malignancies, stones, thrombosis of intramural vessels, increased biliary pressures, use of corticosteroids and systemic diseases such as diabetes mellitus and atherosclerotic heart disease.
- *Idiopathic* is a rare but well-recognized condition in which bile peritonitis occurs without obvious cause, possibly a small perforation due to a calculus, which then becomes sealed.

Biliary peritonitis is associated with high risk of morbidity and mortality, particularly in high-risk elderly patients. The clinical signs and symptoms of bile leakage may be non-specific resulting in delayed recognition and consequent increased risk of complications. The clinical picture is determined by the amount and rate of bile leakage into the abdominal cavity.

Imaging is crucial for establishing an early diagnosis and in guiding treatment.

- *CT and ultrasound* can identify a collection of peri-hepatic fluid.
- *Magnetic resonance cholangiopancreatography (MRCP)* can detect active or contained bile leaks and can help localize the site of leakage, which in turn can help determine if endoscopic management is sufficient, or if surgical management is warranted.
- *ERCP* may provide diagnostic confirmation of a bile leak and also provides the opportunity of concurrent therapy, for example through common bile duct stone removal, or elimination of the transpapillary pressure gradient either by a sphincterotomy, stent insertion or both.

It is important to drain the abdominal contamination caused by infected bilious peritoneal fluid, which can be attempted through radiologically guided drain insertion when non-surgical management is pursued. The gallbladder itself may be drained through a cholecystostomy (drain in the gallbladder). Surgery (with abdominal lavage) is an effective and definitive treatment for biliary peritonitis and can deal with the underlying cause of bile leak. For example, cholecystectomy is the definitive treatment for biliary peritonitis due to gallbladder perforation (see chapter 34).

Mesenteric ischaemia

Pathophysiology

Bowel ischaemia is an important cause of an acute abdomen. Splanchnic ischaemia is caused by a blood supply which is inadequate for the metabolic and oxygen demands of the intra-abdominal visceral organs. The coeliac artery, the superior mesenteric artery (SMA) and the inferior mesenteric artery (IMA) supply the foregut (liver, spleen, stomach to second part of duodenum), midgut (second part of duodenum to splenic flexure of colon) and hindgut (splenic flexure of colon to rectum), respectively. Mesenteric ischaemia is caused by insufficient blood flow through the mesenteric blood vessels which potentially compromises the small and large intestine. The overall prevalence of acute mesenteric ischaemia is 0.1% of all hospital admissions. Ischaemic colitis is caused by inadequate blood supply specifically to the colon and is the most common ischaemic injury of the gastrointestinal tract.

Ischaemia of the small or large bowel leads to bowel wall spasm (causing vomiting or diarrhoea), bowel wall oedema and mucosal sloughing with bleeding into the gut wall, lumen and peritoneal cavity. Injury to the affected bowel may range from reversible ischaemia to transmural infarction with necrosis, gangrene and subsequent perforation.

During bowel ischaemia, the enteric mucosal barrier becomes disrupted, allowing the translocation of bacteria, endotoxins and vasoactive substances into the systemic circulation. A generalized proinflammatory state is produced with release of cytokines by macrophages, with activation of the complement and coagulation systems. This may lead to systemic inflammatory response syndrome, septic shock and multiorgan failure.

Aetiology

Mesenteric ischaemia may result from embolic (50% of cases) or thrombotic (20% of cases) arterial occlusion, thrombotic venous occlusion (10% of cases), or from non-occlusive processes (20% of cases).

Acute mesenteric arterial embolism

Emboli may arise from the left atrium in atrial fibrillation, or from a mural thrombus from a dilated ventricle secondary to myocardial infarction, vegetative endocarditis, valvular disease, mycotic aneurysm, or due to a ruptured atheromatous plaque of the aorta. Rarely, it may be a paradoxical embolus originating in the deep leg veins and crossing the septum of the heart through a patent foramen ovale (see Figure 13.3). The SMA is the most susceptible visceral vessel to emboli due to its size and angle at its origin from the aorta. Embolism has a better overall prognosis than thrombosis.

Acute mesenteric arterial thrombosis

This represents progressive worsening of atherosclerotic vascular disease. It is associated with a history of chronic mesenteric ischaemia where patients complain of 'intestinal angina', i.e., postprandial abdominal pain in which severe abdominal pain follows meals with a resultant fear of eating and consequent weight loss. Minor degrees of occlusion may be overcome by the development of a collateral circulation, particularly if the occlusion develops slowly. Patients may have a history of atherosclerotic disease at other sites (e.g. ischaemic heart disease, cerebrovascular disease and peripheral vascular disease). Thrombosis commonly occurs at the origin of arteries resulting in extensive bowel ischaemia, whereas embolism commonly occurs in more distal arterial branches resulting in more limited bowel ischaemia.

Mesenteric venous thrombosis

In mesenteric venous thrombosis, blood outflow is restricted causing bowel wall oedema and increase in vascular resistance, resulting in bowel ischaemia. Causes of mesenteric venous thrombosis include portal hypertension, post-surgery (e.g. post-splenectomy, portacaval surgery, pelvic surgery), pressure on the superior mesenteric vessels by a tumour, septic thrombophlebitis (e.g. secondary to Crohn's disease), trauma, pancreatitis or intra-abdominal sepsis. It may affect younger patients and may be associated with hypercoagulable states, e.g. due to factor V Leiden deficiency, polycythaemia rubra vera, protein C and S deficiency, antithrombin III deficiency, thrombocytosis, dysfibrinogenaemia, sickle cell disease, cancer, pregnancy and oral contraceptive use.

Low blood flow states

During states of shock or hypoperfusion, the mesenteric blood flow is preferentially reduced in order to maintain blood supply to other vital organs and is one of the last systems to recover blood flow when circulation improves. Non-occlusive ischaemia of the intestine may occur in low blood flow states causing mesenteric ischaemia, such as shock, hypovolaemia, dehydration, sepsis, low cardiac output, congestive cardiac failure, myocardial infarction, transient hypotension (e.g. perioperative) and cardiopulmonary bypass surgery.

Other causes of mesenteric ischaemia

- *Splanchnic vasoconstriction or vasospasm:* caused by reduced blood flow, vasopressors (e.g. vasopressin, α-agonists), digoxin, drugs which produce vasospasm (e.g. cocaine, amphetamines).
- *Intrinsic small vessel disease or vasculitis* due to rheumatoid arthritis, systemic lupus erythematosus, polyarteritis nodosa, dermatomyositis, primary amyloidosis, diabetes mellitus.
- *Luminal bowel obstruction* (e.g. due to strangulated internal hernia, volvulus, tumour, intussusception).
- *Post-angiography complications:* subintimal artery dissection, thrombosis, arterial embolization.
- *Vascular surgery complications* (e.g. aortic surgery, renal allograft recipients).
- *Abdominal compartment syndrome.*
- *Tumour compression.*
- *Aortic dissection.*
- *Blunt or penetrating trauma.*

Clinical features
History

Initially, symptoms and signs are non-specific and are most commonly found in advanced disease. A high index of clinical suspicion should be maintained to avoid delay in diagnosis and treatment. Patients affected tend to be middle-aged or elderly patients with risk factors for thromboembolism and atherosclerotic disease. They may have a history of intestinal angina. There may be some pre-existing factor such as heart valvular disease or liver disease. They may have atrial fibrillation, either as a long-standing finding or of new onset. The classic triad of mesenteric ischaemia is:

- Acute colicky abdominal pain.
- Rectal bleeding.
- Circulatory shock.

Commonly, the patient gives a history of vague, diffuse, colicky or constant abdominal pain, progressively getting worse. The abdominal pain may be severe and disproportionate to physical examination findings. The onset of the abdominal pain may be sudden if the cause is an embolus, or of insidious onset if thrombus is the cause. The patient may have vomiting or diarrhoea due to bowel wall spasm and rectal bleeding due to mucosal sloughing.

Examination

There may be no, or mild-to-moderate, abdominal tenderness initially, until it progresses to perforation or infarction causing peritonitis. The patient then may become generally tender, and a vague, tender mass may be felt, which is the infarcted bowel. Bowel sounds range from hyperactive to absent. The abdomen may be distended, and rectal examination may show blood mixed with stool. Examination may identify atrial fibrillation, heart murmurs or abdominal murmurs (due to arterial stenosis). The patient may have weak peripheral pulses (due to peripheral vascular disease or hypoperfusion) and signs of sepsis (e.g. tachycardia, tachypnoea, pyrexia).

Investigations

- *Blood tests:* Laboratory findings are non-specific but may include leucocytosis, haemoconcentration, elevated serum lactate and metabolic acidosis, elevated liver enzymes (ALT, AST) due to hepatic ischaemia, elevated amylase, elevated lactate dehydrogenase (LDH) and elevated CRP. D-dimer is a sensitive marker for splanchnic ischaemia but is not specific. Blood tests should include coagulation studies (PT, APTT, INR) and screening for coagulopathies.
- *Plain radiographs:* Erect chest and abdominal X-rays often appear normal but may show signs of perforated viscus, ileus, bowel obstruction, thickened bowel wall due to oedema, pneumatosis intestinalis (i.e., submucosal air) and thumbprinting from submucosal oedema.
- *Electrocardiogram (ECG)* may show atrial fibrillation or myocardial infarction.

- *Echocardiography* may identify the source of embolization or demonstrate valvular pathology (e.g. valvular vegetations).
- *Flexible sigmoidoscopy or colonoscopy* can be performed to confirm ischaemic colitis by demonstrating mucosal ulceration, haemorrhage, oedema and fragility consistent with colonic ischaemia.
- *Computed tomography:* A CT angiogram can identify bowel wall oedema, thumbprinting, pneumatosis intestinalis, pericolic stranding, portal venous gas, pneumoperitoneum, lack of bowel wall enhancement and ischaemia of other organs. It can determine the extent of the disease, i.e., how much bowel is affected and whether it is perforated. It demonstrates arterial or venous occlusion and excludes other differential diagnoses. It is non-invasive and readily available. In patients suspected to have mesenteric vessel occlusion, the priority is early diagnosis and treatment to improve chances of survival, justifying the need for an urgent CT scan with intravenous contrast despite the acknowledged risk of contrast-induced renal failure and challenges in the presence of established renal impairment. Renal support in these instances must be discussed with the intensive care team.
- *Diagnostic laparoscopy or laparotomy* can be considered where other investigations have been inconclusive.

Treatment

- Oxygen therapy. Consider invasive ventilation to improve oxygenation.
- Analgesia, with morphine if needed.
- Nasogastric tube for abdominal decompression.
- Optimization of volume status with intravenous fluid resuscitation and optimization of cardiac output. Monitor urine output, arterial pressure and central venous pressure to guide rehydration.
- Use of inotropes if needed, but vasopressors (e.g. adrenaline, noradrenaline, vasopressin, high dose dopamine) may worsen ischaemia.
- Treat underlying conditions (e.g. atrial fibrillation, cardiac failure, myocardial infarction).
- Broad-spectrum antibiotics covering gram-positive, gram-negative and anaerobic bacteria.
- Anticoagulation with intravenous heparin in the short-term, particularly if surgery is to be considered as heparin is more reversible than the low molecular weight heparin alternatives. Anticoagulation is the main treatment for mesenteric venous thrombosis.

In the long term, anticoagulation in the form of warfarin or novel oral anticoagulants (NOACs) should be considered after embolic arterial occlusion or after mesenteric venous occlusion. In addition, long-term therapy should address patient's risk factors, and antiplatelet agents and statins prescribed after thrombotic arterial occlusion.

- Endovascular therapy is an option which may be available through interventional radiology. Endovascular therapy options include intra-arterial thrombolytic therapy (e.g. with tissue plasminogen activator) or intra-arterial vasodilators (e.g. with papaverine). Other endovascular therapy options include aspiration embolectomy of the SMA, or angioplasty and stenting for proximal arterial thrombosis (e.g. origin of SMA).

Surgery

Surgery is the mainstay of treatment especially for patients with signs of peritonitis due to perforation or infarction, and where non-operative therapy fails. Intraoperatively, the extent and severity of intestinal ischaemia is determined by assessing colour and peristalsis of the bowel and pulsations of the mesenteric arteries. Ischaemic or necrotic bowel is resected. Embolectomy, thrombo-endarterectomy or arterial reconstruction (e.g. mesenteric artery bypass) may be required to re-establish arterial blood supply.

After bowel resection, the options are:

- Primary anastomosis, provided the blood supply to both proximal and distal bowel margins is adequate and the patient is not haemodynamically compromised.
- Stoma formation – double-barrelled stoma or end stoma with separate mucous fistula. This is safer and allows assessment of the bowel viability postoperatively.
- Staple off both bowel ends leaving anastomosis or stoma formation for a second-look procedure.

Surgeons may re-explore the abdomen at 24 to 48 hours to reassess bowel viability. The abdomen may be left open (laparostomy) to prevent abdominal compartment syndrome.

For many patients where the entire small bowel is found to be non-viable (due to thrombosis of the SMA origin), resection should not be performed, and palliative treatment may be appropriate. However, in selected cases, such as young patients without significant comorbidities who have undergone extensive resection of the small bowel, long-term total parenteral nutrition and potential intestinal transplantation may be considered.

30

Intestinal obstruction and paralytic ileus

Christopher Watson

Learning objectives

✓ To know the causes of mechanical obstruction in all age groups.

✓ To recognize the four common clinical features of mechanical obstruction, the key points of clinical examination and the management principles.

✓ To know the causes and management of paralytic ileus.

✓ To differentiate mechanical obstruction from paralytic ileus.

The word 'ileus' comes from the Greek verb 'to roll', from which it became applied to colic and hence to obstruction. Obstructions are subdivided into mechanical and paralytic, the latter produced by lack of intestinal motility.

Mechanical obstruction

Classification

Intestinal obstruction (Box 30.1) is a restriction to the normal passage of intestinal contents. It may be divided into two main groups: paralytic and mechanical. Paralytic (or adynamic) ileus is discussed later.

Mechanical intestinal obstruction is further classified according to the following:

- *Speed of onset*: acute, chronic, acute on chronic.
- *Site*: high or low.

Ellis and Calne's Lecture Notes in General Surgery, Fourteenth Edition. Edited by Christopher Watson and Justin Davies.
© 2023 John Wiley & Sons Ltd. Published 2023 by John Wiley & Sons Ltd.
Companion website: www.wiley.com/go/Watson/GeneralSurgery14

- *Nature*: simple versus strangulating.
- *Aetiology*.

Speed of onset

The speed of onset determines whether the obstruction is acute, chronic or acute on chronic.

- *Acute obstruction*: the onset is rapid and the symptoms severe.
- *Chronic obstruction*: the symptoms are insidious and slowly progressive, as, for example, in most cases of carcinoma of the large bowel.
- *Acute on chronic obstruction*: A chronic obstruction may develop acute symptoms as the obstruction suddenly becomes complete, for example when a narrowed lumen becomes totally occluded by inspissated bowel contents.

Site

The site of the obstruction is generally classified according to whether it originates in the small or large intestine.

Nature

The nature of the obstruction is divided into simple or strangulating.

- *Simple obstruction* occurs when the intestine is occluded without damage to its blood supply.
- *Strangulating obstruction* is when the blood supply of the involved segment of intestine is compromised, as may occur, for example, in strangulated hernia, volvulus, intussusception or when a loop of intestine is occluded by a band. Gangrene of the strangulated bowel is inevitable if left untreated.

Aetiology

Whenever one considers obstruction of a tube anywhere in the body, the causes should be classified into the following:

- Causes in the lumen.
- Causes in the wall.
- Causes outside the wall.

This can be applied to intestinal obstruction.

- *In the lumen*: faecal impaction, food bolus, intussusception, gallstone 'ileus', parasites (e.g. ascaris worms in small bowel).

- *In the wall*: congenital atresia, Crohn's disease, tumours, diverticulitis of the colon, carcinoma of the colon.
- *Outside the wall*: strangulated hernia (external or internal), volvulus and obstruction due to adhesions or bands.

It is also useful to think of the common intestinal obstructions that may occur in each age group.

- *Neonatal*: congenital atresia and stenosis (e.g. duodenal atresia), imperforate anus, volvulus neonatorum, Hirschsprung's disease and meconium ileus.
- *Infants*: intussusception, Hirschsprung's disease, strangulated hernia and obstruction due to Meckel's diverticulum.
- *Young adults and middle age*: strangulated hernia, adhesions and bands, Crohn's disease.
- *The elderly*: strangulated hernia, carcinoma of the colon, colonic diverticulitis causing stricture, impacted faeces.

A strangulated hernia is an important cause of intestinal obstruction from infancy to old age. The hernial orifices must, therefore, be carefully examined in every case.

Pathology

When the bowel is obstructed by a simple occlusion, the intestine distal to the obstruction rapidly empties and becomes collapsed. The bowel above the obstruction becomes dilated, partly with gas (most of which is swallowed air) and partly with fluid poured out by the intestinal wall together with the gastric, biliary and pancreatic secretions. There is increased peristalsis in an attempt to overcome the obstruction, which results in intestinal colic. As the bowel distends, the blood supply to the tensely distended intestinal wall becomes impaired and, in extreme cases, there may be mucosal ulceration and eventually perforation. Perforation may also occur from the pressure of a band or the edge of the hernia neck on the bowel wall, producing local ischaemic necrosis, or from pressure from within the gut lumen, for example, by a faecal mass (stercoral perforation).

In strangulating obstruction, the integrity of the mucosal barrier is lost as ischaemia progresses, so bacteria and their toxins can no longer be contained within the lumen. Transudation of organisms into the peritoneal cavity rapidly takes place, with secondary peritonitis. Unrelieved strangulation is followed by gangrene of the ischaemic bowel with perforation.

The lethal effects of intestinal obstruction result from fluid and electrolyte depletion owing to the copious vomiting and loss into the bowel lumen, protein loss into the gut and toxaemia due to migration of toxins and intestinal bacteria into the peritoneal cavity, either through the intact but ischaemic bowel wall or through a perforation.

Clinical features

The four cardinal symptoms of intestinal obstruction are:

1 Colicky abdominal pain.
2 Distension.
3 Absolute constipation.
4 Vomiting.

It is important to note that not all of these four features need necessarily be present in a case of intestinal obstruction. The sequence of onset of symptoms will help localize the obstruction to the upper or lower intestine.

Pain

This is usually the first symptom of intestinal obstruction and is colicky in nature. In small bowel obstruction, it is periumbilical, reflecting the midgut derivation of this bowel; in distal colonic obstruction, it may be more suprapubic in location. In postoperative obstruction, the colic may be disguised by the general discomfort of the operation and by opiates that the patient may be receiving.

Distension

This is particularly marked in chronic large bowel obstruction and also in volvulus of the sigmoid colon. In proximal small bowel obstruction, there may only be a short segment of bowel proximal to the obstruction, and distension will not usually be marked.

Absolute constipation

Absolute constipation is the failure to pass either flatus or faeces. Although it is a usual feature of acute obstruction, a partial or chronic obstruction may be accompanied by the passage of small amounts of flatus. Absolute constipation is an early feature of large bowel obstruction but a late feature of small bowel obstruction as, even when the obstruction is complete, the patient may pass one or two normal stools as the lower bowel empties after the onset of the obstruction.

Vomiting

This usually occurs early in proximal small bowel obstruction, but is often late or even entirely absent in large bowel obstruction. In the late stages of intestinal obstruction, the vomiting becomes faeculent but not faecal.

Faeculent vomiting is due to bacterial decomposition of the stagnant contents of the obstructed small intestine and of the altered blood that may transude into the bowel lumen.

True vomiting of faeces only occurs in patients with gastrocolic fistula (e.g. because of a carcinoma of the stomach, carcinoma of the colon or ulceration of a stomal ulcer into the colon), or in coprophagia.

Clinical examination

The patient may be obviously dehydrated if vomiting has been copious. The patient is in pain and may be rolling about with colic. The pulse is usually elevated, but the temperature is frequently normal. A raised temperature and a tachycardia suggest strangulation. The abdomen is distended and visible peristalsis may be present. Visible peristalsis itself is not diagnostic of intestinal obstruction, as it may be seen in the normal subject if the abdominal wall is very thin.

During inspection, it is important to look carefully for two features: (1) the presence of a strangulated external hernia, which may require a careful search in the case of a small strangulated femoral hernia in a very obese and distended patient, and (2) the presence of an abdominal scar. Intestinal obstruction in the presence of this evidence of a previous operation immediately suggests adhesions as the cause.

Palpation reveals generalized abdominal tenderness. A mass may be present (e.g. in intussusception or carcinoma of the bowel).

Bowel sounds are usually accentuated and tinkling. Rectal examination may reveal an obstructing mass in the pouch of Douglas, the apex of an intussusception or faecal impaction.

Simple obstruction versus strangulating obstruction

Clinically, it is extremely difficult to distinguish with any certainty between simple obstruction and strangulation. The distinction is important, as strangulating obstruction with ensuing peritonitis has a high mortality. Features suggesting strangulation include:

- Toxic appearance, with a rapid pulse and some elevation of temperature.
- Colicky pain, becoming continuous as peritonitis develops.
- Tenderness and abdominal rigidity more marked.
- Bowel sounds becoming reduced or absent, reflecting peritonism.
- Raised white cell count, mostly neutrophils, which is usual with infarcted bowel.

Special investigations

- *Computed tomography (CT) scan*, combined with oral water-soluble contrast (e.g. Gastrografin), is the investigation of choice; it can localize the site of obstruction, detect obstructing lesions and colonic tumours and may diagnose unusual hernias (e.g. obturator hernias). The addition of intravenous contrast allows an assessment of bowel wall perfusion, which is very helpful when assessing for strangulating obstruction.
- *Water-soluble contrast study*. An emergency contrast enema may detect a suspected large bowel obstruction due to carcinoma or diverticular disease. Unlike a normal barium enema, no preexamination laxative is given because of the risk of exacerbating the obstruction, and causing perforation if a closed loop exists. This has been largely superseded by CT scan with rectal contrast.
- *Abdominal X-rays* (erect and supine) were widely used prior to the widespread availability of CT. A loop or loops of distended bowel are usually seen, together with fluid levels on an erect film.
  - *Small bowel obstruction* is suggested by a ladder pattern of dilated loops, their central position and by striations that pass completely across the width of the distended loop produced by the circular mucosal folds (known as valvulae conniventes).
  - *Distended large bowel* tends to lie peripherally and to show the haustrations of the taenia coli, which do not extend across the whole width of the bowel. A small percentage, perhaps 5%, of patients with intestinal obstruction show no abnormality on plain X-rays because the bowel is completely distended with fluid in a closed loop and without the fluid levels produced by co-existent gas.

Treatment

Although the treatment of specific causes of intestinal obstruction is considered under the appropriate headings, certain general principles can be enunciated here.

Chronic large bowel obstruction, slowly progressive and incomplete, can be investigated with less urgency (including sigmoidoscopy or colonoscopy and CT scan) and treated electively.

Acute obstruction, of sudden onset, complete and with risk of strangulation, is invariably an urgent problem requiring emergency surgical intervention.

Preoperative preparation in acute obstruction

1 *Gastric aspiration* by means of nasogastric tube. This helps to decompress the bowel and lessen the risk of inhalation of gastric contents during induction of anaesthesia.
2 *Intravenous fluid replacement*. The large amount of fluid sequestered into the gut, together with losses due to vomiting, means that a lot of fluid may be required. Hartmann's solution or normal saline is given, with potassium if this is low and renal function satisfactory.
3 *Antibiotic therapy* is commenced if intestinal strangulation is likely (or is found at operation).

Operative treatment

The affected bowel is carefully inspected to determine its viability, either at the site of the obstruction (e.g. where a band or the margins of a hernial orifice have pressed against the bowel) or the whole segment of bowel involved in a closed loop obstruction. Loss of viability is determined by four signs:

1 Loss of peristalsis.
2 Loss of normal sheen.
3 Colour (greenish or black bowel is non-viable; purple bowel may still recover).
4 Loss of arterial pulsation in the supplying mesentery.

Doubtful bowel may recover after relief of the obstruction. It should be reassessed after it has been left for a few minutes wrapped up in a warm wet pack. If extensive areas of bowel are of doubtful viability, it may be worthwhile planning a second-look laparotomy in 48 hours to reassess the necessity for an extensive bowel resection.

The general principle is that small bowel in intestinal obstruction can be resected and primary anastomosis performed because of its excellent blood supply. Large bowel obstruction is treated by resection of the obstructing lesion, with a primary ileocolic anastomosis in the case of obstructing lesions proximal to the splenic flexure. Left-sided lesions are managed by excision of the affected segment and either a primary anastomosis with temporary covering stoma or exteriorizing the proximal colon as a temporary end colostomy and either exteriorizing the distal end as a mucous fistula (see Chapter 28), or more commonly, closing the distal large bowel (often the rectum) and leaving it inside the abdomen (Hartmann's procedure[1]). This difference in management of colonic obstruction reflects the intraluminal bacterial flora and poorer blood supply of the large bowel; a colo-colonic or colorectal primary anastomosis has a higher risk of anastomotic leak in the presence of obstruction. Where a primary large bowel anastomosis is performed, a defunctioning loop ileostomy should be considered in order to mitigate the effects of an anastomotic leak. The role of an endoscopically placed colonic stent in the management of acute malignant large bowel obstruction is discussed in Chapter 27.

Conservative treatment

Conservative treatment of obstruction by means of intravenous fluid and nasogastric aspiration ('drip and suck') is indicated *only* under the following conditions.

- When distinction from postoperative paralytic ileus is uncertain and when a period of careful observation is indicated.
- When the obstruction is one of repeated episodes due to extensive intra-abdominal adhesions, rendering surgery hazardous, and when, once again, a short period of observation with conservative treatment is indicated. Gastrografin is given via the NG tube; if it fails to pass through the obstructed bowel, surgery is indicated. It is also indicated if distension is increasing, pain is worsening or there is an increase in abdominal tenderness or a rising pulse.

- When chronic obstruction of the large bowel has occurred. Here, it is reasonable to attempt to remove the obturating faeces by enema, prepare the bowel and carry out further investigation and a subsequent elective operation.

Closed loop obstruction

This is a specific form of mechanical obstruction. It is characterized by increasing distension of a loop of bowel due to a combination of complete obstruction distally and a valve-like mechanism proximally allowing the bowel to fill but preventing reflux back. It is most commonly seen with a left-sided colonic obstruction, in the presence of a competent ileocaecal valve. The caecum, the most distensible part of the large bowel, blows up like a balloon, and perforation of the caecum, with faecal peritonitis, may occur if the obstruction is not rapidly relieved. Diagnosis is most commonly made on CT scan showing characteristic dilation of the caecum and dilated colon down to the site of stricture/obstruction. Other examples of closed loop obstruction include volvulus (gastric, caecal, sigmoid) and stomal obstruction of the afferent loop following Pólya[2] partial gastrectomy.

Adhesive obstruction

Intra-abdominal adhesions are an almost invariable consequence of abdominal or pelvic surgery, although they are less common after minimal access (laparoscopic and robotic) surgery than after open surgery. In most cases, these are asymptomatic, but a small number of patients develop small bowel obstruction as a consequence. This may occur at any time from the immediate postoperative period to many years later. Because abdominal surgery is now so common, adhesions account for about three-quarters of all cases of small bowel obstruction (large bowel obstruction from this cause is extremely rare). Treatment is initially conservative, with nasogastric suction and intravenous fluid replacement. Clinical features of strangulation, peritonitis or failure to respond to the conservative regimen are indications for urgent surgery.

[1] Henri Hartmann (1860–1952), Professor of Surgery, Hôtel Dieu, Paris, France.

[2] Eugen Alexander Pólya (1876–1944), Surgeon, St Stephen's Hospital, Budapest, Hungary.

Volvulus

Definition

A twisting of a loop of bowel around its mesenteric axis, which results in a combination of obstruction together with occlusion of the main vessels at the base of the involved mesentery. Most commonly, it affects the sigmoid colon, caecum and small intestine, but volvulus of the gallbladder and stomach may also occur.

Aetiology

Precipitating factors include:

- An abnormally mobile loop of intestine, for example congenital failure of rotation of the small intestine, or a particularly long sigmoid loop.
- An abnormally loaded loop – as in the sigmoid colon of chronic constipation.
- A loop fixed at its apex by adhesions, around which it rotates.
- A loop of bowel with a narrow mesenteric attachment.

Sigmoid volvulus

This occurs usually in elderly, constipated patients. It is four times more common in men than in women. It is relatively rare in the UK (about 2% of intestinal obstructions) but is much more common in Russia, Scandinavia and central Africa. The loop of sigmoid colon usually twists anticlockwise, from one-half to three turns.

Clinical features

There is a sudden onset of colicky pain with characteristic gross and rapid dilation of the sigmoid loop.

A plain X-ray (or CT scan) of the abdomen shows an enormously dilated oval gas shadow on the left side, which may be looped on itself to give the typical appearance various described as the 'coffee bean' sign or 'bent inner-tube' sign. If left untreated, the strangulated bowel undergoes gangrene, resulting in death from peritonitis. The caecum is usually visible and dilated in the right lower quadrant, distinguishing it radiologically from caecal volvulus.

Treatment

An urgent flexible sigmoidoscopy should be performed. This often untwists an early volvulus and is accompanied by the passage of vast amounts of flatus and liquid faeces. If this method fails, the volvulus is untwisted at surgery (open or laparoscopic) and the bowel is decompressed via a rectal tube threaded upwards from the anus. If gangrene has occurred, the affected segment is excised, the proximal end being brought out as an end colostomy while the distal end is stapled closed (a Hartmann's procedure).

Recurrent sigmoid volvulus is an indication for elective resection of the redundant sigmoid loop, or for percutaneous endoscopic colostomy (PEC) in those who are unfit for major surgery.

Caecal volvulus

Caecal volvulus is usually associated with a congenital malrotation where, in contrast to the incomplete rotation which causes volvulus neonatorum (see later in this chapter), the caecum and proximal ascending colon rotate beyond the right iliac fossa (RIF) during development so that, instead of being fixed in the RIF, it has a persistent mesentery.

Clinically, there is an acute onset of pain in the RIF with rapid abdominal distension. Plain radiograph or CT of the abdomen shows a grossly dilated caecum, which is often ectopically placed and is frequently located in the left upper quadrant of the abdomen.

Treatment

At surgery, the volvulus is untwisted. Right hemicolectomy is necessary, especially if the caecum is infarcted; it is also the most reliable way to prevent recurrence.

Small intestine volvulus in adults

This may occur when a loop of the small intestine is fixed at its apex by adhesions or by a fibrous remnant of the vitello-intestinal duct (often associated with a Meckel's diverticulum). Occasionally, the apex of the volvulus bears a tumour.

In Africa, primary volvulus of the small bowel is relatively common, and may be due to the loading of a loop of gut with large quantities of vegetable foodstuffs. The clinical picture is one of acute intestinal obstruction.

Treatment

Early operation with simple untwisting and treatment of the underlying cause. If gangrene is present, resection must be carried out.

Volvulus neonatorum

This is considered later in this chapter.

Neonatal intestinal obstruction

Classification

- Intestinal atresia.
- Anorectal atresias.
- Hirschsprung's disease.
- Volvulus neonatorum.
- Necrotizing enterocolitis.
- Meconium ileus.

Continuous vomiting in the newborn suggests intracranial injury, infection or obstruction. Bile vomiting in the neonate indicates, almost without exception, intestinal obstruction.

In addition to vomiting, there may be constipation, abdominal distension and visible peristalsis. Plain X-ray of the abdomen shows distended loops of intestine with fluid levels.

Intestinal atresia

This may be a septum, complete or partial, or a complete gap, which may be associated with a corresponding defect in the mesentery. Multiple segments may be involved.

Treatment

Resection of the stricture and anastomosis.

Anorectal atresias

Anorectal atresias are a spectrum of abnormalities from imperforate anus to complete absence of anus and rectum. They result from failure of breakdown of the septum between the hindgut and the invaginating ectoderm of the proctodaeum. Fifty per cent are associated with fistula: in the female into the vagina; in the male into the bladder or urethra. Twenty-five per cent are associated with congenital anomalies elsewhere, and a small proportion are familial.

Clinical features

The anus may be entirely absent or represented by a dimple or a blind canal. Diagnosis may be suspected on prenatal ultrasound by the presence of dilated bowel and intraluminal calcification, but is apparent on the immediate post-natal examination. Since imperforate anus is associated with vertebral and other congenital defects, any child with the diagnosis should have an ultrasound or magnetic resonance imaging of the pelvis, spine and chest (for trachea-oesophageal fistula), and may also need an echocardiogram to look for cardiac anomalies.

Treatment

- If the septum is thin (less than 1 cm), it is divided with suture of the edges of the defect to the skin.
- If there is an extensive gap between the blind end and the anal verge, a colostomy is fashioned with a later attempt at a pull-through operation at about 2 years of age. Some surgeons perform an immediate pull-through procedure in the neonate.
- If a vaginal fistula is present, operation is not urgent, as the bowel decompresses through the vagina. Elective surgery is performed when the child is older.
- If a rectourethral or vesical fistula is present (meconium escaping in the urine), the fistula must be closed urgently, with either colostomy or reconstruction of the anus, in order to prevent ascending infection of the urinary tract.

Hirschsprung's disease[3]

This may present as acute obstruction in the neonate, with an incidence of 1 in 5000. Eighty per cent of the patients are male.

Pathology

This condition, also termed 'congenital or aganglionic megacolon', is produced by faulty development

---

[3] Harald Hirschsprung (1830–1916), Professor of Paediatrics, Queen Louisa Hospital, Copenhagen, Denmark.

of the parasympathetic innervation of the distal bowel. There is an absence of ganglion cells in the submucosal plexus of Auerbach[4] and intermyenteric plexus of Meissner[5] affecting the rectum, which sometimes extends into the lower colon and, rarely, affects the whole of the large bowel. The involved segment is spastic, causing a functional obstruction with gross proximal distension of the colon. There is an association with mutations in the *RET* proto-oncogene, among others, probably interacting with another mutant gene, affecting the migration of neural crest cells in the embryo to the gut, where they normally become ganglia.

Clinical features

In the most severe cases, obstructive symptoms commence in the first few days of life with failure to pass meconium; death results if untreated. Less marked examples present with extraordinarily stubborn constipation in infancy and these children survive into adult life with gross abdominal distension and stunted growth. Many untreated infants develop severe, life-threatening enterocolitis within the first 3 months of life.

Rectal examination reveals a narrow, empty rectum above which faecal impaction may be felt; this examination is usually followed by a gush of flatus and faeces.

Special investigations

- *Abdominal X-ray* shows dilated gas-filled loops of bowel throughout the abdomen except in the pelvis.
- *Barium enema* demonstrates the characteristic narrow rectal segment, above which the colon is dilated and full of faeces.
- *Rectal wall biopsy*, deep enough to include the submucosa, is diagnostic showing complete absence of ganglion cells. In difficult cases, a longitudinal full-thickness biopsy is required.

Differential diagnosis

The differential diagnosis is acquired megacolon, a condition of severe constipation commencing usually

at the age of 1–2 years, often in a child with mental disability. Rectal examination in these cases is typical, impacted faeces being present right up to the anal verge. Biopsy of the rectal wall shows normal ganglion cells. This condition is relieved by regular enemas and aperients.

Treatment

If the child is obstructed in the neonatal period, colostomy is performed. Elective surgery is carried out when the infant is 6–9 months old, or until at least 3 months have elapsed after a colostomy has been established. The aganglionic segment is resected and an abdominoperineal pull-through anastomosis performed between normal colon and the anal canal.

It is important at operation to ensure by frozen section histological examination that ganglion cells are present in the remaining colon.

Volvulus neonatorum

This is due to a congenital malrotation of the bowel. The caecum remains high and the midgut mesentery is narrow, and drags across the duodenum, which may thus also be obstructed. Because of the narrow attachment of mesentery, it readily undergoes volvulus. Untreated, the whole of the midgut becomes gangrenous.

Treatment

Laparotomy is performed as soon as possible. The operative procedure comprises untwisting the volvulus, and widening the narrow mesenteric attachment to the retroperitoneum. Adhesions between caecum and duodenum (Ladd's bands[6]) are divided, and the caecum and ascending colon are placed on the left side or in the midline. An appendicectomy is performed if practical, as the unusual position of the appendix may cause diagnostic difficulty in the future.

Necrotizing enterocolitis

This is a condition seen in premature infants and is due to mesenteric ischaemia, which permits bacterial invasion of the mucosa. Terminal ileum, caecum and distal colon are commonly affected. The condition

---

[4] Leopold Auerbach (1828–1897), Neuropathologist, Breslau, Poland.

[5] Georg Meissner (1829–1905), Professor of Physiology, Göttingen, Germany.

[6] William Edwards Ladd (1880–1967), Professor of Pediatric Surgery, Harvard Medical School, Boston, MA, USA.

probably represents the culmination of a number of disorders, such as hypoxia, hypotension and hyperviscosity, which reduce distal perfusion, together with sepsis and the presence of an umbilical artery cannula.

Clinical features

The infant shows signs of generalized sepsis with vomiting and listlessness. The abdomen is distended and tense. Blood and mucus are passed per rectum in over half the cases. The affected bowel may perforate or the condition resolve with stricture formation.

X-rays of the abdomen show distended loops of intestine, and gas bubbles may be seen in the bowel wall and portal vein. Pneumoperitoneum signifies intestinal perforation.

Treatment

Initially, this is medical. The infant is resuscitated and commenced on total parenteral nutrition and broad-spectrum antibiotics. Indications for surgery are failure to respond, profuse intestinal haemorrhage and evidence of perforation or obstruction due to stricture formation. It comprises resection of the frankly gangrenous or perforated segment or segments of intestine with primary anastomosis when possible to avoid stomas, which are difficult to manage in neonates. Mortality remains around 20%.

Meconium ileus

Eighty per cent of infants with meconium ileus have cystic fibrosis (mucoviscidosis), which is a generalized defect of mucus secretion of the intestine, pancreas (fibrocystic pancreatic disease) and bronchial tree. Because of the loss of intestinal mucus and a blockage of pancreatic ducts with loss of enzymatic digestion, the lower ileum of the foetus becomes blocked with inspissated, viscous meconium. Perforation of the bowel may occur in intrauterine life (meconium peritonitis).

Clinical features

The infant presents with acute obstruction in the first days of life, with gross abdominal distension and vomiting. The loop of ileum impacted with meconium may be palpable. X-ray of the abdomen shows, in addition to distended coils of bowel, the typical mottled 'ground-glass' appearance of meconium.

Treatment

It may be possible to clear the meconium by slow instillation of Gastrografin per rectum under X-ray control. This material is radio-opaque and hyperosmolar (drawing fluid into the bowel lumen) and contains a hydrophilic emulsifying agent (polysorbate 80), which facilitates evacuation of the meconium; n-acetyl cysteine via a nasogastric tube may help solubilize any residual meconium. If this fails, or if the bowel has perforated, surgery is indicated. This comprises enterotomy and removal of the inspissated meconium by lavage. Occasionally, the impacted segment of ileum may show areas of gangrene and require resection. In cystic fibrosis, the presentation with meconium ileus is related to absent pancreatic enzyme secretion, so oral enzyme supplements should be started postoperatively.

The long-term prognosis is dictated by the extent to which the chest is affected since, owing to the lack of mucus secretion of the bronchi, recurrent chest infection is almost inevitable. New agents to manage cystic fibrosis, such as Kaftrio[7], are likely to change the outlook for such patients, and may have a role in preventing bowel complications as well.

Distal intestinal obstruction syndrome

Distal intestinal obstruction syndrome (DIOS) is the equivalent of meconium ileus in older patients with cystic fibrosis or others with pancreatic insufficiency. It is characterized by luminal obstruction by a fat-rich bolus. It may also occur in a patient admitted for other causes after being nil by mouth.

Clinical features

Patients present with colicky abdominal pain and vomiting, with distension; there may be a palpable mass in the RIF. Differential diagnosis includes constipation, appendicitis, intussusception and cholecystitis.

---

[7] Kaftrio, also marketed as Trikafta, is a combination of elexacaftor (a chloride channel opener), tezacaftor and ivacaftor (modulators of the cystic fibrosis transmembrane conductance regulator, CFTR) which has been shown to improve lung function in patients with cystic fibrosis.

Plain abdominal X-ray or CT scan demonstrates faecal loading in the right lower quadrant and dilated proximal bowel.

Treatment

Gastrografin, either orally or via a nasogastric tube, is the first line treatment. If that fails then an iso-osmotic polyethylene glycol (PEG) and electrolyte solution may be effective. Surgery may be indicated if non-operative measures fail.

Subsequent treatment includes encouraging a good fluid intake, optimizing pancreatic enzyme replacement and a stool softener such as lactulose.

Intussusception

Definition

An intussusception is the prolapse of one portion of the intestine into the lumen of the immediately adjoining bowel. The prolapsing or invaginating bowel is called the intussusceptum.

Terminology

Different portions of the intestine may form the apex of the intussusception. The common forms are:

- *Ileoileal*: the ileum is invaginated into the adjacent ileum.
- *Ileocolic*: an ileoileal intussusception that extends through the ileocaecal valve into the colon; this is the most common sort (75%).
- *Ileocaecal*: the ileocaecal valve is the apex of the intussusception.
- *Colo-colic*: the colon invaginates into an adjacent colon (usually because of a protruding tumour of the bowel wall).

Aetiology

Ninety-five per cent occur in infants or young children, in whom there is usually no obvious cause. The mesenteric lymph nodes in these patients are invariably enlarged. It is postulated that the lymphoid tissue in Peyer's patches[8] in the bowel wall undergoes hyperplasia because of an adenovirus; the swollen

---

[8] Johann Peyer (1653–1712), Anatomist, Schaffhausen, Switzerland.

lymphoid tissue protrudes into the lumen of the bowel and acts as a 'foreign body', which is then propelled by peristalsis distally along the gut, dragging the bowel behind.

In adults and in some children, a polyp, carcinoma, intestinal lymphoma or an inverted Meckel's diverticulum may form the apex of the intussusception.

The intussusceptum has its blood supply cut off by direct pressure of the outer layer and by stretching of its supplying mesentery so that, if untreated, gangrene will occur.

Clinical features in infants

Intussusception usually occurs in previously healthy children commonly aged between 3 and 12 months. Males are affected twice as often as females.

The history is of paroxysms of abdominal colic typified by screaming and pallor. There is vomiting and usually the passage of blood and/or slime per rectum, giving the appearance of redcurrant jelly. On examination, the child is pale and anxious, and a typical attack of screaming may be observed. Palpation of the abdomen, after sedation if necessary, reveals a sausage-shaped tumour anywhere except in the RIF. Occasionally, the tumour cannot be felt because it is hidden under the costal margin. Rectal examination nearly always reveals 'redcurrant jelly' on the examining finger and, rarely, the tip of the intussusception can be felt. Ultrasound can confirm the diagnosis.

If neglected, after 24 hours the abdomen becomes distended, faeculant vomiting occurs and the child becomes intensely toxic, owing to gangrene of the intussusception and associated peritonitis.

Treatment in infants

Non-operative

Barium or water-soluble contrast is run in per rectum and X-ray confirmation of the diagnosis is established. If the intussusception is recent, it may be completely reduced hydrostatically by the pressure of the column of barium/contrast and this is confirmed radiologically.

Operative

The intussusception is reduced at laparotomy by squeezing its apex backwards out of the containing bowel. In late cases, reduction may be impossible or the bowel may be gangrenous so that resection may be necessary.

Mortality is very low in the first 24 hours but is very high in the irreducible or gangrenous cases. An intussusception may recur in a small percentage of children.

Paralytic ileus

Paralytic (or adynamic or neurogenic) ileus can be defined as a state of atony of the intestine. Its principal clinical features are:

- Abdominal distension.
- Absolute constipation.
- Vomiting.
- Absence of intestinal movements and, hence, absence of colicky pain.

Aetiology

The state of paralytic ileus may be produced by a large number of factors, sometimes co-existing.

- *Peritonitis:* The bowel in peritonitis becomes atonic, perhaps as a result of toxic paralysis of intrinsic nerve plexuses. There may be an associated mechanical obstruction produced by kinking of loops of bowel by fibrinous adhesions, so that frequently the paralytic ileus is complicated by mechanical obstruction.
- *Metabolic factors:* Severe hypokalaemia, uraemia and diabetic ketoacidosis.
- *Neuropathy:* Acute high spinal cord injury or chronic diabetic autonomic neuropathy.
- *Drugs,* e.g. anticholinergic agents, antiparkinsonian drugs, opiates.
- *Abdominal surgery.*

Postoperative ileus

Some degree of paralytic ileus occurs after every laparotomy, with some bowel segments affected more than others. Its aetiology is complex, including sympathetic overaction, the effects of manipulation of the bowel, potassium depletion (when there has been excessive preoperative vomiting), peritoneal irritation from blood or associated peritonitis and the atony of stomach and the large bowel, which occurs after every open abdominal operation for a period. Minimally invasive (laparoscopic and robotic) surgery is associated with a lower risk of ileus developing.

The distension that occurs on the first and second postoperative day is probably produced by swallowed air. This air passes through the small intestine (where peristalsis usually returns quickly) to the colon, which is atonic and produces a functional hold-up.

Paralytic ileus that persists for more than 48 hours postoperatively probably has some other aetiological factor present.

Sequelae

The deleterious effects of paralytic ileus are similar to those of a simple mechanical obstruction.

- There is severe loss of fluid, electrolytes and protein into the gut lumen and in the vomitus or gastric aspirate.
- Gross gaseous distension of the gut, produced mainly from swallowed air that cannot pass through the bowel, impairs the blood supply of the bowel wall and allows toxin absorption to occur.

Clinical features

Paralytic ileus is most commonly seen in the postoperative stage of peritonitis or of major open abdominal surgery. There is abdominal distension, absolute constipation and effortless vomiting. Pain is not present, apart from the discomfort of the laparotomy wound and the abdominal distension. On examination, the patient is anxious and uncomfortable. The abdomen is distended, silent and tender. CT of the abdomen will show gas distributed throughout the small and large bowel and some fluid levels may be present on an erect abdominal X-ray (although rarely performed now).

The paralytic ileus may merge insidiously into a mechanical obstruction produced by adhesions or bands following abdominal surgery, and an important, often extremely difficult, differential diagnosis lies between these two conditions. The diagnosis is important, since paralytic ileus is treated conservatively whereas mechanical obstruction usually calls for urgent operation.

Differential diagnosis

Differentiation of paralytic ileus from mechanical obstruction is based on the following criteria.

- *Duration.* Paralytic ileus rarely lasts more than 3 or 4 days; persistence of symptoms after this time is suggestive of mechanical obstruction.
- *Bowel sounds.* The presence of bowel sounds is important. An absolutely silent abdomen is

diagnostic of paralytic ileus, whereas noisy bowel sounds indicate mechanical obstruction.

- *Pain.* Paralytic ileus is relatively painless, whereas colicky abdominal pain is present in mechanical obstruction.
- *Timing.* If symptoms commence after the patient has already passed flatus or had a bowel action, it is very likely that a mechanical obstruction has supervened. The other possibility to consider is that there has been a leakage from an anastomosis and that peritonitis is now present.
- *Radiological appearances.* A CT scan of the abdomen showing a localized loop of distended small intestine without gas in the colon or rectum is strongly suggestive of mechanical obstruction, in contrast to the diffuse appearance of gas throughout the distended small and large bowel in paralytic ileus.

Treatment

Prophylaxis

Biochemical imbalance is corrected preoperatively. The bowel is handled gently at operation. Postoperatively, gastric distension due to air swallowing may require nasogastric suction.

In the established case

Nasogastric suction is employed to remove swallowed air and prevent gaseous distension. The aspiration of fluid also helps to relieve the associated gastric dilation. Intravenous fluid and electrolyte therapy is instituted with careful biochemical control. Opiate analgesia should be avoided or minimized if possible. Eventually, recovery from the ileus will occur unless it is secondary to some underlying cause, such as infection. Total parenteral nutrition (TPN) should be instituted until the abdominal distension starts to resolve and the bowels start to work. Gentle introduction of enteral feeding can then be started.

In the absence of any evidence of mechanical obstruction or infection, Gastrografin may stimulate resolution, and a CT following Gastrografin may delineate any new pathology. A prolonged stubborn ileus is occasionally treated pharmacologically. Motility stimulants such as metoclopramide or domperidone, together with erythromycin (which stimulates the motilin receptor), may be tried once a mechanical obstruction has been ruled out. Metoclopramide and domperidone are dopamine D2 antagonists that stimulate gastric emptying and small intestinal transit.

Pseudo-obstruction

Pseudo-obstruction, also known as adynamic ileus or Ogilvie's syndrome[9], is a particular form of paralytic ileus which mainly affects the large bowel. It results from interference with the autonomic supply to the gut in which there is predominant sympathetic activity. It typically complicates fractures of the spine or pelvis, retroperitoneal haemorrhage and retroperitoneal surgery, intestinal ischaemia, ureteric colic and occasionally parturition; Ogilvie described it first in patients with malignant infiltration of the coeliac plexus. Usually, the small bowel is unaffected and peristalsis continues and passes intestinal contents into the colon. The large bowel is atonic, so the colon, in particular the caecum, distends enormously, becomes ischaemic and, if unrelieved, may perforate.

Symptoms are typical of large bowel obstruction, with colicky abdominal pain, distension and absolute constipation. Examination confirms abdominal distension, and digital examination reveals a capacious empty rectum.

CT with rectal contrast will confirm the absence of a mechanical obstruction.

Treatment

The patient is given nothing by mouth and identifiable causes, such as electrolyte imbalances, drugs (e.g. opiates, anticholinergics, calcium channel antagonists) are addressed. The colon is decompressed preferably at colonoscopy, although pharmacological treatment using the cholinesterase inhibitor neostigmine may bring resolution; indications for urgent decompression are a caecal diameter >10 cm and a duration >4 days. Oral laxatives, particularly stimulant laxatives, should be avoided since they are likely to precipitate perforation.

◐ Additional resources

---

[9] Sir William Heneage Ogilvie (1887–1971), Surgeon, Guy's Hospital, London, UK.

31

Hernia

Christopher Watson

✓ To know the common sites of abdominal wall hernias, their anatomy, how they present and their treatment.

Definition

A hernia is the protrusion of an organ or part of an organ through a defect in the wall of the cavity containing it, into an abnormal position. The term is usually used with reference to the abdomen.

Abdominal wall hernias

Most hernias occur as a diverticulum of the peritoneal cavity and, therefore, have a sac of parietal peritoneum. The common varieties of hernias through the abdominal wall are listed below in order of frequency; the incidence of femoral hernias appears to have reduced in the last two decades having previously been the second most common hernia referred for surgery:

- Inguinal (indirect or direct).
- Umbilical and paraumbilical.
- Ventral and epigastric.
- Incisional.
- Femoral.

Aetiology

Hernias occur at sites of weakness in the abdominal wall. This weakness may be congenital, for example

persistence of the processus vaginalis of testicular descent giving rise to a congenital inguinal hernia, or failure of complete closure of the umbilical scar leading to an umbilical hernia. It may occur at the site of penetration of structures through the abdominal wall, for example the femoral canal, or the layers of the abdominal wall may be weakened following a surgical incision (incisional hernia), either by poor healing as a result of infection, haematoma formation or poor technique, or by damage to nerves that results in paralysis of the abdominal muscles.

Hernias should also be thought of as portents of other diseases or conditions, as they are often associated with pathological increases in intra-abdominal pressure by conditions such as:

- *Chronic cough*, secondary to chronic obstructive pulmonary disease.
- *Constipation*, perhaps due to hypothyroidism or colonic carcinoma.
- *Urinary obstruction*, due to prostatic disease.
- *Pregnancy*.
- *Abdominal distension* with ascites.
- *Weak abdominal muscles*, for example in morbid obesity or muscle wasting in cachexia and liver failure.

Varieties

A hernia at any site may be (Figure 31.1):

- Reducible.
- Irreducible.
- Strangulated.

Ellis and Calne's Lecture Notes in General Surgery, Fourteenth Edition.
Edited by Christopher Watson and Justin Davies.
© 2023 John Wiley & Sons Ltd. Published 2023 by John Wiley & Sons Ltd.
Companion website: www.wiley.com/go/Watson/GeneralSurgery14

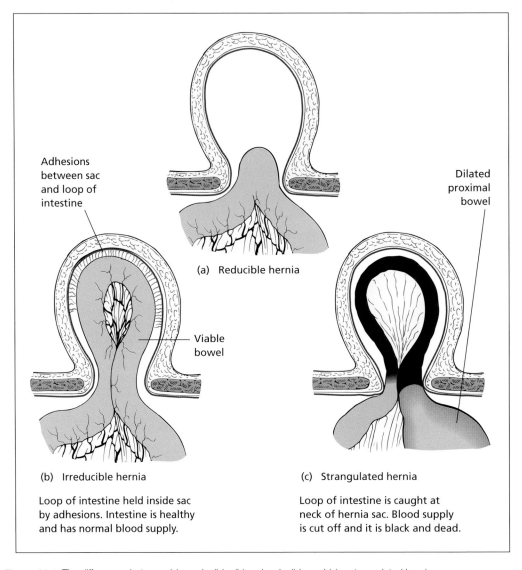

Figure 31.1 The differences between (a) a reducible, (b) an irreducible and (c) a strangulated hernia.

Reducible hernia

The contents of a reducible hernia can be replaced completely into the peritoneal cavity.

Irreducible hernia

A hernia becomes irreducible (incarcerated) usually because of adhesions of its contents to the inner wall of the sac, or sometimes as a result of adhesions of its contents to each other to form a mass greater in size than the neck of the sac. Occasionally, inspissated faeces within the loops of bowel in the hernia prevent reduction.

Strangulated hernia

When strangulation occurs, the contents of the hernia are constricted by the neck of the sac to such a degree that their circulation is cut off. Unless relieved, gangrene is inevitable and, if gut is involved, perforation of the gangrenous loop will eventually occur.

Clinical features

Reducible hernia (Box 31.1)

A reducible hernia simply presents as a lump that may disappear on lying down and that is usually not painful, although it may be accompanied by some discomfort. Examination reveals a reducible lump with a cough impulse.

Irreducible hernia

An irreducible hernia will not reduce on lying, but is painless and there are no other symptoms.

Strangulated hernia

If strangulation supervenes, the patient complains of severe pain in the hernia and also of central abdominal colicky pain. The other symptoms of intestinal obstruction – vomiting, distension and absolute constipation – soon appear. Examination reveals a tender, tense hernia that cannot be reduced and has no cough impulse. The absence of a cough impulse alone does not indicate strangulation, because, for example, the neck of the hernia may be plugged by omentum, which prevents the cough impulse from being felt.

The overlying skin becomes red, inflamed and oedematous and there are other features of intestinal obstruction with abdominal tenderness and noisy bowel sounds. These features are much less marked when omentum rather than intestine is contained within the sac.

The three common types of hernia to strangulate are, in order of frequency, femoral, indirect inguinal and umbilical.

Inguinal hernia

This may be classified into:

- *Indirect*: entering the deep (internal) inguinal ring and traversing the inguinal canal.
- *Direct*: pushing through the posterior wall of the inguinal canal medial to the deep ring, medial to the inferior epigastric vessels.

See Table 31.1 for a summary of the differences between indirect and direct inguinal hernias.

The anatomy of the inguinal canal is the key to the understanding of these hernias.

Anatomy (Figure 31.2)

The inguinal canal represents the oblique passage taken through the lower abdominal wall by the testis and cord in the male and the round ligament in the female. It is 4 cm long and passes downwards and medially, and from deep to superficial, from the deep to the external inguinal rings, lying parallel to, and immediately above, the inguinal ligament.

- *Anteriorly*: skin, superficial fascia and external oblique aponeurosis cover the full length of the canal; the internal oblique covers its lateral third.
- *Posteriorly*: the conjoint tendon (representing the fused common aponeurotic insertion of the internal oblique and transversus abdominis muscles into the pubic crest) forms the posterior wall of the canal medially; the transversalis fascia lies laterally.
- *Above*: the lowest fibres of the internal oblique and transversus abdominis.
- *Below*: lies the inguinal ligament.

The deep ring represents the point at which the spermatic cord pushes through the transversalis fascia; it is demarcated medially by the inferior epigastric vessels as they pass upwards from the external iliac artery and vein.

The external ring is an inverted V-shaped defect in the external oblique aponeurosis and lies immediately above and medial to the pubic tubercle.

The inguinal canal contains the spermatic cord in males and the round ligament in females, and the ilioinguinal nerve.

Indirect inguinal hernia

This passes through the internal ring, along the canal in front of the spermatic cord or round ligament and, if large enough, emerges through the external ring and descends into the scrotum or labia majora. If reducible, such a hernia can be completely controlled by pressure with one fingertip over the deep inguinal ring, which lies 1–2 cm above the point where the femoral artery passes under the inguinal ligament, that is, 1–2 cm above the femoral pulse. This can be felt at the mid-inguinal point, halfway between the anterior superior iliac spine and the symphysis pubis.

If the hernia protrudes through the external ring, it can be felt to lie above and medial to the pubic tubercle here the sac is formed as an outpushing of the abdominal peritoneum.

The narrow internal opening through the deep inguinal ring accounts for two important features of the indirect hernia. First, the hernia often does not reach its full size until the patient has been up and about for a little time, and then does not reduce immediately when the patient lies down, because it takes a little time for the hernial contents to pass in or out of the sac through its narrow neck. Second, the indirect hernia has a distinct tendency to strangulate at the site of this narrow orifice.

Direct inguinal hernia

This pushes its way directly forwards through the posterior wall of the inguinal canal. Because it lies medial to the deep ring, it is not controlled by digital pressure applied over the ring immediately above the femoral pulse. On inspection, the hernia is seen to protrude directly forwards (hence its name), compared with the oblique route downwards towards the scrotum of an indirect inguinal hernia.

Other points that differentiate a direct from an indirect hernia are that the direct is always acquired and is, therefore, extremely rare in infancy or adolescence; it usually has a large orifice and, therefore, appears immediately on standing, disappearing again at once when the patient lies down. Moreover, because of this large opening, strangulation is extremely rare. It is uncommon in women.

Although clinically it is usually quite easy to tell the difference between the two types of inguinal hernia, the ultimate differentiation can only be made at operation. The inferior epigastric vessels demarcate

and is thus differentiated from a femoral hernia, which emerges through the femoral canal below and lateral to this landmark (Figure 31.3).

Indirect hernias may be congenital, due to persistence of the processus vaginalis; these present at or soon after birth or may arise in adolescence. The acquired variety may occur at any age in adult life and

Table 31.1 Characteristic differences that help differentiate indirect and direct inguinal hernias

	Indirect	Direct
Origin	Pass through the deep ring, lateral to the inferior epigastric vessels.	Pass through posterior wall of inguinal canal, medial to inferior epigastric vessels.
Congenital or acquired	May be congenital.	Always acquired, rare in childhood and adolescence.
Control by pressure over deep ring	Yes.	No.
Strangulates	Commonly, because of narrow neck (deep ring).	Rarely, because usually wide-necked.
Extends down into scrotum	Often.	Rarely.
Reduces on lying	Not readily.	Spontaneously.

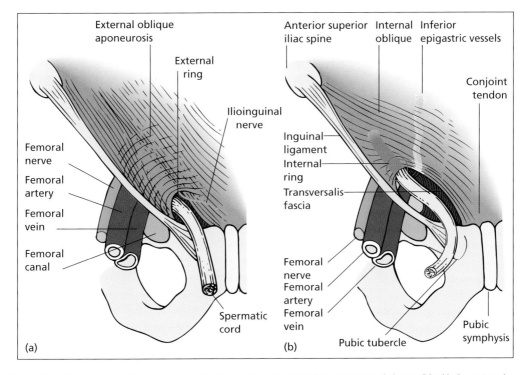

Figure 31.2 The anatomy of the inguinal canal: (a) with the external oblique aponeurosis intact; (b) with the external oblique removed.

the medial edge of the internal ring; therefore, an indirect sac will pass lateral, and a direct hernia medial, to these vessels. Quite often, a direct and an indirect hernia co-exist; they bulge on either side of the inferior epigastric vessels like the legs of a pair of trousers, and are thus known as a 'pantaloon' hernias.

Sixty per cent of inguinal hernias occur on the right side, 20% on the left and 20% are bilateral. The right-sided preponderance may relate to the right testis being the last to descend, and possible persistence of a patent remnant of the processus vaginalis.

Treatment

Investigation is usually unnecessary, since clinical examination should suffice. However, where the hernia is not apparent, it is worth sending the patient away to walk around for 5 min before re-examining afterwards. If the hernia is still not visible, ultrasonography may detect it and ascertain whether direct or indirect, or identify a lipoma of the cord as the culprit.

Congenital inguinal hernias in infants do not obliterate spontaneously; the patent processus

vaginalis is ligated and the hernial sac excised at the age of about one year (herniotomy). In adults, operation is usually advised if the hernia is causing symptoms. This comprises excision of the sac and repair of the weakened inguinal canal, commonly performed by reinforcing the posterior wall with a polypropylene mesh (Lichtenstein repair[1]). An alternative technique is to place a mesh from within the abdomen laparoscopically, covering the hernial orifice. The laparoscopic technique has particular advantages in the treatment of recurrent or bilateral hernias.

A truss is only advised in patients who are in very poor general condition and are unable to withstand an operation, although they often have difficulty keeping a truss correctly in place. Even in such cases, a painful hernia that threatens strangulation is much better repaired as an elective procedure, if necessary under local anaesthesia, rather than as an emergency when strangulation has supervened.

[1] Irving L. Lichtenstein (1920–2000), Surgeon, Cedars-Sinai Medical Center, Los Angeles, CA, USA.

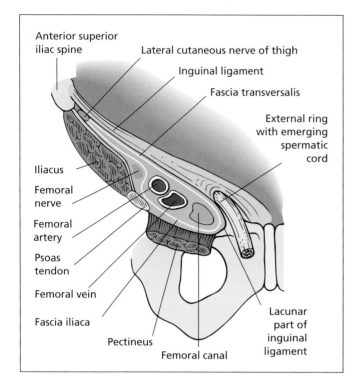

Figure 31.3 The anatomy of the femoral canal and its surrounds to show the relationships of a femoral hernia.

Recurrent inguinal hernias may be caused by, for example, infection, haematoma or poor surgical technique, and also by a failure to appreciate the underlying cause of the increased intra-abdominal pressure that initiated the hernia in the first place (e.g. continuing constipation or bladder neck obstruction by a large prostate).

Femoral hernia

Anatomy

A femoral hernia passes through the femoral canal. This is a gap normally about 1.5 cm in length, which just admits the tip of the little finger and which lies at the medial extremity of the femoral sheath containing the femoral artery and vein. The boundaries of the femoral canal are as follows (see Figure 31.3).

- *Anteriorly*: the inguinal ligament.
- *Medially*: the sharp edge of the lacunar part of the inguinal ligament (Gimbernat's ligament[2]).
- *Laterally*: the femoral vein.

- *Posteriorly*: the pectineal ligament (of Cooper[3]), which is the thickened periosteum along the superior pubic ramus.

The canal contains a plug of fat and a lymph node (the node of Cloquet[4]).

Clinical features

Femoral hernias occur more commonly in women than in men because of the wider female pelvis (but note that indirect inguinal hernias are more common than femoral hernias in women). They are never due to a congenital sac but are invariably acquired; although cases do rarely occur in children, they are usually seen in the middle-aged and elderly.

A non-strangulated hernia presents as a globular swelling below and lateral to the pubic tubercle. It enlarges on standing and on coughing and may disappear when the patient lies down. In most cases, even when the hernia is completely reduced, a swelling

[2] Manuel Gimbernat (1734–1816), Anatomist and Surgeon to King Carlos III of Spain.

[3] Sir Astley Paston Cooper (1768–1841), Surgeon, Guy's Hospital, London, UK.

[4] Jules Germain Cloquet (1790–1883), Professor of Surgery, Paris, France.

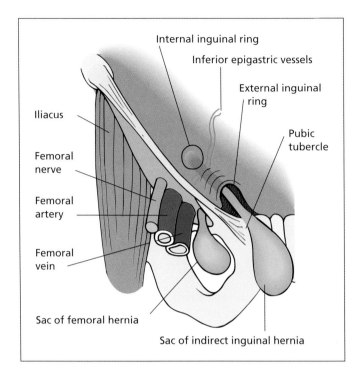

Figure 31.4 The relationships of an indirect inguinal and a femoral hernia compared. The inguinal hernia emerges above and medial to the public tubercle; the femoral hernia lies below and lateral to it.

can still be palpated and this is due to extraperitoneal fat around the femoral sac.

As the hernia enlarges, it passes through the saphenous opening in the deep fascia (the site of penetration of the great saphenous vein to join the femoral vein), and then turns upwards so that it may project above the inguinal ligament. There should not, however, be any difficulty in differentiating between an irreducible femoral and inguinal hernia – the neck of a femoral hernia always lies below and lateral to the pubic tubercle, whereas the sac of an indirect inguinal hernia extends above and medial to this landmark (Figure 31.4).

The neck of the femoral canal is narrow and has a particularly sharp medial border. For this reason, irreducibility and strangulation are extremely common in this type of hernia.

Richter's hernia

A Richter's hernia[5] is particularly likely to occur in the femoral sac. In this type of hernia, only part of the wall of the small intestine herniates through the defect,

[5] August Gottlieb Richter (1742–1842), Surgeon, Göttingen, Germany.

where it is then strangulated. Because the lumen of the bowel is not completely encroached upon, symptoms of intestinal obstruction do not occur, although the knuckle of bowel may become completely necrotic and indeed perforate into the hernial sac and thence into the peritoneal cavity, causing acute peritonitis.

Treatment

All femoral hernias should be repaired by excision of the sac and closure of the femoral canal because of their great danger of strangulation. This may be readily accomplished by open or laparoscopic mesh repair.

Umbilical hernia

Exomphalos

This is a rare condition in which there is failure of all or part of the midgut to return to the abdominal cavity in foetal life. The bowel is contained within a translucent sac protruding through a defective anterior abdominal wall. Untreated, this ruptures with fatal peritonitis, or rupture may occur during delivery. The condition is commonly associated with other congenital anomalies.

Treatment

For small defects less than 4 cm (exomphalos minor) and only containing intestine, immediate surgical repair is undertaken. When the opening is more than 4 cm (exomphalos major) or the liver is within the cord, exomphalos a plastic covering (termed a 'silo') is placed over the viscera and the exomphalos closed in stages over a period of days to weeks, during which the child grows creating more space inside into which the viscera are replaced. While most babies make a full recovery, being very premature or having other physical or genetic conditions are poor prognostic features.

Congenital umbilical hernia

This results from failure of complete closure of the umbilical cicatrix. It is especially common in premature children. The vast majority close spontaneously during the first year of life.

Treatment

Surgical repair should not be carried out unless the hernia persists after the child is 2 years old. The parents of an infant with a congenital umbilical hernia should be reassured that the majority disappear spontaneously. Strapping the hernia or providing a rubber truss are generally not indicated.

Paraumbilical hernia

This is an acquired hernia that occurs just above or below the umbilicus. Although not strictly an umbilical hernia, that term is often used to describe a paraumbilical hernia. It is associated with obesity and is more common in multiparous women. The neck is narrow and, like a femoral hernia, it is particularly prone to become irreducible or strangulated. The contents are nearly always pre-peritoneal fat or omentum; large hernias may contain transverse colon and/or small intestine.

In patients with ascites, a paraumbilical hernia often progresses to one characterized by complete eversion of the cicatrix and appearing as a true umbilical hernia. Repair of such hernias needs careful consideration of the underlying medical condition that caused it.

Paraumbilical incisional hernias are also commonly seen where the hernia has protruded through a defect in the fascia made during laparoscopic surgery, and present in a similar way.

Treatment

The sac is isolated, excised and the edges of the rectus sheath may be opposed or overlapped above and below the hernia (Mayo's operation[6]), or, for defects over 1 cm in size, a polypropylene mesh can be incorporated into the repair via an open or laparoscopic approach.

Divarication of the recti

Divarication of the recti (diastasis recti) is where the fascia between the two rectus sheaths is stretched, leaving a gap between the two rectus abdominis muscles. The result is a midline ridge, predominantly in the upper abdomen between xiphoid and umbilicus, most marked on coughing or raising both legs while lying. It is associated with pregnancy and other causes of abdominal distension. It is not a true hernia, and in the majority of cases requires no treatment.

Epigastric hernia

A particular variety of ventral hernia is the epigastric hernia, which consists of one or more small protrusions through defects in the linea alba above the umbilicus. These usually contain only extraperitoneal fat, but are often surprisingly painful.

Treatment

Simply suturing of the defect is all that is required if it is small. Larger defects are likely to need a mesh repair, and this can be considered via an open or laparoscopic approach.

[6] William Mayo (1861–1939), Surgeon, Rochester, MN, USA. He first described this technique in a presentation to the American Academy of Railway Surgeons in 1895.

Incisional hernia

An incisional hernia occurs through a defect in the scar of a previous abdominal operation. The causes, which are the same as those of a burst abdomen, are given in Chapter 5.

There is usually a wide neck, and strangulation is, in consequence, uncommon.

Treatment

If the general condition of the patient is good and the hernia symptomatic, the hernia is repaired by dissecting out the defect and reducing the sac. Defects are closed with a sheet of mesh, ideally avoiding direct contact of the mesh with bowel which, if it occurs, can result in fistula formation. Surgery can be performed via an open or laparoscopic approach. If operation is considered inadvisable, an abdominal binder may be advised.

Differential diagnosis of midline hernia

Endometrioma of the abdominal wall

Although not a hernia as such, midline endometriomas are often mistaken for hernias. After a Caesarean section through either a Pfannenstiel or lower midline incision, endometrium seeds into the linea alba where it has been divided to allow access to the gravid uterus, where it slowly grows, presenting many months or years after the pregnancy. There may be associated cyclical pain, but this is not common. Examination reveals a non-reducible, midline lump attached deeply. The solid soft tissue mass can be confirmed on ultrasound or computed tomography (CT) scan. Needle core biopsy often reveals fibrotic tissue, but may contain endometrial fragments. Treatment is simple excision.

Unusual hernias

Obturator hernia

These are found particularly in thin, elderly women and usually present with acute intestinal obstruction. The hernia develops through the obturator canal where the obturator nerve and vessels traverse the membrane covering the obturator foramen. Pressure of a strangulated obturator hernia upon the nerve may cause referred pain in its area of cutaneous distribution, so that intestinal obstruction associated with pain along the medial side of the thigh in a thin, elderly woman should suggest this diagnosis. The hernia is often of the Richter type. CT will confirm the diagnosis.

Spigelian hernia

A Spigelian hernia[7] passes upwards through a defect in the transversus abdominis aponeurosis (Spigelian fascia) at the lateral margin of the rectus sheath, usually adjacent to the arcuate (semilunar) line, caudal to which the posterior wall of the rectus sheath is deficient. Typically, it passes laterally through the transversus abdominis fascia and internal oblique, but beneath the external oblique aponeurosis (as such, it is an example of an *interparietal hernia*, one that passes between the layers of the abdominal wall). It presents as a tender mass to one side of the lower abdominal wall, but can be surprisingly difficult to identify clinically. Ultrasound or CT will confirm the diagnosis if doubt exists. Spigelian hernias usually have a narrow neck and thus are prone to obstruct so repair is advised.

Gluteal hernia

Traverses the greater sciatic foramen.

Sciatic hernia

Passes through the lesser sciatic foramen.

Lumbar hernia

A lumbar hernia is most commonly an incisional hernia following an open operation on the kidney, but may rarely occur through the inferior lumbar triangle bounded by the crest of the ilium below, the latissimus dorsi medially and the external oblique on the lateral side.

Parastomal hernia

Passes through the same defect in the abdominal wall that was made to bring the bowel out as a stoma.

---

[7] Adriaan van den Spiegel (Spigelius) (1578–1625), Professor of Anatomy and Surgery, Padua, Italy.

Diaphragmatic hernias

The diaphragmatic hernias can be classified as follows.

1   *Congenital*.
2   *Acquired*:
    a   Traumatic.
    b   Hiatal.

Congenital diaphragmatic hernia

Embryology

These hernias can best be understood by reference to the embryology of the diaphragm (Figure 31.5). The diaphragm is developed by fusion of the following.

- *The septum transversum*, which forms the central tendon, and which develops from mesoderm lying in front of the head of the embryo. With the folding of the head, this mesodermal mass is carried ventrally and caudally to lie in its definitive position at the anterior part of the diaphragm. During this migration, the cervical myotomes and cervical nerves contribute muscle and nerve supply, respectively (C3, 4, 5), thus accounting for the long course of the phrenic nerve from the neck to the diaphragm.
- *The dorsal oesophageal mesentery*.
- *The pleuroperitoneal membranes*, which close the primitive communication between the pleural and peritoneal cavities.
- *A peripheral rim* derived from the body wall.

In spite of this complex story, congenital abnormalities of the diaphragm are unusual. They may manifest as hernias through the following defects:

- The foramen of Morgagni,[8] between the xiphoid and costal origins.
- The foramen of Bochdalek,[9] a defect in the pleuroperitoneal canal.
- A deficiency of the whole central tendon.
- A congenitally large oesophageal hiatus.

[8] Giovanni Battista Morgagni (1682–1771), Professor of Anatomy, Padua, Italy.

[9] Vincent Bochdalek (1801–1883), Professor of Anatomy, Prague, Czech Republic.

Clinical features

Hernias through the foramen of Morgagni are usually small and unimportant. Those through the foramen of Bochdalek or through the central tendon are large and present as respiratory distress shortly after birth. Urgent surgical repair is required.

The congenital hiatal hernias present with regurgitation, vomiting, dysphagia and progressive loss of weight in small children; they usually respond to conservative treatment and nursing the child in a sitting position. If this fails, surgical repair is necessary.

Traumatic diaphragmatic hernias

These are comparatively rare and follow blunt (crush) injuries to the chest or abdomen, or penetrating injuries such as stab wounds, which implicate the diaphragm. The left diaphragm is far more often affected than the right (which is protected by the liver) and is accompanied by herniation of the stomach and spleen into the thoracic cavity. The gas-filled stomach lying in the left chest after a crush injury may be mistaken for a tension pneumothorax on chest X-ray. Passage of a nasogastric tube or ingestion of a small amount of contrast material confirms the diagnosis.

Treatment comprises urgent surgical repair, through either the chest or abdomen.

Acquired hiatal hernias

Classification

These are divided into:

- Sliding (90%).
- Rolling (10%).

In the *sliding* variety, the stomach slides through the hiatus and is covered in its anterior aspect with a peritoneal sac while the posterior part is extraperitoneal. It thus resembles an inguinal hernia *en glissade* (Figure 31.6a). This type of hernia produces both the effects of a space-occupying lesion in the chest and disturbances of the cardio-oesophageal sphincter mechanism.

In the *rolling* (or paraoesophageal) hernia, the cardia remains in position but the stomach rolls up

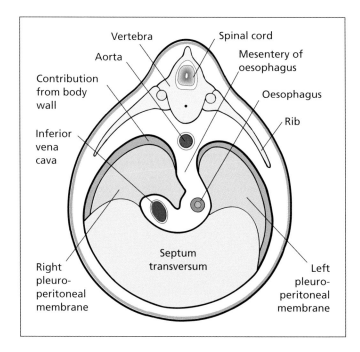

Figure 31.5 The development of the diaphragm. The drawing shows the four contributory elements: septum transversum, dorsal mesentery of the oesophagus, body wall and pleuroperitoneal membrane.

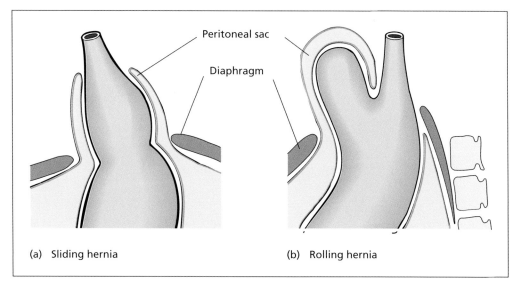

Figure 31.6 (a) Sliding hiatus hernia: the stomach and lower oesophagus slide into the chest through a patulous oesophageal hiatus. (b) Rolling hiatus hernia: the stomach rolls up through the hiatus alongside the lower oesophagus (paraoesophageal hernia).

anteriorly through the hiatus, producing a partial volvulus. Because the cardio-oesophageal mechanism is intact, there are no symptoms of regurgitation (Figure 31.6b).

These hernias probably represent a progressive weakening of the muscles of the hiatus. They occur in the obese, middle-aged and elderly, and are four times more common in women than in men.

Clinical features

Most are symptomless but when they occur, symptoms fall into three groups.

1   *Mechanical*, produced by the presence of the hernia within the thoracic cavity: cough, dyspnoea, palpitations, hiccough.
2   *Reflux*, resulting from incompetence of the cardiac sphincter: burning retrosternal or epigastric pain aggravated by lying down or stooping, and which may be referred to the jaw or arms, thus simulating myocardial ischaemia. Alkalis provide relief. In severe cases, spill over into the trachea may cause pneumonitis.
3   *The effects of oesophagitis*: stricture formation with dysphagia and bleeding, which may be acute or occult.

Treatment

Sliding hiatus hernias are treated symptomatically; if symptoms of reflux and oesophagitis are troublesome, laparoscopic repair is performed, otherwise they may be left. Paraoesophageal (rolling) hernias are usually asymptomatic, but potentially more serious with the risk of complete gastric volvulus into the chest. Should this occur, urgent surgical repair is indicated.

Reflux oesophagitis

This is discussed in Chapter 22.

Additional resources

Case 81: A large swelling in the groin
Case 82: A groin lump in an old woman
Case 83: A lump at the umbilicus
Case 84: A swelling in the abdominal wall

32

The liver

Raaj Kumar Praseedom

Learning objectives

✓ To know the common causes of liver enlargement.

✓ To understand the different causes of jaundice, and how they may be diagnosed and treated.

✓ To have knowledge of cirrhosis, its various manifestations and their management.

Liver enlargement

Physical signs

The normal liver in the adult is impalpable. In contrast, an infant's liver is normally palpable two finger breadths below the right costal margin. The enlarged liver extends downwards below the right costal margin and may fill the subcostal angle or even extend beneath the left costal margin in gross hepatomegaly. The liver moves with respiration, is dull to percussion and the liver dullness may extend above the normal upper level of the fifth right intercostal space.

Causes of hepatomegaly

1 *Congenital*:
   a Riedel's lobe[1] (rare).
   b Polycystic liver disease (which develops in adult life).

2 *Acquired*:
   a Marked steatosis (fatty liver disease, poorly controlled diabetes).
   b Neoplastic – primary or secondary tumour, lymphoma.
   c Cirrhosis.
   d Hepatic venous outflow limitation – congestive cardiac failure and Budd–Chiari syndrome.[2]
   e Liver infiltration – lymphoma, glycogen storage diseases (e.g. Gaucher's disease[3]), amyloid.

Whenever the liver is palpable, the patient must be examined to detect any accompanying splenomegaly, lymphadenopathy or abdominal masses. If the spleen is palpable in addition to the liver, consider cirrhosis, haematological malignancy, amyloid or unusual infections as possible diagnoses. If, in addition, the lymph nodes are enlarged, the diagnosis is often lymphoma.

Jaundice

The normal serum bilirubin is below 17 μmol/L (1 mg/dL). Excess bilirubin becomes clinically

---

[1]Bernhard Riedel (1846–1916), Professor of Surgery, Jena, Germany. Also described Riedel's thyroiditis.

Ellis and Calne's Lecture Notes in General Surgery, Fourteenth Edition. Edited by Christopher Watson and Justin Davies.
© 2023 John Wiley & Sons Ltd. Published 2023 by John Wiley & Sons Ltd.
Companion website: www.wiley.com/go/Watson/GeneralSurgery14

[2]George Budd (1808–1882), Professor of Medicine, King's College, London, UK. Hans Chiari (1851–1916), Professor of Pathology, Prague, Czech Republic.
[3]Phillipe Gaucher (1854–1918), Physician, Hôpital St Louis, Paris, France.

detectable when the serum level rises to over 35 μmol/L (2 mg/dL), and gives a yellow tinge to the sclera and skin, termed 'jaundice' (or 'icterus').

Bilirubin metabolism (Figure 32.1)

Knowledge of bile pigment metabolism and excretion is essential if the pathogenesis, presentation, investigation and treatment of jaundice are to be understood.

When red cells reach the end of their life in the circulation (approximately 120 days), they are destroyed in the reticuloendothelial system. The porphyrin ring of the haemoglobin molecule is disrupted and a bilirubin–iron–globin complex produced. The iron is released and used for further haemoglobin synthesis. The bilirubin–globin fraction reaches the liver as a lipid-soluble, water-insoluble substance. In the liver, the bilirubin is conjugated with glucuronic acid in the hepatocytes and excreted in the bile as the now water-soluble bilirubin glucuronide.

In the bowel lumen, bilirubin is reduced by bacterial action to the colourless urobilinogen. Most of the

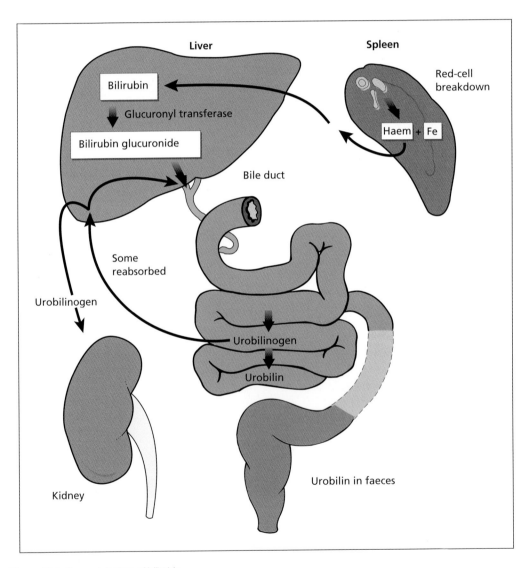

Figure 32.1 The metabolism of bilirubin.

urobilinogen is excreted in the faeces, where it is broken down into urobilin, which is pigmented and which, with the other breakdown products of bilirubin, gives the stool its normal colour.

A small amount of urobilinogen is reabsorbed from the intestine into the portal venous tributaries and passes to the liver, where most of it is excreted once more in the bile back into the gut. Some, however, reaches the systemic circulation and this is excreted by the kidney into the urine. When urine is exposed to air, the urobilinogen it contains is oxidized to urobilin, which is darker.

Physiological neonatal jaundice occurs in 60% of term and 80% of preterm infants. It is explained by the shorter life span of foetal red cells (80–90 days compared to 100–120 days in adults), probably combined with low activity of the enzymes that normally convert unconjugated to conjugated bilirubin; absence of intestinal flora to convert bilirubin to urobilinogen may also play a role, resulting in a high absorption of bilirubin into the circulation.

Classification and pathogenesis

The causes of jaundice are classified according to which was the abnormal stage in the metabolism of bilirubin that resulted in its accumulation.

Prehepatic jaundice

Increased production of (unconjugated) bilirubin by the reticuloendothelial system, as may result from excessive destruction of red cells in haemolysis, exceeds the ability of the liver to conjugate; therefore, the unconjugated bilirubin accumulates in the blood. There is no increase in conjugated bilirubin in the blood, so none is found in the urine. However, there is an increase in the amount of urobilinogen produced in the gut, so more is resorbed and 'overflows' into the systemic circulation, where it is excreted by the kidney.

Hepatic jaundice

In the presence of hepatocellular damage, the liver is unable to conjugate bilirubin efficiently, and less is excreted into the canaliculi. Thus, both unconjugated and conjugated bilirubin accumulate in the blood.

Posthepatic (obstructive) jaundice

Obstruction of the intrahepatic or extrahepatic bile ducts prevents excretion of conjugated bilirubin.

Without pigment, the stools become pale, and the conjugated bilirubin builds up in the blood and is excreted in the urine, turning it dark brown.

Sometimes the hepatic and posthepatic forms coexist. For example, a stone in the common bile duct may produce jaundice partly by obstructing the outflow of bile and partly by secondary damage to the liver (biliary cirrhosis). Similarly, tumour deposits in the liver and cirrhosis may both result in jaundice partly by actual destruction of liver tissue and partly by intrahepatic duct compression.

Causes

Prehepatic jaundice

This is caused by increased production of bilirubin owing to increased red blood cell destruction. The most common cause is haemolysis (e.g. spherocytosis or incompatible blood transfusion), but it may occur during reabsorption of a large haematoma.

Hepatic jaundice

This is a result of impaired bilirubin conjugation owing to the following:

- Hepatitis: viral (hepatitis viruses A, B, C, E), leptospirosis, glandular fever (infectious mononucleosis).
- Cirrhosis.
- Cholestasis from drugs, for example flucloxacillin, chlorpromazine.
- Liver poisons, for example paracetamol overdose, chlorinated hydrocarbons such as carbon tetrachloride, chloroform and halothane; phosphorus.
- Liver tumours, where most of the parenchyma is replaced by deposits.
- Sepsis.

Posthepatic jaundice

This is caused by obstruction to biliary drainage owing to the following.

1 *Obstruction within the lumen*: gallstones.
2 *Pathology in the wall*:
   a Congenital atresia of the common bile duct.
   b Tumour of the bile duct (cholangiocarcinoma).
   c Primary or secondary sclerosing cholangitis.
   d Traumatic stricture (often iatrogenic).
3 *External compression*:
   a Tumour of the head of the pancreas.
   b Tumour of the ampulla of Vater.

c Hilar lymphadenopathy.

d Pancreatitis.

Diagnosis

This is based on history, examination and special investigations.

History

A family history of anaemia, splenectomy or gallstones suggests a congenital red cell defect. Clay-coloured stools, dark urine and itching accompanying the episodes of jaundice indicate hepatic or posthepatic causes. Enquire after recent blood transfusions, intra-muscular/intravenous injections, drugs (antibiotics, chlorpromazine, non-steroidal anti-inflammatories [NSAIDs], methyldopa, repeated exposure to halo-thane, herbal medicines), injections and alcohol consumption. Has there been contact with cases of viral hepatitis? What is the patient's occupation? (Farmers and sewer workers are at risk of leptospirosis – Weil's disease [4]). Enquire about recent travel and unprotected sexual intercourse to rule out infections such as schistosomiasis, hepatitis A and hepatitis B.

Usually, painless jaundice of sudden onset with liver tenderness in a young person is viral in origin. However, painless jaundice associated with weight loss should immediately alert to the possibility of tumour obstructing the bile duct. Attacks of severe colic and intermittent jaundice suggest a stone, with rigors indicating infection. A short, progressive history of jaundice, particularly accompanied by continuous pain radiating to the back, is suspicious of pancreatic cancer. Recent onset of diabetes can also suggest carcinoma of the pancreas.

Examination

The colour of the jaundice is important; a lemon yellow tinge suggests haemolytic jaundice (owing to combined anaemia and mild icterus). Deep jaundice suggests the hepatic or posthepatic types.

Signs of cirrhosis should be sought: spider naevi, gynaecomastia, distended superficial abdominal wall veins, testicular atrophy, encephalopathy, spleno-megaly, liver palms, flapping tremor, leuconychia (white nails) and, occasionally, finger clubbing. There

may also be ascites and leg oedema, but these may be associated with intra-abdominal malignant disease as well as cirrhosis.

Examination of the liver itself is helpful. In viral hepatitis, the liver is slightly enlarged and tender; in cirrhosis, the liver edge is firm and may be irregular, although the liver may be shrunken and impalpable. A grossly enlarged, knobbly liver may also be present in malignant disease.

If the gallbladder is palpable and distended, it is probable that the cause of the jaundice is not a stone (Courvoisier's law;[5] see Chapter 33). The liver may be smoothly enlarged in posthepatic obstructive jaundice.

A separate primary focus of malignant disease may be obvious, inside or outside the abdomen, for example a melanoma.

Splenomegaly suggests cirrhosis of the liver, blood disease or a lymphoma. In the latter, there may also be obvious lymphadenopathy.

Special investigations (Table 32.1)

The prehepatic causes of jaundice are relatively easy to distinguish from hepatic and posthepatic, but the last two are often very difficult to differentiate one from the other and, as already stated, may be associated with each other. Laboratory tests are of some help but are by no means diagnostic. Imaging techniques are valuable in visualizing the liver, gallbladder and pancreas, whereas endoscopic cannulation of the bile ducts or transhepatic duct puncture enables the bile duct system to be outlined. Percutaneous biopsy will usually confirm the hepatic cause of jaundice.

Bilirubin is not excreted by the kidney except in its water-soluble (conjugated) form. It is, therefore, absent from the urine in prehepatic jaundice (hence the old term 'acholuric jaundice'), although present when there is posthepatic obstruction.

In *prehepatic jaundice*, large amounts of bilirubin are excreted into the gut; therefore, the urobilinogen in the faeces is raised, the amount absorbed from the bowel increases and there is, therefore, greater spill over into the urine.

In *hepatic damage*, the urinary urobilinogen may also be raised because of the inability of the liver to re-excrete the urobilinogen reabsorbed from the bowel.

---

[4]Adolf Weil (1848–1916), Professor of Medicine, Berlin, Germany.

[5]Ludwig Courvoisier (1843–1918), Professor of Surgery, Basle, Switzerland.

Table 32.1 Diagnosis of jaundice

Test	Prehepatic	Hepatic	Obstructive
Urine	Urobilinogen.	Urobilinogen.	No urobilinogen. Bilirubin present.
Serum bilirubin	Unconjugated bilirubin.	Conjugated and unconjugated.	Conjugated bilirubin.
ALT (SGPT) and AST (SGOT)	Normal.	Raised.	Normal or moderately raised.
ALP	Normal.	Normal or moderately raised.	Raised.
Blood glucose	Normal.	Low if liver failure.	Sometimes raised if pancreatic tumour.
Reticulocyte count	Raised in haemolysis.	Normal.	Normal.
Haptoglobins	Low due to haemolysis.	Normal or low if liver failure.	Normal.
Prothrombin time	Normal.	Prolonged due to poor synthetic function.	Prolonged due to vitamin K malabsorption; corrects with vitamin K.
Ultrasound	Normal.	May be abnormal liver texture, e.g. cirrhosis.	Dilated bile ducts.

ALP, alkaline phosphatase; ALT, alanine transaminase, formerly known as SGPT, serum glutamic pyruvic transaminase; AST, aspartate transaminase, formally known as SGOT, serum glutamic oxaloacetic transaminase.

In *posthepatic obstruction*, very little bile can enter the gut; therefore, the urobilinogen must be low in both the faeces and the urine.

The important laboratory findings in the various types of jaundice can now be summarized.

- *Urine*: the presence of bilirubin indicates obstructive jaundice, either intra- or posthepatic. Excess of urobilinogen indicates prehepatic jaundice or sometimes liver damage, whereas an absence of urobilinogen suggests obstructive causes. Urine may be easily tested for the above using a dipstick method.
- *Haematological investigations*: red blood cell fragility, Coombs' test[6] and reticulocyte count confirm haemolytic causes.
- *Serum bilirubin* is rarely higher than 100 µmol/L (5 mg/dL) in prehepatic jaundice, but may be

considerably higher in obstructive cases. In late malignant disease, it may exceed 1000 µmol/L.
- *Conjugated bilirubin*: in prehepatic jaundice, bilirubin is present in the unconjugated form. In pure posthepatic obstructive jaundice, the bilirubin is mainly in the conjugated form, whereas in hepatic jaundice it is present in the mixed conjugated and unconjugated forms owing to a combination of liver destruction and intrahepatic duct blockage.
- *Alkaline phosphatase (ALP)* is produced by cells lining the bile canaliculi. It is normal in prehepatic jaundice, raised in hepatic jaundice and considerably raised in posthepatic jaundice, in primary biliary cholangitis and in situations where rapid regeneration of liver is occurring such as following liver resections. A raised ALP level and normal bilirubin are features of obstruction of some, but not necessarily all, of the intrahepatic bile ducts (note that a different isoenzyme of ALP is produced by bone and placenta, and isolated elevated levels should be isotyped to determine origin).
- *Serum proteins* are normal in prehepatic jaundice, have a reversed albumin/globulin ratio with depressed albumin synthesis in hepatic jaundice

[6]Robin Royston Amos Coombs (1921–2006), Professor of Immunology, Cambridge, UK. Described the test for detecting the presence of antibodies to red blood cells. The 'direct Coombs test' involves taking the patient's washed red cells and incubating with an antihuman immunoglobulin; agglutination occurs if the red cells are coated with human immunoglobulin, as occurs in haemolytic anaemia.

and are usually normal in posthepatic jaundice, unless associated with liver damage.

- *Haptoglobin* concentrations are low in haemolysis. Haptoglobin binds free haemoglobin released after haemolysis and, once bound, the complex is catabolized faster than haptoglobin alone. It is also low in severe liver disease owing to impaired synthesis.
- *Serum transaminases* such as alanine transaminase (ALT) and aspartate transaminase (AST) are raised with hepatocyte inflammation such as occurs in viral hepatitis, in the active phase of cirrhosis and in acute hepatocyte damage such as with drugs. γ-glutamyl transferase (GGT) is a more sensitive indicator of liver disease, and is often raised before the transaminases.
- *Prothrombin time* is normal in prehepatic jaundice, prolonged but correctable with vitamin K in posthepatic jaundice (in which functioning liver tissue is still present). It is prolonged, but not correctable in advanced hepatic jaundice, in which not only is absorption of fat-soluble vitamin K impaired, but the damaged liver is also unable to synthesize prothrombin.
- *Ultrasound scanning* is extremely useful in differentiating the causes of jaundice, as well as being non-invasive and should be the imaging modality of choice in the initial investigation of jaundice. Dilation of the duct system within the liver is a good indication of duct obstruction; thus, if the ducts are not dilated, an obstructive cause for the jaundice is unlikely. Dilatation of the intrahepatic biliary tree without concomitant dilatation of the common bile duct suggests a hilar obstruction such as with a hilar cholangiocarcinoma (Klatskin[7] tumour). Gallstones within the gallbladder can be demonstrated with a high degree of accuracy. Unfortunately, stones within the distal bile ducts are often missed because of overlying duodenal gas.
- *Computed tomography (CT)* and *magnetic resonance (MR)* scans are useful in addition to ultrasound in the demonstration of intrahepatic lesions (e.g. tumour deposits, abscess, cyst), which may

then be accurately needle biopsied under imaging control. A mass in the pancreas may also be demonstrated.

- *Abdominal X-ray* may show gallstones (only 10% are radio-opaque and hence not a reliable test).
- *Magnetic resonance cholangiopancreatography (MRCP) along with MRI liver* affords non-invasive high-resolution imaging of the biliary tree and can give valuable information regarding the liver parenchyma.
- *Endoscopic retrograde cholangiopancreatography (ERCP)*, in which the ampulla of Vater[8] is cannulated using an endoscope passed via the mouth, may demonstrate the location and indicate the nature of an obstructing lesion within the bile ducts. A periampullary tumour is also directly visualized at this examination, and can be biopsied. Currently, ERCP is used only for therapeutic purposes such as removing bile duct stones and placing stents to relieve biliary tract obstruction.
- *Percutaneous transhepatic cholangiography (PTC)*, in which a needle is passed percutaneously into the liver substance and a dilated bile duct is cannulated, may be necessary where ERCP is not possible. Both ERCP and PTC should be recommended only after careful deliberation as both are associated with a definite risk of complications and mortality.
- *Endoscopic ultrasound (EUS)*, in which a small ultrasonic transducer fitted to the tip of the endoscope is passed into the duodenum and thus able to be placed close to the pancreas and the biliary tree. This gives excellent definition of the pancreas and the extra hepatic biliary tree. It is currently the most sensitive and specific investigation for conditions such as chronic pancreatitis and stones/debris in the bile duct. EUS can take targeted biopsies for accurate histopathological diagnosis. EUS can also be used therapeutically to drain pseudocysts and ablate coeliac plexus for intractable pain from cancer/chronic pancreatitis.
- *Needle biopsy*. If the ultrasound scan reveals no dilation of the duct system, an obstructive lesion is unlikely and needle biopsy of the liver may give valuable information regarding hepatic pathology (e.g. hepatitis or cirrhosis). If the ultrasound demonstrates focal lesions in the liver, an ultrasound or CT-guided biopsy of one of the lesions can be

[7]Gerald Klatskin (1910–1986), Assistant Professor of Medicine in Yale, where he introduced liver biopsies. In 1963, he described in detail a series of hilar cholangiocarcinomas, himself acknowledging that the first documentation of such tumours was by Altemeier six years earlier. Nevertheless they are now known as Klatskin tumours.

[8]Abraham Vater (1648–1751), Professor of Anatomy, Wittenberg, Germany.

obtained. Needle biopsy is potentially dangerous in the presence of jaundice, particularly where there is biliary dilation or ascites. The prothrombin time, if prolonged, should first be corrected by administration of vitamin K, and fresh frozen plasma and platelet transfusions may also be indicated; a transjugular liver biopsy may be appropriate in the presence of severe coagulopathy. Should bleeding occur following biopsy, angiographic embolization or immediate laparotomy may be necessary.

Summary of investigations of jaundice

The investigations of jaundice may be grouped as follows.

- *Exclusion of prehepatic causes*: haptoglobin level, reticulocyte count, Coombs' test; split bilirubin (conjugated/unconjugated).
- *Liver synthetic function* (hepatocellular dysfunction): prothrombin time, albumin.
- *Liver cell damage*: transaminases, γ-glutamyl transferase.
- *Bile duct obstruction*: alkaline phosphatase, γ-glutamyl transferase, ultrasound of bile ducts, MRCP, PTC, ERCP, EUS and CT for pancreatic lesion.
- *Intrahepatic mass*: cross-sectional imaging, such as ultrasound and CT, with needle biopsy.

Congenital abnormalities

Riedel's lobe

This anatomical variant is a projection downwards from the right lobe of the liver of normally functioning liver tissue. It is a rare condition but may present as a puzzling and symptomless abdominal mass.

Polycystic liver

This is often associated with polycystic disease of the kidneys (and occasionally pancreas), and comprises multiple cysts within the liver parenchyma. The liver may reach a very large size, but functions normally. The most common symptoms are discomfort and awareness of the grossly enlarged liver in the abdomen. Haemorrhage into the cysts, infection and cholangitis are occasional complications.

Liver trauma

This may be due to penetrating wounds (gunshot or stab) or closed crush injuries, often associated with fractures of the ribs and injuries to other intra-abdominal viscera, especially the spleen and the mesentery.

Clinical features

Following injury, the patient complains of abdominal pain. Examination reveals shock (pallor, tachycardia, hypotension) and generalized abdominal tenderness together with the signs of progressive bleeding.

CT is essential to assess the severity of the injury and to identify any additional injuries, such as a ruptured spleen. Occasionally, there is delayed rupture of a subcapsular haematoma, so that abdominal pain and shock may not be in evidence until some hours or days after the initial injury.

Treatment

If the patient's vital observations are stable, and a definite diagnosis made by CT, the patient can initially be managed conservatively with blood transfusion and careful observation. Repeat CT is undertaken to monitor progress. Selective angiography and embolization should be considered in patients where contrast extravasation is seen on a triple phase CT.

If bleeding continues, as denoted by falling blood pressure, rising pulse and falling haemoglobin, and/or there is the risk of overlooking damage to other viscera, a laparotomy is performed. Minor liver tears can be sutured. Packing of the injury with gauze packs, removed after 48 hours, may be life-saving in severe trauma when the patient's condition is deteriorating. If bleeding continues, the relevant main hepatic arterial branch should be tied in addition to packing. It is extremely uncommon for these patients to require emergency resectional surgery.

Antibiotic cover must be given because of the danger of infection of areas of devitalized liver, and is particularly important when packing is used.

Acute infections of the liver

Possible sources of infection are the following:

- *Biliary*, resulting from an ascending cholangitis.
- *Portal*, from an area of suppuration drained by the portal vein, usually diverticular sepsis or appendicitis.
- *Arterial*, as part of a general septicaemia – this is unusual.
- *Adjacent infections* spreading into the liver parenchyma, for example subphrenic abscess or acute cholecystitis.

Pyogenic liver abscess

Pyogenic liver abscess is a consequence of infection in either the portal territory, leading to a portal pyaemia (pyelophlebitis), or the biliary tree. Multiple abscesses are common. Common infecting organisms include *Escherichia coli*, *Streptococcus faecalis* and *Streptococcus milleri*.

Clinical features

The condition should be suspected in patients who develop rigors, high swinging fever, a tender palpable liver and jaundice. A previous history of abdominal sepsis, such as Crohn's disease,[9] appendicitis or diverticulitis, may be obtained. The clinical course is often insidious, with a non-specific malaise for over a month before presentation and diagnosis.

Special investigations

- *Blood culture*, carried out before treatment is commenced, is often positive.
- *Ultrasound or CT* of the liver may identify and localize hepatic abscesses, as well as identifying the source of the pyaemia.
- *MRI of the liver* may be required to differentiate abscesses from tumours.

Treatment

The originating site of sepsis should be dealt with appropriately. Appropriate antibiotic therapy is the first line of treatment. A large liver abscess may need to be drained percutaneously under ultrasound guidance; smaller abscesses are treated by parenteral antibiotic therapy alone.

Portal pyaemia (pyelophlebitis)

Infection may reach the liver via the portal tributaries from a focus of intra-abdominal sepsis, particularly acute appendicitis or diverticulitis. Multiple abscesses may permeate the liver; in addition, there may be septic thrombi in the intrahepatic radicles of the portal vein, and infected clot in the portal vein itself. The condition has become rare since the advent of antibiotics.

Biliary infection

Multiple abscesses in the liver may occur in association with severe suppurative cholangitis secondary to impaction of gallstones in the common bile duct. Clinically, the features are those of *Charcot's intermittent hepatic fever*[10] – pyrexia, rigors and jaundice. (Rigors represent a bacteraemia and are commonly due to infection in either the renal or biliary tract.)

Urgent drainage of the bile ducts is performed, by either endoscopic sphincterotomy or percutaneous transhepatic drainage.

Amoebic liver abscess

This particular type of portal infection is secondary to an *Entamoeba histolytica* infection of the large intestine. From there, amoebae travel via the portal circulation to the liver, where they proliferate. The amoeba produces a cytolytic enzyme that destroys the liver tissue, producing an amoebic abscess, which is sterile, although amoebae may be found in the abscess wall.

CT and ultrasound of the liver are the most valuable special investigations.

Treatment

The majority respond to medical treatment with metronidazole. Ultrasound-guided percutaneous drainage is required infrequently in non-responding cases.

---

[9]Burrill Bernard Crohn (1884–1983), Gastroenterologist, Mount Sinai Hospital, New York, USA. The disease was first described by Morgagni (1682–1771).

[10]Jean-Martin Charcot (1825–1893), First Professor of Neurology, Salpêtrière Hospital, Paris, France.

Hydatid disease of the liver

The liver is the site of 75% of hydatid cysts in humans.

Pathology

Dogs are infected with the ova of *Echinococcus granulosus* (*Taenia echinococcus*) as a result of eating sheep offal. The tapeworms develop in the dog's small intestine from whence ova are discharged in the faeces. Humans (as well as sheep) ingest the ova from contaminated vegetables and the ova penetrate the stomach wall to invade the portal tributaries and thence pass to the liver. Occasionally, the hydatids may pass on to the lungs, brain, bones and other organs. Hydatid disease is, therefore, more commonly seen in sheep-rearing communities, such as in Australia, Iceland, Cyprus, southern Europe, Africa and Wales.

Clinical features

A cyst may present as a symptomless mass. The contents may die and the walls become calcified so that this inactive structure may be a harmless postmortem finding. The active cyst may, however:

- *Rupture* into the peritoneal cavity, pleural cavity, alimentary canal or biliary tree.
- *Become infected.*
- *Produce obstructive jaundice* by pressure on intrahepatic bile ducts, although jaundice is much more often due to intrabiliary rupture and release of cysts into the bile ducts.

Special investigations

- *Ultrasound and CT scan* localize the cyst.
- *Serological tests* depend on the sensitization of the patient to hydatid fluid, which contains a specific antigen, leakage of which induces the production of antibodies.
- *Eosinophil count*: there may be *eosinophilia* which, while not specific, should arouse clinical suspicion.
- *Plain X-ray* of the liver may show a clear zone produced by the cyst, or may show flecks of calcification in the cyst wall, but abdominal radiographs are much less commonly performed nowadays.

Treatment

A calcified cyst should be left alone. Other cysts should be treated to prevent complications. Treatment with albendazole may result in shrinkage or even disappearance of the cysts. Failure to respond to treatment, or the presence of complications, are indications for surgery. The cyst is exposed, aspirated and injected with scolicidal agents such as Savlon. It is then possible to excise the cyst, taking care not to liberate daughter cysts that are present within it.

Cirrhosis

Definition

Cirrhosis of the liver is a consequence of chronic hepatic injury, with healing by regeneration and fibrosis. Fibrosis leads to further cell damage and destruction of hepatic architecture, progressing to liver failure and portal hypertension.

Aetiology

A convenient classification of cirrhosis is as follows.

1. *Toxin related*:
   a. Excess alcohol.
2. *Infectious*:
   a. Hepatitis B.
   b. Hepatitis C.
3. *Autoimmune*:
   a. Autoimmune chronic active liver disease.
   b. Primary biliary cholangitis (PBC, or Hanot's cirrhosis[11]) – an autoimmune disease characterized by raised serum anti-mitochondrial (M2) antibodies.
   c. Primary sclerosing cholangitis (PSC).
4. *Metabolic (acquired and hereditary)*:
   a. Non-alcoholic fatty liver disease.
   b. Iron overload – haemochromatosis.
   c. Copper overload – hepatolenticular degeneration (Kinnier Wilson's disease[12]).
   d. α_1-antitrypsin-associated liver disease.

[11]Victor Charles Hanot (1844–1896), Physician, Paris, France.
[12]Samuel A. Kinnier Wilson (1877–1937), Neurologist, Hospital for Nervous Diseases, London, UK.

5 *Hepatic venous outflow obstruction*:

  a Budd–Chiari syndrome (hepatic venous occlusion).

  b Severe chronic congestive cardiac failure.

6 *Other causes*:

  a Secondary to prolonged biliary obstruction (secondary biliary cirrhosis).

  b Cystic fibrosis.

  c Cryptogenic.

  d Parenteral nutrition related.

In the UK, the most common causes of cirrhosis are excess alcohol, non-alcoholic fatty liver disease and chronic hepatitis C virus infection. Across the developed world, the same aetiological factors predominate, with a higher prevalence of hepatitis C viral cause in southern Europe, though this is on the wane due to the use of newer antiviral agents. In the tropics, schistosomiasis heads the list.

Consequences of cirrhosis

1 Hepatocellular failure:

  a Impaired protein synthesis: prolonged prothrombin time and low albumin.

  b Impaired metabolism of toxins: encephalopathy.

  c Impaired bilirubin metabolism: jaundice.

2 Portal hypertension (see later in this chapter).

3 Ascites due to portal hypertension.

4 Malignant change: hepatocellular carcinoma.

Clinical features of cirrhosis

A number of clinical signs, separate from those of portal hypertension, are seen in cirrhosis. These include gynaecomastia, testicular atrophy, amenorrhoea, spider naevi, finger clubbing and palmar erythema ('liver palms').

Hepatic encephalopathy

A neuropsychiatric condition characterized by mental changes, flapping tremor and hepatic coma. It occurs because the liver is unable to detoxify the nitrogenous breakdown products of protein metabolism combined with portosystemic shunts that divert these products directly into the systemic circulation.

Portal hypertension

The normal portal pressure is between 5 and 10 mmHg. In portal hypertension, this pressure is raised.

Aetiology

Portal hypertension results from an obstruction to portal venous drainage. The causes are classified according to the site of the block.

1 *Prehepatic/presinusoidal* (obstruction of the portal venous inflow into the liver):

  a Congenital malformation.

  b Portal vein thrombosis: often secondary to portal pyaemia, prothrombotic disorders or, in the neonatal period, spreading infection from the umbilicus.

  c Occlusion by tumour or pancreatitis. In adults, there is a special case in which splenic vein thrombosis caused by pancreatic pathology can result in 'segmental portal hypertension' with diversion of the splenic drainage via the short gastric veins, which results in the development of gastric varices.

  d Hepatic sarcoidosis.

  e Portal vein sclerosis.

2 *Hepatic/sinusoidal* (obstruction of the portal flow within the liver): for example, cirrhosis.

3 *Posthepatic/postsinusoidal* (obstruction of the hepatic veins): Budd–Chiari syndrome.

  a Idiopathic hepatic venous thrombosis in young adults of both sexes. This is a manifestation of a prothrombotic tendency, which may be hereditary or acquired, due to myeloproliferative disease, other systemic conditions or drugs.

  b Congenital obliteration.

  c Blockage of hepatic veins by tumour invasion.

By far the most common cause of portal hypertension is cirrhosis, yet there is no strict relationship between the severity of the liver disease and the extent of portal hypertension, which is not, therefore, entirely explained on the basis of mechanical obstruction.

Pathological effects

The four important effects of portal hypertension are:

1 The development of collateral portosystemic venous drainage.

2 Splenomegaly.

3 Ascites (in hepatic and posthepatic portal hypertension only).

4 The manifestations of hepatic failure (in severe cirrhosis).

Porto-systemic collateral channels

Portal obstruction results in the development of collateral channels between the portal and systemic venous circulations (Figure 32.2). The sites of these channels are:

- Between the left gastric vein and the oesophageal veins, forming gastric and oesophageal varices; these are the largest and clinically the most important connections.

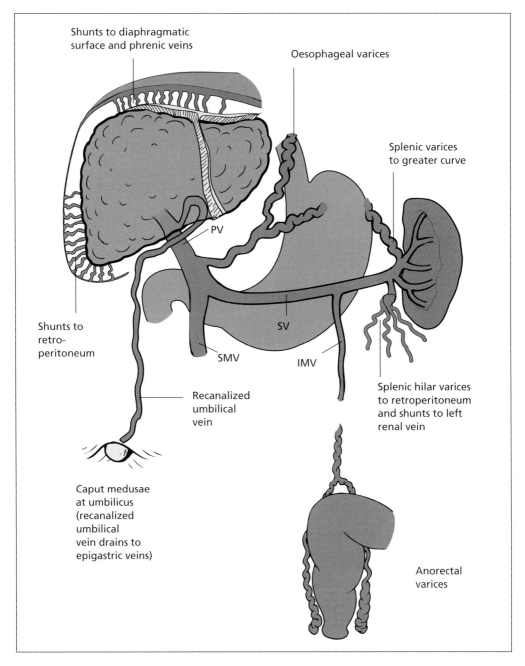

Figure 32.2 The sites of occurrence of portal–systemic communications in patients with portal hypertension. IMV, inferior mesenteric vein; PV, portal vein; SMV, superior mesenteric vein; SV, splenic vein.

- Along the obliterated umbilical vein to the superior and inferior epigastric veins, forming a *caput medusae* around the umbilicus.
- Retroperitoneal and diaphragmatic anastomoses, which present technical hazards to the surgeon at the time of liver transplantation.
- Between the superior and inferior rectal veins with development of anorectal varices.
- Along any adhesions between the visceral and parietal peritoneum due to previous surgery or inflammation.
- At the site of a colostomy or ileostomy.

Gastric and oesophageal varices, and to a much lesser extent anorectal varices, may result in potentially life-threatening gastrointestinal haemorrhage.

Splenomegaly

Progressive splenic enlargement occurs as a result of portal congestion together with some degree of hypertrophy of the splenic substance itself. This is often associated with the haematological changes of hypersplenism: leucopenia and thrombocytopenia. Anaemia accompanying splenomegaly can be accounted for by gastrointestinal bleeding and is not necessarily a result of splenic enlargement.

Ascites

This is due to a combination of factors.

1 Splanchnic vasodilation occurs owing to accumulation of vasoactive mediators in the splanchnic circulation secondary to the liver failure, resulting in pooling of blood. Systemic hypotension is a consequence, with renal hypoperfusion and activation of the renin–angiotensin–aldosterone system, resulting in raised serum aldosterone, which leads to avid salt (sodium) and water retention.
2 The portal venous pressure is raised owing to compression of the portal venous radicles in the liver by the scarred surrounding hepatic tissue.
3 The serum albumin, which is synthesized by the liver, is reduced, resulting in lowering of the serum osmotic pressure.

The build-up of ascites is associated with increased risk of development of hepatorenal failure, due to worsening renal hypoperfusion. This is associated with a high mortality.

The effects of liver failure

- Jaundice.
- Ascites.
- Encephalopathy.

Clinical features

To the surgeon, portal hypertension presents as three problems:

1 As a differential diagnosis of jaundice or hepatomegaly.
2 As a cause of gastrointestinal haemorrhage.
3 As one of the causes of ascites (Box 32.1).

Special investigations

In addition to history and examination (which includes a careful search for the stigmata of liver disease), the following investigations are indicated.

- *Liver function tests*. The degree of jaundice is an important prognostic indicator in cirrhosis.
- *Liver synthetic function tests*, such as prothrombin time and albumin.
- *Ultrasound* can assess focal liver lesions, portal venous flow, splenomegaly and the presence of intra-abdominal varices; it may also detect hepatic venous outflow occlusion.
- *Fibreoptic endoscopy*, which may demonstrate oesophageal varices and differentiate between bleeding from this source and from a peptic ulcer or multiple gastric erosions, all of which are common in patients with cirrhosis.
- *Triple phase abdominal CT or MR scan* gives the best assessment of a focal liver lesion as well as assessing portal vein patency.

In specific situations, further tests can be informative.

> **Box 32.1 The causes of ascites**
>
> - Liver failure and portal hypertension.
> - Carcinomatosis, e.g. ovarian malignancy.
> - Heart failure.
> - Renal failure.
> - Chronic peritonitis, e.g. tuberculous.
> - Pancreatitis.

- *Liver biopsy* – to determine the cause of cirrhosis as well as clinical deterioration.
- *Inferior vena cavagram*, which can demonstrate hepatic venous occlusion.
- *Portal pressure measurement*. This is achieved by means of a catheter passed via the transjugular route into a hepatic vein. The difference between the pressure in the vein with and without an occluding balloon inflated (the hepatic and hepatic wedge pressure) is the portal pressure, a technique akin to pulmonary pressure measurement with a Swan–Ganz catheter.[13] A pressure gradient over 11 mmHg signifies portal hypertension.

Treatment

The treatment of uncomplicated portal hypertension involves treatment of the underlying condition, for example abstinence from alcohol, treatment of underlying viral infection, metabolic condition or autoimmune liver disease. If large oesophageal varices are visible on endoscopy, prophylaxis with medication and/or band ligation of the varices is performed, since the first episode of variceal haemorrhage is associated with a 15–20% mortality.

Management of haemorrhage from gastro-oesophageal varices

Haemorrhage from gastro-oesophageal varices is particularly dangerous, especially in patients with liver damage. In these subjects, the liver is further injured by the hypotension of blood loss, and encephalopathy may be precipitated owing to the absorption of large amounts of nitrogenous breakdown products from the 'meal of blood' within the intestine. Prognosis is better in the small group of patients with normal liver function and portal hypertension due to a prehepatic block, such as portal vein thrombosis.

Prophylaxis against haemorrhage

If varices are detected on screening endoscopy, as above, pharmacological therapy with β-blockers is instituted to reduce splanchnic blood flow and lower

[13]Harold James Charles ('Jeremy') Swan (1922–2005), Cardiologist, Cedars of Lebanon Hospital, Los Angeles, CA, USA. William Ganz (1919–2009), Professor of Medicine, UCLA, and Senior Research Scientist, Cedars of Lebanon Hospital, Los Angeles, CA, USA.

portal venous pressure. Large varices in patients at increased risk of haemorrhage (e.g. severe liver disease) may be treated by endoscopic band ligation (small rubber bands applied to ligate the varices).

Establishing the diagnosis

An attempt must be made to confirm the cause of the bleeding. The presence of established liver disease, an enlarged spleen and proven varices does not necessarily mean that bleeding is from the varices. Such patients are prone to bleeding from gastric erosions and are commonly affected by peptic ulceration. Fibreoptic endoscopy should always be performed in order to determine and, if possible, band ligate the bleeding point. Active bleeding may, however, prevent a satisfactory view at endoscopy.

Immediate treatment

The first priority is airway protection, emergency resuscitation and stabilizing the patient prior to emergency endoscopy.

- *Preventing aspiration*. Patients with liver disease have impaired consciousness and may be at risk of aspirating. They should be managed in conjunction with the critical care team.
- *Resuscitation with fluid and blood*. Blood needs to be cross-matched and transfused as required. Coagulation abnormalities may be corrected with fresh frozen plasma and/or platelet transfusions.
- *Antimicrobial therapy*. Patients are at risk of bacterial infection and benefit from treatment with broad-spectrum antibiotics (e.g. third-generation cephalosporins) to reduce the risk of rebleeding and improve survival.

Stopping the haemorrhage

The bleeding may be arrested by a number of manoeuvres.

- *Intravenous terlipressin*, a vasopressin analogue, is given to reduce portal venous pressure and cause temporary cessation of bleeding by mesenteric arteriolar constriction. In some patients with vascular disease, therapeutic doses cause intestinal colic and myocardial ischaemia, which respond to glyceryl trinitrate infusion.
- *Endoscopic variceal band ligation or sclerotherapy* to oesophageal varices. These procedures can

stop bleeding with minimal trauma to the patient, although there is a risk of perforation of the oesophagus, and repeated injections may produce ulceration or fibrosis and stenosis.

- *Cyanoacrylate injection* into gastric varices.
- *Balloon tamponade*, achieved by passing a Sengstaken–Blakemore tube[14] via the mouth into the oesophagus and cardia. The gastric balloon on the end is inflated, following which gentle traction is applied to the tube such that the balloon impacts on the oesophagogastric junction, which stops flow in the varices. Rebleeding after balloon decompression is common, so it is used to buy time pending definitive treatment.
- *Transjugular intrahepatic portosystemic shunt (TIPS)*: a metal stent is inserted via the jugular vein and, under radiological control, passed through the liver substance to open up a passage between the hepatic vein and the portal vein. The resultant portosystemic shunt decompresses the portal system. TIPS shunts have reduced the necessity for oesophageal transection or operative portosystemic shunt formation.
- *Surgical portocaval shunt*, by surgical anastomosis of the portal vein to the inferior vena cava or the splenic vein to the left renal vein, used to be commonplace. Such procedures have now been superseded by TIPS and endoscopic control of oesophageal varices. Laparotomy should be avoided where possible if a subsequent transplant is planned, as the resulting vascular adhesions will add greatly to the dangers of the transplant operation. The most common complication of shunt procedures (surgical or radiological), in which an anastomosis is made between the portal and systemic circulations, is hepatic encephalopathy.
- *Oesophageal transection*, in which the oesophagus together with the varices are divided at the cardio-oesophageal junction using a circular stapling gun in order to interrupt the communications between the two systems of veins within the wall of the lower oesophagus.

Treatment of ascites

- *Diet*: low-sodium, high-protein diet.
- *Diuretics*: spironolactone often combined with a thiazide or loop diuretic.

[14]Robert Sengstaken (1923–1978), Neurosurgeon, New York, USA. Arthur H. Blakemore (1897–1970), Surgeon, Columbia Presbyterian Medical Center, New York, USA.

- *Paracentesis* gives immediate relief if discomfort is intense, but it has the disadvantage that the patient loses protein, which should, therefore, be replaced at the time (10 g albumin per litre of ascites removed).
- *TIPS shunt*: see earlier in this chapter.

Intractable ascites due to hepatic cirrhosis is an indication for liver transplantation, which is performed after failure of medical therapy.

Hepatorenal syndrome

Renal failure is often associated with ascites and liver failure, particularly alcoholic cirrhosis. It is in part a consequence of depletion of the intravascular volume, as may be caused by diuretic therapy or surgery. There is a reduction in intrarenal blood flow brought about by increased glomerular afferent arteriolar tone, but the cause of this is unknown. The glomerular filtration rate falls as the blood flow is diverted away from the renal cortex. Established renal failure in the presence of liver disease is difficult to treat, and is best avoided by maintaining hydration during surgery.

Renal failure may occur in any patient with jaundice, particularly following surgery. It is best prevented by avoiding fluid depletion and maintaining a good diuresis intraoperatively.

Liver neoplasms

Classification

Benign

- Haemangioma.
- Adenoma.
- Focal nodular hyperplasia.
- Cyst.

Malignant

1 *Primary*:
   a Hepatocellular carcinoma (hepatoma).
   b Fibrolamellar carcinoma, uncommon variant of hepatoma affecting young adults and children.
   c Cholangiocarcinoma.
2 *Secondary* (most common):
   a Portal spread (from alimentary tract).

b Systemic blood spread (from lung, breast, testis, melanoma, etc.).

c Direct spread (from gallbladder, stomach and hepatic flexure of colon).

Hepatocellular carcinoma

Hepatocellular carcinoma (HCC) exhibits marked geographical variation in incidence, being less common in the West but common in central Africa and south-east Asia. This distribution largely reflects the prevalence of hepatitis B and C virus infection. In the UK, the incidence of HCC is increasing, a reflection of the increasing prevalence of viral hepatitis and obesity in particular, and cirrhosis in general.

Eighty per cent of cases of HCC arise in patients with cirrhosis of the liver, and it is most common when cirrhosis is caused by one of the following:

- Hepatitis B infection, the most common cause of HCC worldwide.
- Hepatitis C infection, in which the lead-time from infection to HCC may be 25 years or more.
- Haemochromatosis, in which the degree of iron overload is related to HCC.
- Alcoholic liver disease.
- Non-alcoholic fatty liver disease (NAFLD).

Pathology

The pathogenesis of HCC, when associated with cirrhosis, is related to the chronic inflammatory process within the liver. Macroscopically, the tumour either forms a large, solitary mass or there may be multiple foci throughout the liver.

Spread occurs through the liver substance and into the vessels, so that portal vein thrombosis can be seen adjacent to HCC. Metastasis outside the liver is late and occurs most commonly via haematogenous spread.

Clinical features

The clinical presentation varies depending on the extent of liver disease. In the absence of cirrhosis, the presentation is with massive liver swelling, weight loss and possibly ascites. In the presence of advanced liver disease, malignant change in the liver may be marked by rapid deterioration and decompensation with encephalopathy, ascites and impaired synthetic function. In this instance, survival is more determined by the stage of the underlying cirrhosis rather than the tumour disease.

Special investigations

- *Serum α-fetoprotein (AFP)* may be significantly raised, but it is neither sensitive nor specific for hepatocellular carcinoma and may rise in other diseases such as hepatitis C.
- *Cross-sectional imaging* with ultrasound and contrast-enhanced CT or MR will confirm the presence of a large tumour. Small tumours, 1 cm or less in diameter, are difficult to distinguish from regenerative nodules in the presence of cirrhosis.
- *Selective hepatic angiography* may distinguish regenerative nodules from small HCCs, or may reveal multifocal cancer, though this has largely been replaced by liver MRI.

Treatment

In the absence of cirrhosis, a primary hepatocellular carcinoma confined to one lobe can be treated by hemi-hepatectomy. In the presence of cirrhosis, removal of any liver substance is more likely to precipitate hepatic decompensation and death. Localized treatments such as radiofrequency ablation or transarterial chemoembolization (TACE) may be used, but in this situation the whole liver is 'at risk' and, even after successful destruction of one lesion, further lesions are likely to develop. The only alternative is replacement of the diseased liver by liver transplantation. Results from this procedure are good, providing the tumour load is limited.

Cholangiocarcinoma

This is much less common (20% of primary tumours). It is an adenocarcinoma arising from the bile duct system that usually presents with jaundice and may complicate PSC. Spread occurs directly through the liver substance and regional nodes with a fatal outcome. They can be either mass forming within the liver or present as an infiltrative stricture in the biliary tree.

Some tumours present early and are amenable to resection, which usually involves an extended liver resection (see later in this chapter). For the more usual inoperable cases, it may be possible to relieve the jaundice by passing an expanding metal stent through a percutaneous technique (PTC). This technique is preferred over an ERCP in this condition. This relieves the jaundice, often for many months.

Metastases

The liver is an extremely common site for metastases (secondary deposits), which are often found at autopsy on patients who have died of advanced malignant disease. Necrosis at the centre of metastases leads to the typical umbilication of these tumours.

The clinical effects of secondary deposits in the liver are as follows:

- Hepatomegaly: the liver is large, hard and irregular.
- Jaundice: a late sign due to liver destruction and intrahepatic duct compression.
- Hepatic failure, also a late sign.

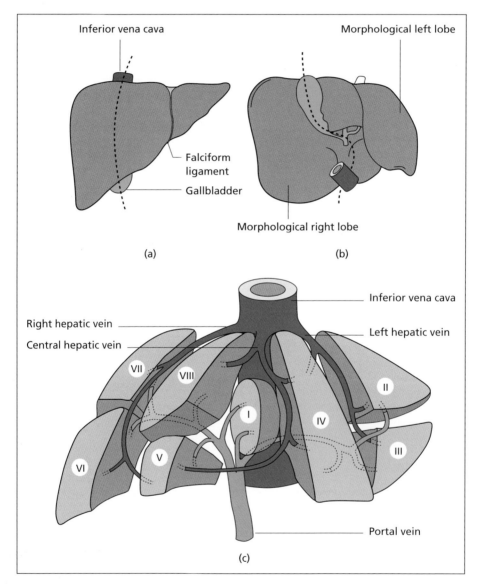

Figure 32.3 (a–c) Segmental anatomy of the liver showing inflow vessels (hepatic artery, portal vein and bile ducts) to the eight liver segments and the hepatic venous drainage via the three main hepatic veins. Reproduced from Ellis H, Mahadevan V (2014) *Clinical Anatomy*, 13th edn. Oxford: Wiley-Blackwell.

- Portal vein obstruction, producing oesophageal varices and ascites.
- Inferior vena cava obstruction, producing leg oedema.

Treatment of secondary tumours

Resection of secondary tumours is not appropriate in the case of disseminated malignancy. However, it may be considered when deposits can be surgically excised leaving an adequate residual liver volume in the absence of any demonstrable and unresectable extrahepatic disease. Following resection, the liver will hypertrophy and regain normal functional capacity. This is mostly applicable to secondary deposits from a previous colorectal carcinoma. For this reason, such patients should have regular surveillance with CT scans postoperatively to detect potentially curable metastatic disease early. Following such a policy, more than 20% of patients who develop colorectal liver metastases can undergo resection with a greater than 40% 5-year survival.

Liver surgery

Anatomical considerations

The liver has remarkable regenerative powers and, as such, will tolerate resection of up to two-thirds of its mass. However, anatomically it is not suited to resection, since the inflow structures (portal vein, hepatic artery and bile duct tributaries) cross the hepatic venous outflow. Nevertheless, there are recognized planes of resection that follow from an understanding of the segmental anatomy of the liver (Figure 32.3).

Surgical resections

The following are the common liver resections performed for primary and secondary (usually, colonic) tumours of the liver:

- Right lobectomy involves removal of segments V–VIII by dividing the liver along a line between the gallbladder fossa and vena cava (Cantlie's line[15]), and leaving the left lobe.
- Left lobectomy involves resection of the left lobe segments II, III and IV; the caudate lobe (segment I) may also be removed.
- Trisegmentectomy is a misnomer, but indicates resection of most of the liver but leaving just the left lateral segments (II and III); since this resection removes the most liver, care has to be taken to ensure that sufficient viable liver remains to sustain life.

If a large resection is required, one option is to embolize the portal vein branch to the area to be resected a couple of weeks before resection in order to promote hypertrophy of the remnant to ensure there is sufficient remaining parenchyma post-resection.

Additional resources

Case 85: A jaundiced and very ill patient
Case 86: A postmortem finding
Case 87: A man with a grossly swollen abdomen
Case 88: A massive haematemesis

---

[15]Sir James Cantlie (1851–1926), Professor of Applied Anatomy, Charing Cross, London.

33

The gallbladder and bile ducts

Anita Balakrishnan

Learning objectives

✓ To know the causes of gallstones, their varying presentations and treatment.

✓ To understand the presentation and principles of management of cancers of the gallbladder and bile duct.

Congenital anomalies

Developmentally, a diverticulum grows out from the ventral wall of the foregut (primitive duodenum), which differentiates into the hepatic ducts and the liver. A lateral bud from this diverticulum becomes the gallbladder and cystic duct (Figure 33.1).

Anomalies are found in 10% of subjects and these are of importance to the surgeon during cholecystectomy.

The principal developmental abnormalities include the following.

- A long cystic duct travelling alongside the common hepatic duct to open near the duodenal orifice. This occurs in 10% of cases.
- Congenital absence (agenesis) of the gallbladder: one in 10000, often associated with other congenital anomalies.
- Duplication of the gallbladder: one in 5000.
- Congenital obliteration of the ducts (biliary atresia, one of the causes of neonatal jaundice): one in 10000.

Ellis and Calne's Lecture Notes in General Surgery, Fourteenth Edition.
Edited by Christopher Watson and Justin Davies.
© 2023 John Wiley & Sons Ltd. Published 2023 by John Wiley & Sons Ltd.
Companion website: www.wiley.com/go/Watson/GeneralSurgery14

- Absence of the cystic duct, the gallbladder opening directly into the side of the common bile duct.
- A long mesentery to the gallbladder, which allows acute torsion of the gallbladder to occur with consequent gangrene and rupture.
- Anomalies of the arrangement of the blood vessels supplying the gallbladder and right-sided bile ducts are common; for example, the right hepatic artery crosses in front of the common hepatic duct instead of behind it in 25% of subjects, and the right anterior or posterior bile ducts can insert into either the left hepatic duct or directly into the common hepatic duct (Figure 33.2). Both arterial and biliary tract anomalies can predispose those structures to injury during cholecystectomy.
- Cystic dilation of the main bile ducts (choledochal cyst): one in 200000, but more common in people of Asian descent (one in 1000 Japanese).

Cholelithiasis (gallstones)

Gallstones are rare in children (although they should still be considered in the differential diagnosis of abdominal pain in children if the diagnosis is not to

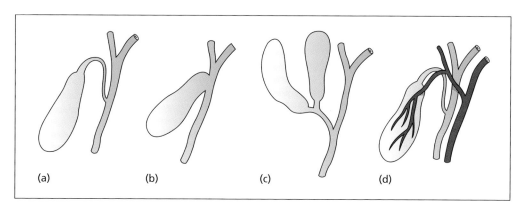

Figure 33.1 Developmental anomalies of the gallbladder. (a) A long cystic duct joining the hepatic duct low down behind the duodenum. (b) Absence of the cystic duct – the gallbladder opens directly into the common hepatic duct. (c) A double gallbladder, the result of a rare bifid embryonic diverticulum from the hepatic duct. (d) The right hepatic artery crosses in front of the common hepatic duct; this occurs in 25% of cases. Reproduced from Ellis H, Mahadevan V (2010) *Clinical Anatomy*, 12th edn. Oxford: Wiley-Blackwell.

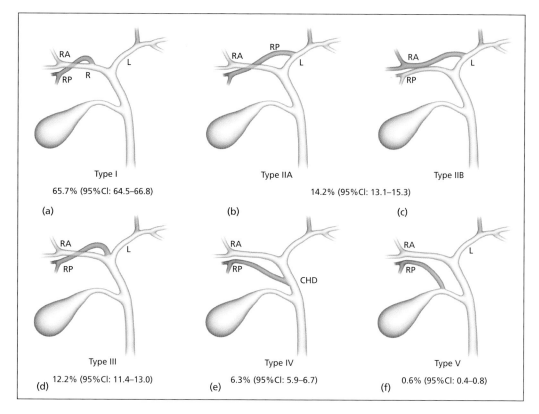

Figure 33.2 Biliary anatomy and anomalies. In the majority of individuals, the right posterior bile ducts (RP) join the right anterior bile ducts (RA) to form the right hepatic duct which then confluences with the left hepatic duct (L) to form the common hepatic duct (a). Other variations of this exist with varying frequency, including drainage of either the RP or RA ducts into the L duct (b, c), or draining directly into the common hepatic duct (d, e) or the cystic duct (f).

be overlooked, and should always be considered in children with spherocytosis or elliptocytosis), the incidence increasing with each decade. The incidence of gallstones is higher in women compared to men and can be more prevalent in those who are overweight. In the UK, they are found in approximately 10% of women in their forties, increasing to 30% after the age of 60 years. They are about half as common in men. Stones are particularly common in the Mediterranean races, and the highest incidence is found among the Indians of New Mexico.

Bile composition and function

To understand gallstones, it is first necessary to understand bile. Bile is a combination of cholesterol, phospholipids (principally, lecithin), bile salts (chenodeoxycholic acid and cholic acid) and water. Bile also contains conjugated bilirubin, the breakdown product of haemoglobin, which is quite distinct from bile salts. Cholesterol is not water soluble and is carried in the bile in water-soluble micelles, in which the hydrophobic cholesterol is carried within a 'shell' of phospholipid and bile salts. Once in the gut, bile salts act as a detergent, breaking up and emulsifying fats to facilitate their absorption.

The bile salts themselves are resorbed in the distal small bowel and pass back via the portal venous system to the liver, from where they are once again secreted in the bile. This circulation of bile salts is termed the *'enterohepatic circulation'*, permitting a relatively small pool of bile salts to circulate up to 10 times a day. Diversion or absence of bile from the gut, as may occur in obstructive jaundice, results in a malabsorption of fat and the fat-soluble vitamins (A, D, E and K).

Gallbladder physiology

Bile flows into the gallbladder when the sphincter of Oddi is closed. Once there, it is concentrated by absorption of water. Fat, in the form of fatty acids, as well as amino acids in the duodenum lead to the release of cholecystokinin, which causes the gallbladder to contract. At the same time, vagal stimulation in response to eating causes relaxation of the sphincter

of Oddi, and also increases the production of bile, as does the hormone secretin. This episodic release of bile aids digestion of fat, but is not essential, although following cholecystectomy many patients may develop loose stools with high-fat meals.

Gallstone types

There are three common varieties of stone (Figure 33.3).

1 *Cholesterol* (20%): these occur as a solitary, oval stone (the cholesterol solitaire) or as two stones, one indenting the other, or as multiple mulberry stones associated with a strawberry gallbladder (see later in this chapter). A cut section shows crystals radiating from the centre of the stone; the surface is yellow and greasy to the touch.
2 *Bile pigment* (5%): small, black, irregular, multiple, gritty and fragile.
3 *Mixed* (75%): multiple, faceted one against the other, and can often be grouped into two or more series, each of the same size, suggesting 'generations' of stones. The cut surface is laminated with alternate dark and light zones of pigment and cholesterol, respectively.

This traditional classification into three groups is an oversimplification; calculi with widely different appearances simply represent different combinations of the same constituents. Importantly, the diagnosis and management of gallstones are not dependent on the type of gallstones, but rather the symptoms and the location of the stone (within the gallbladder versus the bile ducts).

Cholesterol stones

These may be associated with elevated blood cholesterol, but there is little evidence to suggest this as a cause. There is a definite correlation between cholesterol stones and the contraceptive pill and pregnancy, as well as an increase with age. Family history may be contributory in some patients, with the heritability of gallstones varying between 25 and 50% in different ethnic groups, related to multiple heterogenous gene mutations. Low dietary fibre and metabolic abnormalities including obesity, insulin resistance and type 2 diabetes are also risk factors.

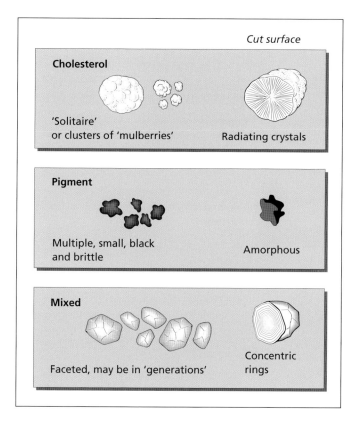

Figure 33.3 The varieties of gallstones.

Four pathophysiological factors have been considered to contribute to the development of cholesterol gallstones.

a Hypersecretion of cholesterol by the liver – this is related to insulin resistance, oestrogen and some genetic mutations.
b Supersaturated bile related to hypersecretion of cholesterol with or without bile salt or phospholipid hyposecretion.
c Gallbladder hypomotility – this can be caused by prolonged fasting or parenteral nutrition and rapid weight loss, and exacerbated by bacteria. The increased fibrosis related to episodes of inflammation can further reduce gallbladder contractility.
d Intestinal factors – enterohepatic recirculation of bile salts is impaired by intestinal resection (e.g. resection of the ileum in treatment for Crohn's disease) or total colectomy, resulting in reduced hepatic secretion of bile salts, reduced cholesterol solubilization and thus supersaturated bile.

Pigment stones

Pigment stones are composed of calcium bilirubinate, with some calcium carbonate. These can occur in any conditions which increase the concentration of systemic bilirubin levels, such as haemolytic anaemias, for example spherocytosis and sickle cell disease, as well as ineffective erythropoiesis and cirrhosis. If such stones are found in the gallbladder of children or adolescents, haemolytic anaemia should be suspected, particularly if there is a family history of calculus. Pigment stones can also form *de novo* in the bile ducts, particularly in conditions of bile stasis and biliary infection.

Mixed stones

It is now considered that the majority of mixed stones have the same metabolic origin as cholesterol stones, that is, some slight alteration in the composition of bile enabling precipitation of cholesterol together with bile pigment.

The pathological effects of gallstones

- *Silent*: gallstones lying free in the lumen of the gallbladder produce no pathological disturbance of the wall and the patient is symptom free.
- *Impaction in gallbladder*, either in Hartmann's pouch[1] or in the cystic duct. Water is absorbed from the contained bile, which becomes concentrated and produces a chemical cholecystitis. Initially, this is usually sterile but may then become secondarily infected. If a stone impacts in Hartmann's pouch when the gallbladder is empty, the wall of the gallbladder may continue to secrete mucus and the gallbladder distends to form a mucocele, which can get secondarily infected to become an empyema of the gallbladder.
- *Choledocholithiasis*: gallstones may migrate into the common bile duct. These may be silent or produce an intermittent or complete obstruction of the common bile duct with pain and jaundice or ascending cholangitis or acute pancreatitis.
- *Mirizzi's syndrome*[2]: a gallstone may impact in the cystic duct or Hartmann's pouch and cause extrinsic compression of the common hepatic duct, also resulting in obstructive jaundice.
- *Gallstone ileus*: this is uncommon, and occurs when a large gallstone ulcerates through the wall of the gallbladder into the adjacent duodenum. The gallstone may pass per rectum or produce a gallstone ileus – this is impaction of the stone in the narrowest part of the small bowel (the distal ileum) with resulting intestinal obstruction. (Note that gallstone ileus is thus a misnomer and is in fact mechanical obstruction by an intraluminal stone, and not a paralytic ileus.) A key feature in such cases is the frequent presence of air in the biliary tree that has entered the bile ducts via the fistula created when the gallstone ulcerates through into the gut and which can be readily seen on computed tomography (CT).

In addition, the presence of gallstones in the biliary tree can be associated with:

- Acute and chronic pancreatitis.
- Carcinoma of the gallbladder.

[1]Henri Hartmann (1860–1952), Professor of Surgery, Hôtel Dieu, Paris, France.
[2]Pablo Luis Mirizzi (1893–1964), Physician, Cordoba, Argentina.

Clinical manifestations of gallstones

The following syndromes can be recognized:

- Biliary colic.
- Acute cholecystitis.
- Chronic cholecystitis.
- Obstruction and/or infection of the common bile duct.

Two or more of these syndromes may occur in the same patient.

Biliary colic

Biliary colic occurs when the gallbladder contracts following cholecystokinin release by the duodenum but its outflow is obstructed, for example by a stone impacted in either Hartmann's pouch or the cystic duct, producing severe pain, which usually comes on 2–3 hours after eating and often wakes the patient. It is a continuous pain, usually rising to a plateau, and may last for many hours, reflecting the release and peak concentration of cholecystokinin. The pain is usually situated in the right subcostal region but may be epigastric, or it may spread as a band across the upper abdomen and be accompanied by vomiting and sweating. Radiation of the pain to the inferior angle of the right scapula is common. In contrast to acute cholecystitis, the patient is usually not systemically unwell.

A variant of biliary colic occurs when a stone impacts in the sphincter of Oddi, in which case the patient is mildly jaundiced, the pain is colicky, and the patient is restless and rolls about in agony. Relief may be sudden as the stone passes into the duodenum.

Differential diagnosis is from the other acute colics, especially ureteric colic (Box 33.1).

Acute cholecystitis

If the stone remains impacted in the gallbladder outlet, the gallbladder wall becomes inflamed owing to the irritation of the concentrated bile contained within it producing a chemical cholecystitis. The gallbladder fills with pus, which is frequently sterile on culture. In these instances, the pain persists and progressively

Box 33.1 Abdominal colic

Colicky pain is the result of smooth muscle contraction against a resistance. The common causes of colic occur in the uterus and fallopian tubes, renal tract, intestinal tract and biliary tract.

Biliary tract

- Stone in Hartmann's pouch.
- Stone in cystic duct.
- Stone in sphincter of Oddi.

Renal tract

- Ureteric colic due to stone, blood clot or tumour.
- Bladder colic in acute retention owing to enlarged prostate.

Intestinal tract

- Mechanical obstruction.
- Appendicular colic as appendix lumen occludes.

Uterus and Fallopian tubes

- Parturition.
- Menstruation.
- Ectopic pregnancy in a fallopian tube.

intensifies. There is a fever in the range of 38–39 °C with marked toxaemia and leucocytosis. The upper abdomen is extremely tender, and a palpable mass may develop in the region of the gallbladder. This represents the distended, inflamed gallbladder wrapped in inflammatory adhesions to adjacent organs, especially the omentum. Occasionally, an empyema of the gallbladder develops or, rarely, gallbladder perforation into the liver or general peritoneal cavity takes place. The swollen gallbladder may press against the adjacent common bile duct and produce a tinge of jaundice, even though stones may be absent from the duct system.

Ninety-five per cent of cases of acute cholecystitis are associated with gallstones. Occasionally, fulminating acalculous cholecystitis may occur and this may be associated with typhoid fever or gas gangrene.

The *differential diagnosis* is from acute appendicitis, perforated duodenal ulcer, acute pancreatitis, right basal pneumonia and coronary thrombosis.

Chronic cholecystitis

This is almost invariably associated with the presence of gallstones. Repeated episodes of inflammation result in chronic fibrosis and thickening of the entire gallbladder wall, which may contain thick, sometimes infected bile.

There are recurrent bouts of abdominal pain owing to mild cholecystitis, which may or may not be accompanied by fever. Discomfort is experienced after fatty meals as the gallbladder contracts onto the stones; there is often flatulence. The picture may be complicated by episodes of acute cholecystitis or symptoms produced by stones passing into the common bile duct.

The *differential diagnosis* is from other causes of chronic dyspepsia, including peptic ulceration and hiatus hernia. Occasionally, the symptoms closely resemble those of angina pectoris. It is as well to remain clinically suspicious – any or all of these common diseases may well occur in association with gallstones.

Stones in the common bile duct (choledocholithiasis)

This may be symptomless. More often, there are attacks of biliary colic accompanied by obstructive jaundice with clay-coloured stools and dark urine, the attacks lasting for hours or several days. The attack ceases either when a small stone is passed through the sphincter of Oddi or when it disimpacts and falls back into the dilated common duct. Above the impacted stone, other stones or biliary sludge may deposit. Occasionally, the jaundice is progressive and, rarely, it is painless.

If the obstruction is not relieved either spontaneously or by ERCP or surgery, superimposed infection develops, or the chronic back-pressure in the biliary system may result in secondary biliary cirrhosis and liver failure.

The *differential diagnosis* of stones in the common bile duct is as follows.

1. With jaundice (75% of cases):
   a. Carcinoma of the pancreas or other malignant obstructions of the common bile duct.
   b. Acute hepatitis.
   c. Other causes of jaundice (see Chapter 32).
2. Without jaundice (25% of cases):
   a. Renal colic.
   b. Intestinal obstruction.
   c. Angina pectoris.

Ascending cholangitis

Infection of the common bile duct can occur in the presence of an obstruction to the normal biliary drainage, usually as a complication of stones in the duct. This is characterized by jaundice, right upper quadrant pain and raised temperatures (known as

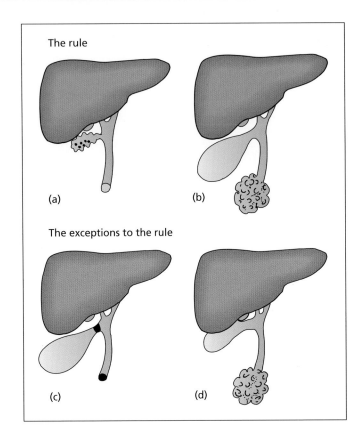

The rule

(a)

(b)

The exceptions to the rule

(c)

(d)

Figure 33.4 Obstructive jaundice due to stone is usually associated with a small, contracted gallbladder (a). Therefore, in the presence of jaundice, a palpable gallbladder indicates that the obstruction is probably due to some other cause, the most common being carcinoma of the pancreas (b). Exceptions are a palpable gallbladder produced by one stone impacted in Hartmann's pouch resulting in a mucocele, another in the common duct causing obstruction (c), which is very rare or, more commonly, the gallbladder is indeed distended but is clinically impalpable (d).

Charcot's[3] triad). In these instances, the duct system is severely inflamed and filled with pus, and the liver may be dotted with multiple small abscesses. Treatment is with appropriate antibiotics and urgent biliary drainage (e.g. endoscopic sphincterotomy).

Courvoisier's law[4] (Figure 33.4)

'If in the presence of jaundice the gallbladder is palpable, then the jaundice is unlikely to be due to stone.' This is an extremely useful rule provided it is quoted correctly. The principle on which it is based is that, if the obstruction is due to stone, the gallbladder is usually thickened and fibrotic and, therefore, does not distend. Moreover, unlike obstruction due to malignant disease, calculus obstruction is not usually complete. There is

usually some escape of bile into the duodenum, with decompression of the gallbladder. Obstruction of the common bile duct due to other causes (e.g. carcinoma of the head of the pancreas) is usually painless, and associated with a normal gallbladder, which can dilate. However, in carcinoma of the bile ducts arising above the origin of the cystic duct, the gallbladder, distal to the obstruction, will be collapsed and empty.

Note that the law is not phrased the other way round – 'If the gallbladder is *not* palpable, the jaundice is due to stone' – as 50% of dilated gallbladders cannot be palpated on clinical examination, owing to either the patient's obesity or overlap by the liver, which itself is usually enlarged as a result of bile engorgement.

Only rarely is the gallbladder dilated when jaundice is due to stone. These circumstances occur when a stone impacts in Hartmann's pouch to produce a mucocele while at the same time jaundice is produced by a second stone in the common duct, or when a stone forms *in situ* in the common bile duct, the gallbladder itself being normal and, therefore, distensible.

[3]Jean Martin Charcot (1825–1893), First Professor of Neurology, Salpêtrière Hospital, Paris, France.
[4]Ludwig Courvoisier (1843–1918), Professor of Surgery, Basle, Switzerland.

Special investigations

- *Ultrasound*: this non-invasive technique gives three pieces of information:
  - The presence of gallstones within the gallbladder, revealed as intensely echogenic foci, which cast a clear acoustic shadow beyond them.
  - The thickened wall of the gallbladder in acute or chronic inflammation.
  - The diameter of the common bile duct which, if over 7 mm, is suggestive of the presence of stones within.

  Unfortunately, ultrasound, like CT, is unreliable in detecting stones in the bile ducts, especially at the lower end where they are obscured by the overlying duodenal gas.
- *Plain abdominal X-ray*, though rarely done these days, reveals radio-opaque gallstones in only 10% of cases. These usually appear as rings due to calcium deposited on a central translucent organic core. Occasionally, the gallbladder may be seen to be calcified ('porcelain gallbladder').
- *Upper gastrointestinal endoscopy* may be advisable to exclude an associated peptic ulcer or hiatus hernia when there is any degree of uncertainty in the clinical picture, even though gallstones have been noted on ultrasound.
- *Liver function tests* are performed whenever jaundice, present or past, is a feature. Raised alkaline phosphatase or alanine transaminase, even in the absence of a raised bilirubin, is suspicious for choledocholithiasis. Prothrombin time should also be checked in the presence of jaundice lest any invasive procedure be required.
- *Computed tomography (CT)* is often performed for investigation of abdominal pain which may arise as a consequence of gallstone-related complications, and is useful in detecting cholecystitis, obstructive jaundice, pancreatitis and rarer complications such as gallstone ileus. The radiolucency of most gallstones means it cannot be used to exclude or confirm the presence of gallstones in the gallbladder.
- *Magnetic resonance cholangiopancreatography (MRCP)* permits visualization of the biliary tree and any contained calculi. This non-invasive procedure provides the same diagnostic information as can be obtained with ERCP but without the small but important risk of complications (perforation, bleeding, pancreatitis) associated with ERCP.

- *Endoscopic ultrasound (EUS)* involves an endoscopic procedure with an ultrasound probe at the tip of an endoscope. This is more sensitive than an MRCP in detecting common bile duct stones or sludge, but also more invasive, carrying a small risk of bleeding and perforation. This procedure may be useful in patients where the differential diagnosis includes a mass lesion (as tissue samples can be taken via this route) or in patients with contraindications to MRI. Unlike ERCP, this investigation does not allow clearance of any ductal stones.
- *Endoscopic retrograde cholangiopancreatography (ERCP)*: endoscopic intubation of the bile ducts through the ampulla of Vater is more invasive than MRCP or EUS, but in addition to visualizing the ducts and contained stones it also permits their extraction, often after first carrying out a diathermy sphincterotomy/balloon sphincteroplasty opening up the sphincter of Oddi[5] to facilitate instrumentation of the bile duct. ERCP has been largely replaced by MRCP for diagnosis but remains an essential part of hepatobiliary management in offering endoscopic therapeutic options and removing the reliance on open surgical procedures.

Treatment

Biliary colic

Most patients with biliary colic are managed in the outpatient setting, but consideration should be given to elective laparoscopic cholecystectomy to control their symptoms and avoid other complications of gallstones.

Acute cholecystitis

At least 90% resolve on bed rest with antibiotics and pain relief. Early cholecystectomy during the same admission is advocated where possible to prevent further attacks; however, the operation may be more technically challenging due to increasing inflammation after the first 48 to 72 hours. Cholecystectomy is routinely performed laparoscopically, with the advantages of minimal scarring of the abdominal wall and rapid convalescence

---

[5]Ruggero Oddi (1864–1913), Surgeon, Genoa, Italy. The sphincter was first described in 1654 by Francis Glisson (1597–1677), Regius Professor of Physic, Cambridge, UK.

compared with an open procedure. Nevertheless, operative difficulties and anatomical aberrations may necessitate conversion to an open operation in approximately 2–5% of cases.

Perforation of the acutely inflamed gallbladder can occur, either into the adjacent liver parenchyma with a resultant liver abscess, or into the peritoneal cavity with biliary peritonitis. The latter is rare and requires urgent surgery, and carries a high mortality.

In patients unfit for surgery, a cholecystostomy (drainage of the gallbladder under ultrasound guidance) may be performed to control symptoms of sepsis and pain. This may also be a temporizing measure in some patients with gallbladder empyema or localized perforation, with a subsequent cholecystectomy once the inflammation has subsided.

Chronic cholecystitis

Cholecystectomy is performed, usually laparoscopically. Intraoperative cholangiography may help ascertain the presence of any stones within the common bile duct, particularly if associated with deranged liver function tests. The cystic duct is intubated and radio-opaque contrast medium is injected into the common duct. If stones are convincingly demonstrated at intra-operative cholangiography, the surgeon may choose between postoperative evacuation of the stones via ERCP, or laparoscopic or open clearance. The stones can be removed either via the cystic duct, or directly through the common bile duct. If the stones are removed through the bile duct, the incision on the bile duct can be either closed primarily (if wide enough to avoid postoperative stricturing) or drained using a latex T-tube inserted into the common duct. The T-tube is removed 10 days postoperatively, provided a check cholangiogram taken through the tube confirms that the ducts are clear and that there is free flow of contrast into the duodenum. If there is any doubt about the presence of ductal stones at the time of surgery, an MRCP can be performed following recovery. Any stones still present can then be removed at ERCP.

Obstructive jaundice due to stones

Impacted stones are removed using a balloon or Dormia[6] basket at ERCP. Subsequent cholecystectomy is performed as soon as possible lest new stones

[6]Enrico Dormia (1928–2009), Professor of Urology, Milan, Italy.

pass into the ducts. The presence of high fever makes removal of the impacted stones and drainage of the obstructed common bile duct imperative as an emergency procedure. Any intervention is preceded by giving intravenous vitamin K, since a lack of bile salts in the gut reduces absorption of this fat-soluble vitamin; hence, serum prothrombin is lowered with consequent bleeding tendency. Rarely ERCP may be unsuccessful, and biliary drainage may require a percutaneous transhepatic external biliary drain to alleviate the sepsis.

Acute or chronic pancreatitis

Gallstones are one of the commonest causes of acute pancreatitis, a condition which can sometimes prove life-threatening particularly for patients with other comorbidities. The diagnosis and management of acute and chronic pancreatitis are discussed in Chapter 34.

Non-surgical treatment of gallstones

There is no satisfactory or effective non-surgical treatment for gallstones. Gallstone dissolution via oral bile salts such as chenodeoxycholic or ursodeoxycholic acid, or lithotripsy (ultrasonic destruction of gallstones) are options that have been previously employed to avoid surgical intervention. However, the high risk of stone migration or recurrence within the gallbladder, and the potential for pancreatitis or biliary obstruction from lithotripsy, are such that these are no longer recommended forms of treatment.

The symptomless gallstone

The incidental diagnosis of gallstones is becoming increasingly common during routine ultrasound examination of the abdomen for a variety of non-biliary reasons. Given the risks of cholecystectomy, there is no evidence at present to support surgery for patients with asymptomatic gallstones, unless conditions associated with an increased risk of gallbladder cancer, such as porcelain gallbladder or large gallbladder polyps, are also present.

Complications of cholecystectomy

There are two special dangers after cholecystectomy, whether performed by laparotomy or laparoscopy.

1   *Leakage of bile.* This may result from:
    a   Injury to bile canaliculi in the gallbladder bed of the liver.
    b   Injury to the common hepatic or common bile duct, or aberrant low inserting right-sided bile ducts.
    c   Slipping of the ligature or clip from the cystic duct.
    d   Leakage from the common bile duct after exploration.

ERCP may identify the site of the leak, and temporary stenting[7] will ensure adequate biliary drainage, thus allowing the bile fistula to close spontaneously; if this does not occur, further exploration may be required. A percutaneous drain is usually placed to prevent generalized biliary peritonitis.

2   *Jaundice.* This may be due to:
    a   Missed stones in the common bile duct.
    b   Inadvertent injury to the common bile duct.
    c   Cholangitis or associated pancreatitis.

Residual stones in the common duct can usually be removed by ERCP; if a T-tube is still present in the common duct, the stone can be removed by means of a Burhenne basket[8] passed along the track formed by the tube under X-ray control.

Gallbladder polyps

Pathology

Gallbladder polyps may be single or multiple and are increasingly being detected by ultrasound examination. They appear as lesions within the gallbladder which do not cast an acoustic shadow (as stones do) and which do not move when the patient rolls onto one side, indicating that they are attached to the gallbladder wall. Polyps may represent a premalignant lesion, the risk of malignancy rising with increasing size of polyp, and becoming significant when the size reaches 1 cm and probable when the size reaches 1.5 cm. Sessile morphology, co-existing primary sclerosing cholangitis and age over 50 years are additional risk factors for malignancy within a polyp.

---

[7]Charles Stent (1845–1901), English dentist.
[8]H. Joachim Burhenne (1925–1996), Radiologist, Vancouver, Canada.

Clinical features

Gallbladder polyps may be entirely asymptomatic and simply represent an incidental finding on an ultrasound examination performed for reasons other than biliary symptoms; if they are situated distally in the gallbladder close to Hartmann's pouch, they may produce symptoms identical to those of gallstones.

Treatment

Cholecystectomy is recommended for polyps associated with gallbladder symptoms or those of greater than 10 mm in diameter. Patients with polyps measuring 6 mm in diameter or greater, and with additional risk factors (over the age of 50, sessile polyps and those with primary sclerosing cholangitis) should also be counselled for cholecystectomy. Patients without additional risk factors or with smaller (<6 mm) asymptomatic polyps should undergo surveillance via annual ultrasound, with surgery advocated if polyps increase in size on imaging.

Carcinoma of the gallbladder

Pathology

This is a relatively uncommon tumour in most countries but shows particularly high prevalence in certain areas including parts of northern India, Chile, China and Korea. The aetiology behind this is unclear and has been proposed to include salmonella infections, dietary factors and other environmental exposures. Gallbladder cancer is strongly associated with the presence of gallstones, pancreatobiliary malfunction and 'porcelain' gallbladders; however, the exact role of these conditions as a cause for cancer development remains uncertain, and may be related to chronic irritation or the carcinogenic effect of cholic acid derivatives. It is 2–3 times more common in women, and 90% of gallbladder cancers are adenocarcinoma with the remaining 10% consisting of squamous carcinoma or neuroendocrine tumours.

This aggressive tumour often invades the adjacent liver parenchyma and bile ducts, and disseminates both via lymphatic spread to nodes in the porta hepatis and beyond, as well as haematogenous spread via the portal vein to the liver.

Clinical features

Carcinoma of the gallbladder may be silent, but can also present with a picture closely resembling chronic cholecystitis, with right upper quadrant pain, nausea and vomiting, in addition to weight loss and, later, progressing to obstructive jaundice. At this stage, a palpable mass may be present in the gallbladder region.

Treatment

Occasionally, cholecystectomy performed for stones reveals the presence of an unexpected early tumour. Under these circumstances, long-term survival may follow depending on the histopathological stage of the tumour. Patients with very early tumours may have good long-term survival with a cholecystectomy alone. Those with tumours invading the muscle layer of the gallbladder and beyond would generally benefit from a radical cholecystectomy incorporating resection of the adjacent liver and removal of local lymph nodes. Surgery yields much more limited survival in patients with involvement of adjacent organs or invasion of the right-sided liver inflow, and is contraindicated in the presence of metastatic disease, where chemotherapy is the more appropriate treatment option.

Cholangiocarcinoma

Pathology

The incidence of cholangiocarcinoma (carcinoma of the bile ducts) is increasing. The disease commonly occurs after 50 years of age and is more common in men. It is associated with primary sclerosing cholangitis, and to a lesser extent, congenital hepatic fibrosis, choledochal cysts and polycystic liver.

Macroscopically, cholangiocarcinomas may occur within the liver substance, or in the larger extrahepatic bile ducts. The confluence of the left and right hepatic ducts, or the common hepatic duct with the cystic duct, are common sites. Microscopically, these are mucin-secreting adenocarcinomas.

Clinical features

The usual presentation is with painless progressive jaundice, with dark urine and pale stools. Epigastric pain, steatorrhoea and weight loss are common. There may be hepatomegaly, usually without a palpable gallbladder because the tumour is proximal to, or at, the cystic duct confluence. Hilar cholangiocarcinoma (Klatskin tumour[9]) should be suspected if there is intrahepatic biliary dilation without common bile duct dilation. Confirmation is often by MRCP, or percutaneous transhepatic cholangiography and brush cytology (poor sensitivity), and EUS biopsy if possible. ERCP examination alone often fails to visualize the intrahepatic biliary tracts, however, when combined with cholangioscopy may be successful in obtaining images of concerning lesions or strictures as well as histological confirmation of malignancy.

Treatment

The tumours are slow growing. Palliation of distal strictures is often achieved by endoluminal stenting at ERCP, and percutaneous transhepatic cholangiography for more proximal strictures, or, less frequently, surgical bypass. The prognosis is poor, and curative resection is only possible in a small percentage of cases with early presentation of hilar tumours (Klatskin tumour[9]). Good results have been reported with extended right hepatectomy (to include the caudate lobe) together with excision of the adjacent portal vein and venous reconstruction. In the rarer cases in which the tumour is located distally in the common bile duct, a Whipple's resection (see Figure 34.2) may be possible.

Additional resources

Case 89: A schoolmistress with attacks of abdominal pain
Case 90: A collection of calculi

[9]Gerald Klatskin (1910–1986), liver Physician, Yale, New Haven, CT, USA. Pioneered the liver biopsy and is considered to be one of the fathers of hepatology.

34

The pancreas

Raaj Kumar Praseedom

Learning objectives

✓ To know the causes and management of acute pancreatitis, and the factors that predict its severity.

✓ To have knowledge of pancreatic cancer, its presentation and the surgical approach to treatment of carcinoma of the head of the pancreas.

Congenital anomalies

The pancreas develops as a dorsal and a ventral bud from the duodenum (Figure 34.1). The ventral bud rotates posteriorly, thus enclosing the superior mesenteric vessels; it forms the major part of the head of the pancreas, and its duct becomes the main duct of Wirsung,[1] which in the great majority of cases has a shared opening with the common bile duct in the ampulla of Vater.[2] The larger dorsal bud becomes the body and tail and its duct becomes the accessory duct of Santorini.[3]

Annular pancreas

The two developmental buds may envelop the second part of the duodenum, producing this rare form of extrinsic duodenal obstruction.

[1]Johann Georg Wirsung (1589–1643), Professor of Anatomy, University of Padua, Italy, where he was murdered.
[2]Abraham Vater (1684–1751), Professor of Anatomy, Wittenberg, Germany.
[3]Giovanni Domenico Santorini (1681–1737), Professor of Anatomy and Medicine, Venice, Italy.

Ellis and Calne's Lecture Notes in General Surgery, Fourteenth Edition. Edited by Christopher Watson and Justin Davies.
© 2023 John Wiley & Sons Ltd. Published 2023 by John Wiley & Sons Ltd.
Companion website: www.wiley.com/go/Watson/GeneralSurgery14

Heterotopic pancreas

This is produced occasionally by an accessory budding from the primitive foregut. A nodule of pancreatic tissue may be found in the stomach, duodenum, jejunum or, rarely, a Meckel's diverticulum. This may produce obstructive or dyspeptic symptoms.

Acute pancreatitis

Acute inflammation of the pancreas is a common cause of acute abdominal pain, with significant morbidity and mortality.

Aetiology

Most cases of acute pancreatitis are associated with either gallstones or alcohol, although a number of less common causes have been identified.

- *Gallstones* are present in half of the cases in the UK.
- *Alcohol*: the majority of cases of non-gallstone pancreatitis are alcohol related. This is particularly common in France and North America. Alcohol is also the most common cause of recurrent pancreatitis. The mechanism is unclear, and it may follow either chronic alcohol abuse or binge drinking.

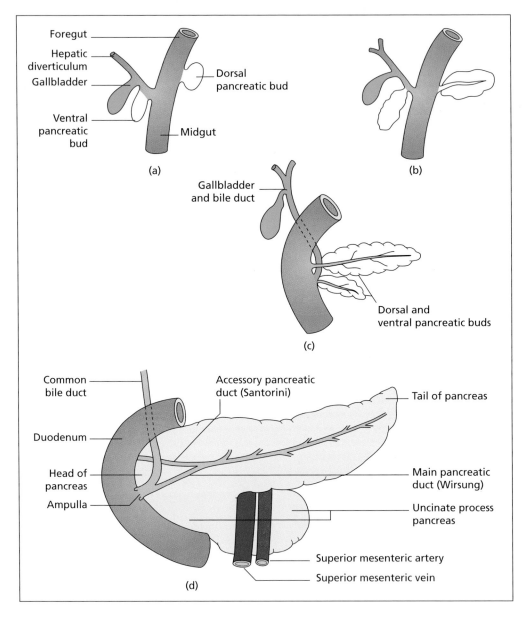

Figure 34.1 (a–d) The development of the pancreas and biliary tree. Reproduced from Ellis H, Mahadevan V (2010) *Clinical Anatomy*, 12th edn. Oxford: Wiley-Blackwell.

Other less common causes of pancreatitis include the following:

- *Postoperative*: particularly after cardiopulmonary bypass or damage to the pancreas during mobilization of the duodenum at partial gastrectomy or splenectomy.
- *Endoscopic retrograde cholangiopancreatography (ERCP)*: particularly if pancreatic duct injection was performed or there was difficulty cannulating the papilla with subsequent oedema and obstruction.
- *Autoimmune* (often characterized by raised serum IgG4 levels) and associated with other autoimmune conditions (e.g. Sjøgren's syndrome).
- *Infection*, for example mumps, cytomegalovirus or coxsackie infection.
- *Trauma*, particularly blunt trauma or crush injury.

- *Drugs*, for example corticosteroids, sodium valproate, azathioprine.
- *Hypothermia*.
- *Hypercalcaemia*.
- *Hyperlipidaemia*.
- *Vascular*: pancreatitis may occur in malignant hypertension, cholesterol emboli and vasculitis such as polyarteritis nodosa, probably as a result of local infarction causing enzyme liberation.
- *Carcinoma of the pancreas (very uncommon)*.
- *Idiopathic*: the cause of some cases of pancreatitis cannot be determined.

Pathology

Acute pancreatitis differs from other inflammatory conditions because of the autodigestion that may result from liberation of digestive enzymes. The pancreas is normally protected from autodigestion by storing its enzymes in intracellular zymogen granules before secreting them as proenzymes. Trypsin, for example, is secreted as trypsinogen and converted to trypsin by the action of enterokinase in the gut. Trypsin itself then cleaves other proenzymes, thus activating them. One such enzyme is phospholipase A which, in pancreatitis, is involved in cell wall damage and fat necrosis along with pancreatic lipase.

The mechanisms initiating autodigestion are multiple. Duodenopancreatic reflux is an important factor that may occur as a result of injury to the papilla following endoscopic cannulation, trauma or surgery in this region, or as a result of damage to the sphincter owing to the recent passage of a stone (hence the strong association of pancreatitis and biliary calculi). Duodenal fluid containing enterokinase then refluxes into the duct, activating the pancreatic proenzymes. Duodenal reflux can be shown experimentally to produce pancreatitis and may be a common factor that underlies many of the aetiological associations mentioned above. As inflammation proceeds, local infarction may occur as arterioles thrombose, and more proenzymes leak out of the necrotic cells to be activated. Once started, pancreatitis can be rapidly progressive, with widespread autodigestion not only confined to the pancreas. There follows multi-system failure secondary to the severe systemic inflammatory response triggered by the local severe inflammation.

As inflammation and autodigestion progress, liquefying necrotic material and inflammatory exudate collect in the lesser sac. This fluid, walled off by the stomach in front and necrotic pancreas behind, forms the so-called 'pseudocyst of the pancreas'. Intra-abdominal fluid collections following acute pancreatitis are classified into the following according to the Revised Atlanta classification.

- Acute peripancreatic fluid collection (<4 weeks).
- Acute necrotizing collection (<4 weeks).
- Pseudocyst (>4 weeks).
- Walled-off necrosis (>4 weeks).

Macroscopic pathology

It is not desirable to operate on patients with acute pancreatitis due to the very high mortality and morbidity associated with it. If surgery has occurred, pancreatitis should be suspected when blood-stained peritoneal effusion and white spots of fat necrosis are seen scattered throughout the peritoneal cavity; these are produced by lipase released from the pancreas, which liberates fatty acids and glycerol from fat; these acids combine with calcium to produce insoluble calcium soaps (saponification). The pancreas is swollen, haemorrhagic or, in severe cases, actually necrotic. Superadded infection of the necrotic tissue is often fatal.

Clinical features

The condition can present at any age but is uncommon in childhood. The patient presenting with gallstone pancreatitis is commonly middle-aged or elderly. By contrast, the alcohol-related form commonly first presents in patients who are younger than 40. Pain is of rapid onset, is severe, constant, usually epigastric and often radiates into the back. The patient typically sits forward, and repeated retching is common. Vomiting is early and profuse. The patient may be shocked with a rapid pulse, cyanosis (indicating circulatory collapse) and a temperature that may be either subnormal or raised up to 39.5 °C (103 °F). Abdominal examination reveals generalized tenderness and guarding.

On rare occasions, a few days after a severe attack, the patient may develop a bluish discoloration in the loins from extravasation of blood-stained pancreatic juice into the retroperitoneal tissues (Grey Turner's sign[4]). The tracking of fluid that results in this sign can often be seen on computed tomography (CT) imaging of patients with acute pancreatitis even when it is not clinically apparent. A bluish discolouration around the umbilicus may also be observed (Cullen's sign[5]).

[4]George Grey Turner (1877–1951), Professor of Surgery, University of Durham, then Foundation Professor of Surgery at the Royal Postgraduate Medical School, London, UK.
[5]Thomas Stephen Cullen (1869–1953), Canadian Professor of Gynaecology, Johns Hopkins, Baltimore. He described the sign in ectopic pregnancy, but it may also occur in acute pancreatitis and with a ruptured abdominal aortic aneurysm.

Differential diagnosis

The less severe episode of acute pancreatitis simulates acute cholecystitis; the more severe attack, with a marked degree of shock, is usually mistaken for a perforated peptic ulcer, leaking abdominal aortic aneurysm or coronary thrombosis. Differentiation must also be made from high intestinal obstruction and from other causes of peritonitis.

Special investigations

The investigation comprises tests to confirm the diagnosis and tests to assess the severity of the disease (i.e. diagnostic and prognostic).

- *Serum amylase.* Amylase is liberated into the circulation by the damaged pancreas, and exceeds the kidney's ability to excrete it, so the serum concentration rises. It is usually significantly raised (fivefold or more) in the acute phase, but returns to normal within 2–3 days; the urinary amylase is elevated for a longer period and may be useful in the diagnosis of cases presenting late. Occasionally, an overwhelming attack of pancreatitis with extensive destruction of the gland, or an attack occurring as an acute exacerbation of chronic pancreatitis, is associated with a normal serum amylase. Other causes of raised serum amylase need to be borne in mind before assuming a diagnosis of pancreatitis (Box 34.1).
- *Serum lipase:* like amylase, serum concentrations of lipase are raised in pancreatitis.
- *Full blood count*: there is a moderate leucocytosis, and anaemia in severe cases.
- *C-reactive protein (CRP)* is often raised in severe cases.
- *Blood glucose* is often raised, with glycosuria in 15% of cases.
- *Arterial blood gases*: hypoxia and acidosis occur in severe cases.
- *Serum calcium* may be lowered, partly as a result of fat saponification.
- *CT* may confirm pancreatitis if the amylase is normal or the diagnosis otherwise is unclear. At a later stage, necrotic pancreas, abscess or pseudocyst may be visualized.
- *Electrocardiography (ECG)* may show diminished T waves, or arrhythmia, and can cause confusion with cardiac ischaemia.

> ### Box 34.1 Raised serum amylase
>
> The causes of raised serum amylase are listed below. Only those marked with an asterisk cause a marked increase in amylase (fivefold or more).
>
> **Impaired renal excretion**
> - Renal failure*.
> - Macroamylasaemia (amylase not cleared by kidneys owing to complexing or protein binding).
>
> **Salivary gland disease**
> - Salivary calculi.
> - Parotitis.
>
> **Metabolic causes**
> - Severe diabetic ketoacidosis*.
> - Acute alcoholic intoxication.
> - Morphine administration (causing sphincter of Oddi spasm[6]).
>
> **Abdominal causes**
> - Acute pancreatitis*.
> - Perforated peptic ulcer.
> - Acute cholecystitis.
> - Intestinal obstruction.
> - Afferent loop obstruction following partial gastrectomy.
> - Ruptured abdominal aortic aneurysm.
> - Ruptured ectopic pregnancy.
> - Mesenteric infarction.
> - Trauma, open or blunt.
> - Inflammatory bowel disease.

- *Abdominal X-rays* often give no direct help. The absence of free gas or of localized fluid levels assists in the differential diagnosis of perforated duodenal ulcer or high intestinal obstruction. In some cases, a solitary dilated loop of proximal jejunum may be seen (the 'sentinel loop sign'). Radio-opaque pancreatic calculi may be present in cases of chronic pancreatitis.
- *Ultrasound* should be carried out in all cases to rule out gallstone-related acute pancreatitis. Patients with acute gallstone pancreatitis should undergo a cholecystectomy prior to discharge from the hospital to prevent relapse.

[6]Ruggero Oddi (1864–1913), Surgeon, Genoa, Italy; he identified the sphincter while a medical student in Perugia, Italy.

Note that each of the three enzymes liberated by the pancreas plays a part in the overall picture of acute pancreatitis.

1 *Trypsin* produces the autodigestion of the pancreas.
2 *Lipase* results in the typical fat necrosis.
3 *Amylase* absorbed from the peritoneal cavity produces a rise in the serum level and is thus a helpful test in diagnosis.

Management

The management of a patient with suspected pancreatitis involves first confirming the diagnosis (serum amylase and/or CT) and determining the severity of the attack. Mortality in severe pancreatitis is high, so severe cases should be managed in a high dependency or intensive care environment where pulmonary, renal and abdominal complications can be promptly diagnosed and treated.

Severe acute pancreatitis

Severe pancreatitis is associated with haemorrhagic necrosis of the pancreas and systemic release of many vasoactive peptides and enzymes, as well as sequestration of large volumes of fluid within the abdomen. Acute lung failure occurs, characterized by increased capillary permeability and reduced oxygen transfer, and the combination of toxins and loss of circulating fluid results in acute renal failure.

Several criteria predictive of the development of severe pancreatitis have been identified (Box 34.2); the presence of three or more is predictive of severe pancreatitis. Both a raised CRP (>140 mg/L) and non-perfusion of areas of the pancreas on a contrast-enhanced CT also predict a poor prognosis. Identification of such high-risk cases enables aggressive intensive management to be instituted at an early stage. Nevertheless, severe acute pancreatitis has a mortality of over 10%.

Supportive treatment

In the established case, treatment is initially *always* non-operative and consists of the following.

- *Analgesia*: relief of pain, traditionally with pethidine to avoid the sphincter spasm associated with morphine.
- *Fluid replacement* with colloid or blood transfusion, to treat shock and establish a diuresis. In less

> **Box 34.2 Glasgow criteria for severe acute pancreatitis**
>
> The factors are assessed over the first 48 hours. Presence of three or more factors indicates severe pancreatitis and are associated with a high mortality.
> - Age over 55 years.
> - Hyperglycaemia (glucose >10 mmol/L in the absence of a history of diabetes).
> - Leucocytosis (>15 × 10^9/L).
> - Urea >16 mmol/L (no response to intravenous fluids).
> - Po_2 <8 kPa (60 mmHg).
> - Calcium <2.0 mmol/L.
> - Albumin <32 g/L.
> - Lactate dehydrogenase >600 IU/L.
> - Raised liver transaminases (aspartate transaminase >100 IU/L).

severe cases, electrolyte and water replacement alone may suffice.
- *Resting the pancreas* by removing stimuli for secretion: the patient is not allowed to take fluid or food by mouth, and nasogastric aspiration is started if the patient is vomiting.
- *Nutrition*: total parenteral nutrition (TPN) may be instituted early in severe cases. There is good evidence that nasojejunal or nasogastric feeding may be superior to TPN in the absence of an ileus, probably because of improved maintenance of the gut mucosal integrity decreasing bacterial translocation and reducing septic complications.
- *Antibiotics:* Use of antibiotics (e.g. co-amoxiclav) is controversial and is associated with infection with resistant bacterial strains and fungal overgrowth. Antibiotics should only be started after careful assessment of the patient and only in severe acute pancreatitis.
- *Prophylaxis against gastric erosions* with sucralfate or an H_2-receptor antagonist (e.g. ranitidine) or proton pump inhibitor (e.g. omeprazole).
- *Endoscopic sphincterotomy* performed early in the admission may be indicated in severe gallstone pancreatitis; a dilated common bile duct on ultrasound associated with deranged liver function tests and cholangitis represents an indication for urgent ERCP and sphincterotomy.

Attempts at treatment with drugs that reduce pancreatic enzyme activation (e.g. aprotinin) or secretion (e.g. probanthine or atropine) are of no proven benefit.

Surgery

Surgery should be avoided early in the acute attack when possible. Later in the disease, percutaneous drainage of collections or abscesses may be indicated, often requiring multiple drains; failure to resolve in spite of adequate drainage may be an indication for operative debridement of the necrotic pancreas (necrosectomy), which should be carried out by minimally invasive techniques. Operative drainage of a pseudocyst may also be required at a later stage (peripancreatic collections in the lesser sac are common in the early stages but usually resolve without intervention). Most pseudocysts can be drained with an endoluminal technique using endoscopic ultrasound (EUS). In the case of gallstone pancreatitis, cholecystectomy should be performed as soon as the patient recovers from the acute attack, preferably during the same admission.

Prognosis

Mortality is in the region of 10% and is directly proportional to the severity of the attack.

Complications

- *Abscess formation* with pancreatic necrosis, characterized by pyrexia and persistent leucocytosis.
- *Peripancreatic collections and pseudocyst formation*, characterized by symptoms attributable to the pressure effect on the stomach with fullness and discomfort commonly associated with a palpable epigastric mass.
- *Intra-abdominal bleeding* from pseudoaneurysms.
- *Gastrointestinal bleeding* from acute gastric erosions or peptic ulceration.
- *Renal failure* associated with shock and pancreatic necrosis.
- *Pulmonary insufficiency*: acute lung injury.
- *Further attacks* (relapsing pancreatitis).
- *Diabetes mellitus*, resulting from a severe attack with pancreatic necrosis, or chronic relapsing pancreatitis.

Chronic pancreatitis

Chronic and acute pancreatitis are clinically distinct entities, although bouts of acute pancreatitis may occur in the course of the development of chronic pancreatitis, and the pathogenesis of chronic pancreatitis has much in common with alcoholic acute pancreatitis. In acute pancreatitis, the gland is normal before the attack; chronic pancreatitis is characterized by gradual destruction of the functional pancreatic tissue.

Aetiology

In the Western world, alcoholism is the main cause of chronic pancreatitis. In parts of Asia and Africa, chronic pancreatitis is associated with malnutrition; hereditary pancreatitis and hypercalcaemia are uncommon causes.

Clinical features

The patient may present with one or more of the following:

- *Asymptomatic*: incidental finding of pancreatic calcification on abdominal X-ray or CT.
- *Recurrent severe abdominal pain* radiating through to the upper lumbar region, relieved by sitting forward.
- *Steatorrhoea* due to pancreatic insufficiency, resulting in malabsorption and weight loss.
- *Diabetes* due to β-cell destruction.
- *Obstructive jaundice*, which even at operation can be very difficult to differentiate from carcinoma of the head of the pancreas.

Special investigations

- *Serum amylase* estimations performed during attacks of pain may be elevated, but in long-standing disease are often normal, there being insufficient pancreatic tissue remaining to cause a large rise.
- *Abdominal X-ray* may show evidence of calcification or biliary calculi.
- *CT* may demonstrate enlargement and irregular consistency of the gland together with calcification and ductal changes, although the ductal changes may be better appreciated by the use of magnetic resonance cholangiopancreatography (MRCP).
- *Endoscopic ultrasound (EUS)* has become the standard technique for examining the head of the pancreas, and aspiration cytology can be carried out from any suspicious areas to help differentiate chronic pancreatitis or areas of focal pancreatitis from carcinoma.

- *ERCP* may show dilation and irregularity of the pancreatic duct and compression of the bile duct by the inflamed pancreatic head.
- *Exocrine function tests*, such as the faecal elastase test, have largely replaced older techniques such as faecal fat estimation.

In spite of preoperative investigation, the differential diagnosis from a pancreatic carcinoma may occasionally only be established following laparotomy and resection when formal histology is obtained.

Treatment

The principal treatment is to remove causative factors such as alcohol consumption. Alcohol should be avoided by anyone with pancreatitis.

- *Analgesics*: the pain is often sufficient to warrant opiate analgesia, but long-term use may result in addiction. Getting the analgesia right is often one of the most difficult aspects of management.
- *Diet*: a low-fat diet with pancreatic enzyme supplements (e.g., pancreatin) by mouth.
- *Insulin* when diabetes mellitus occurs.
- *Surgery* if attacks are very frequent or if there is severe pain. Partial pancreatectomy or, in patients in whom the pancreatic duct is grossly dilated, drainage of the whole length of the pancreatic duct into a loop of small intestine may be required (Puestow procedure[7]) along with coring of the abnormal head of the pancreas (Frey's procedure[8]). Occasionally, total pancreatectomy is required, with consequent diabetes and steatorrhoea. In these patients, the diabetes may be very difficult to control partly because of their poor compliance and partly because of the loss of the glucagon-secreting function when the whole pancreas has been removed.
- *Painless obstructive jaundice* may be relieved by a bypass using a Roux-en-Y reconstruction, usually to the common hepatic duct. However, if diagnostic uncertainty remains or if there is a coincident problem with gastric emptying, a Whipple's pancreaticoduodenectomy operation may be appropriate.

---

[7]Charles Puestow (1902–1973), Professor of Surgery, College of Medicine, University of Illinois, Chicago, IL, USA.
[8]Charles Frederick Frey (b. 1929), Surgeon, UC Davis Medical Center, USA.

Pancreatic cysts

Classification

True cyst

Neoplastic (10%)

Cystic neoplasms can be subdivided according to whether they do or do not communicate with the ductal system.

- *Ductal*: intraductal papillary mucinous neoplasm (IPMN).
- *Non-ductal*: mucinous cystic neoplasm (MCN) and serous cystadenoma.

Non-neoplastic (90%)

- Congenital polycystic disease of pancreas.
- Retention.
- Hydatid.

False cyst

A collection of fluid in the lesser sac:

- After trauma to the pancreas.
- Following acute pancreatitis.
- Owing to perforation of a posterior gastric ulcer (rare).

Clinical features

Cystic lesions of the pancreas are less common than solid lesions, but are increasingly being detected incidentally while they are small and asymptomatic due to higher numbers of CT scans now performed for other reasons. A large pancreatic cyst presents as a firm, large, rounded, upper abdominal swelling. Initially, the cyst is apparently resonant because of loops of gas-filled bowel in front of it, but as it increases in size the intestine is pushed away and the mass becomes dull to percussion.

There are three common cystic neoplasms.

Serous cystadenomas are benign cystic tumours which can grow to a large size and cause symptoms by virtue of their size. Typically, they affect middle-aged women and have a ground glass or 'bunch of grapes' appearance on imaging.

Mucinous cystic neoplasms (MCNs) are cystic tumours that predominantly affect the tail of the pancreas and also occur typically in middle-aged women.

Intraductal papillary mucinous neoplasms (IPMN) arise from ductal epithelium and are characterized by the production of a large amount of mucus. They are slow-growing tumours that may be benign or malignant, and occur more commonly in older men.

Treatment

Treatment of cystic lesions of the pancreas depends on the nature of the cyst. A simple collection of fluid in the lesser sac without communication to the pancreatic duct often requires expectant management only. However, should the lesions fail to settle or cause symptoms, they may be drained either percutaneously under ultrasound control or internally by anastomosis into the stomach (operatively or by EUS control). Cysts which have a true communication with the pancreatic duct will require internal drainage either surgically or under EUS control. Cystadenomas and cystadenocarcinomas are surgically resected by means of a pancreatectomy.

Management of IPMN presents a unique diagnostic challenge. Aspiration and analysis of cyst fluid under EUS guidance (for fluid amylase, fluid carcinoembryonic antigen [CEA], mucin and abnormal cytology) often will give an idea as to the nature of the lesion, and hence its management, premalignant change being suggested by a high CEA and abnormal cytology. Main duct IPMN and large IPMN are also considered precancerous lesions and should be resected by means of a pancreatectomy. Others should be kept under surveillance with regular CT or magnetic resonance (MR) scans for high-risk features such as increasing size, enhancing mural nodules and pancreatic duct dilatation.

Pancreatic tumours

Classification

Benign

1 Adenoma.
2 Cystadenoma.
3 Islet cell tumour:
  a Zollinger–Ellison tumour.
  b Insulinoma (β-cell tumour).
  c Glucagonoma (α-cell tumour).

Malignant

1 *Primary*:
  a Adenocarcinoma.
  b Cystadenocarcinoma.
  c Malignant islet cell tumour.
2 *Secondary*: invasion from carcinoma of the stomach or bile duct.

Pancreatic neuroendocrine tumours

These tumours arise from cell types within the islets of Langerhans and, although rare (less than 2% of pancreatic neoplasms), are of great interest because of their metabolic effects, even from small lesions, which may be difficult to localize even with CT and MR imaging or selective angiography.

Types of tumours

Pancreatic neuroendocrine tumours are derived from amine precursor uptake and decarboxylation (APUD) cells, and are thus sometimes termed 'APUD-omas'. They secrete a number of polypeptides according to the cell type of origin. These may be active hormones and present relatively early, or polypeptides for which no function has been identified; often, more than one polypeptide is secreted. A pancreatic islet contains many cell types of which the alpha (α) cells (producing glucagon), beta (β) cells (insulin) and delta (δ) cells (somatostatin) are best known. In addition, interacinar cells produce pancreatic polypeptide (F cells) and serotonin (enterochromaffin cells). The islet cells may also produce hormones not normally found in the pancreas, such as gastrin (gastrinoma), vasoactive intestinal polypeptide (VIP-oma) and adrenocorticotrophic hormone (ACTH) (Cushing's syndrome[9]).

The islet cell tumours may be associated with other endocrine tumours elsewhere as part of a multiple endocrine neoplasia (MEN) syndrome, often involving the parathyroid and the anterior pituitary gland (see Box 40.1).

---

[9]Harvey Cushing (1869–1939), Professor of Surgery, Harvard Medical School, Boston, MA, USA.

Insulinoma (β-cell tumour)

Ninety per cent are benign, 10% malignant and about 10% are multiple tumours. Because of the high production of insulin by the tumour, two groups of hypoglycaemic symptoms may be produced.

1 *Central nervous system phenomena*: weakness, sweating, trembling, epilepsy, confusion, hemiplegia and eventually coma, which may be fatal.
2 *Gastrointestinal phenomena*: hunger, abdominal pain and diarrhoea.

These symptoms appear particularly when the patient is hungry, or during physical exercise. They are often present early in the morning before breakfast and are relieved by eating. Often, there is excessive appetite with gross weight gain, although once the diagnosis has been made the cause of the symptomatology is clear. However, it is not uncommon for diagnosis to be delayed, and psychiatric diagnoses and referrals to be made during the course of investigations.

Diagnosis: Whipple's triad[10]

The main diagnostic characteristics of the syndrome are as follows.

- The attacks are induced by starvation or exercise.
- During the attack, hypoglycaemia is present.
- Symptoms are relieved by sugar given orally or intravenously.

Differential diagnosis of spontaneous hypoglycaemia in adults includes self-administration of insulin or alcohol, and adrenal, pituitary or hepatic insufficiency.

Special investigations

- *Insulin levels*: raised insulin levels in the presence of hypoglycaemia. The hypoglycaemia can be prompted by a period of prolonged fasting (14–16 hours).

- *C-peptide levels* may be measured to rule out exogenous insulin administration, as these will be high with insulinoma and low when exogenous insulin is administered.
- *Localization tests* include CT, MR, selective angiography and EUS. In recent times, EUS has developed to be a sensitive diagnostic tool with the added advantage of the ability to obtain tissue diagnosis as well. Occasionally, localization is not achieved until laparotomy is performed, when the tumour can usually be located using careful palpation and intraoperative ultrasound.

Treatment

Treatment is excision of the tumour. Depending on the site, this may require either a Whipple's procedure or a distal pancreatectomy, but in patients in whom the insulinoma is well defined and superficial, simple enucleation is often possible.

Gastrinoma (Zollinger–Ellison syndrome,[11] non-β-cell islet tumour)

This tumour of non-β-cells may be benign or malignant, solitary or multiple, and one-quarter are part of the MEN syndrome. Malignant tumours are less common in sporadic forms (30%) than in those related to MEN syndromes (60%); the malignant tumours are also relatively slow growing, although they eventually produce hepatic metastases. The gastrinoma secretes a gastrin-like substance into the bloodstream, which produces an extremely high gastric secretion of hydrochloric acid. Many patients also develop oesophagitis owing to the high acid secretion; diarrhoea is common (probably related to the high acid output). The majority of patients develop fulminating peptic ulceration, presenting with bleeding or perforation, and have multiple duodenal ulcers. Symptoms relapse after cessation of medical therapy.

---

[10]Allen Oldfather Whipple (1881–1963), Professor of Surgery, Columbia University, New York, USA. He also described the operation for carcinoma of the head of the pancreas (Figure 34.2).

[11]Robert Milton Zollinger (1903–1992), Professor of Surgery, Ohio State University, Columbus, OH, USA. Edward Horner Ellison (1918–1970), Associate Professor at the same institution.

Special investigations

- *Serum gastrin* concentration in the blood is 10 times normal.
- *Basal acid output*, measured by nasogastric aspiration, is very high (>15 mmol/h).
- *Localization*: as for insulinoma.

Treatment

Treatment comprises excision of the tumour or, if this is not possible, control of the high acid secretion by means of proton pump inhibitors (e.g. omeprazole) or high doses of histamine H_2-receptor antagonists (e.g. cimetidine). Modern acid suppression therapy has largely replaced surgical treatment by total gastrectomy.

Pancreatic carcinoma

Pathology

Sixty per cent are situated in the head of the pancreas, 25% in the body and 15% in the tail.

Of the tumours of the head of the pancreas, one-third are periampullary, arising from the ampulla of Vater, the duodenal mucosa or the lower end of the common bile duct.

Pancreatic cancer is the 10th most common cancer in the UK, with an incidence of 17 per 100000 population, with men and women now almost equally affected. It affects the middle-aged and elderly, and the disease is more common in those who smoke; half of all new cases occur in those aged 75 and over.

Macroscopically, the growth is infiltrating, hard and irregular; rarer types are characterized by cystic lesions near the tail of the pancreas.

Microscopically, the tumours may be:

- Ductal adenocarcinomas (most common): tumours arising in the cells lining the pancreatic ducts.
- Acinar cell carcinoma.
- Undifferentiated.

Spread

1 *Direct invasion into*:
   a   Common bile duct – obstructive jaundice.
   b   Duodenum – occult or overt intestinal bleeding and duodenal obstruction.
   c   Portal vein – portal vein thrombosis, portal hypertension and ascites.
   d   Superior mesenteric artery – resulting in thrombosis or haemorrhage.
   e   Inferior vena cava – bilateral leg oedema.
2 *Lymphatic*: to adjacent lymph nodes and nodes in the porta hepatis.
3 *Bloodstream*: to the liver and then to the lungs.
4 *Transcoelomic*: with peritoneal seeding and ascites.

Clinical features

Carcinoma of the pancreas may present in a variety of ways.

- *Painless progressive jaundice* is the classic presentation. This form is rather uncommon and is most often found in the periampullary type of tumour where the bile duct is compressed at an early stage, before extensive painful invasion of surrounding tissues.
- *Severe loss of appetite and weight.*
- *Pain*: at least 50% of patients present with epigastric pain of a dull, continuous, aching nature, which frequently radiates into the upper lumbar region. Severe pain usually suggests invasion of peripancreatic nerves and hence is likely to be inoperable.
- *Diabetes*: new onset or worsening of diabetes in the elderly is suspicious.
- *Thrombophlebitis migrans* (Trousseau's sign[12]): the pathogenesis of this is unknown.

Examination

The patient is frequently jaundiced, and around 50% of patients have a palpable gallbladder (Courvoisier's law; see Figure 33.3). If the tumour is large, an epigastric mass may be palpable, although this is very unusual. The liver is frequently enlarged, either because of back-pressure from biliary obstruction or because of secondary deposits.

Special investigations

- *Ultrasound* will confirm dilated bile ducts and a distended gallbladder, but should not be relied on to obtain adequate views of the pancreas.

---

[12]Armand Trousseau (1801–1867), Physician, Hôpital Necker, Hôpital St Antoine and Hôpital Dieu, Paris, France.

- *IV contrast-enhanced CT* usually will demonstrate the tumour mass and detect local vascular invasion and distant metastases.
- *Endoscopy* may visualize a periampullary growth, which can then be biopsied.
- *Endoscopic ultrasound (EUS)*, in which a specialized endoscope is used to obtain ultrasound images of the pancreatic head from within the duodenum, will give detailed information about the location of the tumour and its relationship to the portal vein and superior mesenteric artery and will demonstrate local extent of spread and also visualize enlarged lymph nodes. EUS is thus a key step in defining the operability of a tumour in terms of local invasion and spread.
  - Needle aspiration under EUS control will allow cytological diagnosis of the tumour itself and lymph node metastases.
  - Needle aspiration of cystic lesions may distinguish between pseudocysts (high amylase content) and mucinous tumours (high Ca 19.9 and CEA; see Table 7.2).
- *MRCP and ERCP* will demonstrate an obstruction in the bile duct. These are usually not required in the diagnosis of pancreatic cancer. However, ERCP may be carried out to place a stent in the blocked biliary tree to palliate jaundice.
- *Occult blood* may be present in the stools, especially from a periampullary tumour ulcerating into the duodenum. The stools are pale in the presence of jaundice, and may have a silvery appearance owing to the periampullary bleeding (the silvery stools of Ogilvie[13]).
- *Serum amylase* is rarely elevated; it is not a test for pancreatic cancer.
- *Biochemical analysis* confirms the changes of obstructive jaundice (high bilirubin and alkaline phosphatase). The tumour marker Ca 19.9 may be elevated, but is neither sensitive nor specific for definitive diagnosis of pancreatic cancer.

Differential diagnosis

This is from other causes of obstructive jaundice and from other causes of upper abdominal pain. Carcinoma of the body and tail of the pancreas, in which

obstructive jaundice does not occur, is notoriously difficult to diagnose, the diagnosis often only being made at a late stage when a CT scan is performed following many weeks or months of upper abdominal pain. The tumour is usually inoperable at this stage.

Treatment

Surgical resection may be offered to the 20% of patients who have an operable pancreatic cancer and are also fit to undergo complex major surgery. Accurate staging of the disease and assessment of the patient should be made prior to recommending a pancreatic resection. For the rest, palliative treatment is more appropriate.

- *Curative surgical resection* is possible when disease is confined to the periampullary region. The procedure (Whipple's pancreaticoduodenectomy; Figure 34.2) involves removal of the duodenal 'C' along with the pancreatic head and common bile duct; a gastroenterostomy and biliary drainage using a Roux loop[14] of jejunum are fashioned to restore continuity, together with implantation of the pancreatic duct into the jejunal Roux loop. The 5-year survival for resected pancreatic ductal adenocarcinoma even with adjuvant chemotherapy is only around 25% except in early periampullary tumours and cystic cancers.
- *Palliative surgical bypass* comprises a short circuit between the distended bile duct and a loop of jejunum (hepaticojejunostomy), together with a duodenal bypass by a gastroenterostomy if duodenal obstruction is present. This procedure is only considered in patients where endoscopic placement of biliary/duodenal stents is not possible.
- *Palliative intubation*, by passage of a self-expanding metal stent across the ampulla and through the obstructed common bile duct, is the preferred treatment for obstructive jaundice. This may be performed either endoscopically (ERCP) or transhepatically (percutaneous transhepatic cholangiography). This should allow the terminally ill patient to be spared the additional morbidity of a laparotomy and surgical bypass. Alternatively, laparoscopic

[13]Sir William Heneage Ogilvie (1887–1971), Surgeon, Guy's Hospital, London, UK.

[14]Cesar Roux (1857–1934), Professor of Surgery, Lausanne, Switzerland.

gastroenterostomy can be used to palliate duodenal obstruction.

- *Severe pain* often requires management with opiates, but coeliac plexus block performed either via the percutaneous approach or under endoscopic ultrasound guidance can offer good pain control in some cases.

Prognosis

The outlook for patients with carcinoma of the pancreas itself is gloomy; even if the growth is resectable, the operation has a mortality of about 2–5% and only a small percentage survive for 5 years. Periampullary growths, however, which present relatively early, have a reasonably good prognosis after resection, with about a 40% 5-year survival.

Adjuvant and palliative chemotherapy currently uses protocols based on gemcitabine. The place of radiotherapy is unclear, although some centres do use a combination of radiotherapy and chemotherapy in selected patients. Recent trials have shown a definite survival benefit in patients who have undergone attempted curative resection and who receive postoperative chemotherapy.

Occasionally, a patient has a surprisingly prolonged survival after a palliative bypass operation. In such a case, the diagnosis should be revisited and rare conditions such as IgG4 disease and chronic pancreatitis should be ruled out.

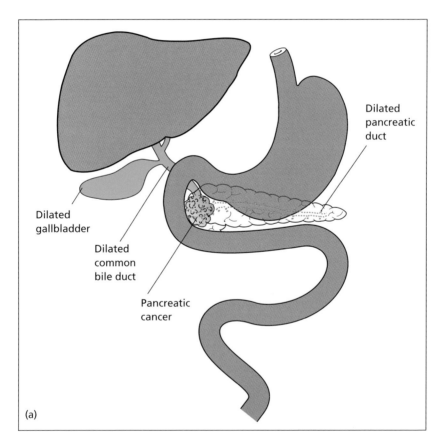

Dilated pancreatic duct

Dilated gallbladder

Dilated common bile duct

Pancreatic cancer

(a)

Figure 34.2 Whipple's pancreaticoduodenectomy. (a) The initial appearance characterized by a distended gallbladder, dilated bile duct and pancreatic duct, and mass in the head of the pancreas. (b) Following resection, the stomach remnant is anastomosed to the proximal jejunum as a gastrojejunostomy; the common hepatic duct is anastomosed to a Roux-en-Y loop of jejunum, the end of which is anastomosed to the pancreatic duct.

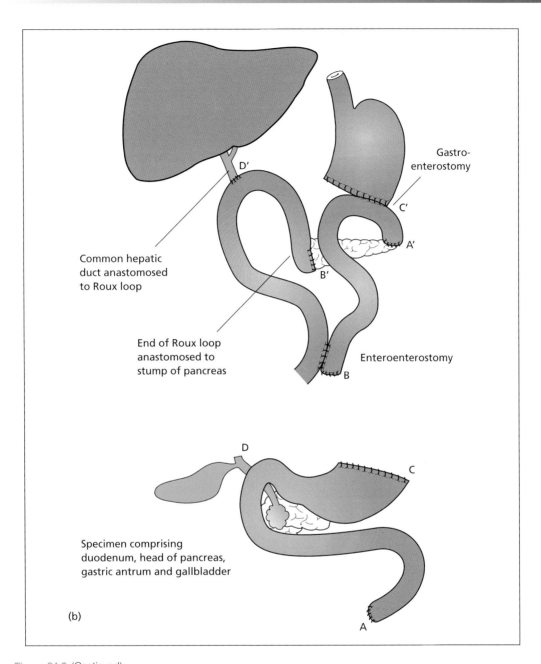

Gastro-
enterostomy

D′

C′

Common hepatic
duct anastomosed
to Roux loop

A′

B′

End of Roux loop
anastomosed to
stump of pancreas

Enteroenterostomy

B

D

C

Specimen comprising
duodenum, head of pancreas,
gastric antrum and gallbladder

(b)

A

Figure 34.2 (*Continued*)

🖰 Additional resources

Case 91: A patient with jaundice and interesting
physical signs

Case 92: The patient in case 91 has surgery
Case 93: A giant abdominal mass

35

The spleen

Christopher Watson

Learning objective

✓ To know the common causes of splenomegaly, the presentations of a ruptured spleen and the prophylaxis and treatment of post-splenectomy syndrome.

Splenomegaly

Physical signs

The spleen must be enlarged to about three times its normal size before it becomes clinically palpable. It then forms a swelling that descends below the left costal margin, moves on respiration and has a firm lower margin, which may or may not be notched. The mass is dull to percussion, the dullness extending above the costal margin.

There are three important differential diagnoses.

1 An enlarged left kidney; unless this is enormous, there is resonance over the swelling anteriorly, as it is covered by the gas-containing colon.
2 Carcinoma of the cardia or upper part of the body of the stomach; by the time such a tumour reaches palpable proportions, there are usually symptoms of gastric obstruction, which suggest the site of the lesion.
3 An enlarged left lobe of the liver.

Classification

It is essential to have a working classification of enlargements of the spleen.

1 *Infections.*
   a Viruses: glandular fever (Epstein-Barr virus).
   b Bacterial: typhus, typhoid, septicaemia ('septic spleen').
   c Protozoal: malaria, kala-azar, schistosomiasis (Egyptian splenomegaly).
   d Parasitic: hydatid.
2 *Haematological diseases.*
   a Leukaemia: chronic myeloid and chronic lymphocytic.
   b Lymphoma: Hodgkin's and non-Hodgkin's lymphoma.
   c Myelofibrosis, idiopathic thrombocytopenia, polycythaemia rubra vera.
   d Haemolytic anaemias, for example spherocytosis, β-thalassaemia.
3 *Portal hypertension.* Increased pressure in the portal system causes progressive enlargement of the spleen and may lead to hypersplenism with overactivity of the normal splenic functions such as removal of platelets, erythrocytes and leucocytes, resulting in thrombocytopenia, anaemia and leucopaenia.
4 *Metabolic and collagen disease.*
   a Amyloid: secondary to rheumatoid arthritis, collagen diseases, chronic sepsis.
   b Storage diseases, for example Gaucher's disease.[1]
5 *Cysts, abscesses and tumours of the spleen*: all uncommon.

Ellis and Calne's Lecture Notes in General Surgery, Fourteenth Edition. Edited by Christopher Watson and Justin Davies.
© 2023 John Wiley & Sons Ltd. Published 2023 by John Wiley & Sons Ltd.
Companion website: www.wiley.com/go/Watson/GeneralSurgery14

[1] Phillipe Gaucher (1854–1918), Physician, Hôpital St Louis, Paris, France.

Massive splenomegaly in the UK is likely to be due to one of the following: chronic myeloid leukaemia, myelofibrosis, lymphoma, polycythaemia or portal hypertension.

If the spleen is palpable, special attention must be paid to detecting the presence of hepatomegaly and lymphadenopathy (see Chapter 32).

Splenectomy

Splenectomy is indicated under the following circumstances.

- *Rupture*: either from closed or open trauma or from accidental damage during abdominal surgery.
- *Haematological disease*: haemolytic anaemia, thrombocytopenic purpura.
- *Tumours and cysts*.
- *Part of another operative procedure*, for example radical excision of carcinoma of the stomach, distal pancreatectomy, splenorenal anastomosis for portal hypertension.

Complications of splenectomy

Gastric dilation

Following splenectomy, there may be a gastric ileus. Swallowed air causes rapid dilation of the stomach, which may tear ligatures on the short gastric vessels on the greater curve of the stomach, which were tied during splenectomy; haemorrhage results. To prevent this, a nasogastric tube is placed and regularly aspirated.

Thrombocytosis

Following splenectomy, the platelet count rises, often to a level of $1000 \times 10^9/L$ (normal is $<400 \times 10^9/L$). In time, the count falls but while it is high, the patient is at a greater than normal risk of deep vein thrombosis and pulmonary embolus. Antiplatelet agents such as aspirin are given as prophylaxis in addition to low molecular weight heparin.

Post-splenectomy sepsis

One of the spleen's functions is to clear capsulated micro-organisms (such as *Streptococcus pneumoniae*, *Neisseria meningitidis* and *Haemophilus influenzae*)

from the bloodstream after they have been opsonized by the binding of host antibodies to their surface as part of the normal immune response. The spleen also has important phagocytic properties, as well as being the largest repository of lymphoid tissue in the body.

Splenectomy predisposes the patient, especially a child, to infection with capsulated organisms such as the *Pneumococcus*. The clinical course is of a fulminant bacterial infection, with shock and circulatory collapse, termed 'overwhelming post-splenectomy infection' (OPSI).

Prophylactic immunization with pneumococcal, meningococcal and *H. influenzae* type B vaccines should be administered, at least 2 weeks preoperatively when possible, or prior to hospital discharge as part of an emergency splenectomy. In addition, children should have prophylactic daily low-dose penicillin at least until they reach 16 years of age. Adults should have penicillin for at least the first 2 years after splenectomy, and lifelong once over 50 years of age. Other high-risk groups who should receive daily antibiotic prophylaxis include those who are immunosuppressed, have had splenic irradiation, or have previously had invasive pneumococcal disease, or who fail to develop an antibody response following immunization. Annual flu immunizations are also recommended to minimize the additional risk of bacterial superinfection and special care is required if the patient is to travel to malarial areas.

Patients presenting with infections who have previously had a splenectomy should be treated immediately with amoxicillin (or erythromycin if penicillin allergic).

Ruptured spleen

This is the most common internal injury produced by non-penetrating trauma to the abdominal wall. It usually occurs in isolation, but may co-exist with fractures of the ribs or rupture of the liver, the left kidney, the diaphragm or the tail of the pancreas.

Clinical features

Rupture of the spleen manifests in one of the following ways.

1 *Immediate massive bleeding* with rapid death from shock. This results from a complete shattering of the spleen or its avulsion from the splenic pedicle,

and death from exsanguination may occur in a few minutes. Fortunately, this is rare.

2 *Peritonism from progressive blood loss.* Following injury, there are the symptoms and signs of progressive blood loss together with evidence of peritoneal irritation. Over a period of several hours after the accident, the patient becomes increasingly pale, the pulse rises and the blood pressure falls. There is abdominal pain, which is either diffuse or confined to the left flank. The patient may complain of pain referred to the left shoulder tip or admit to this only on direct questioning.

On examination, the abdomen is generally tender, particularly on the left side. There may be marked generalized rigidity, or it may be confined to slight guarding in the left flank. Bruising of the abdominal wall is often absent or only slight.

3 *Delayed rupture.* This may occur from hours up to several days after trauma. Following the initial injury, the concomitant pain soon settles. Then, following a completely asymptomatic interval, the signs and symptoms described above become manifest. This picture is produced by a subcapsular haematoma of the spleen, which increases in size and then ruptures the thin overlying peritoneal capsule with a resultant sudden, brisk haemorrhage.

4 *Spontaneous rupture.* A spleen diseased by, for example, malaria, glandular fever or leukaemia, may rupture spontaneously or after only trivial trauma.

Special investigations

The diagnosis of a ruptured spleen is a clinical one, and an unstable patient must be resuscitated aggressively and the surgeon proceed at once to laparotomy. In the less acute situation, and only after resuscitation has begun, the following investigations are useful.

- *Focused abdominal sonography for trauma (FAST) (ultrasound)* may reveal free fluid, an intrasplenic

haematoma or a laceration of the capsule, although the latter may be overlooked. Ultrasound is increasingly used as a diagnostic tool in the emergency department for such cases.
- *Computed tomography* is the investigation of choice in all cases of abdominal trauma, and will demonstrate the laceration of the spleen and the presence of intra-abdominal fluid and identify traumatic injuries to other organs.
- *Chest X-ray* may reveal associated rib fractures, rupture of the diaphragm or injury to the left lung.
- *Urinalysis* showing haematuria will suggest associated coincidental renal damage.

Treatment

Resuscitation is commenced with plasma expanders initially and blood replacement as soon as blood is available. Haemodynamically unstable patients with positive FAST or CT scans should undergo immediate laparotomy. If the spleen is found to be avulsed or hopelessly pulped, emergency splenectomy is required. If there is minor laceration of the spleen, an attempt may be made to preserve it, especially in children and young adults, in whom there is a greater risk of post-splenectomy sepsis. This may be carried out by using argon beam coagulation, sutures, fibrin glues and/or topical haemostatic fibrin patches. Having controlled the bleeding at laparotomy, it is important to carry out a full examination to exclude injury to other organs.

In haemodynamically stable patients with minor injuries not requiring surgery and evidence of on-going splenic bleeding, a non-operative approach with angiographic embolization to control bleeding may be considered.

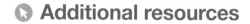 **Additional resources**

Case 94: A severe abdominal injury

36

The lymph nodes and lymphatics

Christopher Watson

Learning objectives

✓ To know the causes of lymphadenopathy and the appropriate management.

✓ To have knowledge of lymphoedema and its causes.

Enlarged lymph nodes are a common diagnostic problem, so it is important to have a simple classification and clinical approach to their assessment.

The lymphadenopathies

The lymphadenopathies can be conveniently divided into those due to local disease and those due to generalized disease.

Classification

Localized

1   *Infective*:
    a   Acute, for example a cervical lymphadenopathy secondary to tonsillitis.
    b   Chronic, for example tuberculous nodes of neck.
2   *Neoplastic*: due to secondary spread of tumour.

Generalized

1   *Infective*:
    a   Acute, for example glandular fever (mononucleosis), septicaemia.
    b   Chronic, for example human immunodeficiency virus (HIV), secondary syphilis.
2   *The reticuloses*: Hodgkin's disease,[1] non-Hodgkin's lymphoma, chronic lymphocytic leukaemia.
3   *Sarcoidosis*.

Clinical examination

The clinical examination of any patient with a lymph node enlargement is incomplete unless the following three requirements have been fulfilled.

1   The area drained by the involved lymph nodes has been searched for a possible primary source of infection or malignant disease. There are four important points to remember.
    a   *Cervical lymphadenopathy*. In addition to examining the skin of the head and neck, the inside of the oropharynx together with the

Ellis and Calne's Lecture Notes in General Surgery, Fourteenth Edition.
Edited by Christopher Watson and Justin Davies.
© 2023 John Wiley & Sons Ltd. Published 2023 by John Wiley & Sons Ltd.
Companion website: www.wiley.com/go/Watson/GeneralSurgery14

[1]Thomas Hodgkin (1798–1866), Curator of Pathology, Guy's Hospital, London, UK.

larynx should be examined for chronic sepsis or malignant disease.

b *Inguinal lymphadenopathy.* If a patient has an enlarged lymph node in the groin, the skin of the leg, buttock and lower abdominal wall below the level of the umbilicus must be scrutinized, together with the external genitalia and the anal canal.

c *Testicular tumours* drain along their lymphatics, which pass with the testicular vessels to the para-aortic lymph nodes, and not to the inguinal lymph nodes.

d *Virchow's node*[2] is a prominent node in the left supraclavicular fossa arising from malignant disease below the diaphragm, such as gastric carcinoma, with secondaries ascending the thoracic duct to drain into the left subclavian vein (Troisier's sign[3]). A supraclavicular node may also signify spread from intrathoracic, testicular or breast tumours.

2 The other lymph node areas are examined, as enlarged lymph nodes elsewhere would suggest a generalized lymphadenopathy.

3 The liver and spleen are carefully palpated; their enlargement will suggest a lymphoma, sarcoid or glandular fever.

Special investigations

In many instances, the cause of the lymphadenopathy will by now have become obvious. The following investigations may be required in order to elucidate the diagnosis further.

- *Examination of a blood film* may clinch the diagnosis of glandular fever or leukaemia.
- *Chest X-ray* may show evidence of enlarged mediastinal nodes or may reveal a primary occult tumour of the lung, which is the source of disseminated deposits.
- *Serological tests*: an HIV antibody test is performed if infection is suspected; syphilis may be confirmed by specific treponemal antigen tests.

- *Ultrasound* of a lymph node may be able to determine whether it has a normal morphology or is suggestive of malignant infiltration.
- *Lymph node biopsy*: ultrasound-guided needle core biopsy, or surgical removal of one of the enlarged lymph nodes, may be necessary for definite histological proof of the diagnosis. This is particularly so in Hodgkin's disease and non-Hodgkin's lymphoma.
- *Computed tomography (CT) scan* of the neck, chest, abdomen and pelvis may be required to determine the stage of any lymphoma, or to identify the primary tumour.
- *X-ray of cervical nodes* may show spotty calcification typical of tuberculous nodes.

Lymphoedema

Lymphoedema results from the obstruction of lymphatic flow, owing to inherited abnormalities of the lymphatics, their obliteration by disease or their operative removal. It is characterized by an excessive accumulation of interstitial fluid. Affected individuals are prone to infections (cellulitis) in the affected areas together with lymphangitis. The causes of lymphoedema may be divided into primary and secondary.

Primary lymphoedema

There are two autosomal dominant inherited forms of lymphoedema, both are more common in women.

- *Type 1* (also known as Milroy disease,[4] Nonne–Milroy[5] disease and primary congenital lymphoedema) is very uncommon and is often associated with a mutation in the *FLT4* gene, which encodes vascular endothelial growth factor receptor 3 (VEGFR-3), VEGF being important in lymphangiogenesis. It is characterized by onset soon after birth with lower limb swelling.
- *Type 2* (also known as Meige syndrome[6]) is the most common primary lymphoedema, and is associated with mutations in *FOXC2*, a forkhead family transcription factor gene. It is characterized

[2]Rudolf Ludwig Karl Virchow (1821–1902), Professor of Pathology in Würzburg and later Berlin, Germany. He described the nodes in association with gastric carcinoma (1848).
[3]Charles Émile Troisier (1844–1919), Professor of Pathology, Paris, France. He described the sign in connection with other types intra-abdominal cancer (1889).

[4]William Forsyth Milroy (1855–1942), Professor of Medicine, University of Nebraska, Omaha, NE, USA.
[5]Max Nonne (1861–1959), Neurologist, Hamburg, Germany.

by lymphoedema that is particularly severe below the waist. It has been arbitrarily divided into *lymphoedema praecox*, which develops between puberty and the age of 35, and the less common *lymphoedema tarda*, which develops in adult life.

There are three principal pathological processes affecting the lymphatic channels in congenital lymphoedema: aplasia, hypoplasia and varicose dilation (megalymphatics).

Secondary lymphoedema

Secondary lymphoedema develops where a previously normal lymphatic system has been damaged. It affects more than 200000 people in the UK, with one in 6000 having primary lymphoedema

- *Post-inflammatory*: the result of fibrosis obliterating the lymphatics following repeated attacks of streptococcal cellulitis, particularly when the lymphatic drainage is already compromised.
- *Filariasis*: *Filaria bancrofti*[7] infects lymphatics; a chronic inflammatory reaction is set up with consequent lymphatic obstruction. There is gross lymphoedema, especially of the lower limbs and genitalia, often called elephantiasis.
- *Following radical surgery*, particularly after block dissection of the axilla, groin or neck in which extensive removal of lymphatics is performed.
- *Post-irradiation fibrosis*.
- *Malignant disease*: late oedema of the arm after axillary clearance and radical mastectomy is often indicative of massive recurrence of tumour in the axilla occluding the residual lymphatic pathways.
- *Obesity* is also a cause of secondary lymphoedema.

Special investigations

- *Lymphoscintigraphy* involves injecting a radiolabelled protein subcutaneously and monitoring its movement through the lymphatics. It will confirm lymphatic obstruction.
- *Magnetic resonance imaging* may be used to confirm the cause of obstruction in secondary cases.
- *CT scan* may also detect disease in proximal lymphatics.

[6]Henri Meige (1866–1940), Professor of Medicine, Hôpital de Salpêtrière, Paris, France.
[7]Joseph Bancroft (1836–1894), Physician and Public Health Officer, Brisbane, Australia.

> ### Box 36.1 A swollen leg
>
> **Generalized disease**
> - Cardiac failure.
> - Nephrotic syndrome.
> - Liver failure.
>
> **Venous disease**
> - Venous thrombosis*.
> - Deep venous insufficiency.
> - Arteriovenous fistula,* e.g. Klippel–Trenaunay syndrome[8].
>
> **Lymphatic disease**
> - Primary lymphoedema*.
> - Secondary lymphoedema,* e.g. filariasis, malignant infiltration, following surgery or irradiation to lymphatics.*
>
> *Also may cause unilateral upper limb swelling.

Differential diagnosis

The diagnosis of lymphoedema depends first of all on the exclusion of other causes of oedema, for instance venous obstruction, cardiac failure or renal disease, and, second, on demonstration of one of the causes mentioned above (Box 36.1). It was previously taught that lymphoedema could readily be differentiated from other forms of oedema on the simple physical sign of absence of pitting in the lymphoedematous limb. However, lymphoedema of acute onset will initially pit on pressure, although it is true that, when it becomes chronic, the subcutaneous tissues become indurated from fibrous tissue replacement and pitting will not then occur. However, oedema of any nature, if chronic, will have this characteristic.

Treatment of lymphoedema
Conservative

The recommended treatment is decongestive lymphatic therapy (DLT). This involves four components:

[8]Maurice Klippel (1858–1942), French Neurologist, Salpêtrière Hospital, Paris, France. Paul Trenaunay (b. 1875), French Neurologist and junior colleague of Klippel at the time of its description. The syndrome involves multiple congenital venous malformations producing varicose veins together with hypertrophy of bones and soft tissues and extensive cutaneous haemangiomas, usually affecting the lower limbs.

- *Exercise*, using muscles in the affected limb to promote fluid drainage. It is also important to reduce weight if overweight.
- *Manual lymphatic drainage*, a massage technique to stimulate the flow of lymph to reduce swelling.
- *Compression garments*, custom made, to move fluid out of the affected limb and prevent it reaccumulating.
- *Skin care* to avoid any infection that may worsen the lymphatic compromise. This includes avoiding insect bites, careful nail care, wearing gloves for manual tasks, avoiding phlebotomy and venous cannulation in affected limbs, avoiding sun burn, hot baths, saunas, steam rooms and sun beds.

Surgery

In severe cases, surgery may be appropriate. There are three options:

- *Debulking*, removing excess skin and subcutaneous tissue.

- *Liposuction*, removing subcutaneous fat. This is not a cure, but rather debulks the limb after which compression garments should be worn again.
- *Provision of alternative lymphatic drainage*, bypassing obstructions, such as by tunnelling a tongue of omentum down to the inguinal nodes, to provide drainage along mesenteric lymphatics to the thoracic duct, bypassing obstructed iliac nodes. Unfortunately, the results are poor. Other techniques, such as lymphovascular anastomoses, have also been disappointing.

Additional resources

Case 95: A painless lump in the neck
Case 96: Swollen legs in a young woman

37

The breast

Eleftheria Kleidi

Learning objectives

✓ To know about benign and malignant breast disease.

✓ In particular, to be able to recognize the features of breast cancer and have knowledge of its management.

Developmental anomalies

Accessory nipples and breasts

Extra nipples or breasts may develop along the milk line extending from the axilla to the groin. Accessory nipples, called polythelia, are usually found just below the normal breast. Accessory breast tissue, called polymastia, is most commonly found at the axilla. They are influenced by circulating hormones, and the nipples may discharge during lactation.

Hypoplasia or absence of the breast

Although asymmetry of the breasts is normal, complete failure of development of the breast, called amastia, may occur and is often associated with chest wall defects. Bilateral developmental failure may be associated with ovarian failure or Turner syndrome.[1]

Unilateral failure is associated with Poland[2] syndrome, which presents with concurrent underdevelopment of the pectoralis muscle and is more common in males. Asymmetry can be treated by a combination of ipsilateral breast augmentation and contralateral breast reduction.

Tuberous breasts

This can be unilateral or bilateral and consists of a narrow breast base with a relatively wide areola, so that the breast looks like an hourglass. Cosmetic surgery might be considered for correction of this anomaly in adulthood.

Nipple inversion

This may be primary (present since birth) or secondary to duct ectasia or a carcinoma of the breast. If of recent onset (see later in this chapter), then the process is more appropriately called nipple retraction. Primary indrawn nipples may cause problems during lactation but are of no other significance.

---

[1] Henry Hubert Turner (1892–1970), Endocrinologist and Professor of Medicine, University of Oklahoma, Norman, OK, USA

Ellis and Calne's Lecture Notes in General Surgery, Fourteenth Edition. Edited by Christopher Watson and Justin Davies. © 2023 John Wiley & Sons Ltd. Published 2023 by John Wiley & Sons Ltd. Companion website: www.wiley.com/go/Watson/GeneralSurgery14

[2] Sir Alfred Poland (1822–1872), Surgeon to Guys and latterly Moorfields Hospitals. He described the condition when he was still a student based on his dissection of the body of a convict.

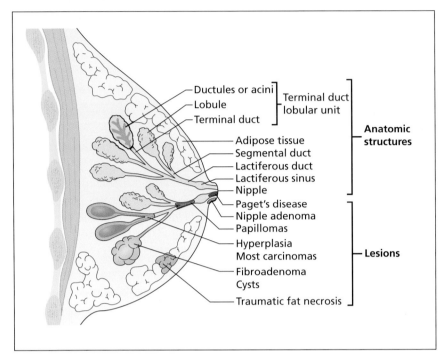

Figure 37.1 Anatomical features of the breast. Adapted from Koeppen BM, Stanton BA (2008) *Berne and Levy Physiology*, 6th edn. St Louis, MO: Mosby (Elsevier).

Symptoms of breast disease

There are five common symptoms of breast disease that warrant urgent attention:

- New, discrete lump.
- Nipple discharge – blood-stained, or spontaneous single duct, or persistent.
- Nipple retraction or distortion of recent onset.
- Altered breast contour or dimpling.
- Nipple changes suspicious of Paget's disease.

Other common symptoms that require further investigation include persistent asymmetrical nodularity, pain (mastalgia), and a family history of breast cancer.

A lump in the breast

When considering the different pathologies of the breast, it is helpful to think in terms of its anatomy and the pathology which is associated with the different structures (Figure 37.1). Ninety per cent of all lumps in the breast will be one of the following:

1 *Cyst.*
2 *Fibroadenoma.*
3 *Carcinoma of the breast.*

In addition, the following less common causes need to be considered.

1 *Trauma*: fat necrosis.
2 *Other cysts:*
    a Galactocele.
    b Abscess.
    c Cystadenoma.
    d Retention cyst of the glands of Montgomery.[3]
    e Fibrocystic changes (presenting as prominent nodularity).
3 *Other tumours:*
    a Ductal papilloma.
    b Sarcoma (extremely rare).

[3]William Featherstone Montgomery (1797–1859), Professor of Midwifery, Dublin, Ireland

c Hamartoma.

d Lipoma.

Uncommon chest wall swellings may rarely be confused with breast swellings. Examples of such are rib swellings (e.g. tumour, Tietze's syndrome or tuberculosis), superficial thrombophlebitis (Mondor's disease[4]) and abscesses.

Management

The diagnosis of discrete breast lumps is based on a triple assessment that comprises the following.

1 Clinical examination.

2 Radiological imaging:

   a *Mammography*, usually in patients over 40 years.

   b *Ultrasound*, both diagnostic and to guide biopsy.

   c *Magnetic resonance imaging*, useful in symptomatic patients with breast implants in whom ultrasound is not diagnostic. It is also used when there is discrepancy on the findings between clinical examination and mammogram and/or ultrasound. MRI is usually performed as a second-line investigation.

3 Biopsy, usually ultrasound-guided:

   a Core biopsy: investigation of choice for the assessment of breast and axillary abnormalities.

   b Vacuum-assisted biopsy (VAB), mostly used in areas of microcalcification to obtain a larger amount of tissue and optimize the possibility of adequate sampling of the area.

   c Punch biopsy: when the abnormality is on the skin, i.e. ulcerating lesion or rash/eczema.

   d Fine-needle aspiration cytology, is hardly ever used to assess breast abnormalities; it is still used in some units to assess the axillary nodes.

The predictive value for benign disease when all three components of the triple assessment are benign is 99%. If there is discordance between any of the three tests, open biopsy or further investigations are considered.

Discharge from the nipple

1 *Blood-stained*:

   a Benign intraductal papilloma, when blood arises from a single duct.

   b Intraductal carcinoma; (ductal carcinoma *in situ*, DCIS).

   c Trauma.

   d Paget's disease (rare).

   e Invasive carcinoma (very rare).

2 *Clear, single duct*: benign intraductal papilloma.

3 *Multicoloured (often multiductal)*: duct ectasia (discharge commonly yellow, brown or green).

4 *Milky*: galactorrhoea: may follow lactation but can also be drug induced or a manifestation of hyperprolactinaemia (or, occasionally, hypothyroidism).

5 *Purulent*: breast abscess, periductal mastitis.

Management

Nipple discharge is usually physiological when non-spontaneous. The majority of cases of spontaneous nipple discharge are benign, and this symptom is rarely a presenting feature of breast cancer, even when blood-stained. Spontaneous, clear, single-duct or blood-stained discharge requires further investigation; if a lump is present, it should be managed by triple assessment (see earlier in this chapter). In the absence of a lump, the management of discharge is as follows:

Multicoloured, multiductal discharge

If clinical examination and imaging are normal, a diagnosis of duct ectasia is likely and no further treatment is required. If the symptoms are distressing, total duct excision (Hadfield's procedure[5]) can be considered.

Clear single-duct discharge

If triple assessment is normal, the diagnosis is likely to be an intraductal papilloma and excision of the affected duct (a microdochectomy) is indicated.

Bloody nipple discharge

When blood is present, a focused central breast ultrasound is performed and a mammogram (for women over 40 years). If imaging is normal, and the discharge persists, a microdochectomy is recommended if a single duct can be identified; a total duct excision is

---

[4]Henri Mondor (1885–1962), Professor of Surgery, Hôpital Salpêtrière, Paris, France.

[5]Geoffrey John Hadfield (1923–2006), Surgeon, Stoke Mandeville Hospital, Aylesbury, UK.

performed if a single duct cannot be clearly identified. Cytology of the nipple discharge is no longer recommended, as the results do not impact management.

Bloody nipple discharge can be seen in up to 20% of women in pregnancy and lactation, due to the hypervascularity of the ducts. This is usually benign and resolves spontaneously. Triple assessment is still warranted: if bloody discharge persists, the recommended management is the same as above, usually after delivery.

Pain in the breast (mastalgia)

It can be separated into true and extramammary breast pain. True breast pain is further divided into cyclical and non-cyclical. Mastalgia is rarely a symptom of breast cancer.

Extramammary breast pain

It is likely the most common cause of breast pain and is usually unilateral. Any irritation of the intercostal nerves that innervate the breast (T3-T5) can cause referred pain. Careful clinical examination, also in the lateral positions, can differentiate extramammary from true breast pain. Common causes include:

- *Musculoskeletal chest wall pain*, usually derives from the pectoralis major muscle or the ribs. *Tietze's syndrome*,[6] which is costochondritis of the cartilage of the second, to fourth costochondral junctions is another cause of chest wall pain.
- *Intercostal neuralgia* due to trauma or underlying pleuritic pain, gallbladder disease or herpes zoster can be a less common causes of extramammary pain.
- *Spinal disorder* like arthritis or spondylitis, is also a less common cause.

Patients with extramammary breast pain are reassured once the cause is identified and their treatment is symptomatic and cause directed.

Cyclical mastalgia

Cyclical mastalgia is caused by hormonal changes during the menstrual cycle. It is usually bilateral, diffuse, worse premenstrually and relieved following menstruation. It is more common in younger women. Risk factors include hormonal preparations (oral contraceptive pill [OCP] or hormone replacement

[6] Alexander Tietze (1864–1927), Surgeon, Breslau, Germany.

therapy [HRT]) and other medications. Diet high in caffeine and/or in fat had been previously considered a risk factor but convincing evidence is lacking. In the absence of any focal findings on clinical examination, mammography may be offered for screening for patients over 40 years old.

Management

Initial management consists of reassurance and primary measures, which include a supportive bra and local or oral anti-inflammatory agents. Adjustment of hormonal medications might also be required, such as an alteration to, or introduction of, the OCP or HRT. Evening primrose oil containing γ-linolenic acid (GLA), and/or dietary modifications are no longer recommended, as they have not proven effective in trials; however, some clinicians still use them due to the small benefit in some women.

Second-line management for cyclical mastalgia, if symptoms persist after 6 months may be considered, taking into account the potential side effects:

- *Tamoxifen*, an oestrogen receptor antagonist; at low dose for 3 months.
- *Danazol*, an androgen with antigonadotrophic and anti-oestrogenic effects.

Non-cyclical mastalgia

In one-third of women with true breast pain, this will be non-cyclical. Causes include:

- *Breast infection:* mastitis and abscess.
- *Benign breast conditions:* breast cysts, duct ectasia, Mondor's thrombophlebitis.
- *Trauma or prior breast surgery.*
- *Hormonal therapies,* usually HRT.
- *Carcinoma of the breast*: an uncommon presenting symptom.

Management is directed towards the precipitating factor, along with the primary measures mentioned earlier in this chapter for cyclical mastalgia, if indicated.

Traumatic fat necrosis

Aetiology

Fat necrosis may be associated with a history of trauma and is a common result of seat belt injury or surgical trauma. Its importance lies in its ability to mimic breast carcinoma; conversely, many women presenting with a lump in the breast attribute this to injury when it is, in fact, cancer.

Clinical features

Fat necrosis commonly presents with a painless, irregular, firm lump in the breast and there may be a previous history of trauma. It is often associated with skin thickening or retraction and as a result is often difficult to distinguish from carcinoma on clinical examination. The lump usually decreases in size with time, but following resolution may leave an oil cyst within the breast, which is a collection of liquified fat.

Treatment

Although mammography may demonstrate non-specific changes, or show a spiculate, dense mass that mimics carcinoma, ultrasound will often reveal characteristic features. The diagnosis can be confirmed by core biopsy and the mass should resolve. In the absence of a firm diagnosis, an open biopsy is recommended.

Acute inflammation of the breast (mastitis)

There are two common causes of acute breast inflammation in children and adults:

- *Acute bacterial mastitis*: may be lactational or non-lactational.
- *Periductal mastitis*.

Two less common conditions are worthy of mention:

- *Mondor's disease*: superficial thrombophlebitis in the anterior chest, characterized by the presence of painful, cord-like lumps.
- *Post-irradiation oedema*: irradiation may be associated with oedema (peau d'orange), warmth and a heavy sensation, mimicking inflammation.

Acute bacterial mastitis

It is the most frequent acute inflammation of the breast; the majority of cases occur during lactation. It initially presents as cellulitis and progresses to an abscess in 5–10% of cases. A microorganism is isolated in 60–80% of cases.

Lactational mastitis is more common during the first months of breastfeeding mainly due to stagnation of the milk or cracking of the nipples. *Staphylococcus aureus* is the most common pathogen but *methicillin-resistant S. aureus (MRSA)* should be considered in refractory cases.

Non-lactational (non-puerperal) mastitis and abscess may be associated with systemic conditions such as diabetes, steroid therapy and rheumatoid arthritis. The common organisms include *staphylococci, enterococci*, α-haemolytic *streptococci, proteus* and *bacteroides*.

Clinical features

Common symptoms include pain, swelling and tenderness of the breast. The inflammation may be localized, with erythema and tenderness of a segment of the breast or may spread to involve the entire breast. In the later stages, there may be a fluctuant mass and patients may have signs of sepsis with pyrexia, tachycardia and leucocytosis.

The possibility of an inflammatory breast cancer should be considered if the inflammation fails to resolve on treatment or if there is an associated mass lesion. In these cases, a core biopsy should be obtained.

Treatment
Cellulitis

In the early phase of mastitis, appropriate antibiotics can prevent abscess formation. In lactational mastitis, suppression of lactation is not required and breast-feeding or pumping should be highly encouraged, as this will speed up recovery.

Abscess

Patients with clinical or radiological evidence of pus should have ultrasound-guided aspiration performed in addition to appropriate antibiotic therapy. Repeat aspiration may be necessary and resolution of the abscess can be monitored with sequential ultrasound examinations. If the abscess fails to resolve, or the overlying skin is thin or necrotic, incision and drainage should be performed.

Severe or refractory infection

Admission for intravenous antibiotic administration might be required if there is progression on oral antibiotics or in the presence of sepsis. Intraoperative surgical drainage and debridement may be indicated in advanced stages.

Periductal mastitis

This is an inflammatory process that occurs around dilated milk ducts near the nipple. Cellular debris and keratin plugs block the lactiferous ducts, leading to duct dilation and secondary infection, often with mixed flora (e.g. *staphylococci*, *enterococci*, anaerobic *streptococci* and other anaerobes). Occasionally, the infected ducts may result in a subareolar abscess beneath the nipple which discharges to form a fistula, often at the margin of the areola. It is much more common in smokers, and nipple piercing increases the risk of infection. It occurs mostly in premenopausal women, in contrast to duct ectasia.

Clinical features

Common features include pain and thick, pasty nipple discharge. There may be cellulitis, nipple retraction or a mass deep to the nipple. An associated mammary duct fistula may be present in the periareolar region. Ultrasound may confirm a thickened or dilated duct or abscess formation.

Treatment

Initial treatment is with appropriate antibiotics and smoking cessation advice. Nipple rings should be removed if present. Patients with recurrent periareolar inflammation and ductal discharge should be treated with total duct excision. A mammary duct fistula is treated by total duct excision combined with excision of the fistulous track between the duct and the skin.

Duct ectasia

An involutional change in the ducts associated with the menopause. The terminal ducts behind the nipple become dilated (ectasia) and engorged with secretions. Secondary infection may lead to retroareolar abscess, and fibrosis may result in nipple inversion.

Chronic inflammatory conditions of the breast

There are two uncommon chronic inflammatory conditions of the breast.

1 *Granulomatous mastitis* may be secondary to systemic conditions (sarcoidosis), infections (tuberculosis, fungi), foreign material (silicone) or be idiopathic. Idiopathic mastitis presents with peripheral masses or abscess and it might take months to resolve; surgery is avoided due to poor wound healing. Management includes treatment of any organisms cultured and exclusion of malignancy.
2 *Lymphocytic lobulitis* occurs in patients with autoimmune diseases, particularly type 1 diabetes mellitus (diabetic mastopathy), and usually presents with a firm, mass. The diagnosis is made on core biopsy, with fibrosis and lymphoid infiltrate on microscopy. No further treatment is required.

Benign breast disease

At the start of the menstrual cycle, increasing amounts of oestrogen stimulate the growth of breast ducts. After ovulation, increasing amounts of progesterone stimulate lobular development. When implantation fails, these changes regress and the levels of progesterone and oestrogen fall, corresponding to the onset of menstruation. Benign epithelial breast disease is a consequence of aberrations of these hormonal effects on the breast; the incidence decreases following the menopause.

Benign breast disease is characterized by cystic and solid lesions and is divided into:

- *Nonproliferative* (the most common), including cystic disease and duct ectasia.
- *Proliferative,* including sclerosing adenosis, radial scars, fibroadenomas and ductal papillomas.

Cystic disease

Simple cysts are dilations of the ducts and acini, as a result of the obstruction of the terminal duct-lobular unit caused by metaplasia of the epithelial lining. They are more common in women aged 35 to 50 years old but uncommon after the menopause.

Clinical features

Cysts often present as a smooth and often tender lump in the breast. The lump may be fluctuant, but tense cysts may mimic a solid lump on clinical examination. Cysts may be multiple and/or bilateral. They appear as well-defined, rounded opacities with characteristic halo on mammography, and are clearly differentiated from a solid lump by ultrasound. Ultrasound can also identify the presence of internal debris (complicated and complex cysts) and/or thick walls (complex cysts).

Treatment

Newly diagnosed simple cysts do not require aspiration to dryness unless they are symptomatic. If the fluid is blood-stained, core biopsy of the cyst wall is indicated.

Core biopsy or fine-needle aspiration cytology (FNAC) is also indicated for complex and complicated cysts, where there is evidence of septae or a solid area in the cyst wall or if the palpable mass persists following aspiration.

The presence of simple cysts does not increase the risk of breast cancer. The risk of breast cancer following a complicated or complex cyst depends on the results of the biopsy.

Sclerosing adenosis

Sclerosing adenosis is characterized by an increase in the number of acini in the breast lobules, and is thought to be the result of an abnormality in breast involution.

Patients may present with pain or lumpiness in the breast, or increased density or microcalcifications on screening mammography which may be indistinguishable from *in situ* carcinoma. Definitive diagnosis can be made with stereotactic core biopsy. Once the diagnosis is confirmed, no further treatment or follow-up is required.

Radial scars

Radial scars are mostly radiological findings, appearing as an area of distortion, which is often difficult to distinguish from carcinoma, with lines radiating out from a central scar. A number of radial scars will be associated with atypical hyperplasia or carcinoma *in situ;* thus, a radial scar should be adequately sampled either with large-gauge core biopsies or diagnostic

excision in order to rule out these pathologies. If atypia is found during assessment, then surveillance with mammogram for 5 years is indicated; otherwise the risk of subsequent malignancy is small.

Fibroadenoma

Fibroadenomas are the most common benign breast tumours and are considered as an aberration of normal development. Fibroadenomas are proliferative lesions arising from an entire lobule. There is no increased risk of malignancy with simple fibroadenomas and about one-third will decrease in size or resolve over time.

Clinical features

Fibroadenomas are more common in women under 30 years old and are also known as 'breast mice'. They usually present as a discrete, firm, mobile lump, or as multiple or bilateral lumps. Fibroadenomas can grow rapidly during pregnancy. Apart from 'simple', fibroadenomas can also be:

- *Complex*: when there are other features in pathology, such as sclerosing adenosis or calcifications. These can slightly increase future breast cancer risk.
- *Giant*: when they measure more than 5 cm.
- *Juvenile*: when found in teenage girls.

Treatment

Like all solid breast lumps, fibroadenomas must be investigated by triple assessment. In those patients with multiple fibroadenomas, the largest lump should undergo core biopsy, as should any lump increasing in size. Excision is recommended only in large (over 4 cm) or symptomatic fibroadenomas.

Intraductal papilloma

A papilloma occurs in the large subareolar ducts and is a result of epithelial proliferation. They can be single or multiple and may present with intermittent clear or blood-stained nipple discharge from a single duct. If the papilloma is large, there may be a palpable mass in the periareolar area. Multiple papillomas (papillomatosis) are associated with an increased lifetime risk of breast cancer. Papillomas can sometimes harbour areas of atypia and rarely DCIS.

In the presence of atypia or nipple discharge, treatment involves surgical excision of the affected duct (microdochectomy).

Hamartoma

These rare lesions may present clinically as a breast lump or may be incidental findings on screening mammography, when they have the appearance of a 'breast within a breast'. They have a well-defined capsule and comprise a variable mixture of breast lobules, stroma and fat. Once the diagnosis is confirmed, no further treatment is necessary.

Gynaecomastia

A benign condition arising from proliferation of breast tissue in males of all ages. It is caused by an imbalance of oestrogens and androgens and must be distinguished from carcinoma of the male breast. Common causes include:

- *Drugs*: digoxin, spironolactone, cimetidine, oestrogens or androgens; anabolic steroids or drugs of abuse (alcohol, methadone, heroin, etc.).
- *Cirrhosis* of the liver.
- *Renal failure.*
- *Hypogonadism.*
- *Adrenal tumours.*
- *Testicular tumours.*
- *Malnutrition.*
- *Idiopathic.*

Clinical features

Gynaecomastia presents as a bilateral or unilateral diffuse, soft swelling or mass behind the areola. In patients with any suspicious features (firm or eccentric lump or skin changes), carcinoma must be excluded. Particular care should be taken not to miss a testicular tumour in a young man presenting with otherwise unexplained gynaecomastia.

Treatment

The majority of idiopathic cases will resolve with no intervention. Secondary gynaecomastia usually reverses with management of the precipitating factor. A trial of low-dose tamoxifen can be considered in selected cases. Surgery in specialist centres can be discussed if the gynaecomastia does not settle, is symptomatic or has significant psychological impact.

Phyllodes tumour

Phyllodes tumour is a rare neoplasm of the breast that arises from stromal cells. According to its microscopic features it is classified as low, intermediate or high grade. Although phyllodes[7] tumours have clinical features similar to fibroadenomas, they can have benign, borderline or malignant behaviour. Malignant phyllodes tumours rarely metastasize and can recur locally if inadequately excised. Benign and borderline phyllodes tumours rarely recur after complete excision.

Clinical features

These lesions usually present as a firm, discrete lump and patients may note a recent increase in size. They should be investigated by triple assessment to confirm the diagnosis.

Treatment

All phyllodes tumours should be treated by excision to achieve a clear margin around the tumour. In large lesions, this may require mastectomy with immediate reconstruction. Some units might also offer radiotherapy after excision of borderline or malignant tumours. The role of chemotherapy is still debatable and it is not routinely indicated.

Carcinoma of the breast

Breast cancer is the most common cancer in the UK, accounting for 15% of all new cancers (2016–2018), with around 56000 new cases and about 11500 deaths annually. One in eight women will develop breast cancer during their lifetime. The incidence has increased by 3% in the last 10 years. Average survival is continuously improving with 5-year survival being at 90% and 10-year survival at 76%. Less than 1 in 10 breast lumps referred to a breast clinic will prove to be malignant.

[7] Phyllodes means 'leaf-like', a reference to the lobulated appearance of the cut surface of the tumour.

Aetiology

There is an increased incidence of breast cancer with age and, although any age may be affected, it is extremely rare below the age of 30 years and 80% of cases occur in women aged 50 years and over. A previous history of invasive or *in situ* breast cancer are all associated with an increased risk of invasive carcinoma. In addition, the following have been identified as important risk factors.

Hormonal factors

An increase in breast cancer risk mostly correlates with increased oestrogen exposure:

- *Gender*: 99% of breast cancers occur in women, with fewer than 1% in men.
- *Menarche and menopause*: early age at menarche (under 13 years) and late menopause (over 50 years) are associated with a twofold higher risk.
- *Parity*: nulliparous women have a higher risk than multiparous women; later age at first pregnancy also increases the risk. Breastfeeding reduces overall risk, which is greater with a longer duration of breastfeeding.
- *Hormone replacement therapy (HRT)*: the risk of breast cancer is increased while women take combined oestrogen/progesterone HRT but reverts 5 years after discontinuation; it is thought to account for 3 additional cases per 1000 women with the risk being proportional to the length of treatment. There is little or no change in the risk with oestrogen-only HRT. Both types of HRT increase the breast density and can make a breast cancer harder to visualize on mammograms.
- *Oral contraceptive pill (OCP)*: the combined oestrogen-containing pill, and for up to 10 years from discontinuation, is associated with a slight to no increase in breast cancer risk.
- *Obesity* in postmenopausal women results in a twofold increase in breast cancer risk, likely due to increased oestrogen deriving from the adipose tissue. In premenopausal women, obesity slightly decreases the risk, for reasons yet unclear.
- *IGF-1*: raised levels of insulin growth factor-1 are associated with an increased risk of breast cancer, though it is not clear why this is the case.

Genetic factors

The majority of breast cancers are sporadic in nature, with up to 10% being due to genetic predisposition.

- *Family history*. The risk increases by twofold with one first-degree relative (mother or sister) and threefold with two first-degree relatives with breast cancer. The risk is higher with younger age at diagnosis of the affected relative.
- *Gene carriage* accounts for 5% of breast cancer cases. Mutations in the *BRCA1* and *BRCA2* genes are the most common. They are autosomal dominant inherited gene mutations and translate to a 50–70% lifetime risk of breast cancer. They also confer an increased risk of ovarian and other cancers. Less common mutations in other genes, such as *TP53, PTEN* and *PALB2*, are also associated with an increased susceptibility to breast cancer.

Other factors

- *Breast density:* when increased, results in four- to five-fold increase in breast cancer risk.
- *Benign breast disease:* history of proliferative lesions slightly increases breast cancer risk. The presence of atypia, though, can confer an up to four- to five-fold increase.
- *Bone mineral density:* when increased, increases breast cancer risk.
- *Lifestyle factors: i*ncreased risk is associated with increased alcohol intake, whereas smoking does not seem to be related to breast cancer risk. Even moderate physical activity is known to reduce breast cancer risk.
- *Radiation exposure:* irradiation in adolescence or early adulthood can markedly increase breast cancer risk. Young women treated with mantle radiotherapy for lymphoma have a 1 in 3 to 1 in 7 risk of breast cancer in the following 25 years.

Classification

1 *Primary*:
  a Ductal carcinoma *in situ* (DCIS).
  b Invasive ductal carcinoma.
  c Lobular carcinoma *in situ* (LCIS).
  d Invasive lobular carcinoma.
  e Inflammatory carcinoma.
  f Rare invasive carcinoma types.
  g Paget's disease of the nipple.

h Lymphoma.

i Sarcoma.

2 *Secondary*:

  a Direct invasion from tumours of the chest wall.

  b Metastatic deposits, for example from melanoma or ovarian cancer.

Pathology

Breast cancers arise from the epithelium of the terminal duct-lobular unit. The characteristic growth pattern and not their anatomic location at the duct-lobular system determines the categorization in ductal and lobular carcinomas. Carcinomas which have not penetrated through the basement membrane are known as carcinomas *in situ* or *non-invasive* (Figure 37.2).

Ductal carcinoma *in situ*

Ductal carcinoma *in situ* (DCIS) is the most common type of non-invasive breast cancer. According to its histologic appearance, it is classified as low, intermediate and high grade, which impacts prognosis. It usually occurs in localized areas of the breast but may be extensive; untreated, it will become invasive. DCIS is generally asymptomatic, appearing as a mammographic finding, usually as microcalcifications. Because of its malignant potential, treatment is wide local excision of the disease; extensive disease or multiple areas of DCIS may necessitate advanced oncoplastic surgery or mastectomy. Adjuvant radiotherapy is indicated for high-grade DCIS after breast conservation surgery.

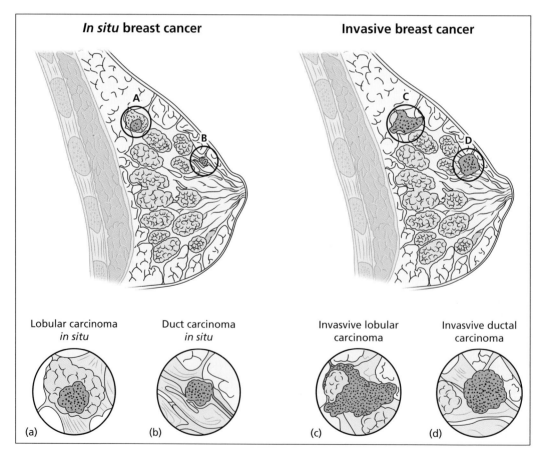

In situ breast cancer

A

B

Lobular carcinoma *in situ*

(a)

Duct carcinoma *in situ*

(b)

Invasive breast cancer

C

D

Invasvive lobular carcinoma

(c)

Invasvive ductal carcinoma

(d)

Figure 37.2 The different origins of *in situ* and invasive ductal and lobular carcinomas.

Lobular carcinoma *in situ*

Lobular carcinoma *in situ* (LCIS) is an uncommon entity not visible on mammography; it is usually an incidental finding on a biopsy. LCIS is a marker of increased risk of future breast cancer (approximately 7- to 11-fold increase). According to its histologic appearance, it is classified as classic and non-classic. Incidental classic LCIS on a core biopsy or at the margins of a breast excision requires no further treatment if the findings are concordant. Annual 5-year surveillance with mammography is recommended. Incidental non-classic LCIS should be excised to clear margins, as it might be upgraded to DCIS or invasive lobular carcinoma.

Invasive ductal carcinoma

This is the most common type of breast cancer, accounting for about 70–80% of all breast cancers. It is often described as being of 'no special type' (NST) to distinguish it from 'special types' of cancer such as invasive lobular cancer or rarer tumours described below.

Invasive lobular carcinoma

Invasive lobular carcinoma accounts for about 8% of breast cancers. It does not always form a firm lump but rather an area of thickening, so tends to present late, and is more likely to be bilateral or multicentric than ductal carcinoma. Prognosis may be more favourable for lobular cancers compared to ductal. Mixed ductal/lobular cancers account for another 7% of breast cancers and have got mixed histologic characteristics.

Rare types of breast cancer

There are several less common types accounting for under 5% of breast cancers. Presentation and management are generally similar to those required for the more common invasive cancers, such as ductal carcinoma. These types are named after their distinct histopathologic characteristics and compared to ductal carcinoma they can have:

- *Favourable prognosis*: usually mucinous, medullary, tubular, papillary and cystadeno-carcinomas.
- *Worse prognosis*: mostly associated with metaplastic and micropapillary subtypes.

Spread

- *Direct extension*. Involvement of skin and subcutaneous tissues leads to skin dimpling, retraction of the nipple and eventually ulceration. Extension deeply involves pectoralis major, serratus anterior and, eventually, the chest wall.
- *Lymphatic*. The main lymph channels pass directly to the axillary – that receive 95% of drainage – and the internal mammary lymph nodes (Figure 37.3). Later, spread occurs to the supraclavicular and rarely to contralateral axillary or distant nodes. Blockage of dermal lymphatics leads to cutaneous oedema pitted by the orifices of the sweat ducts, giving the appearance of *peau d'orange* (orange peel). Dermal lymphatic invasion produces daughter skin nodules and if untreated, 'cancer *en cuirasse*',[8] the whole chest wall becoming a firm mass of tumour tissue.
- *Bloodstream*. Blood-borne spread is most commonly to the bones (at the sites of red bone marrow, i.e. skull, vertebrae, pelvis, ribs, sternum, etc.), the lungs, the brain and the liver. Ovaries and adrenals are also frequent sites of secondary deposits.

Prognostic factors

A number of prognostic factors are routinely determined following breast cancer surgery to help predict the outcome of an individual patient and plan adjuvant systemic therapy.

- *Axillary node spread* is a strong and independent determinant of prognosis; the greater the number of ipsilateral nodes involved, the worse the prognosis.
- *Tumour size*. The size of a tumour has a positive correlation with the metastatic potential. Larger tumours are, therefore, more likely to be lymph node positive and to have a worse survival.
- *Tumour grade*. Breast carcinoma is graded as I, II or III according to the level of differentiation. Grade I tumours (well differentiated) have a better prognosis than grade III tumours (poorly differentiated) and this is an independent prognostic factor.

Additional prognostic factors in invasive breast cancer include:

- *Lymphovascular invasion* by the tumour: is an indicator of poor prognosis, even in the absence of nodal involvement.

---

[8] A cuirass was an armour breastplate.

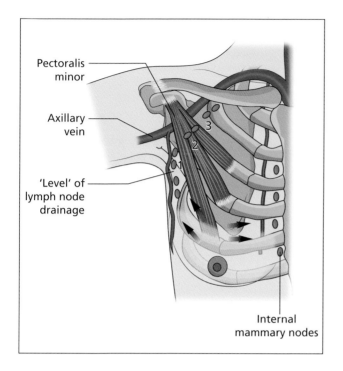

Pectoralis minor

Axillary vein

'Level' of lymph node drainage

Internal mammary nodes

Figure 37.3 The lymphatic drainage of the breast.

- *Hormone receptor expression* refers to the oestrogen (ER) and progesterone (PR) receptors. It implies a less aggressive, hormone-responsive tumour. Prognosis is worse in singly hormone receptor positive cancers (ER positive and PR negative).
- *Human epidermal growth factor receptor 2 (HER2) is a protein found in the breast tissue.* HER2 is overexpressed in 15–20% of all breast cancers. HER2 positive disease is associated with a more aggressive tumour.
- *Histological type*: different types have better or worse prognosis (see earlier in this chapter).
- *Genomic assays*: analyse different breast cancer gene expression in breast tumours. These emerging prognostic tools provide valuable information on the recurrence risk, for suitable patients, that help guide adjuvant treatments. Most widely used tools are the Oncotype DX, Prosigna, Mammaprint and EndoPredict.
- *Risk calculators*: different calculators, based on many of the above factors, have been developed to assess prognosis. Tools like PREDICT[9], MD

Anderson Calculators and CancerMath[10] are widely used to estimate benefit from adjuvant treatments in patients with early breast cancer and assist in guiding treatment recommendations. Results should always be used in conjunction with all other clinical and pathological parameters of the patient, and in conjunction with discussion at a local multidisciplinary team (MDT) meeting.

Clinical features

The majority of patients with invasive carcinoma will present with a lump in the breast. Other features that warrant urgent investigation include altered breast contour, recent nipple inversion, blood-stained nipple discharge and unilateral nipple eczema (Paget's disease).

The breasts are inspected with the patient both lying supine and sitting with the arms elevated. The latter often accentuates any skin tethering or dimpling. Any evidence of nipple inversion or eczema should be noted.

[9] Predict: https://breast.predict.nhs.uk/tool

[10] CancerMath http://cancer.lifemath.net/index.html

Palpation should be with the flat of the hand with the patient lying flat and the head supported. Both breasts and both axillae should be examined as well as the supraclavicular fossae. Any lump should be carefully examined for evidence of skin or muscle fixation and the clinical size and position in relation to the nipple noted. Large, firm nodes in the axilla may suggest metastatic disease. In patients with suspected tumour, liver palpation and chest auscultation should also be performed.

Special investigations

Diagnostic investigations

The diagnosis of breast carcinoma is made by triple assessment comprising clinical examination, imaging (mammography and/or ultrasound) and biopsy (see earlier in this chapter). In the vast majority of cases, the diagnosis has been confirmed prior to surgery.

Staging investigations

Depending on the local extent of the tumour and the presence of other symptoms, the following investigations may be indicated to assess the potential of distant disease:

- *Full blood count*: anaemia and leucopenia suggest widespread bone marrow involvement.
- *Liver function tests*: raised alkaline phosphatase may signify liver or bone metastases.
- *Chest X-ray.*
- *Isotope bone scan.*
- *Staging CT scan of chest and abdomen +/-pelvis.*
- *Positron emission tomography-CT (PET-CT)*: might be indicated if whole body imaging is required.

Cancers are staged using the TNM classification (see Chapter 7). The TNM staging for breast cancer is shown in Table 37.1.

Treatment

The treatment of breast cancer involves a multimodality approach comprising the following elements:

1 Surgery.
  a *Tumour excision* either with breast conservation surgery or mastectomy.
  b *Surgery to the axilla* according to the nodal involvement.
  c *Breast reconstruction.*

Table 37.1 Pathologic TNM staging for breast cancer, AJCC UICC 2010[11]

Stage	Description
T	**Primary tumour.**
TX	Primary tumour cannot be assessed.
T0	No evidence of primary tumour.
Tis	Carcinoma *in situ* (DCIS, LCIS or Paget's disease with no invasive tumour).
T1	Tumour 2 cm or less in greatest dimension.
T2	Tumour >2 cm but ≤5 cm in greatest dimension.
T3	Tumour >5 cm in greatest dimension.
T4	Tumour of any size with direct extension to the chest wall or skin. T4a – extension to the chest wall, apart from pectoralis major muscle only. T4b – extension to the skin (ulceration or skin nodules or and/or oedema). T4c – both T4a and T4b. T4d – inflammatory carcinoma.
N	**Regional lymph nodes.**
NX	Regional lymph nodes cannot be assessed (e.g. previously removed).
N0	No regional lymph node metastasis.
N1	Micrometastases or metastases in 1–3 axillary lymph nodes and/or in internal mammary nodes but not clinically detected.
N2	Metastases in 4–9 axillary lymph nodes or in clinically detected internal mammary lymph nodes in the *absence* of axillary lymph node metastases.
N3	Metastases in ≥10 axillary or ipsilateral infraclavicular (level III) or supraclavicular lymph nodes or both axillary and clinically detected internal mammary nodes.
M	**Distant metastasis.**
MX	Distant metastasis cannot be assessed.
M0	No distant metastasis.
M1	Distant metastasis.

DCIS, ductal carcinoma *in situ*; LCIS, lobular carcinoma *in situ*.

[11] AJCC: American Joint Committee on Cancer; UICC: Union for International Cancer Control. These two organisations revise staging for cancers. The version in this table was published in 2010.

2 Systemic therapy.
   a *Hormonal therapy.*
   b *Chemotherapy* with or without HER2-directed treatment.
   c *Bisphosphonate treatment.*
3 Locoregional therapy.
   a *Radiotherapy* to the breast or chest wall with or without nodal irradiation.

Some of these treatments are recommended, either after surgery (adjuvant) or before surgery (neoadjuvant). The order depends on multiple clinicopathological factors discussed later in this chapter.

Surgical management

The aims of surgery are to remove the primary tumour and any involved lymph nodes, in order to determine prognosis and plan systemic therapy. Small tumour/breast ratio is an indication for breast-conserving surgery (wide local excision). Increased tumour/breast ratio or multifocal tumours (multiple foci in one quadrant) might require oncoplastic procedures or mastectomy. Mastectomy, with or without breast reconstruction, is also indicated in:

- *Multicentric tumours* (multiple foci in more than one quadrant).
- *Inflammatory breast cancer.*
- *Patients with gene mutations*, i.e. breast cancer in BRCA-positive patients.
- *When radiotherapy is contraindicated* such as during pregnancy or in most circumstances of previous radiotherapy to the breast or chest wall (previous breast cancer or previous Hodgkin's lymphoma).
- *Patient preference.*

Tumour excision

Breast-conserving surgery (BCS)

There is good evidence that BCS followed by radiotherapy is equally as effective as mastectomy with regards both to local control and to survival.

a *Wide local excision.* A cylinder of breast tissue is excised usually from skin down to the pectoral muscle, in order to achieve complete excision ('clear resection margins').
b *Oncoplastic breast surgery.* When larger amounts of breast tissue need to be removed, then oncoplastic techniques can be applied to provide the optimal cosmetic outcome. These aim to either reshape the breast (level I and II oncoplasty) or

replace the breast volume with local chest wall perforator flaps.

Mastectomy

A simple mastectomy involves excision of the breast tissue, including the nipple, leaving a flat chest wall. If combined with immediate breast reconstruction, then a skin-sparing or a nipple-sparing technique should be performed.

Complications

Common complications after surgery to the breast include:

- Infection.
- Seroma.
- Haematoma.
- Delayed wound healing.
- Pain.
- Numbness.
- Asymmetry.

These are more common after mastectomy compared to BCS. Additional risks of BCS include further surgery if margins are involved (ranging from 10 to 20%) and fat necrosis or nipple complications which increase with the greater volume of breast tissue that is removed.

Surgical management of the axilla

Axillary node status is an important prognostic indicator in the treatment of invasive breast cancer. As a result, axillary surgery should be performed on all patients with invasive operable breast cancer, but is not generally required for *in situ* disease.

Negative axillary nodes at presentation

For patients *with negative axillary nodes* at presentation, the following is performed:

- *Sentinel lymph node (SLN) biopsy*, in which the first axillary lymph node(s) draining the cancer field is identified, excised and examined for metastatic tumour. Different techniques can be used to identify the sentinel node(s) that include a radioisotope, and/or a blue dye injection under the nipple or around the tumour before surgery. New techniques for SLN localization are also being developed.

- *Axillary node sampling (ANS)* is indicated if the sentinel node cannot be identified, either because of failure of the localizing injections or due to previous surgery in the axilla. A sample of a minimum of four lymph nodes are removed for histological analysis.

When the sampled nodes are free of tumour, no further axillary surgery is required. If there are positive nodes following SLN biopsy or ANS, then further treatment to the axilla might be required in the form of axillary radiotherapy or axillary clearance.

Positive axillary nodes at presentation

Positive axillary nodes at presentation implies the possibility of onward nodal spread. There are two surgical options for such patients:

- *Axillary node clearance (ANC),* removing all the nodes lateral and deep to the pectoralis minor muscle (a level I and II clearance) (see Figure 35.3).
- *Targeted axillary dissection (TAD)* is an evolving approach for patients with 1–2 positive nodes at presentation undergoing neoadjuvant chemotherapy. If there is evidence of good response to neoadjuvant chemotherapy, then the previously positive nodes can be removed along with the sentinel nodes. If all the nodes are now negative for cancer cells, then no further treatment is required for the axilla.

Complications

Complications of axillary surgery include the risk of lymphoedema, which is increased with the greater extent of dissection (20% after ANC vs 6% after SLN biopsy) along with the risks of pain, numbness, shoulder stiffness and damage to the axillary nerves and vessels (e.g. winged scapula following damage to the long thoracic nerve).

Breast reconstruction

Breast reconstruction may be performed either at the time of mastectomy (immediate) or as a delayed procedure. The combination of skin- or nipple-sparing mastectomy and immediate breast reconstruction may produce better cosmetic results. Reconstruction does not appear to impede the ability to detect local recurrence and is of psychological benefit.

The choice of reconstruction for a suitable individual patient will depend on several factors, including breast size, the adequacy of skin flaps, whether radiotherapy is planned or has previously been used, abdominal size and previous abdominal operations, smoking status, lifestyle, comorbidities, body mass index and the patient's preference. Common reconstructions include the following:

1 *Implant based*: a breast implant containing either silicone, saline or both, is used to replace the excised breast tissue. It is placed either above (prepectoral) or below (subpectoral) the pectoralis major muscle. It can be done as one or two stages. The latter involves a tissue expander to increase the skin envelope, which is later on replaced by a permanent implant.

   Common complications of implants include the risk of rupture and infection that can result in implant loss, as well as the risks of rotation, animation and capsular contracture that may require a revision. A very rare entity called breast implant associated anaplastic large cell lymphoma (BIA-ALCL) is also included in the consent process.

2 *Autologous flaps*: skin and fat with or without the underlying muscle is used to replace the breast, based on its own vascular pedicle. A flap may be pedicled (swung around on its existing blood supply) or free (pedicle removed and anastomosed to vessels in the mastectomy site). These can be one of the following:

   a *Latissimus dorsi myocutaneous flap:* pedicled flap based on the thoracodorsal artery (a continuation of the subscapular artery).

   b *Deep inferior epigastric artery perforator (DIEP) flap:* the most commonly used free flap, where an island of skin and fat from the lower abdominal wall is used to reconstruct the breast. It includes an abdominoplasty for flap harvesting and microsurgery for the anastomosis of the flap to the chest wall. The amount of harvested tissue is usually sufficient for bilateral breast reconstruction, if indicated.

   c *Transverse rectus abdominis myocutaneous (TRAM) flap:* based on the inferior epigastric vessels, a transverse skin ellipse with underlying fat and a portion of the rectus abdominis muscles. It can be pedicled or free. However, due to the implications to abdominal wall weakening this flap is now less frequently used.

   Complications of autologous reconstructions include the scarring, infection and weakening of the donor sites, as well as site-related complications. The risk of postoperative thrombo-embolism is also increased with these operations.

3 *Combination of flap and implant.*

Systemic therapy

Adjuvant systemic therapy (after the operation) using cytotoxic agents and/or endocrine therapy improves survival and reduces recurrence, with greatest benefit in those women at greatest risk of relapse. Treatments are continuously evolving and have contributed in a dramatic increase in disease-free and cancer-specific survival over the years.

The choice of adjuvant systemic therapy is individualized and based on disease factors, patient overall status and patient preferences. Prognostic factors that predict relapse and risk calculators, like PREDICT, may help to categorize this risk and select appropriate adjuvant therapy (see earlier in this chapter on prognostic factors).

1 *Endocrine therapy* is recommended in all patients with ER-positive breast cancer. Duration of treatment is debatable; usual recommendation is for at least 5 years if tolerated, with potential extension to 10 years for high-risk tumours.
   a *Tamoxifen*, an oestrogen receptor antagonist in the breast tissue, is mainly used in premenopausal women. It is commonly associated with menopausal symptoms, such as hot flushes.
   b *Aromatase inhibitors (AIs)*, like letrozole and anastrozole, block extra-ovarian oestrogen production in postmenopausal women. They may result in bone loss and joint pains due to oestrogen deficiency, which requires monitoring.
   c *Ovarian function suppression* by drug therapy (LHRH inhibition, e.g. goserelin), or by oophorectomy and rarely irradiation, may be indicated for premenopausal women with high-risk ER-positive tumours, in addition to tamoxifen or AIs.
2 *Combination chemotherapy*, with anthracyclines and taxanes is used in different schemes. Regimen choice varies according to institution and clinicians. Due to treatment toxicity, suitable patients for chemotherapy should be carefully assessed.
3 *Monoclonal antibody therapy:* directed to the HER2 improves prognosis in HER2-positive breast cancer. These agents are *Trastuzumab (Herceptin)* with or without *Pertuzumab* (Perjeta).
4 *Bisphosphonates:* like zoledronic acid and clodronate, may reduce the risk of the breast cancer spreading to the bones and improve survival in high-risk postmenopausal women.

A suggested outline for adjuvant systemic therapy is as follows.

1 Premenopausal women.
   a *Low-risk disease*: tamoxifen if ER positive.
   b *Intermediate-risk disease and ER-positive tumours*: tamoxifen possibly with ovarian function suppression. Chemotherapy discussion or genomic assays if indicated. Anti-HER2-directed treatment, if HER2 positive.
   c *High-risk disease and ER-positive tumours*: tamoxifen with ovarian function suppression, likely extended duration. Chemotherapy. Anti-HER2-directed treatment, if HER2 positive.
   d *Low/Intermediate/high-risk disease which is ER negative*: chemotherapy.
2 Postmenopausal women.
   a *Low-risk disease*: AIs, usually Letrozole, if ER positive. Tamoxifen, if *AIs* not tolerated or contraindicated.
   b *Intermediate-risk disease and ER-positive tumours*: letrozole. Chemotherapy discussion or genomic assays if indicated. Anti-HER2-directed treatment, if HER2 positive.
   c *High-risk disease and ER-positive tumours*: letrozole, likely extended duration chemotherapy and bisphosphonates. Anti-HER2-directed treatment, if HER2 positive.
   d *Low/Intermediate/high-risk disease which is ER negative*: chemotherapy and bisphosphonates.

Neoadjuvant systemic therapy (before any operation) usually refers to chemotherapy with or without anti-HER2-directed treatment; however, the role of neoadjuvant endocrine therapy is also expanding. Neoadjuvant systemic therapy is indicated for:

• *Downstaging the disease:* this can allow for less extensive surgery to the breast and axilla in locally advanced disease. This can lead to improved cosmesis and decreased risk of postoperative complications i.e. can allow breast conservation versus mastectomy or TAD versus axillary clearance.
• *Assessing the response*: this can determine the prognosis; pathologic complete response (*pcr*) signifies the best prognosis It can also allow the selection of different agents, if there is only partial or no response to neoadjuvant treatment.

HER2 positive breast cancers have the highest *pcr* rates and neoadjuvant chemotherapy with anti-HER2 treatment is also indicated in early-stage disease.

Adjuvant radiotherapy

- *Following wide local excision.* Following BCS, such as wide local excision for invasive cancer, radiotherapy to the breast significantly reduces the risk of recurrence within the breast.
- *Following mastectomy.* Post-mastectomy radiotherapy decreases the risk of local recurrence in high-risk patients. These include patients with large tumour size, high-grade, nodal involvement, lymphatic invasion and/or involvement of deep margins.
- *Following axillary surgery.* After axillary sampling, the axilla can be irradiated if low volume node positive disease (1–2 nodes). After axillary clearance, the axilla is not routinely irradiated. Addition of radiotherapy to regional nodes, like the internal mammary and the supra/infra clavicular nodes, is usually indicated in extensive disease.

Survival

Several factors are thought to have contributed to increased survival rates for breast cancer, including breast screening, specialist multidisciplinary teams and more individualized treatment plans that optimize each aspect of patient treatment. The overall 10-year survival is now 76%, with 64% of all women surviving for 20 years, although survival for individual tumours depends on stage and type, as discussed.

Cancers detected by screening have a better prognosis (83% at 15 years), due to detection of early cancers and less aggressive forms of breast cancer.

Paget's disease of the nipple

Presentation

Paget's disease[12] of the nipple mostly occurs in middle-aged and elderly women and is present in around 2% of breast cancers. It presents as a unilateral red, scaly or bleeding, eczematous lesion of the nip-

ple and areola, often accompanied by a burning sensation. Diagnosis is confirmed by punch biopsy.

Histologically, the epithelium of the nipple contains numerous 'Paget cells': large cells with clear cytoplasm and small eccentric nuclei. It is associated with an intraductal carcinoma of the underlying breast in 50% of cases, and DCIS in many of the others; a mammogram with or without a breast MRI should be part of the workup.

Treatment

Treatment will be determined by any underlying breast carcinoma detected on clinical or radiological investigation. Surgical management may include mastectomy and axillary surgery if associated with invasive cancer. In the absence of invasive disease, or if a small central tumour lies close to the nipple, cone excision of the nipple and underlying tissue followed by breast radiotherapy may be considered.

Inflammatory breast cancer

Inflammatory breast cancer is a rare, aggressive disease, representing only 0.5–2% of breast cancers. The breast appears swollen, red, firm and warm to touch, all cardinal features of inflammation. Symptoms appear quite quickly as cancer cells block the small lymphatics in the breast, and produce the peau d'orange appearance. The majority of these tumours will be ER negative. Treatment involves a combination of neoadjuvant chemotherapy, surgery (usually, mastectomy and axillary clearance) and chest wall radiotherapy. Prognosis is poorer; 5- and 10-year survival rates of the order of 50% and 30%, respectively, although improvements are being made with the introduction of new systemic treatments.

Patients unfit for surgery

These will usually be elderly patients with significant comorbidity, and some may have locally advanced tumours. The principles of management are closer to those for metastatic disease, the aim of therapy being to control the primary tumour while maintaining the best quality of life. Many patients will respond to an aromatase inhibitor or other hormonal therapy.

---

[12]Sir James Paget (1814–1899), Surgeon, St Bartholomew's Hospital, London, UK. He also described diseases of the bone and penis, and discovered the parasite of trichinosis in humans while a first-year medical student.

Metastatic disease

The aim of treatment is to prolong survival and control symptoms while maintaining a good quality of life. All patients with metastatic disease should be considered for some form of systemic therapy. Receptors for ER and HER2 should be repeated at the metastatic site and treatment should be directed accordingly. Hormone therapy, chemotherapy and HER2-directed treatment can be used alone or in combination. With the current advances, patients can live for many years with metastatic breast cancer. Prognosis is worse if the relapse is within 2 years from initial diagnosis and if it involves visceral disease (i.e. liver metastases).

As the disease progresses, patients may require referral to palliative care specialists for control of symptoms and to enhance support for patients and carers.

Carcinoma of the male breast

This accounts for less than 1% of all cases of breast cancer. In men, breast cancer affects an older age group than in women, with a peak incidence at 60 years. Clinically, it usually presents as a firm, painless, subareolar lump, although gynaecomastia and breast tenderness may also be present. Most aspects of management have many similarities to that of women.

Treatment usually consists of a mastectomy due to the limited amount of breast tissue, but a wide local excision can also be performed if feasible. SLN biopsy or axillary lymph node clearance is performed for node negative and node positive disease, respectively.

Most tumours are oestrogen receptor positive, and the recommended agent is tamoxifen for men if there are no contra-indications. Chemotherapy and HER2-directed treatments, as well as radiotherapy, mirror the indications applied to women.

Due to the rarity of male breast cancer, genetic testing is recommended for all newly diagnosed cases.

The prognosis for men is worse than for women, probably because of the sparse amount of breast tissue present, which allows rapid dissemination of the growth into the regional lymphatics.

Breast screening

Screening women aged 50–70 years with mammography every 3 years results in detection of early breast cancers and DCIS and a reduction in mortality, estimated to be 1300 patients a year in the UK. Screen-detected cancers tend to be smaller and node negative with an increasing detection rate of *in situ* disease. Screening may also detect some cancers that are very early and slow growing that would probably not be problematic in the woman's lifetime, but this is outweighed by the many other significant cancers that are detected (2 to 2.5 lives saved for every over diagnosed case).

The success of the screening programme has led to it being expanded to include women aged 47–73 in England, whereas emerging data suggest this to be beneficial for women aged 40–49 years as well. Screening may also start at an earlier age in women who have a higher risk, due to family history or are known carriers of high-risk genes; these patients are offered yearly MRI scans from the age of 30 to 40 to avoid repeated irradiation and improve accuracy due to the increased breast density at this age.

Prophylactic mastectomy

Women at high and very high risk for developing a breast cancer may be offered prophylactic mastectomy. This includes women with a strong family history of breast cancer with or without a confirmed inherited mutation (like *BRCA1/2, TP53 genes*). In these cases, bilateral mastectomy can be discussed, whereas contralateral prophylactic mastectomy can be offered to women with a history of breast cancer that remain high risk. The procedure may be either a simple mastectomy or a subcutaneous nipple or skin-sparing mastectomy with or without breast reconstruction. It is rarely possible to remove all breast tissue so surveillance for this and other *gene-mutation*-related cancers is necessary.

⊘ Additional resources

38

The neck

Ekpemi Irune

Learning objectives

✓ To understand the different causes of neck lumps.

✓ To know about the origin, presentation and management of branchial cysts.

The thyroid gland is considered separately in Chapter 39, and the parathyroids in Chapter 40. A summary of the possible causes of a lump in the neck is given in Box 38.1.

Branchial cyst and sinus

Anatomy

There are six arches and five clefts in the branchial system (Figure 38.1). The first arch forms the lower face, its external cleft the external auditory meatus, and its internal cleft the Eustachian tube. The second arch grows down over the third and fourth arches to form the skin of the neck. Normally, there is no external cleft, while the internal cleft forms the tonsillar fossa.

Aetiology

Persistence of remnants of the second branchial arch may lead to formation of a branchial cyst, sinus or fistula. The external cleft remnants open just anterior to the sternocleidomastoid, at the junction of the upper one-third and lower two-thirds. A sinus or fistula

represents a patent second branchial arch sinus, which passes between the internal and external carotid artery to the tonsillar fossa. That a branchial cyst is a remnant of the second branchial arch has been questioned, based on the observation that the cysts are lined with stratified squamous epithelium rich in lymphatic tissue. This countertheory suggests that the cyst arises from cystic degeneration of lymphoid tissue in the neck and is thus better termed a 'lateral cervical cyst'.

Clinical features

A *branchial cyst* usually presents in early adult life and forms a soft swelling 'like a half-filled hot water bottle', which bulges forward from beneath the anterior border of the sternocleidomastoid. It is lined by squamous epithelium and contains pus-like material, which is in fact cholesterol. It often presents following an upper respiratory tract infection. Clinical diagnosis can be clinched by aspirating a few drops of this fluid from the cyst and demonstrating cholesterol crystals under the microscope. Occasionally, the cyst may become infected.

Differential diagnosis is from a tuberculous gland of the neck or from an acute lymphadenitis.

The rare *first branchial arch cyst* may present just below the external auditory meatus at the angle of the jaw, with extension closely related to the VII nerve.

A *branchial sinus* presents as a small orifice, discharging mucus, which opens over the anterior

Ellis and Calne's Lecture Notes in General Surgery, Fourteenth Edition. Edited by Christopher Watson and Justin Davies.
© 2023 John Wiley & Sons Ltd. Published 2023 by John Wiley & Sons Ltd. Companion website: www.wiley.com/go/Watson/GeneralSurgery14

> **Box 38.1 A lump in the side of the neck**
>
> When considering the swellings that may arise in any anatomical region, one enumerates the anatomical structures lying therein and then the pathological swellings that may arise from them. The side of the neck is an excellent example of this exercise.
>
> **Skin and superficial fascia**
> - Sebaceous cyst.
> - Lipoma.
>
> **Lymph nodes**
> - Infective.
> - Malignant.
> - Lymphoma, lymphatic leukaemia (see Chapter 36).
>
> **Lymphatics**
> - Cystic hygroma.
>
> **Artery**
> - Carotid body tumour.
> - Carotid artery aneurysm.
>
> **Neural elements**
> - Neuroma – greater auricular neuroma.
> - Paraganglioma.
>
> **Salivary glands**
> - Submandibular salivary tumours or sialectasis or sialadenitis.
> - Tumour of the parotid gland.
>
> **Pharynx**
> - Pharyngeal pouch.
>
> **Branchial arch remnant**
> - Branchial cyst.
>
> **Bone**
> - Cervical rib.
>
> **Other soft tissue and cartilaginous structures**
> - Thyroid mass – goitre, thyroid cancer.
> - Parathyroid mass – adenoma or carcinoma.
> - Mass arising from the laryngeal cartilages – laryngeal cancer.

behind at operation. The sinus extends upwards between the internal and external carotid arteries to the sidewall of the pharynx. It may open into the tonsillar fossa (which represents the second internal cleft) to form a branchial fistula.

Investigation

In patients over the age of 40 years, cystic lymph node metastases should be considered. It is also not uncommon for squamous cell carcinomas of human papilloma virus (HPV) type to present with cystic cervical lymph nodes in younger patients. Caution should be paid to obtaining a full clinical history, thorough oropharyngeal examination and flexible nasolaryngoscopy. Cross-sectional imaging of the neck (by CT or MRI scan), ultrasound characterization of the neck lump combined with fine-needle aspiration cytology or core-biopsy are essential to exclude malignancy in this patient group.

Treatment

Where no evidence of tumour is found on imaging and biopsy of the branchial cyst, the patient may undergo a neck dissection alone. Where there remains *suspicion* of malignancy, the neck dissection is undertaken in conjunction with a pharyngoscopy to examine the upper aero-digestive tract for a primary cancerous lesion, bilateral tonsillectomy and a tongue base mucosectomy. All specimens from surgery are sent for histological analysis to confirm the pathological diagnosis.

Tuberculous cervical adenitis

Once an extremely rare disease in the UK, a diagnosis of tuberculosis (TB) was made in over 8 900 people in the year 2011. Actively raising awareness, surveillance and comprehensive treatment in affected individuals has ensured that new cases of TB in the UK have fallen to the lowest levels since records began in 1960: dropping to approximately 4458 cases in 2020. Individuals at risk of contracting TB include the elderly, the immunocompromised, non-immunized migrants from countries with high a incidence of TB, deprived individuals residing in crowded conditions, those with high risk lifestyles such as drug and alcohol

border of the sternocleidomastoid in the lower part of the neck. The majority are present at birth but a secondary branchial sinus may form if an infected branchial cyst ruptures, or if part of the cyst is left

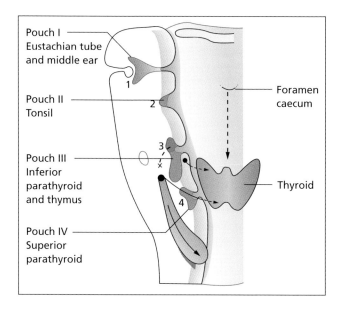

Pouch I
Eustachian tube
and middle ear

Pouch II
Tonsil

Pouch III
Inferior
parathyroid
and thymus

Pouch IV
Superior
parathyroid

Foramen
caecum

Thyroid

Figure 38.1 The derivatives of the branchial pouches and clefts. Reproduced from Ellis H, Mahadevan V (2010) *Clinical Anatomy*, 12th edn. Oxford: Wiley-Blackwell.

dependence, and cases that arise due to unexpected contact with infected individuals.

Cervical nodes are usually secondarily involved from a focus originating in the upper aero-digestive tract such as the tonsils and adenoids. The dental roots may occasionally be the primary source of infection. The organisms may be human or bovine, and occasionally the disease is secondary to active pulmonary infection (pulmonary TB). The upper jugular chain of lymph nodes is most commonly affected in pulmonary and extra-pulmonary TB.

Clinical features

At first, the nodes are small and discrete; then, as they enlarge, they become matted together and caseate with abscess formation, which eventually bursts through the deep fascia into the subcutaneous tissues. This results in a pocket of pus deep to and another superficial to the deep fascia, both connected by a small track: a 'collar stud' abscess. Left untreated, this discharges onto the skin, resulting in a chronic tuberculous sinus.

Differential diagnosis

Extra-pulmonary TB commonly affects lymph nodes, especially in the neck. Solid nodes must be differentiated from acute lymphadenitis, lymphoma or secondary malignant deposits. The abscess originating from a necrotizing lymph node must be differentiated from a branchial cyst (see earlier in this chapter).

Diagnosis may be facilitated with the use of ultrasound scan, as the chronic tuberculous nodes show flecks of calcification and core needle biopsy samples may be obtained simultaneously for microbiological and histological analysis.

Treatment

The mainstay of TB treatment is non-surgical. Input from Infectious Diseases clinicians and the respiratory physicians should be sought in the management of these patients. Most institutions have a specialist team dedicated to overseeing the investigation and management of patients with suspected tuberculosis within a multidisciplinary setting. The decision to treat is taken by experts in TB management and includes a full course of multi-drug anti-tuberculous chemotherapy. Small nodes are treated conservatively and the patient is kept under observation. Significantly enlarged nodes greater than 3 cm with significant abscess burden and/or fistula may be treated surgically with neck dissection in tandem with ongoing TB chemotherapy. This should only be offered in selected cases in discussion with the primary TB team due to the risk of creating a non-healing wound in an already immunocompromised patient.

Carotid body tumour (chemodectoma)

Pathology

Also called carotid glomus tumours or carotid para-gangliomas, these are slow-growing tumours that arise from the chemoreceptor cells in the carotid body at the carotid bifurcation. Most behave in a benign fashion; in a few patients, the tumour becomes locally invasive and may metastasize. There is a familial tendency to development of the tumour. They may also occur sporadically.

Macroscopically, it is a lobulated, yellowish tumour closely adherent to the internal and external carotid arteries at the bifurcation.

Microscopically, it is made up of large chromaffin polyhedral cells in a vascular fibrous stroma.

Clinical features

The tumour presents as a slowly enlarging mass in a patient over the age of 30 years, which transmits the carotid pulsation. The mass itself may be so highly vascular that it too demonstrates pulsation with a bruit on auscultation. Occasionally, pressure on the carotid sinus from the tumour produces attacks of faintness. Extension of the tumour may lead to cranial nerve palsies (VII, IX, X, XI and XII), resulting in dysphagia and hoarseness.

Special investigations

- *Duplex ultrasound* gives precise localization of the tumour and its relation to the carotid and its bifurcation.
- *Magnetic resonance imaging* and *computed tomography* show the tumour and its relation to the carotid artery, the bifurcation of which is splayed open by a richly vascularized mass.
- *Genetic Testing* for the patient and family members should be carried out via referral to the Medical Genetics team. This is specifically aimed at uncovering tendency to and diagnosis of further paraganglioma in patients found to have genetic mutations. Approximately a quarter of paragangliomas are hereditary, with mutations in genes associated with succinate dehydrogenase.

Treatment

These cases are usually managed within a multidisciplinary team (MDT) of surgeons, geneticists, radiologists, pathologists, endocrinologists and other allied healthcare professionals.

Where surgery is offered, it is often possible to dissect the tumour away from the carotid sheath. If the carotid vessels are firmly involved, resection can be performed with graft augmentation or replacement of a segment of the artery. There is a risk of up to 5% of cerebrovascular complications, including a higher risk of damage to adjacent cranial nerves. Thus, patients must be counselled appropriately and the option of conservative management with surveillance scanning may even be offered.

In the elderly, slow-growing tumours can be left untreated. In other cases, stereotactic radiosurgery may be offered to arrest the growth of the tumour. This may be by way of targeted radiotherapy in more recent times, with the benefits being the avoidance of surgery and its potential life-changing complications.

Additional resources

Case 102: A painless lump in the neck
Case 103: A young immigrant with a lump in the neck

39

The thyroid

Brian Fish

Learning objectives

✓ To know the embryological course of the thyroid and related remnants.
✓ To understand the management of benign and malignant thyroid conditions.

Congenital anomalies

Embryology

The thyroid gland forms as a diverticulum originating in the floor of the pharynx, and descends through the tongue, past the hyoid bone, to its position in the neck. The diverticulum usually closes, leaving a pit at the base of the tongue (the foramen caecum, which lies in the midline at the junction of the anterior two-thirds and the posterior third of the tongue). Failure of the thyroid to descend or incomplete descent along the track may result in ectopic thyroid tissue (Figure 39.1). Incomplete obliteration of the track may result in fistula or sinus formation. In all cases of unexplained midline nodules in the neck, thyroid tissue should be suspected. A neck ultrasound with or without a thyroid uptake scan should be considered before removal of any ectopic thyroid tissue to ensure that there is normal thyroid tissue present in the correct place before the ectopic thyroid tissue is removed.

Lingual thyroid

Rarely, the thyroid fails to descend into the neck. Such a patient presents with a lump at the foramen caecum

of the tongue. This is termed a 'lingual thyroid', and usually represents the sum total of thyroid tissue. Treatment may not be required, although it can cause obstructive symptoms and rarely can undergo malignant change. Treatment with levothyroxine may suffice if associated with hypothyroidism and occasionally excision may be required.

Thyroglossal cyst

A thyroglossal cyst forms in the embryological remnants of the thyroid and presents as a fluctuant swelling in or near the midline of the neck. It is diagnosed by its characteristic physical signs.

1 It moves upwards when the patient protrudes the tongue, because of its attachment to the tract of the thyroid descent.
2 It moves on swallowing, because of its attachment to the larynx by the pretracheal fascia.

Treatment

Such cysts should be removed surgically, together with remnants of the thyroglossal tract, up to the foramen caecum and the body of the hyoid bone, to which the tract is closely related (Sistrunk's procedure[1]).

Ellis and Calne's Lecture Notes in General Surgery, Fourteenth Edition. Edited by Christopher Watson and Justin Davies.
© 2023 John Wiley & Sons Ltd. Published 2023 by John Wiley & Sons Ltd.
Companion website: www.wiley.com/go/Watson/GeneralSurgery14

[1]Walter Ellis Sistrunk (1880–1930), Associate Professor of Surgery, Mayo Clinic, Rochester, MN. Described the procedure in 1928.

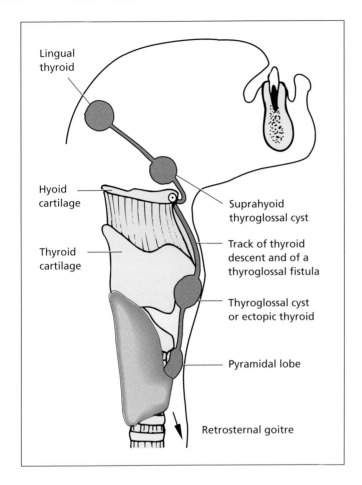

Hyoid cartilage

Lingual thyroid

Thyroid cartilage

Suprahyoid thyroglossal cyst

Track of thyroid descent and of a thyroglossal fistula

Thyroglossal cyst or ectopic thyroid

Pyramidal lobe

Retrosternal goitre

Figure 39.1 The descent of the thyroid, showing possible sites of ectopic thyroid tissue or thyroglossal cysts, and also the course of a thyroglossal fistula. (The arrow shows the further descent of the thyroid that may take place retrosternally into the superior mediastinum.)

There is an associated risk of malignancy of approximately 1%. Infection of the cyst or incomplete excision can lead to a thyroglossal fistula.

Thyroid physiology

The thyroid gland is concerned with the synthesis of the iodine-containing hormones thyroxine (tetra-iodothyronine, T4) and tri-iodothyronine (T3), which control the metabolic rate of the body; T3 is the active hormone and T4 is converted to T3 in the periphery. The thyroid gland also secretes calcitonin from the parafollicular C cells, which reduces the level of serum calcium and is, therefore, antagonistic to parathormone.

Iodine in the diet is absorbed into the bloodstream as iodide, which is taken up by the thyroid gland. After entering the follicle, the iodide is converted into organic iodine, which is then bound with the tyrosine radicals of thyroglobulin to form the precursors of the thyroid hormones. The colloid within the thyroid vesicles is composed of thyroglobulin, which is synthesized in the follicular cells, and T3 and T4. These hormones are released into the bloodstream after being separated from thyroglobulin within the follicular cells. In the general circulation, about 99% of T3 and T4 is bound to protein, and it is the minute amount of unbound 'free' thyroid hormones in the circulating blood that produces the endocrine effects of the thyroid gland.

Physiological control of secretion

The immediate control of synthesis and liberation of T3 and T4 is by thyroid-stimulating hormone (TSH) produced by the anterior pituitary. TSH is secreted in response to the level of thyroid hormones in the blood by a negative feedback mechanism. The secretion of TSH is also under the influence of the hypothalamic thyrotrophin-releasing hormone (TRH).

Pharmacological control of secretion

The production of thyroid hormones can be inhibited by thionamide antithyroid drugs such as carbimazole, propylthiouracil and methimazole which block the binding of iodine but do not interfere with the uptake of iodide by the gland.

High doses of iodine (e.g. Lugol's[2]) given to patients with excessive thyroid hormone production result in an increase in the amount of iodine-rich colloid, and a diminished liberation of thyroid hormones; the gland also becomes less vascular. The effects of iodide treatment are maximal after 2 weeks of treatment and then diminish. This can be useful in preparing hyperthyroid patients for surgery when antithyroid drugs have been ineffective.

Lack of iodine in the diet prevents the formation of thyroid hormones, and excess pituitary TSH is produced, which may result in an iodine-deficient goitre. Thiocyanates prevent the thyroid gland from taking up iodide.

Pathology of goitre

The term 'goitre' is used to describe any enlargement of the thyroid gland irrespective of the underlying pathology. It can be diffuse or nodular and non-toxic or toxic.

Multinodular goitre

The aetiology of multinodular goitre is unclear but several contributing factors have been identified. The principal cause is believed to be a functional heterogeneity of follicular cells, with some having a higher growth potential than normal follicular cells, some of

[2]Jean Guillaume Auguste Lugol (1788–1851), Physician, Hôpital Saint-Louis, Paris. He proposed a solution of iodine as a treatment for tuberculosis, for which it was ineffective. Its use in treating thyrotoxicosis was pioneered by Henry Stanley Plummer (1874–1936).

which may replicate even in the absence of TSH. The difference in areas of excessive activity and other areas of regression results in a varied appearance of the gland. Some follicles are lined with hyperactive epithelium and others with flattened atrophic cells. Some contain no colloid, others an excessive amount. The thyroid interstitium is excessive, with some fibrosis and mononuclear cell infiltration. Factors which are associated with the development of a multinodular goitre include female gender and elevated TSH secondary to iodine deficiency or natural goitrogens. Nodular goitres may produce a normal amount of T4, but sometimes excessive T4 production results in hyperthyroidism in this condition (toxic nodular goitre). Radioactive iodine-131 is the treatment of choice in such cases.

The thyroid is usually enlarged, irregular and nodular and, although one lobe often predominates at presentation, the condition does affect the entire gland.

Symptoms

The enlarging thyroid can produce a number of 'pressure' symptoms including dysphagia, breathlessness, orthopnoea, hoarseness and facial swelling.

Investigation of multinodular goitre

Patients require a few specific investigations.

- *TSH* concentration is low in the few patients with hyperthyroidism in association with multinodular goitre.
- *Ultrasound* of the gland to exclude any suspicious nodules.
- *Computed tomography (CT) of the neck and thoracic inlet* may be required to define the size of the goitre, the extent of the goitre including any retrosternal extension, and to identify the presence of tracheal compression (Box 39.1).

Complications

- Tracheal displacement or compression.
- Haemorrhage into a cyst, producing pain and increased swelling (which may produce sudden tracheal compression).
- Toxic change.
- Malignant change (rare).

> **Box 39.1 Symptoms of multinodular goitre**
>
> - *Dysphagia*: usually of solids, worse with certain food, for example meat.
> - *Breathlessness*: worse on exertion, bending forward (especially, retrosternal extension).
> - *Orthopnoea*: owing to the weight of the gland pressing on the trachea when lying flat.
> - *Stridor*: from significant tracheal compression.
> - *Hoarseness*: from pressure on one recurrent laryngeal nerve (rare).
> - *Facial congestion*: venous engorgement especially on raising arms (Pemberton's sign[3]).

Clinical features in thyroid disease

Patients may present complaining of a lump in the neck and/or with symptoms due to excessive or diminished amounts of circulating thyroxine.

The thyroid swelling

The characteristics of an enlarged thyroid are a mass in the neck on one or both sides of the trachea, which moves on swallowing, since it is attached to the larynx by the pretracheal fascia.

Colloid goitre

All diseases of the thyroid are more common in geographical locations in which the water and diet are low in iodine. In the UK, the most notorious district historically was Derbyshire, and the frequency of goitres in this region gave rise to the term 'Derbyshire neck'. Iodination of table salt has all but abolished this state of affairs. Switzerland, Nepal, Ethiopia and Peru are also areas where natural iodine is very scarce in the diet and water, and thyroid disease is more common. The most common lesion of the thyroid gland due to iodine deficiency is the colloid goitre, in which the gland is enlarged and the acini are atrophic with a large amount of colloid. This can also occur in physiological goitres (pregnancy and puberty). This accumulation of colloid is probably due to over secretion of TSH from the anterior pituitary, acting on the thyroid, which is unable to produce T4.

Hyperplasia

In primary hyperthyroidism (Graves' disease[4]), the thyroid is uniformly enlarged and there is hyperactivity of the acinar cells with reduplication and infolding of the epithelium. The gland is very vascular and there is little colloid to be seen. Lymphocyte infiltration is usually a predominant feature.

Retrosternal goitre

Evidence of retrosternal enlargement of the thyroid should be sought by palpation and percussion with the neck fully extended. A retrosternal thyroid can block the venous return to the superior vena cava and result in engorgement of the jugular veins and their tributaries and in oedema of the upper part of the body – a cause of the superior mediastinal syndrome. In such cases, CT imaging of the thoracic inlet should be performed to assess its extent.

Tracheal displacement

The trachea should be examined to determine displacement or compression by the thyroid enlargement; the patient should be asked to take a deep breath with the mouth open, when stridor may become apparent.

Vocal cord integrity

The vocal cords should be examined by flexible nasendoscopy or indirect laryngoscopy, as thyroid carcinoma may infiltrate the recurrent laryngeal nerves and cause vocal cord paralysis. If surgery is contemplated, it is important to know whether or not the cords are functioning normally before operation.

Regional nodes

As with any other lump, the regional lymph nodes must be examined in any case of thyroid swelling. The draining nodes of the thyroid lie along the carotid

---

[3]Hugh Spear Pemberton (1890–1956), Physician, Liverpool, UK.
[4]Robert Graves (1796–1853), Physician, Meath Hospital, Dublin, Ireland.

sheath on each side. Hard enlarged nodes strongly suggest malignant disease of the thyroid.

The physiological state of the patient

Determine whether the patient is euthyroid, hyperthyroid or hypothyroid. In the majority of patients, this can be determined from the clinical features.

Hyperthyroidism

Clinical features of hyperthyroidism are determined by examination of the eyes and the hands, as well as from the history and examination of the neck. Thyroxine potentiates the actions of adrenaline (epinephrine), and many of the features of hyperthyroidism represent increased activity of the sympathetic nervous system.

History

The patient is irritable and nervous, and cannot keep still. The appetite is increased and yet there is loss of weight; diabetes mellitus is the other condition in which this paradox occurs. Diarrhoea is occasionally a feature. The patient prefers cold environments rather than warm. Palpitations due to tachycardia or atrial fibrillation may occur.

Examination

The thyroid gland

The thyroid itself is usually smoothly enlarged but not invariably so. It may be highly vascular and demonstrate a bruit and thrill.

Eye signs

- *Exophthalmos* is present in most patients with hyperthyroidism of Graves' disease, owing to oedema and infiltration by mononuclear cells of the orbital fat and extrinsic muscles of the eye.
- *Lid retraction*: the innervation of the levator palpebrae superioris is partly under sympathetic control. In hyperthyroidism, it is tonically active, retracting the upper lid, giving the appearance that the patient is staring.
- *Lid lag*: ask the patient to follow your finger as you move it from over the head downwards – the

upper lid does not immediately drop, revealing the white sclera above the cornea.
- *Dilated pupils* owing to increased sympathetic pupil dilator tone.
- *Double vision* following the examiner's finger to the upper outer quadrant. This is due to infiltration of the extrinsic muscles of the eye, which causes exophthalmic ophthalmoplegia.

Exophthalmos is an extremely distressing condition for the patient and, if severe, the patient is unable to close the eyelids; the eyes are then susceptible to corneal ulceration and eventual blindness. This condition is difficult to treat, but may respond to high-dosage corticosteroids; surgical decompression of the orbit with suture of the eyelids across the eyeball (tarsorrhaphy) may be required.

The hands

- *Sweating*: the hands are warm and moist.
- *Tachycardia*: a rapid pulse is almost invariable and typically the sleeping pulse is also raised. There may be atrial fibrillation and indeed the patient may present with heart failure. A rapid sleeping pulse rate permits differentiation of hyperthyroidism from an acute anxiety state; such patients when sleeping will have a normal pulse rate whereas, in patients with hyperthyroidism, the sleeping pulse rate will remain elevated.
- *Fine tremor* of the outstretched hands is present and reflects the increased sympathetic activity.
- *Finger clubbing*, more accurately termed 'thyroid acropachy'.
- *Onycholysis*: the nail lifts off the nail bed, a condition also seen in psoriasis and with some fungal infections.
- *Pretibial myxoedema*, thickening of the subcutaneous tissues in front of the tibia, is a rare feature.

Aetiology

Patients with hyperthyroidism fall into two groups: primary (Graves' disease) and secondary.

Primary hyperthyroidism (Graves' disease)

This occurs usually in young women with no preceding history of goitre. The gland is smoothly enlarged and exophthalmos common. Symptoms are primarily those of irritability and tremor; exophthalmos and ophthalmoplegia are often quite marked. Primary hyperthyroidism is due to the action of autoantibodies which bind to, and stimulate, the TSH receptor. These thyroid-stimulating antibodies have a prolonged stimulatory effect compared with TSH; hence the traditional name of 'long-acting thyroid stimulators'.

Secondary hyperthyroidism

Secondary hyperthyroidism is overactivity developing in an already diseased and hyperplastic gland. It is a disease of middle age, occurring in patients with a pre-existing non-toxic (euthyroid) goitre. The gland is nodular and there are no eye changes. Symptoms fall more on the cardiovascular system, the patient often presenting in heart failure with atrial fibrillation, although nervousness, irritability and tremor may also be present.

Hypothyroidism

Congenital hypothyroidism

Congenital hypothyroidism (or cretinism) is a condition in which the child is born with little or no functioning thyroid. The infant is stunted and mentally subnormal, with puffy lips, a large tongue and protuberant abdomen, often surmounted by an umbilical hernia.

Adult hypothyroidism

In adults, hypothyroidism (or myxoedema) usually affects women, and most often occurs in the middle aged or elderly. These patients have a slow, deep voice and are usually overweight and apathetic, with dry, coarse skin and thin hair, especially in the lateral third of the eyebrows. In contrast with hyperthyroidism, myxoedematous patients usually feel cold in hot weather, have a bradycardia and are constipated. They are often anaemic and may suffer from heart failure owing to myxoedematous infiltration of the heart.

Hashimoto's disease

Hashimoto's disease[5] is an uncommon thyroid disease that was the first of the autoimmune diseases to be elucidated. The patient is usually a middle-aged woman with clinical evidence of hypothyroidism. The gland is uniformly enlarged and firm, although it may occasionally be asymmetrical and irregular.

Macroscopically, its cut surface is lobulated and greyish yellow. Microscopically, there is diffuse infiltration with lymphocytes, increased fibrous tissue and diminished colloid. It is an autoimmune disease in which the patient has developed both a humoral and cell-mediated autoimmune reaction to elements within their own thyroid. Thyroglobulin and microsomal antibodies can be demonstrated in about 90% of patients.

It is important to diagnose the condition correctly by demonstrating the presence of thyroid antibodies and, if necessary, by biopsy, because thyroidectomy will precipitate severe hypothyroidism in these cases. Occasionally, lymphoma occurs in such glands.

Treatment

Thyroxine replacement therapy with levothyroxine will shrink the gland and treat the symptoms of myxoedema.

Riedel's thyroiditis

Riedel's thyroiditis[6] is an extremely rare disease of the thyroid in which the gland may be only slightly enlarged, but is woody hard with infiltration of adjacent tissues. It is a chronic inflammatory condition that is associated with elevated IgG4 levels and IgG4-positive plasma cell infiltrates, supporting an autoimmune aetiology.

It may be mistaken clinically for a thyroid carcinoma due to its hard texture and apparent infiltration of the neighbouring muscles, but histologically the

[5]Hakaru Hashimoto (1881–1934), Surgeon, Kyushu University, Kyushu, Japan.
[6]Bernhard Riedel (1846–1916), Professor of Surgery, Jena, Germany.

gland is replaced by fibrous tissue containing a dense lymphoplasmacytic infiltrate. It is associated with other IgG4-related conditions (Box 39.2).

Treatment with high-dose steroids may be effective, but resection of a portion of the gland may be required if symptoms of tracheal compression develop.

De Quervain's thyroiditis

De Quervain's thyroiditis[8] is a rare condition usually affecting young women. It often follows a viral infection of the upper respiratory tract. The gland is slightly enlarged, firm and tender. It is generally self-limiting, and rarely leads to hypothyroidism.

Investigations in thyroid disease

- *Serum free T4 and free T3*. Measurement of the biologically active unbound fraction is more accurate than measurement of total T3 and T4; elevation suggests hyperthyroidism.

[7]Jan Mikulicz-Radecki (1850–1905). Professor of Surgery in Krakow and Königsberg.
[8]Fritz de Quervain (1868–1940), Professor of Surgery, Bern, Switzerland.

- *TSH concentration*: raised in myxoedema; suppressed in hyperthyroidism, in which the gland secretes T4 autonomously.
- *Thyroid scintigram*: radioiodine studies of the thyroid gland can provide very useful information. A small tracer dose of γ-ray-emitting iodine-131 is injected intravenously and the gland scanned with a γ-ray detector to map areas of high uptake reflecting high activity. A nodule in the thyroid gland that is hyperactive can be pinpointed by this method, a so-called 'hot nodule'. Similarly, a nodule that is not producing T4 will not take up the radioiodine, for example a cyst or tumour ('cold nodule').
- *Thyroid antibodies*, anti-thyroglobulin antibodies or antithyroid peroxidase antibodies, indicate an autoimmune pathology such as Hashimoto's thyroiditis, or primary hyperthyroidism; other autoantibodies are often present.
- *Ultrasound* of the thyroid gives valuable information as to whether a mass is solid or cystic, unifocal or multifocal. Certain radiological features can be markers of increased risk for malignancy and there are now grading systems to aid the identification of nodules which should have a needle biopsy.
- *Fine-needle aspiration and core biopsy* allow material to be obtained for cytological and histological examination. It is now the principal investigation for all solitary nodules, often under ultrasound guidance.
- *Serum cholesterol* is usually raised in myxoedema and may be normal or a little low in hyperthyroidism.
- *Electrocardiogram (ECG)*: in myxoedema, cardiac involvement will show low electrical activity with small complexes. Atrial fibrillation complicating hyperthyroidism will be confirmed.
- *CT scan*: allows definition of size and extent of goitre, particularly any retrosternal extension and the presence of tracheal compression.

Clinical classification of thyroid swellings

The clinical assessment of a patient with a thyroid swelling has two components.

1 The physical characteristics of the gland itself. Is it smoothly enlarged? Is there a single nodule present? Is it multinodular?
2 The endocrine state of the patient. Is the patient euthyroid, hyperthyroid or hypothyroid?

A synthesis of these two observations gives a simple clinical classification of the vast majority of thyroid swellings, as follows.

- *Smooth, euthyroid enlargement of the thyroid gland*: this is the 'physiological' goitre, which tends to occur at puberty and pregnancy.
- *Nodular, euthyroid gland*: this is the common nodular goitre, there being either a solitary nodule or multiple nodules.
- *Smooth, hyperthyroid goitre*: primary hyperthyroidism (Graves' disease).
- *Nodular hyperthyroid goitre*: toxic nodular goitre.

The less common findings are as follows.

- *Smooth, firm enlargement with myxoedema*: Hashimoto's disease. Usually in a middle-aged woman, and the gland is sometimes asymmetrical and irregular.
- *Invasive enlargement, hard*: carcinoma.

Riedel's thyroiditis and acute thyroiditis are uncommon.

Outline of treatment of goitre

Euthyroid nodular enlargement

Multinodular goitre

Thyroidectomy is advised in patients with an enlarged, euthyroid, nodular goitre when there are symptoms of tracheal compression and dyspnoea. In addition, in younger patients, it is reasonable to advise surgery because of the danger of haemorrhage into a thyroid cyst with the risks of acute tracheal compression. If there is retrosternal extension in a younger patient, then surgery should be advised as delay will only make surgery more challenging. The patient may also be concerned with the cosmetic appearance of the swollen neck.

In elderly patients with a long-standing goitre that is symptomless, it is good practice to pursue a non-operative approach.

T4 replacement (levothyroxine) may be effective by reducing TSH secretion, and so suppressing further enlargement. It is best given following thyroidectomy to suppress enlargement of the remaining gland tissue.

Single euthyroid nodule

In the patient with a single nodule in the thyroid, this may be a solitary benign adenoma, a malignant tumour or, most likely of all, a cyst or nodule in a thyroid showing the histological changes of a nodular goitre. Half of all solitary nodules are in fact prominent areas of multinodular goitres.

Historically all solitary nodules were excised to make a diagnosis. Nowadays, ultrasound combined with fine-needle aspiration cytology can usually differentiate nodules that should be excised from benign lesions. Cysts are aspirated and checked at an interval to ensure that they do not re-collect. Cytology cannot distinguish benign follicular adenomas from follicular carcinomas, so these are often excised to provide definitive histology.

Hyperthyroidism

The available therapy comprises:

- Antithyroid drugs, of which carbimazole is the drug of choice.
- β-adrenergic blocking drugs.
- Antithyroid drugs combined with subsequent thyroidectomy.
- Radioactive iodine-131.

Antithyroid drugs

Carbimazole and propylthiouracil are the most commonly used antithyroid drugs in the UK. Carbimazole is used as the first-line treatment with propylthiouracil being used in pregnancy or in patients intolerant to carbimazole. There is rapid regression of symptoms, the patient beginning to feel better and to gain weight with reduction of tachycardia within 1–2 weeks. Treatment is continued for 12 months and may be combined with levothyroxine (so-called 'block and replace therapy'). If symptoms recur, a further 6 months' treatment is given, after which surgery is advised. Unfortunately, a high relapse rate (up to 60%) occurs after terminating the treatment, even if this is prolonged for 2 or more years. Medical treatment alone is, therefore, usually confined to the treatment of primary hyperthyroidism in children and adolescents.

The toxic effects of carbimazole include a rash, fever, arthropathy, lymphadenopathy and agranulocytosis; the last is a dangerous and potentially lethal complication but occurs in well under 1% of patients. The first symptom is a sore throat and patients on carbimazole must be warned to discontinue treatment immediately if this occurs and to report to hospital. Granulocyte colony-stimulating factor may be required.

β-Adrenergic blocking drugs

In patients with severe hyperthyroidism, propranolol induces rapid symptomatic improvement of the cardiovascular features by blocking sympathetic overactivity, while the hyperthyroidism comes under control with specific antithyroid therapy.

Drugs and surgery combined

The majority of adult patients in the UK are treated with preliminary carbimazole until euthyroid; relapse after medical therapy is an indication for radioactive iodine or thyroidectomy. Most patients will be euthyroid following a course of drug therapy although 50% will relapse and require further drug treatment at a later stage. Radioiodine is associated with a higher relapse rate than surgery, and a high incidence of late-onset hypothyroidism, but may be more suitable for treating older patients. It is not associated with increased malignancy.

The surgical management of primary hyperthyroidism (Graves' disease) is now usually limited to younger patients in their late teens or early twenties who have relapsed following their second course of drug treatment and who are looking for a long-term cure for their disease. The historical operation for primary hyperthyroidism had been subtotal thyroidectomy in an attempt to render the patient euthyroid with no need for exogenous thyroxine. Unfortunately, most patients will require thyroxine replacement in time, and, by leaving too much thyroid tissue *in situ*, there is a risk of recurrence. As a result, total thyroidectomy has become the operation of choice for these patients in the same way as for patients with multinodular goitre.

Radioactive iodine

From the patient's point of view, this is the most pleasant treatment, as all the patient has to do is swallow a glass of water containing the radioiodine. There is no need for prolonged treatment with drugs or the risk of operation; it is particularly useful in recurrence of hyperthyroidism after thyroidectomy. It usually takes 2–3 months before the patient is rendered euthyroid. Antithyroid drugs, with or without a β-blocker, may be used to control symptoms during this time.

There is a theoretical risk of malignant change in the irradiated gland, although it is very uncommon. There is no convincing evidence of an increased risk of developing an unrelated cancer in the long term with the dose of radioactive iodine administered. Nevertheless, it is current practice not to use radioiodine in young women who may become pregnant during treatment, as there is a very real danger of affecting the infant's thyroid. It is also not used when there is thyroid eye disease or there are concerns about tracheal compression. Another disadvantage of this treatment is the high incidence of late hypothyroidism, which requires replacement therapy with T4.

Complications of thyroidectomy

In addition to the hazards of any surgical operation, there are special complications to consider following thyroidectomy. These can be divided into hormonal disturbances (the thyroid itself and the adjacent parathyroid glands) and injury to closely related anatomical structures.

1 *Hormonal*:
   a Paraesthesiae, owing to coincidental parathyroid removal or bruising.
   b Tetany (parathyroid removal or bruising).
   c Thyroid crisis.
   d Hypothyroidism, owing to extensive removal of thyroid tissue.
   e Late recurrence of hyperthyroidism owing to inadequate excision of the hyperthyroid gland.
2 *Damage to related anatomical structures*:
   a Recurrent laryngeal nerve injury.
   b Injury to trachea.
   c Pneumothorax.

3 *The complications of any operation, especially*:
   a Haemorrhage.
   b Sepsis.
   c Postoperative chest infection.
   d Hypertrophic scarring (keloid).

Some of these complications require further consideration here.

Hypoparathyroidism

This may result from inadvertent removal of the parathyroids or their injury during operation. The patient may develop paraesthesiae or tetany (see Chapter 40) a few days postoperatively with typical carpopedal spasms, which may be induced by tourniquet around the arm (Trousseau's sign, see Chapter 40), and a positive Chvostek's sign (see Chapter 40); this is elicited by tapping lightly over the zygoma, when the facial muscles will be seen to contract.

Treatment

Treatment consists of giving oral calcium together with vitamin D derivatives (ergocalciferol or alfacalcidol) or 10 mL of 10% calcium gluconate intravenously if symptoms are severe. Often, the tetany is transient and the injured parathyroids recover; in other cases, permanent treatment with alfacalcidol is required. Parathormone is not used.

In addition to frank tetany, which occurs in about 1% of cases, milder degrees of hypoparathyroidism may occur and may present with mental changes (depression or anxiety neurosis), skin rashes and bilateral cataracts. Low postoperative calcium is treated by the administration of oral calcium and/or vitamin D daily by mouth.

Thyroid crisis

An acute exacerbation of hyperthyroidism seen immediately postoperatively is now extremely rare because of the careful preoperative preparation of these patients. It is a frightening phenomenon, with mania, hyperpyrexia and marked tachycardia, which may lead to death from heart failure. The cause is not fully understood, but it may be due to a massive release of thyroxine from the hyperactive gland during the operation.

Treatment

Treatment comprises heavy sedation, propranolol, antithyroid medication, iodine and cooling by means of ice packs.

Recurrent laryngeal nerve injury

The recurrent laryngeal nerve lies in the groove between the oesophagus and trachea in close relationship to the inferior thyroid artery (Figure 39.2). Here it is at risk of division, injury from stretching or compression by oedema or blood clot.

If one nerve alone is damaged, the patient may have little in the way of symptoms apart from slight hoarseness because the opposite vocal cord compensates by passing across the midline during phonation.

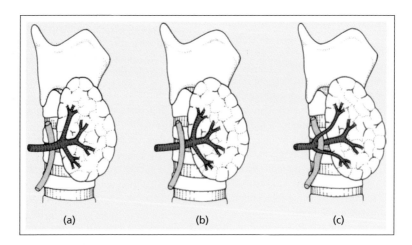

(a)   (b)   (c)

Figure 39.2 The relationship of the recurrent laryngeal nerve to the thyroid gland and the inferior thyroid artery.

However, if both recurrent nerves are damaged there is almost complete loss of voice and serious narrowing of the airway; a temporary tracheostomy may be required, although an incomplete injury may recover in time. It is estimated that the nerve is injured in about 2–3% of thyroidectomies.

Vocal cord assessment by flexible nasendoscopy should be performed prior to thyroid surgery, and is essential for patients with known malignancy, previous neck surgery and for patients with hoarseness or stridor.

It is also possible to injure the external branch of the superior laryngeal nerve resulting in a lower, less powerful voice.

Haemorrhage

If this occurs shortly after thyroidectomy, it can be life-threatening, as bleeding into the thyroid bed and haematoma formation cause respiratory distress by causing venous congestion and laryngopharyngeal oedema. Symptoms and signs include dysphagia, odynophagia, respiratory distress, neck swelling, oozing from the wound and pain.

Treatment

This may be an extreme emergency and must be dealt with at once by decompressing the neck in the ward. The skin and the subcutaneous sutures are removed, the wound is opened and the blood clot expressed. The patient can then be transferred to theatre, anaesthetized, bleeding points secured and the wound resutured.

Thyroid tumours

Classification

Benign

- Follicular adenoma.

Malignant

1 *Primary* (five main types):
   a Papillary adenocarcinoma.
   b Follicular adenocarcinoma.
   c Anaplastic.
   d Medullary carcinoma.
   e Lymphoma (rare).
2 *Secondary*:
   a Direct invasion from adjacent structures, for example, oesophagus.
   b Rare site for blood-borne deposits e.g. from renal carcinoma.

Benign adenoma

Although benign encapsulated nodules in the thyroid gland are common, the majority are part of a nodular colloid goitre. A small percentage represent true benign adenomas, of which 10% are 'hot nodules', that is, they produce excess thyroxine. Thyroid adenomas are four times more common in women.

Thyroid carcinoma

Thyroid carcinoma affects women three times as often as men and the incidence is rising. Risk factors include endemic goitre, radiation exposure in childhood, familial, Hashimoto's thyroiditis (lymphoma), familial adenomatous polyposis and Cowden syndrome[9]. It has an incidence of around 6 per 100000 and long-term survival rates following treatment are excellent. Ten-year survival rates for papillary and follicular cancer are over 90% and 80%, respectively. Papillary and follicular cancer, together referred to as 'differentiated thyroid cancer', account for approximately 90% of all thyroid cancers.

Differentiated thyroid cancer is usually curable when detected at an early stage. The high cure rate can be attributed to a multidisciplinary approach, including specialist surgery, radioiodine ablation, TSH suppression and, finally, the use of thyroglobulin as a thyroid-specific tumour marker (see later in this chapter). Despite this management strategy, a small number of patients will develop recurrence. Half of all thyroid cancer deaths are due to respiratory failure secondary to either pulmonary metastasis or airway obstruction.

[9]Cowden syndrome: Autosomal dominant condition caused by mutation in *PTEN* tumour suppressor gene characterised by the development of multiple hamartomas in skin and mucous membranes, but also cancers of the thyroid, breast and uterus, among others. Named after the Cowden family in whom it was first described.

Pathology

Papillary carcinoma

This is the most common type of thyroid cancer, constituting 80% of thyroid cancers. It occurs in young adults, adolescents or even children. It is a slow-growing tumour and lymphatic spread occurs late. Deposits in the regional lymph nodes may be solitary and in the past have been mistakenly regarded as lateral aberrant thyroid tissue. However, a careful search of the thyroid gland will reveal a well-differentiated tumour in the ipsilateral lobe.

Follicular carcinoma

This occurs in young and middle-aged adults, the incidence peaking in the fifth decade, and accounts for 10% of thyroid cancers. It is more common in areas where endemic goitres are common. It has a tendency to spread via the bloodstream particularly to bones and lungs; lymph node spread is uncommon.

Medullary carcinoma

This arises from the parafollicular C cells and secrete calcitonin.[10] It may occur at any age and, unlike other thyroid tumours, has a roughly equal sex distribution; it accounts for 5% of thyroid cancers. It may be familial (in 25% of cases) and may be associated with other cancers in the multiple endocrine neoplasia syndrome (type II, associated with phaeochromocytoma and either parathyroid tumours or neurofibromas; see Chapter 40). The characteristic finding is deposits of amyloid between the nests of tumour cells.

The disease is usually multicentric and bilateral in all familial forms, and is associated with C cell hyperplasia. In contrast, the sporadic form is usually unifocal with no associated hyperplasia. The tumour cells produce calcitonin, which acts as a tumour marker and can be used as a screening test in syndromic families or to detect recurrence in follow-up of patients after surgery. Fine-needle aspiration cytology of medullary thyroid carcinoma may be diagnostic.

[10]Calcitonin acts to lower serum calcium, stimulating osteoblast and inhibiting osteoclastic activity in bones, among other actions.

Anaplastic carcinoma

This occurs in the elderly, thus reversing the usual state of affairs, in that the more malignant tumours of the thyroid occur in the older age group. Rapid local spread takes place with compression and invasion of the trachea. There is early dissemination to the regional lymphatics and bloodstream spread to the lungs, bone and brain. It accounts for around 2% of thyroid cancers.

Lymphoma

Rarely a thyroid tumour may be a non-Hodgkin's lymphoma.

Clinical features

Tumours may present like other goitres as a lump in the neck, often more rapidly growing. Dysphagia is uncommon, and suggestive of an anaplastic tumour; more common is the complaint that swallowing is uncomfortable. Pain may occur with local infiltration, and hoarseness is suggestive of infiltration of the recurrent laryngeal nerve. Lateral cervical lymph nodes may be palpably enlarged. The patients are usually euthyroid. Ultrasound-guided core needle biopsy or fine-needle aspiration cytology is used to confirm the diagnosis.

Treatment of differentiated thyroid cancer

Surgery

The management of a patient with thyroid cancer should be the responsibility of a multidisciplinary team. Well-differentiated tumours can be treated by a combination of surgery, thyroid suppression by levothyroxine and radioiodine.

Total thyroidectomy is recommended for patients with tumours greater than 4 cm in diameter (pT3), or tumours of any size in association with any of the following characteristics: multifocal disease, bilateral disease, extra-thyroidal spread (pT4a), familial disease, and those with clinically or radiologically involved nodes and/or distant metastases. Furthermore, radioiodine ablation is facilitated by total thyroidectomy.

Thyroid lobectomy is, therefore, appropriate surgery for unifocal, papillary tumours less than 4 cm in diameter in the absence of lymph node metastasis. In addition, it may also be adequate for follicular tumours with minimal capsular invasion, small tumour size and no metastatic disease. Most other patients with differentiated thyroid cancer will require total thyroidectomy and possible radioiodine therapy.

Radioiodine ablation (RAI)

Iodine-131 ablation of the thyroid bed and remnant is an essential component of the treatment of differentiated thyroid cancer. The majority of differentiated thyroid cancers retain the capacity to take up and concentrate iodine. This permits radioactive isotopes of iodine to be used both for the localization and treatment of residual or metastatic thyroid carcinoma. By removing and then ablating all thyroid tissue, follow-up using thyroglobulin is possible (see later in this chapter).

Complications of ^{131}I therapy include oedema and swelling, or thyroiditis in those patients with a large thyroid remnant. In addition, radiation sialadenitis affecting the parotid or submandibular glands may present with painful swelling of the affected salivary gland(s) after eating. There are few long-term sequelae from radioiodine providing that the cumulative dose is kept to a minimum.

TSH suppression

Recurrence rates are reduced by postoperative levothyroxine therapy. Patients who have not required RAI do not need TSH suppression and the serum TSH should be maintained in the low-normal range between 0.3 and 2.0 mU/l. Following initial treatment with total thyroidectomy and RAI, and before evaluation of the patient's response to treatment after 9–12 months, TSH should be suppressed to below 0.1 mU/l in all patients. Following evaluation of response after 9–12 months after total thyroidectomy and RAI, the risk of thyroid cancer recurrence should be reclassified according to the criteria for Dynamic Risk Stratification. This restratification should enable the degree of TSH suppression to be adjusted accordingly.

Thyroglobulin

Serum thyroglobulin is the best way of detecting the presence of normal or malignant thyroid tissue and most patients who are free of disease will have undetectable levels. In patients in whom the thyroglobulin rises during follow-up, careful clinical examination and whole-body scanning should be performed to look for local or systemic recurrence.

Medullary carcinoma

Phaeochromocytoma and hyperparathyroidism should be excluded. All patients with medullary carcinoma require total thyroidectomy and central lymph node dissection. Radical neck dissection may be required when cervical lymphadenopathy is present.

Prophylactic thyroidectomy is indicated in unaffected kindred members with the germline *RET* mutation, even in childhood.

Anaplastic carcinoma

This condition has a very poor prognosis with a 1-year survival of <15%. The main aim of treatment following diagnosis is local control of the disease. Useful palliation may be achieved with external beam radiotherapy, and tracheostomy should be avoided if at all possible.

🕐 Additional resources

Case 104: A lump in the neck that moves on swallowing
Case 105: A woman with an obvious endocrine disease
Case 106: A mass of cervical lymph nodes
Case 107: A rapidly enlarging mass in the neck

40

The parathyroids

Ekpemi Irune

Learning objective

✓ To understand the presentations of both hypoparathyroidism and hyperparathyroidism and their management.

Anatomy and development

The parathyroids are four endocrine glands (sometimes three or five) about the size of peas, which usually lie in two pairs behind the lateral lobes of the thyroid gland. The superior parathyroids arise from the fourth branchial pouch and owing to their short migration can usually be found posterior to the upper two-thirds of the thyroid. The inferior glands arise from the third pouch in association with the developing thymus (see Figure 39.1). The inferior parathyroids may lie almost anywhere in the neck or superior mediastinum although the majority lie within 1 cm of the lower thyroid pole.

Physiology

The parathyroids produce parathormone (PTH), which has a profound influence on calcium and phosphate metabolism. There are three main effects.

1 It increases the excretion of phosphate from the kidney by inhibiting its tubular reabsorption (phosphaturic effect); active tubular reabsorption

of calcium (and magnesium) from the distal tubules is reciprocally increased.
2 It activates the 1α-hydroxylase enzyme in the kidney, which converts the inactive 25-hydroxy-cholecalciferol (25-hydroxy-vitamin D) into 1,25-dihydroxycholecalciferol. The resultant activated 1,25 form of vitamin D facilitates intestinal absorption of calcium.
3 It stimulates osteoclastic activity in the bones, resulting in the decalcification and liberation of excessive amounts of calcium and phosphate in the blood.

Effects of increased PTH production

- A raised serum calcium and a lowered serum phosphate.
- An increased excretion of phosphate in the urine (phosphaturic effect of PTH).
- An increased excretion of calcium in the urine. The large amount of calcium filtered (owing to the hypercalcaemia) exceeds the capacity of the tubules to reabsorb it all, so increased calcium excretion occurs.
- In the longer term, it causes increased osteoclastic activity, with a raised serum alkaline phosphatase associated with decalcification of the bones.

Ellis and Calne's Lecture Notes in General Surgery, Fourteenth Edition.
Edited by Christopher Watson and Justin Davies.
© 2023 John Wiley & Sons Ltd. Published 2023 by John Wiley & Sons Ltd.
Companion website: www.wiley.com/go/Watson/GeneralSurgery14

Hypoparathyroidism

Lack of PTH results in low serum calcium. This leads initially to paraesthesiae (perioral and fingertips) then hyperirritability of skeletal muscle with carpopedal spasms, the syndrome being called *tetany*. The most common cause of this is removal or bruising of the parathyroids during thyroidectomy (see Chapter 39). Tetany is liable to occur if the serum calcium falls below 1.5 mmol/L.

Clinical features

Spasms may affect any part of the body, but typically the hands and feet. The wrists flex and the fingers are drawn together in extension, the so-called '*main d'accoucheur*'. This spasm may be induced by placing a tourniquet around the arm for a few minutes (Trousseau's sign[1]). Hyperirritability of the facial muscles may be demonstrated by tapping over the facial nerve, which results in spasm (Chvostek's sign[2]).

Note that clinical tetany may occur with a normal level of serum calcium in alkalosis (e.g. overbreathing, excessive prolonged vomiting) because of a compensatory shift of ionized calcium to the unionized form in the serum.

Hyperparathyroidism

There are four distinct types of pathologically increased PTH secretion: primary, secondary, tertiary and that due to ectopic PTH production by tumours.

Primary hyperparathyroidism

The diagnosis of primary hyperparathyroidism is made following the detection of hypercalcaemia in the presence of inappropriately normal or elevated circulating PTH levels; the PTH should be low if calcium is raised. The hypercalcaemia is usually discovered on routine screening of patients who have either no symptoms or non-specific symptoms including fatigue, depression and weakness; less commonly, it is detected during the investigation of nephrolithiasis or osteopenia (e.g. on dual-energy X-ray absorptiometry [DEXA] testing), the two main complications of hyperparathyroidism. Many 'asymptomatic' patients feel much better after treatment. The annual incidence is highest among women in the 5th and 6th decade of life (2 per 1000 population).

Pathology

In 85–90% of patients, primary hyperparathyroidism is due to a solitary hyperfunctioning parathyroid adenoma. The lower glands are affected more commonly than the upper ones. In 10% of cases, the cause of primary hyperparathyroidism is familial with the presence of multiglandular hyperplasia. This may be associated with multiple endocrine neoplasia (MEN) type I, MEN type II and MEN type IV (Box 40.1) or may be sporadic or induced by long-term lithium intake, radiotherapy to the neck and calcium supplementation. More rarely, hyperparathyroidism-jaw tumour syndrome is an inherited cause of hyperparathyroidism, which is also linked with maxillary and antral fibro-osseous tumours and renal and uterine tumours.

Parathyroid carcinoma

Parathyroid carcinoma is a very rare condition and accounts for less than 1% of all cases of primary hyperparathyroidism. Patients often have higher serum calcium and PTH levels and are more likely to have a palpable neck mass than those with benign hyperparathyroidism. There is an association with previous neck irradiation and the MEN type 1 syndrome.

Surgery is the only effective treatment. Malignancy should be considered with any gland that is firm, has a grey appearance or that is adherent to surrounding structures. If malignancy is confirmed, surgery may involve simple excision or *en bloc* resection, including excision of local structures such as ipsilateral thyroid, lymph nodes, thymus, strap muscles and the recurrent laryngeal nerve. Approximately 30% of tumours will metastasize, but death from the disease is usually attributable to hypercalcaemia and its effects on the heart, pancreas and kidney, rather than metastatic tumour burden.

---

[1]Armand Trousseau (1801–1867), Physician, Hôpital Necker, Hôpital St Antoine and Hôpital Dieu, Paris, France. Also described thrombophlebitis migrans associated with cancer.
[2]Frantisek Chvostek (1835–1884), Physician, Josefs-Akademie, Vienna, Austria.

Box 40.1 Multiple endocrine neoplasia (MEN) syndromes

These syndromes are characterized by the development of tumours in two or more endocrine structures in the same patient. These may be endocrine adenomas or adenocarcinomas. Some, such as medullary carcinoma of the thyroid, may be familial, with autosomal dominant inheritance.

MEN type I
- Pancreatic tumour: islet cell tumours except β-cell tumours (insulinoma).
- Hyperparathyroidism.
- Pituitary tumour, e.g. prolactinoma.
- Adrenocortical tumour.

MEN type II
- Medullary carcinoma of the thyroid.
- Phaeochromocytoma.
- Hyperparathyroidism.

MEN type III (also known as type IIB)
- Medullary carcinoma of the thyroid.
- Phaeochromocytoma.
- Neurofibromas of tongue, lips and eyelid.
- Marfanoid appearance.

MEN type IV
- Hyperparathyroidism.
- Anterior pituitary tumours.
- Adrenocortical tumours and renal tumours.
- Tumours of the reproductive organs (e.g. neuroendocrine tumour of the cervix and uterine tumours).

Secondary hyperparathyroidism

In some 10% of patients with hyperparathyroidism, the condition is found to be due to hyperplasia of all four parathyroid glands. This occurs most commonly in patients with renal failure maintained by dialysis, in whom renal conversion of 25-hydroxycholecalciferol (calcidiol) to 1,25-dihydroxycholecalciferol (calcitriol) is impaired. This active form of vitamin D is required for absorption of calcium from the gut; deficiency results in hypocalcaemia, which chronically stimulates PTH production. The parathyroid glands undergo hyperplasia in response. To prevent this, dialysis patients are routinely given 1α-hydroxycholecalciferol (alphacalcidol), so bypassing renal 1α-hydroxylase.

Tertiary hyperparathyroidism

Prolonged secondary hyperparathyroidism leads to autonomous PTH production, which continues even after renal transplantation replaces the previously deficient renal 1α-hydroxylase conversion step. Total parathyroidectomy is required.

Ectopic PTH production

Hyperparathyroidism is occasionally due to ectopic PTH production by tumours, such as squamous carcinoma of the bronchus.

Clinical features of hyperparathyroidism

These depend on the results of excessive production of PTH by the tumour (see earlier in this chapter). Presenting symptoms may include the following.

- *Renal effects*: renal stones, infection associated with renal calculi, calcification in the renal substance (nephrocalcinosis) or uraemia. Urinary tract calculi are the most common clinical manifestation of hyperparathyroidism. It is important to remember that chronic renal disease with impaired excretion of phosphate may result in secondary hyperplasia of the parathyroid glands with features similar to those of a primary adenoma of the parathyroid.
- *Bone changes*: spontaneous fractures or pain in the bones. X-ray will show decalcification of the bones with cyst formation. The weakened bones may be deformed; this condition is known as osteitis fibrosa cystica or von Recklinghausen's disease[3] of bone. There may be metastatic calcification in soft tissues, arterial walls and the kidneys.
- *Abdominal pain*: constipation is common. Dyspepsia or frank peptic ulceration is also

[3]Friederich Daniel von Recklinghausen (1833–1910), Professor of Pathology, successively at Königsberg, Germany; Würzburg, Germany; and Strasbourg, France. He also described neurofibromatosis.

sometimes associated with parathyroid adenoma, as is pancreatitis. If ulcer symptoms persist after treatment of the adenoma, the presence of a gastrinoma should be excluded by serum gastrin assay (there is an MEN syndrome association).

- *Vague ill health associated with high serum calcium*: the patient very often complains of lassitude, mental disturbances, weakness, anorexia and loss of weight. Thirst and polyuria are common.
- *Cardiovascular*: hypertension may be noted at the initial diagnosis and is often associated with left ventricular hypertrophy. Although serum PTH correlates strongly with left ventricular mass, the reduction in left ventricular mass following parathyroidectomy is not associated with a similar reduction in mean blood pressure. Primary hyperparathyroidism appears to be associated with an increased rate of premature death owing to cardiovascular disease, although early surgical intervention may result in improved survival.
- *Asymptomatic*: an increasing number of patients with very few or no symptoms are now being diagnosed on routine biochemical screening. Despite this, the majority of these patients feel better following parathyroidectomy and this, combined with a recognition that up to 25% of patients will have progressive disease, has led to support for early surgical intervention following initial diagnosis.

A careful family history should also be taken to exclude MEN and this, or presentation of primary hyperparathyroidism at an early age, should raise the suspicion of hyperplasia rather than an adenoma.

The main effects have historically been summarized as: 'stones, bones, abdominal groans, mental moans'.

Special investigations

Diagnostic investigations include the following.

- *Serum calcium and PTH*. A high serum calcium, corrected for plasma albumin, in the presence of detectable serum PTH should raise a strong suspicion of primary hyperparathyroidism. The PTH may be normal or elevated but in either case is *inappropriately elevated* for the level of serum calcium.
- *Serum phosphate* may be low (hypophosphataemia) and *phosphaturia* may also be present.
- *24-hour urine collection for calcium* should be taken to exclude familial hypocalciuric hypercalcaemia (FHH).

- *Serum urea and creatinine* should be measured to assess renal function.
- *Tc99m-Sestamibi (methoxyisobutylisonitrile [MIBI]) parathyroid scintigraphy* will identify a solitary parathyroid adenoma and highlight an ectopic retrosternal location. Sestamibi is technetium-99-labelled MIBI and, following injection, is taken up by parathyroid glands and retained by adenomas.
- *Ultrasound of the neck* is also effective in localizing an adenoma. In clinical practice, surgeons look for concordance between two imaging modalities to improve the preoperative localization of parathyroid tumours. This is often by pooling ultrasound and sestamibi imaging outcomes.
- *Renal ultrasound* may be implemented to exclude kidney stones.
- *Computed tomography (CT) scan*, with images before and repeated several times after contrast administration, may also show up ectopic adenomas, which take up contrast rapidly.
- *4-Dimensional-CT (4D-CT) scanning* is a modern imaging technique that has higher reported sensitivity of up to 79.8% in detecting single, multiple and ectopic parathyroid gland disease.
- *Genetic Testing* is an essential part of diagnostic screening in all patients with a family history of hyperparathyroidism, patients < 35 years of age presenting with hyperparathyroidism or those < 45 years with evidence of multigland disease, suspected jaw tumour syndrome and/or gland hyperplasia. There are specific national guidelines that underpin genetic testing in this population.

Medical management

Patients with primary hyperparathyroidism may be managed medically with oral medication such as Cinacalcet. This is a calcimimetic that is a calcium sensing receptor (CaSR) agonist. Stimulation of CaSR results in inhibition of PTH synthesis and secretion thus leading to a reduction in serum calcium concentrations.

Fracture risks in patients can be managed using a bisphosphonate taken orally. This approach is especially suitable in patients who are not medically fit for surgery or where surgery has been unsuccessful. Medical management must be directed under the care of an endocrinologist.

Indications for surgery

Surgery should be considered in any patient once a diagnosis of primary hyperparathyroidism has been confirmed and even patients with mild hypercalcaemia get symptomatic benefit following surgery. This is subject to the patient being medically fit enough to undergo general anaesthesia.

Bilateral neck exploration

This procedure is normally carried out using endotracheal intubation and neck extension to facilitate access to the neck. Bilateral neck exploration is carried out through a transverse (Kocher's[4]) incision just above the clavicle to provide access to both retrothyroid spaces to detect and remove one or more enlarged glands.

If a single gland is enlarged, it is likely to be an adenoma and is removed once the remaining glands have been visualized and confirmed to be normal. Frozen section of the gland, or urgent 'near patient' estimation of PTH levels, will confirm the tissue removed during surgery contains parathyroid tissue. Frozen section will not distinguish between an adenoma or a carcinoma. Robust pathological assessment of the entire gland is required to achieve this.

Unilateral neck exploration

Most (95%) patients with primary hyperparathyroidism have a single affected gland. Preoperative localization of the adenoma by ultrasound of the neck and/or sestamibi scanning (or where available 4D-CT) enables unilateral neck exploration. Patients with multigland disease, MEN-related hyperplasia, FHH and renal disease are not suitable for this approach. In addition, patients with a short neck and previous neck surgery or irradiation may also not be suitable.

Focused parathyroidectomy

Following accurate preoperative localization of single gland disease, exploration is carried out through a small incision lateral in the neck which may be per-

[4]Theodore Kocher (1841–1917), Professor of Surgery, Bern, Switzerland. He won a Nobel Prize in 1909 for work on the thyroid gland. In addition to the thyroid incision, he also described a subcostal incision for open cholecystectomy and a posterior approach to the hip.

formed under either general anaesthesia or local anaesthetic cervical block as a day case. This technique can be combined with intraoperative PTH measurement, a fall of at least 50% indicating removal of all hyperfunctioning parathyroid tissue.

Minimally invasive parathyroidectomy

This relies on the use of an incision of about 2.5 cm in the neck. In some cases, access is gained through a remote site such as in the transaxillary approach. Specially designed ports are inserted in strategic locations to avoid placing a scar in the neck and endoscopes may be used in the case of video-assisted parathyroidectomy. These procedures are comparable to open procedures in terms of achieving curative outcomes in parathyroid surgery. Patient selection and surgeon experience are crucial to success. In some cases, a minimally invasive procedure may be converted to an open neck procedure when challenges that cannot be remedied using a minimally invasive approach arise intraoperatively.

Complications of parathyroid surgery

The main complications of parathyroid surgery include:

- *Recurrent laryngeal nerve palsy*: occurs in under 1% of patients.
- *Hypocalcaemia*: the remaining parathyroid glands are suppressed by the high PTH levels and may take some time to recover.
- *Persistent hypercalcaemia*: residual parathyroid tissue remains, possibly a fifth gland or an ectopic gland within the anterior mediastinum.

Management of persistent or recurrent primary hyperparathyroidism

Despite careful initial surgery, a number of patients will not be cured following initial surgery or will relapse at a later stage. This is most often due to a failure to diagnose multigland disease or the presence of an ectopic parathyroid gland. Failure of primary surgery often raises the prospect of revisional surgery. These patients require extensive imaging (ultrasound, sestamibi, CT and MRI scans) prior to surgery to localize and remove the abnormal gland(s). Selective venous sampling, with PTH measurement by catheterization of the venous tributaries in the neck, may also help localization and is often combined with arteriography.

Additional resources

Case 108: A patient with colic and its underlying endocrine cause

41

The thymus

Christopher Watson

Learning objective

✓ To have knowledge of the tumours of the thymus and their association with myasthenia gravis.

The thymus gland controls the development of T lymphocytes in the embryo and neonate and lies in the anterior mediastinum between the sternum in front and great vessels and pericardium posteriorly.

Following puberty, the thymus involutes and becomes a fat-infiltrated remnant but to the surgeon, it is of importance in having an ill-understood connection with myasthenia gravis and being a rare site of mediastinal tumour.

Tumours

Tumours of the thymus are of complex pathology; they may arise either from the epithelium (Hassall's corpuscles[1]) and are termed 'thymomas', or from lymphoid tissue, or a mixture of both. Thymic tumours typically have solid and cystic components, and may be benign thymomas, or malignant and rapidly invasive thymic carcinomas. Peak incidence is between the fifth and seventh decades. The thymus may also be involved in cases of lymphoma, particularly Hodgkin's disease. Neuroendocrine tumours may occasionally originate

in the thymus and may produce vasoactive substances akin to those produced in carcinoid syndrome.

Clinical features

There are three modes of presentation:

1 *A mediastinal mass:* Incidental finding on chest imaging.
2 *Local symptoms of a mass in the mediastinum:* Chest pain, breathlessness, phrenic nerve palsy or obstruction of the superior vena cava.
3 *Paraneoplastic syndromes:* Autoimmune conditions such as myasthenia gravis and pure red cell aplasia, or immunodeficiency syndromes.

Treatment

Treatment is by thymectomy via median sternotomy, combined with radiotherapy and/or chemotherapy if malignant, to prevent mediastinal recurrence.

Early invasion, with no more than pleural and mediastinal fat involvement (stage 1), carries a good prognosis (90% at 5 years); involvement of the pericardium, great vessels or lung has a poor prognosis.

Myasthenia gravis

This condition is characterized by weakness of skeletal muscle caused by autoantibodies directed against the postsynaptic nicotinic acetylcholine receptors at the neuromuscular junction, as a consequence of

---

[1] Arthur Hassall (1817–1894), Physician, Royal Free Hospital, London, UK. He published the first textbook on histology in English.

Ellis and Calne's Lecture Notes in General Surgery, Fourteenth Edition. Edited by Christopher Watson and Justin Davies.
© 2023 John Wiley & Sons Ltd. Published 2023 by John Wiley & Sons Ltd.
Companion website: www.wiley.com/go/Watson/GeneralSurgery14

which the motor endplate becomes refractory to the action of acetylcholine. About 15% of cases are associated with a tumour of the thymus, whereas thymic hyperplasia is present in most of the remaining cases.

Clinical features

Women are twice as commonly affected as men, and the disease usually commences in early adult life. The extrinsic ocular muscles are most often affected and may indeed be the only ones involved, with ptosis, diplopia and squint. The affected muscles become weak with use and recover, partially or completely, after rest. The voice is weak and death may eventually occur from respiratory muscle failure.

Treatment

The majority of cases are controlled by choline esterase inhibitors, for example pyridostigmine, with immuno-suppression also having a role in resistant cases.

If a thymoma is present, it is excised, although such tumours are often locally invasive. Thymectomy is otherwise indicated if the disease is progressive and the prognosis is best in young women (under the age of 40 years) with a history of 5 years or less.

42

The adrenal glands

Vasilis Kosmoliaptsis

Learning objective

✓ To know the physiology of the adrenal (suprarenal) glands and functional and non-functional tumours that derive from the separate parts of the gland, and their management.

The adrenal glands are paired glands situated above and medial to the upper pole of each kidney. The cortex derives from the mesoderm of the urogenital ridge, while the medulla derives from neural crest ectoderm. These different origins account for the different physiology of medulla and cortex, and the different pathology encountered surgically.

Physiology

Adrenal cortex

The adrenal cortex secretes three groups of steroids:

1 *Glucocorticoids (from the zona fasciculata)*, which regulate carbohydrate metabolism, protein breakdown and fat mobilization.
2 *Androgenic corticoids (from the zona reticularis)*, which are virilizing.
3 *Mineralocorticoids (from the zona glomerulosa)*, which regulate mineral and water metabolism. Aldosterone acts to retain sodium and water and to excrete potassium.

Glucocorticoids and androgens are under hypothalamic control via adrenocorticotrophic hormone (ACTH) secreted by the anterior pituitary gland;

Ellis and Calne's Lecture Notes in General Surgery, Fourteenth Edition. Edited by Christopher Watson and Justin Davies.
© 2023 John Wiley & Sons Ltd. Published 2023 by John Wiley & Sons Ltd.
Companion website: www.wiley.com/go/Watson/GeneralSurgery14

mineralocorticoids are under the control of the renin–angiotensin system (see Chapter 13). As the steroids share a similar biochemical structure, it is not surprising that there is some overlap in actions; thus, hydrocortisone (cortisol), a glucocorticoid, also affects salt and water metabolism and has sex steroid effects (acne, hirsutism) if given in large amounts.

Adrenal medulla

The adrenal medulla is richly innervated with sympathetic preganglionic fibres, and produces the catecholamines adrenaline (epinephrine) and noradrenaline (norepinephrine) in response to autonomic stimulation.

Pathology

The main pathologies affecting the adrenal gland can be categorized based on whether they lead to increased function, owing to tumour or hyperplasia; decreased function, owing to atrophy, infarction or removal; or abnormal function, owing to enzyme disorders.

Increased function

- *Glucocorticoids* (Cushing's syndrome): adrenocortical adenoma; ACTH-producing pituitary adenoma; ectopic ACTH production (paraneoplastic).
- *Androgenic corticoids*: virilism (the adrenogenital syndrome).
- *Mineralocorticoids*: primary hyperaldosteronism (Conn's syndrome).
- *Catecholamines*: phaeochromocytoma.

Decreased function

Hypoadrenalism is most commonly a sequel of prolonged corticosteroid therapy, in which endogenous steroid production is suppressed, followed by abrupt steroid withdrawal. It may also be due to the following:

- *Congenital* adrenal hypoplasia.
- *Autoimmune* destruction: Addison's disease.[1]
- *Adrenal infarction*: a rare consequence of stress or sepsis (notably, meningococcal sepsis).
- *Bilateral adrenalectomy*: intentionally (to treat Cushing's syndrome) or secondary to bilateral nephrectomy.
- *Adrenal infiltration* by secondary tumours from primaries in bronchus and breast.
- *Bilateral tuberculosis* of the adrenals.

Enzyme disorders

Congenital adrenal hyperplasia, the collective description for the adrenal hyperplasias resulting from increased ACTH secretion, may result from certain enzyme disorders. ACTH is produced in excess because glucocorticoids, the end point in the pathway of steroid hormone synthesis, are not produced as a result of one of many possible enzyme deficiencies. Instead, all the substrate synthesized is turned into an intermediate hormone, such as an androgen.

Cushing's syndrome

Cushing's syndrome[2] is produced by increased circulating corticosteroids. Excepting therapeutic exogenous steroid administration, the majority of cases result from a pituitary adenoma producing ACTH, resulting in hyperplasia of the adrenal cortex (the disease that Cushing first described); 10 to 20% are due to benign or malignant adrenocortical tumours and another 10 to 15% are due to ectopic ACTH production by a distant tumour, such as carcinoma of the bronchus. Cushing's syndrome due to bilateral macronodular adrenal hyperplasia is very rare.

Clinical features

The syndrome usually affects young adults (occasionally, children), women more often than men. The nature and relative severity of symptoms depend on the degree and duration of hypercortisolism; when the latter is severe, the appearance is characteristic: adiposity with central distribution, abdominal striae, a red moon face and diabetes. There may be osteoporosis, leading to vertebral collapse, hypertension, with increased cardiovascular risk, and thromboembolic events. Associated androgenic corticoid oversecretion occurs only in females with adrenal cancer or with ACTH-driven stimulation (the adrenal gland is the major source of androgen production in females whereas it is the testes in males) and can produce varying degrees of hirsutism, acne and oligomenorrhea. Most adrenal adenomas secrete only glucocorticoids.

Special investigations

These may be thought of as investigations to confirm the diagnosis, and investigations to identify the cause. The diagnosis is usually established when at least two different first line tests are abnormal:

- *Urinary 24-h cortisol level*: a level above three times the upper limit of normal is considered positive.
- *Late night salivary cortisol level*: the normal evening nadir is lost in patients with Cushing's syndrome. This test in non-invasive and can easily be performed on two or more separate occasions to increase accuracy (the levels of cortisol in Cushing's may be variable).
- *Late night serum cortisol*: similar principle to the salivary cortisol test, but less convenient; hence it is not used routinely.
- *Dexamethasone suppression test (DST)*, in which the steroid dexamethasone is administered. The overnight low-dose DST (1 mg dexamethasone orally between 11 pm and midnight followed by serum cortisol measurement at 8 am the next morning) is commonly used as a screening test to differentiate patients who have Cushing's syndrome from those that do not. As an alternative test, or when the overnight test is equivocal, a two-day low-dose DST can be performed (total of 4 mg dexamethasone).

  Careful interpretation of the tests is required and physiological causes of hypercortisolism may need to be excluded (e.g. obesity, pregnancy, and

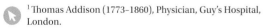
[1] Thomas Addison (1773–1860), Physician, Guy's Hospital, London.
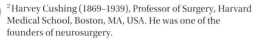
[2] Harvey Cushing (1869–1939), Professor of Surgery, Harvard Medical School, Boston, MA, USA. He was one of the founders of neurosurgery.

physical or psychological stress). After establishing the presence of hypercortisolism, further investigations can help determine the cause:

- *Plasma ACTH* is usually performed on two separate days. ACTH is raised in the presence of ectopic or pituitary ACTH-driven disease; its secretion is suppressed in ACTH-independent disease (ACTH can be normal in cyclic or mild hypercortisolism).
- *Abdominal computed tomography (CT) and magnetic resonance (MR) scans* are the best imaging modalities for localization of a tumour in the adrenal gland. Pituitary MR can also detect corticotroph adenomas.

Treatment

ACTH-independent Cushing's syndrome

In cases of ACTH-independent Cushing's syndrome due to bilateral adrenal hyperplasia, bilateral adrenalectomy is performed and the patient placed on glucocorticoid replacement. Removal of the affected adrenal gland is carried out in cases of adenoma or carcinoma. Prolonged hypercorticolism will result in suppression of the contralateral adrenal which may necessitate glucocorticoid replacement, often for several months post-surgery.

ACTH-dependent Cushing's disease

Cases due to basophil adenoma of the pituitary (the disease Cushing described) can be treated with transsphenoidal adenomectomy, when a clear adenoma can be identified at surgery, or with subtotal resection of the anterior pituitary (anterior hypophysectomy). Medical therapy with adrenal enzyme inhibitors, pituitary irradiation and bilateral adrenalectomy are further treatment options, especially when surgery is unsuccessful or contra-indicated.

Primary hyperaldosteronism (Conn's syndrome)

Once considered to be rare, it is now acknowledged that the prevalence of Conn's syndrome[3] is much higher and the condition often underdiagnosed. The aetiology

---

[3] Jerome Conn (1907–1994), Physician, University of Michigan, Ann Arbor, MI, USA.

most commonly involves an aldosterone-secreting adenoma or bilateral hyperplasia of the adrenal cortex. Unilateral adrenal hyperplasia and familial hyperaldosteronism are relatively rare. Characteristically, there is unexplained hypokalaemia (which may result in episodes of muscle weakness or paralysis), metabolic alkalosis and hypertension. However, most patients are normokalaemic. Drug-resistant or severe hypertension and hypertension presenting at a young age should raise suspicion of primary aldosteronism.

The condition is interesting because aldosterone-producing adenomas represent a curable cause of hypertension.

Special investigations

- *Serum electrolytes*: hypernatraemia and hypokalaemia.
- *Plasma aldosterone concentration (PAC) and plasma renin concentration (PRC) or activity (PRA)*: High PAC (typically, >555 pmol/L) and undetectable PRC establish the diagnosis, especially in the presence of spontaneous hypokalaemia. Otherwise, aldosterone suppression testing is required (e.g. with administration of intravenous sodium chloride and measurement of PAC). Interfering drugs, such as mineralocorticoid receptor antagonists and angiotensin-converting enzyme inhibitors, may have to be discontinued.

Once the diagnosis of Conn's syndrome is established, it is important to determine whether this is due to a unilateral adrenal adenoma or bilateral hyperplasia. Most commonly, this involves:

- *Abdominal CT*: this may show a solitary unilateral adenoma or bilateral adrenal thickening or micronodules.
- *Selective adrenal vein sampling*: this can confirm the presence of unilateral disease and lateralize the side of the tumour. It is particularly important when surgery is considered and in cases where the adenoma is less than 1 cm (when it may be missed by CT) or both adrenals are abnormal (e.g. bilateral adrenal nodularity but unilateral source of excess aldosterone). A PAC/cortisol ratio between abnormal and normal side of >4:1 often indicates unilateral excess aldosterone production (cortisol corrected aldosterone ratio).
- *Metomidate positron emission tomography (PET) CT*: increased tracer avidity at the site of an adrenal nodule may help lateralize the disease. Although

not fully established in clinical practice, this investigation may be particularly helpful in cases of inconclusive adrenal vein sampling results, especially in the presence of bilateral adrenal nodularity.

Treatment

Laparoscopic adrenalectomy has become the standard procedure for unilateral lesions; it has the advantage of lower morbidity and a shorter hospital stay than the traditional open procedure. Medical treatment is the usual standard of care for bilateral

adrenal hyperplasia, with mineralocorticoid receptor antagonists being the first line.

The adrenogenital syndromes (Figure 42.1)

These rare syndromes result from the hypersecretion of adrenocortical androgens, due either to a defect in the enzyme pathway of steroid production,

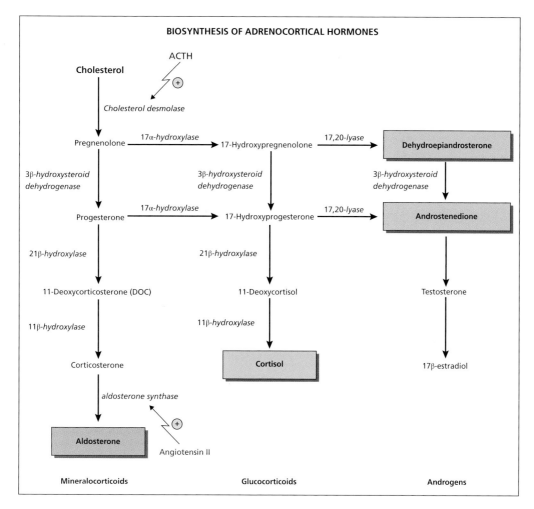

Figure 42.1 Adrenocortical steroid synthesis

commonly 21-hydroxylase deficiency (the congenital form), or to an autonomous tumour producing androgens (the acquired form).

Congenital adrenogenital syndrome

Also known as congenital adrenal hyperplasia, this is due to an inborn defect of normal steroid synthesis (especially, hydrocortisone) by the adrenal cortex. Excessive ACTH production by the pituitary then occurs with resulting hyperplasia of the cortex and hypersecretion of cortical androgens.

Acquired adrenogenital syndrome

In children, it is always due to an adrenocortical tumour, which is usually malignant. In young adults, the condition may be caused either by a tumour or by cortical hyperplasia in cases of Cushing's syndrome, in which androgen production is excessive.

Clinical features

These are conveniently divided into three varieties depending on age of onset.

Infancy

In the congenital variety of the adrenogenital syndrome, the newborn female child has a large clitoris and is often mistaken for a male (female pseudohermaphrodite). Growth is initially rapid, but the epiphyses fuse early so that the final result is stunted growth. There may be episodes of acute adrenocortical insufficiency, especially with stress or infection.

Childhood

Virilization occurs in the female child and precocious sexual development, particularly of the penis, in the male child.

Adults

Amenorrhoea, hirsutism and breast atrophy in women, often associated with other features of Cushing's syndrome. In men, feminization is seen, but this is extremely rare.

Differential diagnosis

The diagnosis is based on detecting the excessive amount of steroid precursors, such as 17α-hydroxyprogesterone, which is raised in the most common congenital form, 21-hydroxylase deficiency.

Differentiation must be made from the masculinizing tumour of ovary, in which the 17-ketosteroid urinary excretion is normal, and also the common condition of simple hirsutism in women.

Treatment

Bilateral cortical hyperplasia in infancy is treated by suppressing the excess ACTH secretion with exogenous steroids (e.g. hydrocortisone); on this regimen the virilizing features clear and growth progresses normally. In the acquired variety, when a tumour is present it can be removed by laparoscopic adrenalectomy, and hyperplasia can be treated by bilateral adrenalectomy with hydrocortisone maintenance treatment.

Non-functioning tumours of the adrenal cortex

Small non-secreting adenomas of the adrenal cortex are common postmortem findings of no significance; they are increasingly detected by modern cross-sectional imaging techniques such as CT and MR (see later in this chapter). Lesions less than 4 cm in diameter with benign characteristics on imaging studies, which are proven to be non-secreting and which do not change on repeated imaging over a 6-month interval can be safely left *in situ*. Adrenal cysts and myelolipomas are relatively uncommon and usually are easily characterized on cross-sectional imaging. Myelolipomas may grow over time and cause local mass-effect symptoms; surgery can be considered when they exceed 6 cm in diameter.

Adrenocortical carcinoma

Carcinomas of the adrenal cortex are rare with an incidence of one to two per million population per year. They are highly malignant and most cases are sporadic.

Most patients present with clinical symptoms related to hormone excess, commonly Cushing's syndrome and less frequently with virilization syndrome or hyperaldosteronism. Non-functioning tumours present with abdominal or flank pain and/or constitutional symptoms, such as anorexia and weight loss.

Special investigations

- *Hormonal evaluation*: carcinomas secrete large amounts of adrenal steroid precursors. Urine steroid profiling of metabolites of glucocorticoid, androgen, and aldosterone steroids and their precursors is a valuable diagnostic tool that can help differentiate benign (e.g. lipid-poor adenomas) and secondary (e.g. metastases or lymphoma) from malignant tumours and can serve as tumour markers.
- *CT and MRI* are both used for diagnostic evaluation and to plan surgery (e.g. evidence of local invasion). FDG-PET CT scanning is used to stage the disease.
- *Fine-needle aspiration biopsy* should **not** be performed when adrenal cancer is suspected as it is poor at differentiating benign from malignant adrenocortical tumours and can lead to needle track seeding.

Treatment

The only potential curative option is complete surgical resection that often has to include *en bloc* removal of involved organs. Tumour stage and resection margin status are the most important prognostic factors.

Adrenomedullary tumours

Classification

Primary

- Neuroblastoma.
- Phaeochromocytoma.
- Ganglioneuroma.

Secondary (metastasis)

A common site, especially from breast and bronchus.

Neuroblastoma

A highly heterogeneous tumour of sympathetic cells occurring in children under the age of 5 years, and the most common malignant tumour in neonates and infants under 1 year old. It may be bilateral, and up to 80% are associated with chromosomal abnormalities.

Macroscopically, it varies from a small nodular tumour to a large retroperitoneal mass, containing areas of haemorrhage and necrosis. Microscopically, it arises from neuroblasts of the adrenal medulla, or within any cells of neuroectodermal origin along the spine.

Neuroblastomas are clinically diverse and their behaviour can range from spontaneous regression, to maturation to a ganglioneuroma, to aggressive disease. They can invade adjacent tissues and spread to regional nodes and by the blood to bones and the liver.

Special investigations

- *CT, MR, ultrasound and bone scan* are all used to stage the disease.

Treatment

A combined approach with surgical removal of local disease together with chemotherapy and/or radiotherapy is necessary.

Prognosis

Early disease, localized to the area of origin and in the absence of distant or lymph node spread, carries a favourable prognosis, as do absence of chromosome abnormalities, and age under one year together with histologically well-differentiated tumour.

Phaeochromocytoma and paraganglioma (PPGL)

A physiologically active tumour of chromaffin cells, which secretes adrenaline and noradrenaline in varying proportions. Ten per cent are malignant and 10% are multiple; 10% arise outside the adrenal gland (the '10% tumour') from the sympathetic or parasympathetic ganglia from the skull base to the pelvis or the organ of Zuckerkandl[4] near the aortic bifurcation (paragangliomas). Until recently, it had been thought that 10% of cases are familial, however, molecular genetics studies have now shown that around 40% of

---

[4] Emil Zuckerkandl (1849–1910), Professor of Anatomy in Graz, and later Vienna, Austria. The organ he described is important in the regulation of blood pressure in early foetal life, but regresses in the third trimester. It is composed of cells of neural crest origin and its remnant typically lies near the aortic bifurcation or inferior mesenteric artery.

patients harbour a germline mutation in an inherited PPGL gene.

Any age may be affected, but the tumour is most common in the fourth to fifth decade. The sexes are equally affected.

Clinical features

These are produced by excess circulating adrenaline and noradrenaline.

There is hypertension, which is paroxysmal or sustained, and which may be accompanied by palpitations, headache, blurred vision, fits, papilloedema and episodes of pallor, sweating and anxiety. There may be hyperglycaemia with glycosuria. Attacks may be infrequent, or occur several times a day.

The diagnostic triad, with high specificity and sensitivity, is as follows:

- *Headache*, sudden in onset, and pounding.
- *Tachycardia* and/or palpitations.
- *Sweating*.

Familial cases can be multifocal. The tumour may co-exist with neurofibromas and café-au-lait spots (neurofibromatosis type 1, NF1), medullary carcinoma of the thyroid or a parathyroid adenoma as part of a multiple endocrine neoplasia (MEN2) syndrome and von Hippel–Lindau disease (see Chapter 38). Germline mutations in the various succinate dehydrogenase subunit genes (SDHX) are relatively common but mutations in multiple other genes have been described.

Special investigations

Identifying the presence of a phaeochromocytoma

- *Plasma metanephrines*: measurement of plasma metanephrine and nor-metanephrine is a useful first line test. Specificity and sensitivity depend on upper cut-off limits used in the assay (specificity can reach 100%). Some medications are implicated in false positive results (e.g. beta- and alpha-blockers, tricyclic antidepressants, caffeine, SSRIs).
- *Twenty-four-hour urine metanephrines*: highly accurate, especially when the index of suspicion for identifying catecholamine-secreting tumours is low.

Locating a phaeochromocytoma

- *CT or MR* may demonstrate the site and size of the tumour.

- *Fluorodeoxyglucose (FDG) PET scan*: this is the imaging modality of choice in patients with suspected metastatic disease and has largely superseded the meta-iodobenzylguanidine (^{131}I-MIBG [meta-iodobenzylguanidine]) scan, although this is still useful in patients considered for MIBG therapy. A ^{68}Gallium (Ga-68)-dotatate PET scan is more sensitive than other imaging modalities for detection of metastatic disease.

Treatment

Surgical excision is performed, usually laparoscopically but larger tumours may require an open operation. Prior to surgery, the patient receives α-adrenergic blockade (e.g. phenoxybenzamine or alternatively doxazosin) to negate the hypertensive effects of catecholamines, which are released as a consequence of manipulation of the tumour during the operation. Beta-blockade (e.g. propranolol) is not routinely required unless significant tachycardia is noted in a euvolaemic patient (no significant postural blood pressure drop).

The catecholamines produced by phaeochromocytomas cause marked vasoconstriction; hence, patients with phaeochromocytomas are relatively volume depleted. Immediately after removal of the tumour, the blood pressure may fall to very low levels; this is countered by volume replacement, although a vasopressor infusion is sometimes required.

Histological examination cannot differentiate benign from malignant PPGL. Patients who are less than 60 years old or any patients with extra-adrenal or metastatic disease should be referred for genetic testing. Patients should be followed up for a minimum of 10 years or sometimes for life (e.g. familial cases). Surveillance is based on plasma or urinary metanephrine testing and/or cross-sectional imaging.

Ganglioneuroma

A benign, slow-growing tumour of sympathetic ganglion cells, which only becomes clinically manifest if it reaches a large size. Only about 15% arise in the adrenal; the rest arise elsewhere along the sympathetic chain.

Adrenal 'incidentaloma'

Adrenal masses are increasingly being recognized as incidental findings on imaging performed for other

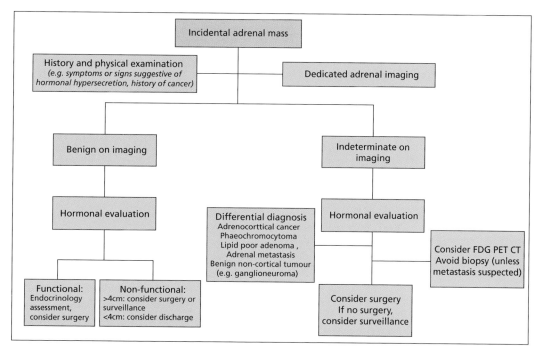

Figure 42.2 Scheme for investigation of incidental adrenal lesion on imaging.

indications. Their prevalence is increasing and is higher among older adults. The majority are non-functional benign tumours but approximately 25% represent functional tumours and/or primary or secondary adrenal malignancies. Assessment should focus on establishing whether incidentalomas are functional and whether they are malignant.

Special investigations

- *Hormonal evaluation*: this should focus on testing for phaeochromocytoma (plasma metanephrines), hyperaldosteronism if the patient is hypertensive or has episodes of hypokalaemia (paired PAC and PRC, potassium level), and for hypercortisolism (e.g. overnight low-dose DST). If primary adrenal malignancy is suspected, a urinary steroid profile should be added.
- *Dedicated adrenal imaging (CT or MRI)*: a low attenuation, homogeneous adrenal mass on non-contrast CT (<10 Hounsfield Units, HU) is very likely to be an adrenal adenoma. Over 10 HU on unenhanced attenuation and delayed contrast washout on contrast enhanced CT (<60% absolute washout or <40% relative washout) indicate an indeterminate adrenal mass.

A simplified algorithm for the assessment of adrenal incidentalomas is shown in the above Figure 42.2.

Hypertension

This section summarizes some surgical aspects of raised blood pressure.

Classification

- Primary (cause unknown).
- Secondary (causes at least partially understood).

Primary hypertension

Primary hypertension is a disease of middle-aged and elderly patients, which tends to run in families. It is a very common condition and may be compatible with few symptoms and a long life. There is an increase in the peripheral resistance due to arteriolar thickening or spasm but, as arteriolar thickening is a consequence of hypertension, the argument as to which is the primary factor has not been resolved in this disease.

The kidney may be an important contributor to the hypertension when its blood supply is impaired owing to arteriolar narrowing. There is a vicious circle of arteriolar spasm, arteriolar thickening, renal ischaemia and further hypertension, which leads to a progressive increase in the severity of this condition.

Secondary hypertension

This should be suspected mainly in patients with drug-resistant hypertension, young patients (e.g. under 30 years), hypertension associated with electrolyte abnormalities and patients with malignant hypertension. It may be due to the following factors:

1 Renal disease.
2 Coarctation of the aorta (see Chapter 13).
3 Endocrine causes:
   a Phaeochromocytoma (see earlier in this chapter).
   b Cushing's syndrome (see earlier in this chapter).
   c Conn's syndrome (see earlier in this chapter).
4 Raised intracranial pressure (see Chapter 17).
5 Toxaemia of pregnancy.
6 Obstructive sleep apnoea.

Renovascular hypertension

Mechanism of renal hypertension (Figure 42.3)

Ever since the experiments of Goldblatt,[5] it has been known that impairment of blood perfusion to the kidneys can result in hypertension which, if the renal perfusion remains impaired, may become permanent, owing to the vicious circle that has already been mentioned. The mechanism of renal hypertension appears to be the release of the hormone renin from the juxtaglomerular cells in the renal cortex. Renin acts on the serum protein angiotensinogen to give rise to a physiologically inactive decapeptide, angiotensin I. Angiotensin I is then converted to the octapeptide angiotensin II by the action of angiotensin-converting enzyme (ACE). Angiotensin II is a potent vasoconstrictor and causes an increase in peripheral resistance

[5] Harry Goldblatt (1891–1977), Professor of Experimental Pathology, University of Southern California, Los Angeles, California.

(and thus hypertension) and acts on the adrenal cortex to release aldosterone (which causes sodium retention). The features of hypertension are thus set in motion. This renin mechanism is protective as far as the kidney is concerned and is one method by which the kidney maintains its circulation. How important renin is in the maintenance of normal blood pressure has not been established. All forms of renal parenchymal disease are likely to produce hypertension. Especially common are chronic glomerulonephritis and chronic pyelonephritis.

ACE inhibitors, such as captopril, are effective at reducing blood pressure in patients with renal disease. However, when renal insufficiency is due to renal artery stenosis, their use will exacerbate the impaired perfusion and may result in deterioration in renal function.

Unilateral renal diseases producing hypertension

These are of particular surgical importance, as they may sometimes be amenable to curative treatment either by nephrectomy or by reconstructive procedures on the kidney or on its blood supply.

Unilateral pyelonephritis

Rarely, pyelonephritis may affect one kidney only, especially if this kidney has been the site of previous trauma or of congenital malformation, if the ureter on that side has been blocked or if there is unilateral hydronephrosis. If the condition is diagnosed early, before the hypertension has reached the chronic established stage and before hypertensive changes have taken place in the opposite kidney, removal of the affected kidney may result in a return to normal blood pressure. Presence of a functioning contralateral kidney must be confirmed first.

Renal artery stenosis

This is a fairly common cause of secondary hypertension. It occurs in two age groups: the elderly (70%), in whom the cause of the narrowing is atherosclerosis, and young people, especially women, in whom the cause appears to be the thickening of the intima and media by hyperplasia of collagen and muscle – fibro-muscular dysplasia.

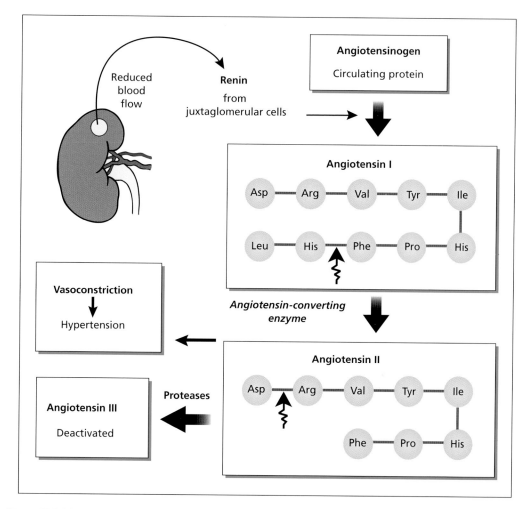

Figure 42.3 Mechanism of renal hypertension.

Special investigations

- *Arteriography* should be performed in young patients, in whom fibromuscular dysplasia characteristically shows up as a string of beads in the distal part of the renal artery and is bilateral.
- *Duplex scanning* may permit diagnosis of a significant stenosis.
- *Renin estimation* should be performed by selective renal vein catheterization. Renin concentration is at least 1.5 times higher on the affected side. It is mostly informative in the presence of bilateral renal artery stenosis where the test can help lateralize the side that contributes most to the hypertension.

- *Diethylene-triamine-penta-acetic acid (DTPA) radionuclide scan* will show renal blood flow difference, especially if the patient has been given an ACE inhibitor such as captopril to exaggerate the condition. It helps determine the relative function of each kidney when therapeutic nephrectomy is considered.

Treatment

- *Angioplasty with or without stent placement.* In suitable cases, a localized stenosis can be dilated by a balloon angioplasty. This is particularly successful in fibromuscular dysplasia.

- *Renal artery bypass.* If the stenosis is fairly proximal and the distal vessels relatively healthy, it may be possible to remove the stenotic portion of the artery or bypass it, for example on the left side by joining the splenic artery to the renal artery distal to the blockage.
- *Autotransplantation* of the kidney may be performed after excising the stenosed portion of the artery.
- *Unilateral nephrectomy* may be appropriate when the small intrarenal branches of the renal artery are also diseased or to remove a small atrophic kidney with almost complete renal artery occlusion.

Other lesions of the renal arteries, for instance aneurysm and congenital bands, may also result in hypertension, which can be cured by unilateral nephrectomy or direct arterial surgery.

It should be noted that, since the introduction of effective antihypertensive drugs (in particular ACE inhibitors), enthusiasm for surgery in unilateral renal disease has waned, apart from patients in whom the kidney's function is grossly impaired.

Other unilateral renal diseases can cause hypertension, including hydronephrosis, tuberculosis of the kidneys or tumours of the kidney; nephrectomy is indicated in these conditions.

Additional resources

Case 109: A girl with hirsutes

43

The kidney and ureter

Alexandra J. Colquhoun

Learning objectives

✓ To understand the congenital renal anomalies and polycystic kidney disease.

✓ To understand the causes of haematuria and its investigation and management.

✓ To understand the causes, presentations and management of urinary tract infections.

✓ To outline the causes of renal failure, its investigation and treatment.

Congenital anomalies

Embryology (Figure 43.1)

The embryology of the kidney involves three separate stages with all tissues being derived from the urogenital ridge. Initially, a pronephros develops in the posterior wall of the coelomic cavity in the cervical region. This is replaced by the mesonephric system, which comprises a long ridge of intermediate mesoderm in the thoraco-lumbar region, the mesonephros, along with its duct, the mesonephric (Wolffian[1]) duct. The mesonephros itself then disappears except that, in men, some of its ducts become the efferent tubules of the testis; it is replaced by the metanephros. At the lower end of the mesonephric duct a diverticulum develops. This diverticulum becomes the ureteric bud, on top of which a cap of tissue develops, the metanephric mesenchyme. The metanephric mesenchyme gives rise to the glomeruli and the proximal part of the renal duct system. The ureteric bud forms the ureter, renal pelvis, calyces and distal part of the renal duct system. The mesonephric duct atrophies in women but the remnants persist in the broad ligament as the epoöphron, paraoöphron and ducts of Gartner.[2] In men, it gives rise to the epididymis and the vas deferens.

The kidney originally develops in the pelvis of the embryo and then migrates cranially, acquiring a progressively more proximal arterial blood supply as it does so. This complex developmental process explains the high frequency with which congenital anomalies of the kidney, the ureter and the renal blood supply are found.

Common renal anomalies (Figure 43.2)

- *Pelvic kidney*: owing to failure of cranial migration of the developing kidney. It occurs in 1 in 500–1000 subjects.

---

[1] Kaspar Friedrich Wolff (1733–1794), born in Berlin, Germany; Professor of Anatomy, St Petersburg, Russia.

Ellis and Calne's Lecture Notes in General Surgery, Fourteenth Edition. Edited by Christopher Watson and Justin Davies.
© 2023 John Wiley & Sons Ltd. Published 2023 by John Wiley & Sons Ltd.
Companion website: www.wiley.com/go/Watson/GeneralSurgery14

[2] Hermann Treschow Gartner (1785–1827), Danish Surgeon and Anatomist.

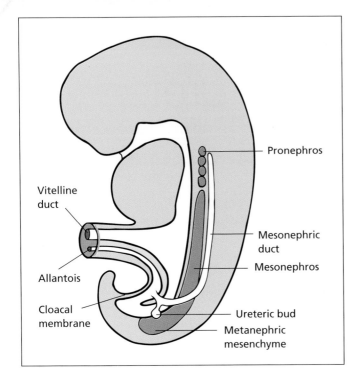

Vitelline
duct

Allantois

Cloacal
membrane

Pronephros

Mesonephric
duct

Mesonephros

Ureteric bud

Metanephric
mesenchyme

Figure 43.1 Development of the
pro-, meso- and metanephric systems
(after Langman).

- *Horseshoe kidney*: produced by fusion of the two metanephric masses across the midline (see later in this chapter). It occurs in 1 in every 400 subjects.
- *Duplex system*: double ureters and/or kidneys owing to duplication of the metanephric bud.
- *Congenital absence* of one kidney (1 in every 2500 subjects). Congenital absence of a kidney is rare, but should be borne in mind whenever the possibility of nephrectomy arises, for instance after kidney trauma.
- *Polycystic kidneys*: multiple cyst formation throughout both kidneys, caused by a variety of gene mutations (see later in this chapter). It occurs in 1 in 500–1000 subjects.
- *Congenital hydronephrosis*: produced by failure of normal smooth muscle contraction at the pelviureteric junction.
- *Aberrant renal arteries*: one or more arteries supplying the upper or lower pole of the kidneys are very common; they represent the persistence of aortic branches that pass to the kidney in its lower embryonic position.

Polycystic disease, the various types of reduplication of the renal pelvis and the abnormal fusions are all associated with an increased incidence of infection when compared with kidneys that are anatomically normal.

Horseshoe kidney

The kidneys may fuse during their ascent from their pelvic position as the metanephros in the embryo. The most common example is fusion of the lower poles across the midline, forming one large horseshoe-shaped kidney. The linked lower ends of the kidneys usually lie in front of the aorta in the region of the fourth or fifth lumbar vertebra and the ureters descend from the front of the fused kidneys.

A horseshoe kidney may present clinically as a firm mass in the abdomen or with recurrent urinary tract infections. Pelviureteric obstruction occurs in 10% of people with a horseshoe kidney and kidney stones are

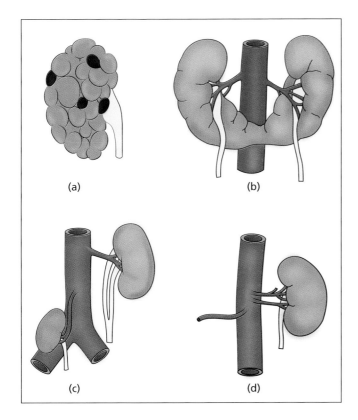

Figure 43.2 Renal abnormalities: (a) polycystic kidney; (b) Horseshoe kidney, (c) Pelvic kidney (right) and double ureter (left); (d) additional renal artery.

common. Computed tomography (CT) will show rotation of the two renal pelvises with the ureters arising anteriorly close to the midline. Each renal pelvis is usually directed laterally.

Duplex system

Instead of a single metanephric mass draining via a single ureter into the bladder, part of the system may be duplicated. The most common finding is separation of the renal pelvis into a double pelvis draining the upper and lower pole separately. This may extend distally as a bifid ureter, which unites to form a single ureter in its distal third, entering the bladder by a common ostium. A second diverticulum grows occasionally from the mesonephric duct, producing a double ureter. In this circumstance, the upper pole ureter always enters the bladder below and medial to the lower pole ureter, which enters the bladder in the normal position. The upper pole ureter may, rarely, drain in an ectopic position directly into the urethra below

the external sphincter in men, or into the vagina or perineum in women.

Duplex anomalies are usually asymptomatic, but may present as a cause of hydronephrosis (see later in this chapter) or urinary tract infection. Ectopic ureters may present with infection owing to reflux up the abnormal ureteric orifice, resulting in reflux nephropathy (chronic pyelonephritis) of the upper pole. Ectopic ureters opening into the urethra or onto the vagina or perineum are a cause of incontinence.

Polycystic disease

Pathology

The condition is characterized by multiple cysts throughout the renal substance, nearly always in both kidneys. These cysts are surrounded by attenuated renal tissue. The condition is usually inherited as an autosomal dominant form presenting in middle age; a more uncommon autosomal recessive form also exists, presenting in childhood with renal failure. The dominant form may result from a number of different gene mutations, the most common being in the *PKD1* and *PKD2* genes; it is thought that a second, spontaneous somatic mutation is required for a cyst to form, accounting for the appearance of cysts in adulthood.

There may be associated multiple cysts in other viscera, particularly the liver (30%), lungs, spleen or pancreas (10%). There is also a strong association with intracranial 'berry' aneurysms and a history of subarachnoid haemorrhage. Diverticulosis of the colon is also more common in people with polycystic kidneys.

Presentation of adult polycystic kidney disease

Polycystic kidney disease usually presents between 30 and 60 years of age with one of the following:

- *Abdominal mass*: asymptomatic, bilateral, lobulated renal swellings found on routine examination.
- *Haematuria*.
- *Loin pain*, usually aching.
- *Urinary tract infection*.
- *Renal failure*: presenting with headache, lassitude, vomiting and refractory anaemia.
- *Hypertension*.
- *Intracranial haemorrhage*, as a result of hypertension or 'berry' aneurysm.

On examination, the enlarged lobulated kidneys are usually readily palpable. There may be clinical features of chronic uraemia, and the blood pressure is often raised.

Special investigations

- *Ultrasound scan* is very accurate in detecting the multiple cysts in adults, but is less so in children because of the smaller size of the cysts.
- *Creatinine* rises as renal function deteriorates.
- *CT scan* demonstrates the replacement of renal substance by multiple cysts.

Treatment

Many people with polycystic kidney disease who are untreated may survive in reasonable health well past middle age. Medical treatment is required in the management of the complicating hypertension and renal failure (dialysis and transplantation). Nephrectomy is considered if recurrent pain, infection and haematuria

affect quality of life or, with very large kidneys, to provide enough room in an iliac fossa to accommodate a renal transplant; bilateral nephrectomy may rarely be required to treat uncontrollable hypertension.

Renal cysts

Simple unilocular cysts of the kidney are common, the incidence increasing with age such that 50% of 50-year-olds will be affected. A simple cyst may be small or may reach a very large size. Several cysts may be present and both kidneys may be affected. The cause is unknown, but may relate to two spontaneous somatic mutations in a tubular cell.

Clinical features

The cyst may be asymptomatic and may be found as a mass on routine clinical examination. If very large, it may present as an aching pain in the loin. Haematuria is absent, and this is an important point in differentiation from a renal carcinoma.

Special investigations

- *Urine* is clear on dipstick testing.
- *Ultrasound* confirms a cystic mass.
- *CT scan* shows one (or more) fluid-filled cysts, which do not enhance with intravenous contrast.

Ultrasound and CT are used to differentiate a simple cyst (thin wall, sharp and distinct border, homogeneous contents, non-enhancing) from a complex cyst that may be a renal cancer.

Treatment

Once an asymptomatic simple cyst has been delineated by imaging, no treatment is required. Aspiration may be performed if infection is present. Pressure symptoms can be alleviated by laparoscopic cyst deroofing.

Haematuria

Classification

Haematuria is best classified as either visible or non-visible, depending on whether it can be appreciated by eye. Alternative descriptions for visible haematuria include frank, gross and macroscopic, whereas non-visible haematuria may be described as dipstick or microscopic.

Two useful rules are as follows.

1 When considering the causes of bleeding from any orifice in the body, always remember the general causes due to bleeding diatheses.
2 When considering any local cause of symptoms in the genitourinary tract, always think of the whole tract from the kidneys to the urethra.

Haematuria is an excellent example of these two general rules and the causes can be classified as follows (Figure 43.3).

General

Bleeding diatheses, for example anticoagulant drugs, thrombocytopenic purpura. However, most patients with haematuria and a bleeding diathesis have underlying renal tract pathology.

Local

- *Kidney*: cancer, stone, infection, glomerulonephritis, trauma, polycystic disease, tuberculosis and infarction (e.g. from emboli in infective endocarditis).
- *Ureter*: cancer and stone.
- *Bladder*: infection (cystitis), cancer, stone, trauma and, in affected areas, bilharzia.
- *Prostate*: benign prostatic enlargement, cancer.
- *Urethra*: trauma, stone and cancer.

Management

Blood in the urine is an alarming symptom and usually brings the patient rapidly to the doctor. It requires full history, examination and appropriate special investigations.

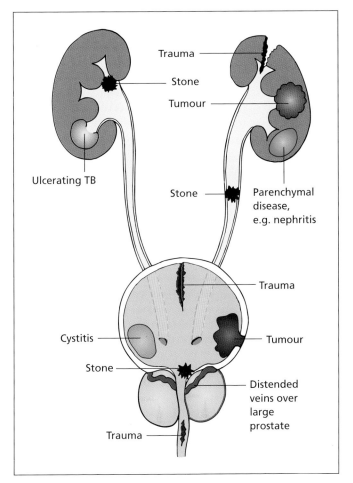

Figure 43.3 Some important causes of bleeding in the urinary tract.

History

Haematuria accompanied by pain in one or the other loin suggests renal origin, and intermittent pain indicates a stone in the renal pelvis or ureter, or partial ureteric obstruction by clot or necrotic papilla. Terminal bleeding with severe pain and frequency indicates a bladder cause, usually infection. Prostatic bleeding is more likely to be initial or terminal and usually painless. Dribbling of blood from the urethra independent of micturition is typical of a urethral origin for the blood. Completely painless and otherwise symptomless haematuria is suggestive of a tumour in the urinary tract.

A history of recent sore throat, especially in a child, would make a diagnosis of acute nephritis a possibility. Always check whether the patient is on anticoagulant or antiplatelet therapy or if there is a history of bleeding tendencies; haematuria while on anticoagulation is still more commonly due to urinary tract pathology, which the anticoagulation has made symptomatic – full investigation is always warranted.

Examination

One or other kidney may be palpable. An enlarged prostate, particularly if the patient is hypertensive, may suggest a prostatic source of bleeding, although other causes must be excluded before this diagnosis is made.

Special investigations

- *Urine microscopy*. The presence of red cells will exclude haemoglobinuria and beeturia (red coloured urine following ingestion of beetroot). The presence of casts will indicate nephritis; pus cells and organisms suggest infection.
- *Urine cytology* is performed looking for evidence of malignancy; cytology is best at detecting high-grade tumours.
- *Ultrasound* detects parenchymal tumours, renal calculi and lesions in the collecting system and bladder.
- *Contrast-enhanced CT* is the principal imaging modality for investigation of visible haematuria.
- *Cystoscopy* will show any intravesical lesion in addition to bleeding from the prostate or blood emerging from one or the other ureter. Flexible cystoscopy may be performed under local anaesthetic at the initial clinic visit.

Injury to the kidney

The kidney may be injured by a direct blow in the loin or by a penetrating wound. The degree of damage varies from slight subcapsular bruising to complete rupture and fragmentation of the kidney or its avulsion from its vascular pedicle. Each kidney is contained within its own compartment of extraperitoneal fascia – the renal fascia. A closed rupture of the kidney usually undergoes tamponade within this compartment; hence, almost all closed renal injuries can be treated conservatively.

Clinical features

There is usually local pain and tenderness and haematuria is a common finding. Retroperitoneal haematoma may cause abdominal distension due to ileus. There may be associated injury to other viscera, especially the spleen or liver, depending on the side of the renal injury.

Special investigations

- *Urine*: macroscopic haematuria is common.
- *CT scan*: the investigation of choice for abdominal trauma, defining renal tract injuries as well as injuries to other solid viscera.

Imaging in renal trauma is indicated in anyone with penetrating trauma to the flank, back or abdomen, and in blunt trauma in patients with visible haematuria, or non-visible haematuria and shock.

Treatment

Associated injuries and shock will require appropriate treatment.

Penetrating injuries may be managed with interventional radiology assistance to embolize bleeding and with retrograde ureteric stenting if the pelvicalyceal system is breached. Cardiovascular instability that cannot be managed with embolization is the main indication for surgical exploration after imaging, but usually results in nephrectomy. Blunt injuries can normally be managed conservatively, with bed rest, serial observations of the urine to determine whether or not the haematuria is clearing, and careful monitoring of blood pressure and pulse rate.

Nephrectomy is required in renal trauma in the following circumstances:

- *Continued bleeding*, which threatens life.
- *Severe hypertension* persisting after renal injury.
- *Lack of function* in the affected kidney after several months, but only if symptomatic (e.g. recurrent infections, stone formation).

Hydronephrosis

Pathology

Hydronephrosis is a dilation of the renal pelvis and calyces. The causes may be classified according to whether or not the hydronephrosis was consequent on obstruction of the renal tract, as follows.

1 *Hydronephrosis secondary to obstruction*:
   a Within the lumen, for example ureteric calculus.
   b In the wall, for example urothelial carcinoma, congenital pelviureteric junction (PUJ) obstruction owing to neuromuscular incoordination.
   c Outside the wall, for example retroperitoneal fibrosis, extrinsic tumour such as cervical cancer.
2 *Hydronephrosis without obstruction*: vesicoureteric reflux.

Obstruction may be unilateral (e.g. calculus impacted in one ureter) or bilateral (e.g. prostatic enlargement, urethral stricture, posterior urethral valve in newborn) with resultant bilateral hydronephrosis. It is important not to use the terms 'hydronephrosis' and 'obstruction' interchangeably.

Aberrant renal vessels were considered to be a common cause of hydronephrosis, because they frequently cross the dilated renal pelvis at its junction with the ureter. It is probably unusual for these aberrant vessels actually to initiate the hydronephrosis; more probably, they snare the congenitally dilated pelvis and act as a secondary constrictive factor.

Clinical features

An uncomplicated hydronephrosis on one side may be symptomless or may produce a dull, aching pain in the loin often mistaken for mechanical back pain. People, usually young adults, with congenital PUJ obstruction may suffer acute attacks of pain resembling ureteric colic, particularly after drinking large volumes of fluid, known as a Dietl crisis.[3]

Associated infection may present with fever, pyuria, rigours and severe loin pain. Bilateral hydronephrosis may present with the clinical features of uraemia. Very often, it is the underlying cause, for example the ureteric calculus, the enlarged prostate or the urethral stricture, that manifests itself clinically.

On examination, the enlarged kidney may be palpable. The size of this may vary according to the degree of distension of the renal pelvis.

Complications

- *Infection*: resulting in pyonephrosis (see later in this chapter).
- *Stone formation*: calculi readily form in the infected stagnant urine.
- *Hypertension*: secondary to renal ischaemia.
- *Renal failure*: where there is extensive atrophy and bilateral destruction of renal tissue.
- *Traumatic rupture* of the hydronephrotic pelvis.

Special investigations

- *Ultrasound* shows a dilated collecting system (calyces and pelves).
- *CT scan* may be required to determine the cause.
- *Diuretic renography (MAG3 renogram-*mercapto-*a*cetyl triglycine*)*, in which a furosemide injection is given at the time of, or 15 min before, MAG3 injection, will differentiate between an obstructed and non-obstructed dilated system, and will also provide information concerning the relative function of each kidney, which is important if reconstruction is being considered.
- *Retrograde pyelogram*, via a catheter inserted into the ureter at cystoscopy, may be required to show the exact anatomy of the hydronephrosis and to demonstrate any obstructive cause in the ureter.

Treatment

Obstruction of a kidney may warrant percutaneous drainage (nephrostomy) or retrograde passage of a double pigtail ureteric stent. Obstruction with infection

---

[3] Jósef Dietl (1804–1878), Austro-Polish Physician, Professor at Jagiellonian University, Kraków.

and obstruction in a solitary kidney are indications for emergency drainage.

Subsequent treatment is directed at removal of any underlying cause of the hydronephrosis. When the cause is a neuromuscular incoordination, an operation to widen the pelviureteric junction (pyeloplasty) may save the kidney from progressive damage.

A symptomatic, poorly functioning (particularly an infected) kidney is an indication for nephrectomy, provided that the other kidney has reasonable function.

Urinary tract calculi

Aetiology

Knowledge of stone formation within the urinary tract is still incomplete and many stones form without apparent explanation. Predisposing factors may be classified into four main groups:

1 Inadequate drainage.
2 Excess of normal constituents in the urine.
3 Lack of inhibitors of stone formation.
4 Presence of abnormal constituents in the urine.

Inadequate drainage

Calculi may form whenever urine flow is poor, for example within a hydronephrotic kidney or in a diverticulum of the bladder.

Excess of normal constituents

Increased concentration of solutes in the urine, because of either a low urine volume or increased excretion, may result in precipitation from a supersaturated solution.

- *Inadequate urine volume*: renal stones are particularly common in people from temperate climates who go to live in the tropics, where dehydration produces extremely concentrated urine.
- *Increased excretion of calcium* (hypercalciuria) may be secondary to hypercalcaemia or, more commonly, idiopathic. Common causes of an increase in serum calcium are hyperparathyroidism (see Chapter 40) and prolonged immobilization (e.g. a paraplegic person confined to bed).
- *Increased serum uric acid* may be accompanied by uric acid stone formation. The most common

cause is gout, but it may also occur following chemotherapy for leukaemia, lymphoma or polycythaemia.
- *Increased oxalate excretion* results from increased dietary intake, with strawberries, rhubarb, leafy vegetables and tea containing high levels of oxalate. Hyperoxaluria is also a complication of loss of the terminal ileum (e.g. in Crohn's disease or after surgical resection), which results in increased oxalate absorption by the colon.

Lack of inhibitors of stone formation

Low levels of citrate and magnesium in the urine make calcium complexes less soluble, which promotes calcium oxalate and phosphate stone formation.

Presence of abnormal constituents

- *Urinary infection*, particularly in the presence of obstruction, for example hydronephrosis or chronic retention, produces epithelial cell sloughing, and this may act as a nidus for stone formation. In addition, infection may alter the urine pH, favouring precipitation of certain solutes. A high pH, brought about by the presence of urea-splitting organisms such as *Proteus*, favours calcium phosphate stone formation, for example.
- *Foreign bodies*, such as non-absorbable sutures inserted at operation, ureteric stents, sloughed necrotic renal papilla or a urinary catheter, may act as a nidus for stone formation.
- *Vitamin A deficiency*, which may occur in malnourished patients, alters the composition of urine, with increased saturation of stone promotors (e.g. calcium and oxalate), and decreased levels of stone inhibitors (e.g. glycosaminoglycans)
- *Cystinuria*, caused by a mutation in one of two different genes responsible for amino acid transfer in the kidney, may result in cystine stone formation.

Composition of urinary calculi

The three common stones are oxalate, phosphate and urate.

- *Oxalate stones* (calcium oxalate) are the most common (60%). They are hard with a sharp, spiky surface, which traumatizes the urinary tract epithelium; this causes bleeding that usually colours the stone a dark brown or black.

- *Phosphate stones* (34%) are composed of a mixture of calcium, ammonium and magnesium phosphate ('triple phosphate stone'). They are hard, white and chalky. They are nearly always found in an infected urine and produce the large 'staghorn' calculus deposited within a pyonephrosis.
- *Uric acid and urate stones* (5%) are moderately hard and brown in colour with a smooth surface. Pure uric acid stones are radiolucent but, fortunately for diagnosis, most contain enough calcium to render them opaque to X-rays.
- *Cystine stones* account for about 1% of urinary calculi.

Note that a stone found in the lower urinary tract may have arisen there primarily or it may have migrated there from a primary source within the kidney.

Clinical features (Figure 43.4)

Pain is the presenting feature of the great majority of kidney stones but if the calculus is embedded within the parenchyma of the kidney, it may be entirely symptom free. If the stone lies within the minor or major calyx system, it produces a dull loin pain. Impaction of the stone at the pelviureteric junction, or migration down the ureter itself, produces the dreadful agony of ureteric colic; the pain radiates from loin to groin, is of great severity and the patient is unable to find a comfortable position. The pain is usually continuous, although quite often with sharp exacerbations. The pain is often accompanied by vomiting and sweating.

Haematuria, either visible or non-visible, is present in 90% of people with ureteric colic.

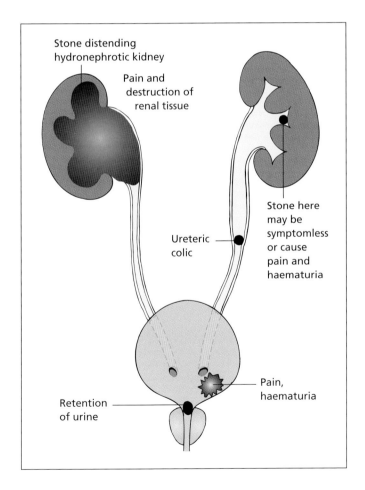

Figure 43.4 Diagram of the effects of urinary calculi.

Special investigations

These are usefully divided into investigations to confirm the diagnosis, and others to elucidate the aetiology of the stone.

Diagnostic investigations

- *Urine* is tested for the presence of blood.
- *Plain abdominal X-ray* specifically looking at kidneys, ureters and bladder (a 'KUB') will show the presence of stone in 90% of cases.
- *CT scan* is the investigation of choice to determine whether pain is due to a urinary tract stone or other pathologies (e.g. torted ovarian cyst, ruptured aortic aneurysm), and to confirm the size and site of the stone.
- *MAG3 renography* may also be used to determine the presence of obstruction and impairment of function.

Investigation of the underlying cause

- *Urine microscopy and culture*: the urine is cultured for bacteria and examined microscopically for the presence of cystine crystals.
- *Analysis of the stone* should be performed.
- *Uric acid estimation*: the serum uric acid is raised in gout with its associated uric acid stones.
- *Serum calcium estimation* is carried out. About 1% of stone formers have hypercalcaemia, occasionally due to a parathyroid adenoma.

Complications

- *Hydronephrosis*: see earlier in this chapter.
- *Infection*: pyelonephritis, pyonephrosis.
- *Anuria* due to either impaction of calculi in the ureter on each side, blockage of the ureter in a solitary kidney, or impaction of calculi within the urethra.

Treatment

Acute ureteric colic

Analgesia, ideally a non-steroidal anti-inflammatory agent, is given to relieve the severe pain. The great majority of small stones within the ureter (up to 5 mm) pass spontaneously. These ureteric stones tend to lodge at one of three places:

1 The pelviureteric junction.
2 The point at which the ureter crosses the pelvic brim.
3 The entrance of the ureter into the bladder (vesicoureteric junction).

The lower and smaller the stone, the more likely it is to pass spontaneously.

Ureteric calculi

If the stone remains in the ureter following an episode of acute colic and cannot or will not pass despite a trial of conservative management, intervention is necessary to avoid renal impairment due to obstruction. Depending on stone size and location, and patient factors (e.g. body habitus, concomitant anticoagulant therapy, presence of abdominal aortic aneurysm) extracorporeal shock-wave lithotripsy (ESWL) or ureteroscopy with stone disintegration by holmium laser may be used to fragment the stone and promote its passage.

Renal calculi

A small calculus lodged in the solid substance of the kidney without symptoms can be left alone but kept under periodic survey. Depending on stone size and location, either ESWL or ureteroscopy and laser can be employed to shatter the stone. The small fragments generated are passed spontaneously, and may cause acute colic as they pass. For larger stones, a ureteric stent may be required to prevent this.

Stones that are large, for example staghorn calculi, or those that do not respond to ESWL or ureteroscopy and laser may be removed percutaneously using a nephroscope (percutaneous nephrolithotomy). Ultrasonic, electrohydraulic or laser energy is used via the nephroscope to fragment the stone.

Acute calculous anuria

This may be due to blockage of both ureters by stones, obstruction of a solitary kidney or blockage of the urethra by stone. It is best treated by percutaneous nephrostomy, although retrograde ureteric stenting is an alternative. A urethral stone may be bypassed by urethral catheterization, but often impacted urethral stones need extraction after laser fragmentation under general anaesthesia. Temporary renal replacement therapy (haemofiltration) may also be required. The stone is then removed as indicated above.

Treatment of the cause

In every case of renal stone, an attempt is made to determine the underlying cause and eliminate it. Thus, renal infection is dealt with and surgical correction of any obstructive lesion performed. A small percentage of recurrent and bilateral stones are found to be due to parathyroid tumour (see Chapter 40), removal of which will prevent further recurrences. In every case of renal calculus disease, the patient should be instructed to drink plenty of fluid in order to encourage the production of dilute urine.

Urinary tract infections

The urinary tract may be divided into the upper tract, comprising ureter and kidney, and the lower tract, comprising bladder and urethra. Lower tract infections arise from infection via the urethra. Upper tract infection may be due to either haematogenous infection of the kidney or an ascending infection from the lower urinary tract.

Cystitis

Cystitis is usually an ascending infection which is more common in women, presumably because the urethra is shorter, and therefore, bacterial access to the bladder is easier than in men; it may be temporally associated with sexual activity. In men, it is commonly the consequence of urethral or prostatic obstruction. Urethral catheterization for more than 48 hours invariably results in bacterial colonization of the bladder.

The principal symptoms are stinging/burning pain on passing urine (dysuria), with increased frequency and urgency. Haematuria may be present, and examination may show a low-grade pyrexia and suprapubic tenderness. Loin pain suggests renal infection (pyelonephritis).

Special investigations

In women, recurrent infections are an indication for investigation. In men and children, a single episode is unusual and merits investigation.

- *Urine microscopy and culture* to identify the causative organism (invariably bowel flora, usually *Escherichia coli*). The presence of pus cells with no growth of bacteria on culture (sterile pyuria) is most often due to incompletely treated infection, but can be seen in bladder cancer and tuberculosis of the urinary tract (see Chapter 44).
- *Ultrasound scan* of the bladder and kidneys may demonstrate a large residual volume of urine within the bladder, or hydronephrosis.
- *Plain abdominal X-ray* will exclude a bladder stone as a source of recurrent infection.
- *Cystoscopy* may be necessary to exclude bladder cancer, stone or bladder diverticula.

Treatment

Antibiotics are given according to sensitivity of the infecting organism. A high oral fluid intake is encouraged. Alkalinizing the urine with potassium citrate or utilization of D-mannose sugar supplements may be helpful.

- *Postcoital urinary infection* is an indication for postcoital antibiotic therapy.
- *Recurring urinary infection* is an indication for low-dose antibiotic prophylaxis, or an alternative is a self-start regimen of antibiotics whereby antibiotics are taken as soon as symptoms develop, without the need for further urine culture. This latter approach is less likely to result in antibiotic resistance.

Any underlying cause, such as calculus or prostatic obstruction, must be dealt with.

Reflux nephropathy

Reflux nephropathy, formerly termed 'chronic pyelonephritis', is the consequence of ureteric reflux in the presence of infected urine, due to recurrent infections. It results in shrunken, scarred kidneys. It usually presents in childhood, as the growing kidney seems most susceptible. Reflux nephropathy accounts for almost 20% of chronic renal failure in adults. It is believed that two factors are important: vesicoureteric reflux and intrarenal reflux.

Vesicoureteric reflux

When the normal flap valve mechanism at the vesicoureteric junction is deficient, urine can pass back up the ureter during bladder contraction. This flap valve failure can occur as an isolated finding or with an ectopic ureter in a duplex system.

Intrarenal reflux

The collecting ducts enter the calyx of the renal pelvis on a renal papilla. There are two types of renal papillae; in simple (convex) papillae the ducts open at an oblique angle, so that as the pressure within the calyx increases, the ducts close, preventing urine from refluxing into the kidney (intrarenal reflux). The other type of papilla is the compound papilla, commonly seen in the polar regions of the kidney. In compound papillae, the ducts open perpendicular to the surface of the calyx, and do not close as intrarenal pressure rises; intrarenal reflux occurs. If the urine is infected, the resulting inflammation leaves a permanent scar and loss of nephrons. In addition, neighbouring papillae are distorted by the scarring, allowing further intrarenal reflux, hence repeated episodes of infection result in major damage and loss of function.

Clinical features

While the typical features of urinary infection, namely dysuria, frequency and pyrexia, may be present, subclinical infection, often only signified by urinary incontinence at night, is common, particularly in children. In infants, it may be impossible to elicit symptoms *per se*, so the diagnosis may be difficult to make until after significant renal damage has been done.

Special investigations

- *Micturating cystogram*: contrast is first introduced into the bladder via a catheter, the patient voids, and reflux of urine during voiding can be seen with the aid of an image intensifier.
- *Indirect micturating cystogram*: an isotope (MAG3) study in which differential function of the kidneys can be assessed, and scanning during micturition allows any reflux of the isotope to be demonstrated. This avoids the need for urethral catheterization, and is, therefore, less intrusive for the patient. It is commonly used in children.
- *DMSA (dimercaptosuccinic acid) scan* is used to demonstrate the degree of renal scarring as a result of reflux.

Treatment

The cause of the reflux nephropathy should be treated when identified. Long-term low-dose antibiotic prophylaxis is given to patients with asymptomatic or frequent infections. Surgical reimplantation is very seldom indicated.

Pyonephrosis

This is an infected hydronephrosis so that the renal pelvis is full of pus. If the ureter is obstructed, there may be little to find on examining the urine although, more commonly, pyuria is a marked feature. Usually, the enlarged tender kidney is easily palpable. The substance of the kidney is destroyed rapidly thus this is a urological emergency.

Special investigations

- *Ultrasound* of the kidneys to confirm hydronephrosis.
- *CT scan* confirms the diagnosis, and excludes stone.
- *DMSA scan* will quantify the residual function in the kidney after treatment.

Treatment

There should be urgent drainage by percutaneous nephrostomy, and intravenous antibiotic therapy, with critical care support as needed. The nephrostomy will allow a subsequent nephrostogram, which may identify the cause of the problem, if CT has not already done so. If there is no residual renal function, deferred nephrectomy is usually advised.

Renal abscess

Haematogenous spread of *Staphylococcus* was previously the cause of renal abscess, albeit an uncommon condition. In current practice, however, renal abscess is usually a consequence of sepsis from infected urine.

Clinical features

There is pain and tenderness in the loin, fever, possibly tachycardia and hypotension, and the kidney may be palpable.

Special investigations

- *Urine culture* may show the infecting organism.
- *Blood culture* is the most likely means of identifying the infecting organism.

- *Full blood count*: there is a leucocytosis.
- *CT scan* should confirm the diagnosis.
- *Ultrasound* may be useful to monitor response to treatment.

Treatment

Percutaneous drainage and intravenous antibiotics, with critical care support as needed.

Renal tuberculosis

Pathology

The kidney may be involved either as part of a generalized miliary spread of tuberculosis or more commonly as a focal lesion representing haematogenous spread from a distant site in the lungs (25% of patients have pulmonary tuberculosis), the bone or gut. The original focus may be quiescent at the time of active renal disease.

Early lesions are found near the junction of the cortex and medulla. These enlarge, caseate and then rupture into a calyx, eventually producing extensive destruction of renal substance. The ureter becomes infiltrated and thickened and may take on a 'corkscrew' configuration; its obstruction leads to tuberculous pyonephrosis. A pyonephrosis may rarely become completely walled off as a symptomless, caseating and calcified mass ('autonephrectomy').

Spread of infected urine down the ureter frequently produces a tuberculous cystitis and may result in infection of the epididymis and seminal vesicles.

If the infection is not treated, the contralateral kidney often becomes involved, but this probably represents separate haematogenous spread.

Clinical features

The patient is usually a young adult, often with a present or previous history of tuberculosis elsewhere, or an immunosuppressed individual (e.g. secondary to HIV infection). Symptoms in the early stages are mild and indeed may be entirely absent. There may be dysuria, frequency, pyuria or haematuria, which may be visible but is more usually slight or non-visible. There may be loin pain on the affected side.

In more advanced cases, the dysuria and frequency become intense because of extensive involvement of the bladder, and then constitutional symptoms of tuberculosis, with fever, night sweats, loss of weight and anaemia, may be present. In some cases, a tuberculous epididymitis is the presenting feature (see Chapter 48).

Examination is usually negative, but the kidney may be tender and palpable. The epididymis and seminal vesicles may be enlarged and thickened if involved. The epididymis often feels craggy owing to calcification.

Special investigations

- *Urine* is commonly sterile to ordinary culture but contains pus cells and is acid in reaction ('sterile acid pyuria'); protein and usually red cells are also found. Acid-fast bacilli may be present on Ziehl–Neelsen[4] staining of a spun deposit from an early morning specimen of urine. Three early morning specimens of urine (250 mL each) are sent for culture, which takes 6 weeks for a result.
- *CT scan* will show destruction of the kidney and thickening of the wall of the ureter and bladder.
- *Chest X-ray* may show a primary lung focus.
- *Cystoscopy* may reveal a decreased capacity of the bladder, an oedematous mucosa on which tubercles may be seen, and perhaps a 'golf hole' ureteric orifice, the ureter being held rigidly open by surrounding fibrosis.

Treatment

Anti-tuberculous therapy should not be commenced until the diagnosis has been confirmed as, once undertaken, treatment must be prolonged. Treatment usually involves isoniazid, rifampicin and pyrazinamide, with ethambutol unless the organism is known to be fully sensitive. Healing occurs with the production of fibrous tissue, which in early cases merely produces a small scar. In an advanced stage of the disease, this fibrous tissue may lead to stricture formation at the neck of a calyx or at the pelviureteric junction with a secondary hydronephrosis. Similar scarring of the heavily involved bladder may produce gross contraction on healing.

Surgery is indicated in only a minority of patients with advanced disease or where complications occur.

---

[4] Franz Heinrich Paul Ziehl (1825–1898), Neurologist, Lübeck, Germany. Friedrich Karl Adolf Neelson (1854–1894), Professor of Pathology in Rostock, later Prosector in the State Hospital, Dresden, Germany.

Renal failure

Acute kidney injury

Acute kidney injury (previously known as acute renal failure) is characterized by a reduced glomerular filtration rate (GFR), retention of nitrogenous waste (urea and creatinine rise), impaired acid–base balance (acidosis develops) and, usually, a reduced urine output.

An absence of urine production is termed '*anuria*', whereas production of less than 400 mL/day in the adult is *oliguria*.

Aetiology

In the surgical context, acute kidney injury may be a consequence of surgery or may be due to a surgically treatable lesion.

The causes of acute kidney injury may be usefully divided into prerenal, renal and postrenal, in a similar way to the causes of jaundice relative to the liver. The presence of two kidneys means that the pathology must affect both kidneys in order to manifest, unless one kidney has previously failed or been removed.

Prerenal causes

Prerenal factors involve reduction in the blood flow to the kidney, resulting in decreased glomerular filtration.

1 *Fluid loss*:
   a   Blood loss, for example haemorrhage.
   b   Plasma loss, for example burns, generalized peritonitis.
   c   Electrolyte loss, for example vomiting, diarrhoea, fistula, inadequate replacement.
2 *Impaired circulation*:
   a   General factors, for example hypotension due to sepsis, cardiac failure.
   b   Local factors, for example aortic dissection in which the renal arteries are excluded from the circulation.

Renal perfusion is maintained in the presence of mild hypoperfusion by a number of regulatory mechanisms: vasoconstriction of splanchnic, muscular and cutaneous vascular beds, and alteration of afferent and efferent renal arteriolar tone. The GFR is normally maintained even if the mean arterial pressure falls to 60–80 mmHg. In hypertensive patients, the elderly and patients with pre-existing renal disease (e.g. diabetic nephropathy), autoregulation may be impaired and the GFR maintained only at higher mean pressures. Some drugs, particularly non-steroidal anti-inflammatory drugs (NSAIDs) and angiotensin-converting enzyme (ACE) inhibitors, also impair the normal compensatory mechanisms and make the kidney more sensitive to hypovolaemia.

Renal causes

Renal causes of acute kidney injury include factors directly acting upon the glomerular apparatus and tubules:

- Acute tubular necrosis (ATN).
- Acute cortical necrosis, due to severe ischaemia.
- Myoglobin secondary to rhabdomyolysis (e.g. following a crush injury or reperfusion of an ischaemic limb).
- Drugs (e.g. antibiotics such as gentamicin, or NSAIDs such as diclofenac).
- Acute nephritis — interstitial nephritis or glomerulonephritis.

Postrenal (obstructive) causes

An obstructing lesion occurring at any level from the tubules to the urethra may cause renal impairment. Only in patients with a solitary kidney will an upper tract obstruction cause acute renal failure; otherwise, the obstruction is likely to be in the lower tracts and affect both kidneys.

Clinical features

The majority of cases of acute kidney injury are prerenal in aetiology, which means that the kidneys will recover as soon as the circulation is restored. The diagnosis is usually clear: the patient has failed to pass urine and bladder catheterization reveals no urine or a mere trickle. It should be remembered that the most common cause of apparent oliguria while catheterized is a blocked catheter, and this should always be excluded.

Special investigations

Initial investigation should be quickly performed, since rapid treatment may prevent life-threatening sequelae, and the shorter the period of renal failure, the more quickly renal function will be restored.

- *Serum electrolytes*: urea and creatinine are raised; potassium may be very high and demands immediate treatment (see later in this chapter). Comparison to previous creatinine readings is useful in determining pre-existing renal function.

- *Renal tract Doppler ultrasound*: are there two kidneys, and are they perfused? Are they of normal size or is one small, suggesting prior renal disease? Is there evidence of hydronephrosis/hydroureter? Is the bladder full or empty? If obstruction is documented, it should be rapidly relieved and this may require bladder catheterization or nephrostomy.
- *Urine microscopy and stick test* for blood and protein. Some blood may be present as a consequence of urethral catheterization. Rhabdomyolysis is suggested by a positive stick test for blood without red cells on microscopy. Acute nephritis should be considered when blood and protein are present.

Management

Replenish the intravascular volume

Initial management requires a clinical assessment of the intravascular volume to determine the extent of volume depletion. The best signs are the following.

- *Jugular venous pressure* (JVP): is it visible and is it raised?
- *Postural hypotension*: is there a fall in blood pressure when the patient stands up? (If the patient cannot stand, the blood pressure should be measured lying and sitting up in bed.)

Depletion of intravascular volume is suggested by a postural fall in blood pressure and a low (not visible) JVP. Treatment requires rapid infusion of a fluid that remains in the intravascular compartment (blood, colloid or saline, but not dextrose). Infusion is continued until the JVP is visible and postural hypotension corrected. Potassium additives should not be given until a diuresis is established since patients are likely to be hyperkalaemic.

A *central venous catheter* may be inserted at this stage to accurately measure the central venous pressure; the target pressure is 10 cmH$_2$O measured relative to the mid-axilla. Persistent low central venous pressure readings may indicate the requirement for inotropes such as noradrenaline (norepinephrine),

which will be guided by measures of cardiac output and systemic vascular resistance (see Chapter 8).

Once volume repletion is achieved, the infusion is stopped until the urine output picks up. Further infusion would result in fluid overload, and would require dialysis to remove the excess fluid in the absence of renal function.

Diuretics

If rehydration is unsuccessful in inducing a diuresis, a bolus of furosemide (100–500 mg over 30 min) should be given. If these measures fail to induce a diuresis, it is likely that either ATN or, less commonly, acute cortical necrosis has occurred.

Hyperkalaemia

A potassium level of over 6.5 mmol/L should be treated immediately to avoid life-threatening ventricular arrhythmias. The electrocardiogram (ECG) changes with increasing potassium: first, the T waves become peaked (tenting); next, the P waves disappear and, finally, the ECG becomes sinusoidal. Resolution of these appearances can be monitored with treatment. However, patients may have significant hyperkalaemia without ECG changes.

Calcium gluconate (10 mL of 10% intravenously) should be given over a few minutes to stabilize the myocardium. Insulin and dextrose (5–10 units of soluble insulin in 50 mL of 50% dextrose) is given as an infusion over 10–20 minutes. This drives potassium into the cells, and lowers serum potassium by 1–2 mmol/L. Because these measures do not remove potassium from the body, a more definitive treatment is necessary before the potassium rises once more. This is best achieved by establishing a diuresis but, if this fails, urgent dialysis is indicated. Potassium exchange resins (e.g. sodium zirconium), taken by mouth, may give good interim potassium control.

Acute tubular necrosis

Persistence of acute kidney injury after correction of hypovolaemia is usually due to the development of ATN. This is characterized by a prolonged period of oliguria lasting anywhere from a few days to 3–6 weeks.

Pathology

The condition usually follows ischaemia to the kidneys. The blood supply to a nephron passes first to the glomerulus via afferent arterioles, and exits via the efferent arterioles to supply the tubules. In response to hypotension, the efferent arterioles constrict to maintain blood flow to the glomerulus, but in so doing further reduce the blood flow to the tubules. Hence, although the glomerular apparatus is usually preserved, the tubules, especially the proximal tubules, suffer patchy ischaemic damage. The kidneys become enlarged and oedematous. As this damage recovers, renal function returns.

Clinical features

The features are of a persistent oliguria, unresponsive to replenishment of the intravascular circulating volume. The symptoms are those of acute kidney injury described above.

Treatment

If ATN is established, the patient should be managed by regular dialysis until function returns. Recovery of function is characterized by a stepwise increase in urine output, although there may be a short polyuric phase during which maintenance of fluid balance can be difficult.

If function fails to return, it is more likely that acute cortical necrosis occurred with necrosis of glomeruli in addition to tubules.

Chronic renal failure

Chronic renal failure may be classified into three groups, like acute kidney injury. Most causes are non-surgical, but some surgically correctable causes are given below.

1 *Prerenal*: renal artery stenosis.
2 *Renal*: there are no surgical causes.
3 *Postrenal (obstructive)*:
   a Congenital posterior urethral valves.
   b Prostatic enlargement/carcinoma, which causes chronic retention and upper tract dilation.
   c Urethral stricture.
   d Cervical carcinoma, infiltrating the ureters.

e Urothelial tumour affecting the bladder base or both ureters.
f Bilateral ureteric strictures, such as occurs after pelvic radiotherapy treatment.

Symptoms are of malaise, weakness, confusion, hiccoughs with pallor, hypertension and fluid overload (e.g. pulmonary oedema, ankle oedema) on examination. The investigations are those of acute kidney injury, and are directed at finding a treatable cause such as prostatic enlargement. In the absence of a treatable lesion, established renal failure is managed by renal replacement therapy with either peritoneal dialysis or haemodialysis, with a view to renal transplantation in the future.

Renal tumours

Tumours of the kidney are divided into those arising from the kidney substance itself and those originating from the renal pelvis.

Classification

Of the kidney itself

1 *Benign.*
   a Adenoma (small and symptomless).
   b Oncocytoma (uncommon tumour, characterized by a 'stellate scar' on CT).
   c Angiomyolipoma (uncommon hamartoma, characteristic CT appearance).
   d Haemangioma (a rare cause of haematuria).
2 *Malignant.*
   a Primary: nephroblastoma, renal cell carcinoma.
   b Secondary: the kidney is an uncommon site for deposits of carcinoma although it may be involved in advanced cases of lymphoma and leukaemia, as well as tumours of breast and bronchus.

Of the renal pelvis

• Papilloma.
• Urothelial carcinoma.
• Squamous carcinoma.

The two principal malignant tumours of the kidney are nephroblastoma in children and renal cell carcinoma in adults.

Nephroblastoma (Wilms' tumour[5])

Pathology

This is a rare and extremely anaplastic tumour, which usually arises in children under the age of 5 years, although it occasionally affects older children and adolescents. It probably originates from embryonic mesodermal tissue. Bilateral tumours are present in 5–10% of cases, and there is an association with congenital anomalies (aniridia, hemihypertrophy, macroglossia) in a few patients.

Macroscopically, the tumours are large and may be difficult to distinguish from neuroblastoma (see Chapter 42). They are pale on cut section and contain areas of haemorrhage.

Microscopically, there is a mixture of mesenchymal and epithelial components, with spindle cells, epithelial tubules and smooth or striated muscle fibres.

The regional lymph nodes are soon involved, and spread occurs via the bloodstream to the lungs and liver.

Clinical features

Rapid growth produces a large mass in the loin, although involvement of the renal pelvis is late and, therefore, haematuria relatively uncommon. Other features include weight loss and anorexia, fever and hypertension. Children may also present on account of metastases, which occasionally involve bone.

Special investigations

- *Ultrasound scans* may distinguish the solid tumour from a cystic or hydronephrotic mass.
- *CT scan* is useful for staging and preoperative assessment, in particular to look at the contralateral kidney.

Treatment

When possible, nephrectomy is performed. In early disease, with no residual tumour following surgery,

chemotherapy alone will give prolonged survival. For more extensive disease, radiotherapy is given. When the tumour is unresectable, chemotherapy is given and nephrectomy performed once the tumour regresses. With such therapy, 90% of children with the condition survive 5 years.

Renal cell carcinoma

Pathology

This tumour accounts for 80% of all renal tumours. Men are affected twice as often as women. The patients are usually 40 years of age or over. It may be associated with familial conditions such as tuberous sclerosis and von Hippel–Lindau disease,[6] and can be bilateral.

The tumour appears as a large, vascular, golden yellow mass, usually in one or the other pole of the kidney (hence its earlier name of hypernephroma).

The microscopic appearance of the tumour cells is typically large with an abundant foamy cytoplasm and a small, central, densely staining nucleus. The tumour originates from the renal tubules. There are three common subtypes:

- Clear cell (80%) – very pale or clear looking cytoplasm.
- Papillary (15%) – cancers cells form projections like papillae.
- Chromophobe (5%) – larger cells, also clear cytoplasm, often pink coloured.

Spread

- *Directly* throughout the renal substance with invasion of the perinephric tissues.
- *Via lymphatics* to the para-aortic lymph nodes.
- *Via the bloodstream* with growth along the renal vein into the inferior vena cava (IVC), from which it may shower emboli. Metastases in the lungs and bones are common. Occlusion of the IVC results in a typical appearance with bilateral leg oedema.

Renal cell carcinoma is a tumour that may occasionally produce a solitary blood-borne metastasis,

---

[5] Max Wilms (1867–1918), Professor of Surgery, first in Basle, Switzerland, and then in Heidelberg, Germany. He died of diphtheria after operating on the throat of an infected French prisoner of war.

[6] Eugen von Hippel (1867–1939), Professor of Ophthalmology, Göttingen, Germany; Arvid Lindau (1892–1958), Pathologist, Lund, Sweden.

so that removal of the primary together with this metastasis *may* be followed by prolonged survival.

Clinical features

The patient may present with symptoms either of local disease or of one of the paraneoplastic syndromes with which it may be associated.

Local disease

The most common presentation is as an incidental finding on imaging done for other reasons. This is often the so-called 'small renal mass'. The management of this is somewhat controversial, with the role of biopsy not clearly established.

The classic triad of symptoms of a renal cell carcinoma, present in well under 10% of cases, is:

1 Haematuria, present in half the cases – it may produce clot colic.
2 Loin pain, aching, present in 40%.
3 Loin mass, presenting in 25%.

Rarely, a left varicocele may occur (1%) as a consequence of tumour spread along the left renal vein occluding the confluence with the testicular vein on that side.

General features

In addition to local symptoms, the patient may present with the general features of malignancy, namely anaemia, loss of weight and occasionally a pyrexia of unknown origin, or as a consequence of metastases, for example a pathological fracture.

Paraneoplastic syndromes

A number of hormones may be released from renal cell carcinoma. The clinical consequences may be hypertension (renin production), polycythaemia (erythropoietin) and hypercalcaemia (ectopic parathormone production).

On examination, the diseased kidney may be palpable.

Special investigations

- *Urine* nearly always contains either visible or non-visible haematuria.
- *Ultrasound scans* will differentiate cystic from solid mass.
- *CT scan* is the investigation of choice, providing accurate visualization of the tumour, as well as showing spread to lymph nodes and the chest, and demonstrating caval invasion.
- *MR imaging* may be utilized to determine the extent of any vascular involvement.
- *Bone scan*, looking for metastatic disease, is indicated in the presence of a raised serum calcium or alkaline phosphatase.

Treatment

The slow growth of small renal tumours has led to a trend towards active monitoring of small renal masses and also of presumed cancers in the frail or elderly.

For small tumours, partial nephrectomy is considered. Alternatively, in less fit patients, radiofrequency ablation or cryotherapy can be considered. Central and larger tumours are treated by radical nephrectomy unless there is reduced function in the contralateral kidney or if there is no contralateral kidney, in which case the indications for nephron preserving treatments are broadened. Laparoscopic and robotic surgery are widely used, and open nephrectomy is now mainly reserved for large cancers with lymph node or vascular involvement.

Medical therapy is commonly used in the management of locally advanced or metastatic renal cell carcinoma, including the use of anti-angiogenic tyrosine kinase inhibitors that target the vascular endothelial growth factor (VEGF) receptors, mechanistic target of rapamycin (mTOR) inhibitors and systemic immunotherapies.

The 5-year survival rate after successful resection is about 50%, but metastases may occur many years after nephrectomy. Poor prognostic factors include perinephric and lymphatic invasion.

Tumours of the renal pelvis and ureter

Urothelial carcinoma of the renal pelvis is an uncommon cancer: distinguishing it from renal cell carcinoma may be difficult sometimes. Upper tract urothelial cancer has a sinister reputation because the tumour frequently extends through the wall of the renal pelvis or ureter at the time of presentation, so the prognosis is then poor.

A squamous carcinoma of the renal pelvis may occur when there has been squamous metaplasia of the epithelium; one-third of these cases are associated with renal calculus. Some may be associated with analgesic abuse and analgesic-associated nephropathy.

Clinical features

Patients present usually either with haematuria or with hydronephrosis due to ureteric obstruction. The tumour may seed down the ureter and even involve the bladder.

Treatment

Treatment is nephroureterectomy, increasingly done using laparoscopic techniques. The ureter must be removed *en bloc* with the kidney in its entirety. This can be achieved by endoscopically detaching the ureter from within the bladder ('rip and pluck'), or excising a cuff of bladder in continuity with the specimen, through a separate pelvic incision. Postoperative platinum-based chemotherapy improves survival rates.

Additional resources

Case 110: Congenital disease of both kidneys
Case 111: Haematuria of sinister origin

44

The bladder

Alexandra J. Colquhoun

Learning objectives

✓ To understand congenital anomalies of the bladder including urachal defects and bladder exstrophy.

✓ To understand the classification of bladder trauma and its management.

✓ To know about bladder stones and bladder diverticula, their causes and management.

✓ To know the causes, presentation and management of bladder cancer.

Congenital anomalies

Embryology

The bladder and urethra are formed from the cloaca, which is the distal end of the hindgut. During development, the urogenital septum divides the cloaca into anterior and posterior compartments (Figure 44.1). The anterior compartment subsequently divides into three sections with the bladder forming from the most cranial part. The urethra and some of the reproductive tract in females, and the prostatic and membranous urethra in males, form from the middle section, while the caudal section becomes the remaining reproductive organs in females and the spongy urethra in males. The posterior section forms the anal canal.

The urinary bladder is drained *in utero* by the allantois. This structure fibroses during development eventually forming the median umbilical ligament, also known as the urachus.

Ellis and Calne's Lecture Notes in General Surgery, Fourteenth Edition.
Edited by Christopher Watson and Justin Davies.
© 2023 John Wiley & Sons Ltd. Published 2023 by John Wiley & Sons Ltd.
Companion website: www.wiley.com/go/Watson/GeneralSurgery14

Urachal anomalies

Urachal defects may result from anomalies of the primitive urachal connection. There are three principal anomalies:

1 *Urachal fistula*: a persistent urachal tract, which leads from the bladder to the umbilicus in the foetus, results in a urinary discharge at the umbilicus.
2 *Urachal diverticulum*: an outpouching of the bladder, the urachal equivalent of a Meckel's diverticulum and the vitellointestinal duct.
3 *Urachal cyst*: where the urachus persists but is closed above and below. The cyst often becomes infected in later life, presenting with periumbilical pain and inflammation.

Treatment

In all cases, treatment is excision.

Bladder exstrophy (ectopia vesicae)

Failure of fusion of the structures forming the anterior abdominal wall may cause a number of anomalies.

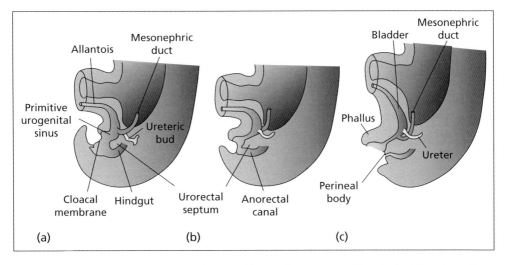

Figure 44.1 Embryological development of the bladder and lower urinary tract. a: at 5 weeks; b at 7 weeks; c at 8 weeks.

Lower urinary tract changes include bladder exstrophy, where the ureters together with the bladder trigone open directly onto the anterior abdominal wall below the umbilicus. This is usually associated with a failure of fusion of the pubic bones and, in men, there is an associated epispadias (opening of the urethra on the dorsal penile shaft rather than the glans penis). There is often a widened pelvis with a waddling gait.

The infant is completely incontinent of urine, with excoriation of the abdominal skin and a permanent unpleasant ammoniacal smell of infected urine. If the condition is untreated, the child may die of pyelonephritis, or develop a stratified squamous carcinoma of the bladder rudiment after initial metaplastic change.

Treatment

Reconstructive surgery is highly specialist, the need for which can usually be predicted before birth, enabling appropriate planning of the optimal time and place of delivery. Corrective surgery is usually staged, and may require correction of defects of formation of the bony pelvis, as well as the urinary tract.

Rupture of the bladder

Bladder rupture may be either intraperitoneal or, more commonly, extraperitoneal.

Intraperitoneal rupture

This follows a penetrating wound (e.g. a bullet wound) or crush injury to the pelvis when the bladder is distended. Occasionally, it occurs during transurethral resection of a tumour, and, very rarely, the over-distended bladder of retention may rupture spontaneously.

Extraperitoneal rupture

This happens most commonly during transurethral urological surgery, typically resection of a bladder tumour, or evacuation of clot retention. It may also occur by injury from a spicule of bone in a pelvic fracture or occasionally may be caused during a hernia operation or repair of a cystocoele.

Clinical features

Intraperitoneal rupture produces the typical picture of peritonitis with generalized abdominal pain, marked rigidity and a silent abdomen.

Extraperitoneal rupture is associated with extraperitoneal extravasation of blood and urine producing a painful swelling that arises out of the pelvis. When associated with pelvic fracture, differentiation must be made from rupture of the membranous urethra (see Chapter 46), although this may not be possible until surgical exploration is carried out. A urethral tear is, however, typically accompanied by anterior displacement of the prostate, which can be detected on rectal examination.

In either circumstance, traumatic bladder rupture causes haematuria.

Special investigations

- *Computed tomography (CT) scan* demonstrates extravasation and any associated pelvic injury.
- *Cystography* will confirm rupture.
- *Urethrography* will demonstrate a urethral injury.

Treatment

Extraperitoneal ruptures are usually managed conservatively, with indwelling urethral (Foley[1]) catheter drainage of the bladder and percutaneous drainage of the suprapubic space; larger leaks may necessitate exploration and repair, with drainage of the retropubic space and antibiotic therapy.

Intraperitoneal ruptures are sutured and the bladder drained by means of a urethral and/or suprapubic catheter.

Diverticulum of the bladder

The aetiology of diverticula of the bladder is unclear. It is no longer assumed that they are simply secondary to bladder outflow obstruction, and a small number are congenital in origin. About 95% of diverticula occur in men and this was the basis of the belief that bladder outlet obstruction was invariably the cause. Congenital diverticula have all the layers of the bladder wall; acquired diverticula contain only the urothelium.

Complications

- *Urinary infection* because of urinary stasis.
- *Calculus formation* because of a combination of infection and stasis.

Clinical features

The majority of diverticula remain silent unless they undergo one of the complications listed above. Some are found incidentally during investigation of the underlying obstructive lesion, for example a prostatic

[1] Frederick Foley (1891–1966), Urologist, St Paul, MN, USA.

enlargement or urethral stricture. Occasionally, a large, uninfected diverticulum gives the strange symptom of double micturition (*'pis en deux'*). In this circumstance, the patient empties the bladder but a substantial amount of the urine passes into the distensible diverticulum. No sooner does micturition end than the diverticulum passively empties again into the bladder, giving the surprised patient the desire once again to empty their bladder.

Special investigations

- *Ultrasound*: this defines the size of the diverticulum.
- *Cystoscopy*: the neck and body of the diverticulum can be visualized.

Treatment

Excision of a diverticulum is very seldom indicated. Associated bladder outflow obstruction may require treatment, but the diverticulum will remain.

Bladder stone

The varieties of bladder calculi are the same as renal stones, namely phosphate, oxalate, urate and rarely cystine (see Chapter 43).

Aetiology

Bladder stones either originate in the kidney and pass down the ureter into the bladder, where they remain and grow, or originate *de novo* in the bladder. Stones that arise in the bladder are due to the following.

- *Stasis and infection*: bladder stones commonly arise as a consequence of outflow obstruction (e.g. urethral stricture or prostatic enlargement). They may be secondary to an atonic bladder in a paraplegic person, and may have arisen first within a bladder diverticulum.
- *Foreign body*: a calculus will deposit on a long-term indwelling catheter or on any foreign body inserted into the bladder.

Clinical features

The typical triad of bladder stone symptoms is frequency, pain and haematuria. In addition, patients sometimes complain of intermittent stopping of the urinary flow as the stone blocks the internal urinary meatus like a ball valve, and occasionally actual retention of urine may occur if the stone impacts in the urethra.

- *Frequency* is more troublesome during the day than at night, probably because, in the upright position, the stone lies over, and irritates, the bladder trigone.
- *Pain* is felt in the suprapubic region, in the perineum and the tip of the penis; it particularly occurs at the end of micturition, when the bladder contracts down upon the calculus.
- *Haematuria* tends to occur as the last few drops of urine are passed.

Special investigations

- *Plain abdominal X-ray* (specifically, a 'KUB' to show kidneys, ureters and bladder): the majority of bladder stones are radio-opaque and are readily visible.
- *Cystoscopy* allows stones to be seen, and to be fragmented and retrieved.

Treatment

Unless the stone is very small, when there is a possibility that it will pass spontaneously, it should be removed either by crushing with an endoscopic lithotrite under direct vision or by endoscopic disintegration with laser.

Bladder tumours

Pathology

Nearly all bladder tumours are malignant. Bladder cancer may be classified as follows, together with the relative incidence.

1 *Primary*:
   a Urothelial carcinoma (90%).
   b Squamous cell carcinoma arising in an area of metaplasia (7%).
   c Adenocarcinoma (may occur in urachal remnants) (2%).
   d Neuroendocrine tumours (small cell carcinoma) (~1%).
   e Sarcomas (rare).

2 *Secondary*: direct invasion from adjacent tumours, that is, colorectal, renal, ovarian, uterine, prostatic tumours.

Urothelial carcinoma

Urothelial carcinoma (UC) is most commonly found in middle-aged and elderly patients. Men are more frequently affected than women.

Aetiology

Risk factors include cigarette smoking (four-fold increase in incidence compared to non-smoker) and workers in the aniline dye, rubber and plastics industry, because of the excretion of carcinogens such as β-naphthylamine in the urine. The manufacture of many of the more dangerous dyes and chemicals has been abolished in most countries. In addition, exposure to polycyclic hydrocarbons, as happens in industries working with carbon and crude oil, has been associated with bladder cancer. Other occupations associated with chemical exposure, such as leather workers, hairdressers and painters, have increased risk.

There is a high incidence of malignant change in the exposed bladder epithelium of untreated bladder exstrophy (see earlier in this chapter), and in the bladder infected with schistosomiasis. It can also occur in association with long-term catheterization in paraplegic patients and in the presence of bladder stones; in these cases, characterized by chronic inflammation and urothelial metaplasia, development of squamous cell dysplastic change is common.

Pathology

Although any part of the bladder may be involved, tumours are particularly common at the base, trigone and around the ureteric orifices. They are often multiple, signifying a field change throughout the urothelium with the tendency for tumours to develop anywhere from the renal pelvis to the urethra.

Macroscopic appearance

The low-grade tumours form fine fronds, which resemble seaweed floating in the urine. High-grade tumours are sessile, solid growths, which infiltrate the bladder wall, then ulcerate, often with marked surrounding cystitis. Carcinoma *in situ* may produce a suspicious red patch of urothelium.

Microscopic appearance

Urothelial carcinoma may be well, moderately or poorly differentiated. Keratinizing squamous cell carcinoma or adenocarcinoma may be seen.

Spread

- *Local* with infiltration of the bladder wall, the prostate, urethra or, in women, the pelvic viscera. The ureteric orifices may be occluded, producing hydronephrosis and ultimately renal failure.
- *Lymphatic*, to the obturator, iliac and para-aortic lymph nodes.
- *Blood-borne* spread occurs late to the liver, lungs and bones.

Clinical features

Bladder cancer usually presents with painless haematuria (visible or non-visible). It may also cause dysuria, frequency and urgency of micturition. The patient may present with hydronephrosis caused by ureteric obstruction or with retention of urine caused either by clot or by tumour growth involving the urethra. In late cases, there may be severe pain from pelvic invasion or uraemia from bilateral ureteric obstruction.

Examination is usually negative, but tumours invading muscle may be palpable bimanually at the time of cystoscopy.

Special investigations

- *Urine examination* usually reveals blood, either to the naked eye or microscopically.
- *Urine cytology* is usually positive in high-grade (G3 and carcinoma *in situ*) cancers; a positive urine test always indicates urothelial cancer in the urinary tract, but negative cytology does not exclude it.
- *CT or MRI scans* are done to stage high-grade cancers and may demonstrate ureteric obstruction or hydronephrosis. At the same time, the presence of pelvic bony secondaries may be revealed.
- *Flexible cystoscopy* under local anaesthesia in the clinic is the most valuable investigation.

Treatment

Initial assessment of all tumours involves bimanual examination and transurethral resection under general anaesthesia; further treatment depends on the grade and stage of the tumour.

Staging

Staging is generally according to the TNM system (see Chapter 6). The local staging (T) involves both bimanual palpation and histological examination to ascertain the depth of invasion through the bladder wall, and the grade of the tumour (G1, well differentiated, to G3, poorly differentiated). Carcinoma *in situ* (CiS) is a high-grade (G3) tumour confined to the urothelium.

Low-risk non-muscle-invasive cancers

Well-differentiated (G1 and low-grade G2) tumours that do not invade the bladder wall (pTa) are treated by endoscopic resection followed by intravesical chemotherapy (mitomycin C) to prevent recurrence. Follow-up cystoscopy is required to detect and treat recurrence. This severity of disease has a low chance (<5%) of progression to muscle-invasive disease.

High-risk non-muscle-invasive cancers

High-risk non-muscle-invasive disease (G3pTa, G3pT1 and CiS) has a much greater chance of progression to muscle invasion (30–60%). The treatment options are intravesical bacille Calmette–Guérin (BCG) therapy[2] or early cystectomy.

Muscle-invasive cancers

Muscle-invasive cancers (pT2 and greater) have a poor prognosis, with approximately 50% 5-year survival. Treatment is initially with platinum-based chemotherapy if possible (depending on adequate renal function and performance status), followed by cystectomy or radiotherapy. After radiotherapy, cystoscopic follow-up is undertaken, with consideration

---

[2] Léon Calmette (1863–1933), Director of the Pasteur Institute, Paris, France. Camille Guérin (1872–1961), Veterinary Surgeon, Lille, France.

of cystectomy if recurrence is diagnosed – so-called 'salvage cystectomy'.

At cystectomy, the bladder and distal ureters are removed, along with the prostate or gynaecological organs. Urinary drainage is fashioned with either implantation of the ureters into a tube of ileum brought out as a stoma (an ileal conduit) or bladder reconstruction (avoiding an external stoma), using bowel to create a substitute bladder or reservoir that can be catheterized.

Chemotherapy and immunotherapy may be used for metastatic disease, but tends to be palliative rather than curative.

◗ Additional resources

Case 112: A gross congenital abnormality
Case 113: A bladder stone found at autopsy
Case 114: An insidious cause of lumbago

45

The prostate

Arthur McPhee

Learning objectives

✓ To know the causes and treatment of benign prostatic enlargement.

✓ To know about the presentation of urinary retention and its treatment.

✓ To know the causes and treatment of prostate cancer.

There are two common conditions of the prostate that require consideration: benign enlargement and cancer.

Benign prostatic enlargement

Pathology

Benign prostatic enlargement is the clinical finding of an enlarged prostate due to the underlying histological process of benign prostatic hyperplasia (BPH).

Some degree of enlargement of the prostate is extremely common from the age of 45 onwards, but this enlargement often produces either no or only minor symptoms. A UK study suggested that 14% of 40–49-year-olds, and 43% of 60–69-year-olds have symptomatic BPH.

The prostate, like the breast and thyroid, is composed of glandular tissue, stromal tissue and epithelium. Growth regulation in the prostate is complex with androgens playing a role as well as multiple growth factors from autocrine, endocrine and paracrine systems. The gland may become enlarged during periods of change, with excessive micronodule formation and proliferation of both stromal and epithelial tissue.

Enlargement of the lateral lobes of the prostate results in encroachment on the prostatic urethra. The median lobe may also enlarge as a rounded swelling overlying the posterior aspect of the internal urinary meatus. The three lobes may then obstruct the urethral lumen, impeding the passage of urine.

Complications of benign prostatic enlargement

The obstruction to bladder outflow which results from progressive BPH is associated with the following.

- *Lower urinary tract symptoms (LUTS).*
- *Bladder diverticula,* which form from saccules between muscle bands.
- *Bladder stones* form as a consequence of urinary stasis, particularly in diverticula. Stone formation occurs due to significant urinary stasis with supersaturation and eventual crystallization. These crystals then enlarge over time to become stones, which can eventually become too large to pass.
- *Urinary infection* may occur (especially after catheterization).
- *Renal impairment,* with or without hydronephrosis, a result of back-pressure on the ureters. It is commonly referred to as 'obstructive nephropathy'.

Ellis and Calne's Lecture Notes in General Surgery, Fourteenth Edition.
Edited by Christopher Watson and Justin Davies.
© 2023 John Wiley & Sons Ltd. Published 2023 by John Wiley & Sons Ltd.
Companion website: www.wiley.com/go/Watson/GeneralSurgery14

Clinical features

There are three types of symptoms that result from prostatic hyperplasia.

- *Storage symptoms* due to associated bladder overactivity.
- *Voiding symptoms* due to bladder outlet obstruction.
- *Symptoms of the sequelae*, such as infection or renal failure.

It is important to realize that LUTS such as those associated with BPH may be due to bladder overactivity, or other conditions; indeed, they also occur commonly in women. Urinary tract infection may exacerbate the symptoms or precipitate acute retention (see later in this chapter).

Lower urinary tract symptoms

Voiding symptoms

- Weak urinary stream.
- Hesitancy – delay in starting to pass urine.
- Prolonged voiding.
- Intermittency – stopping and starting several times during micturition.
- Terminal and post-void dribbling.
- Incomplete bladder emptying and retention.

Storage symptoms

- Nocturia.
- Frequency.
- Urgency and urge incontinence.
- Incontinence.
- Enuresis.

Symptoms of the sequelae

Urinary retention

Urinary retention can present as either an acute episode, typically characterized by suprapubic pain, a palpable bladder and the urge to pass urine, or as chronic retention.

Chronic urinary retention has been defined as a nonpainful bladder that remains palpable after voiding, with renal impairment a consequence. Acute-on-chronic presentations may involve worsening LUTS with small volumes of voided urine. This can be associated with episodes of incontinence (referred to as 'overflow incontinence') and may also present with a degree of renal impairment.

Urinary tract infection

Urinary tract infection may occur as a consequence of urinary stasis due to incomplete bladder emptying. UTIs and/or renal impairment in men should result in an assessment of bladder emptying looking for a palpable bladder and/or enlarged prostate.

Symptoms of renal failure

The obstruction to the outflow of the bladder may result in renal failure, with nausea, lethargy, drowsiness, headache and confusion.

Confusion can be a presenting symptom of either UTI or renal impairment, and thus it is wise to examine the bladder for enlargement and to check the serum creatinine in men with confusion.

Examination

Examination of the abdomen may reveal a large bladder, which may reach to the umbilicus or above. The swelling has the typical globular shape of the bladder arising from the pelvis, and is dull to percussion. If there is acute retention, the bladder will be tender to palpation.

On digital rectal examination, the prostate may be enlarged. Typically, in benign enlargement, the lateral lobes are enlarged and a sulcus is palpable between them in the midline. Palpable nodularity, loss of palpable sulcus or a globally hard craggy mass should raise suspicion for prostate cancer.

Special investigations

- *Medication review,* to identify any medication being taken that may contribute to LUTS.
- *Assessment of LUTS:*
  - *Urinary frequency/volume chart.* The patient records when passed urine, and how much is passed.
  - *International prostate symptom score (IPSS)* is a questionnaire tool for classifying the severity of LUTS. Marks are given according to the frequency with which the patients suffers from incomplete emptying, frequency, intermittency, urgency, weak stream, straining and nocturia. Scores will define mild, moderate or severely symptomatic patients.
  - *Urine flow rate assessment.* A voided volume of at least 150 mL is required for adequate assessment of maximum flow rate. A maximum flow rate of

less than 12 mL/sec indicates obstruction or weak bladder contractility. A flow rate over 15 mL/sec makes bladder outlet obstruction unlikely. Urodynamics (pressure flow assessment) can be used to distinguish outflow obstruction from poor detrusor contraction, which will not improve following prostate surgery.

- *Urine sample:*
  - *Urinalysis* for the presence of leucocytes, protein, blood and glucose.
  - *Urine culture* is performed if urinalysis is positive. Most patients with prostatic disease do not have infected urine until the bladder and urethra have been instrumented.
- *Serum creatinine* to assess renal function.
- *Prostate-specific antigen* (PSA) is an indicator of prostate cancer. A PSA concentration below 4.0 ng/mL is usually deemed normal, but age-adjusted upper limits of normal may be used. Refinements in PSA include measurement of the free/total PSA ratio, which is over 0.15 in normal men.
- *Ultrasound* to assess post-void residual urine volume, retention or hydronephrosis. Normally, there is no significant residual volume; however, in the presence of bladder outflow obstruction, the bladder cannot be completely emptied.

Treatment

This depends on whether presentation is with LUTS (nocturia, frequency, urgency, etc.) or acutely with urinary retention (see later in this chapter).

Conservative management

If there are few symptoms, lifestyle measures, such as adjusting fluid intake and reducing caffeine intake, as well as the use of containment products (e.g. pads) may be helpful.

Medical therapy

This is indicated for those who are moderately symptomatic.

- *Selective α_1-adrenergic antagonists* (α-blockers, e.g. tamsulosin or alfuzosin) are the mainstay of treatment for lower tract symptoms.
- *5α-reductase inhibition* (e.g. finasteride or dutasteride) blocks the conversion of testosterone to its active metabolite, dihydrotestosterone, in the prostate. The beneficial effect may take up to 6 months to appear.

In addition, anticholinergics may help symptoms of an overactive bladder, and an afternoon loop diuretic or oral desmopressin may help with nocturnal polyuria, but needs careful monitoring of sodium.

Surgical therapy

Surgery is offered to symptomatic patients in whom medical therapy has failed and who have bladder outflow obstruction on flow rate and pressure/flow assessment or have presented with urinary retention with renal impairment or have had recurrent urinary retention after removal of catheter.

Endoscopic prostatectomy

The prostate can be removed endoscopically by means of an operating cystoscope, using a diathermy cutting loop (TURP) or laser fibre (most commonly, holmium laser prostatectomy, HoLEP). Removal of too much gland may damage the urethral sphincter mechanism. Newer techniques have been developed to offer less invasive surgery to address some of the risks surrounding erectile dysfunction and retrograde ejaculation. Morbidity and mortality from these procedures is typically low and minimally invasive approaches now exist even for significant prostatic enlargement (over 100 grams).

Novel therapies

Newer therapies include:

- Prostate artery embolization – super selective catherization of the prostatic artery via a femoral artery approach to embolize the prostate's blood supply causing necrosis and shrinkage.
- Rezum – a transurethral steam vapour therapy, causing thermal ablation of the prostate.
- Urolift – a small device like a treasury tag is inserted through the prostatic lobe, and the implant retracts the enlarged prostate.
- Aqua-ablation uses a high pressure jet of saline to hydro-dissect away the obstructing prostate.

Complications of prostatectomy

Transurethral prostatectomy and HoLEP have a low morbidity and mortality, particularly in view of the elderly population in which surgery is usually performed.

- *Haemorrhage*: primary haemorrhage is more common with malignant glands, with large resections, and in patients on aspirin or clopidogrel.

- *Transurethral resection (TUR) syndrome*: absorption of large volumes of the irrigating fluid through open prostatic veins may result in hyponatraemia and confusion.
- *Infection* is particularly common in patients who are catheterized before surgery; prophylactic antibiotics are given.
- *Retrograde ejaculation* is almost certain after TURP.
- *Erectile dysfunction* occurs in 5–15% of patients, depending on the level of preoperative potency.
- *Bladder neck stenosis*, due to stricturing of the bladder neck following resection, may occur and presents with outflow obstruction.
- *Urinary incontinence* is uncommon but may occur if the resection is extended below the verumontanum with damage to the urethral sphincter.
- *Recurrent LUTS*: late recurrence may be due to either regrowth of an adenoma or malignant change.

Urinary retention

Urinary retention is generally divided into acute and chronic.

- *Acute retention* presents with inability to pass urine, suprapubic pain and a suprapubic mass.
- *Chronic urinary retention* is a more insidious process with gradual enlargement of the bladder, dribbling incontinence and little or no pain. However, there can be an abrupt shift to acute urinary retention referred to as 'acute-on-chronic retention'.

Causes of urinary retention

Causes of urinary retention may be divided into general and local:

1 *General causes* (no organic obstruction to urinary flow):
   a Postoperative.
   b Neurological causes, such as diabetes, stroke or spinal tumour.
   c Drugs, for example anticholinergics, tricyclic antidepressants.
2 *Local causes*:
   a In the lumen of the urethra, for example stone or blood clot.
   b In the wall, for example stricture.
   c Outside the wall, for example prostatic enlargement (benign or malignant), faecal impaction, pelvic tumour, pregnant uterus.

General causes of retention of urine must always be borne in mind: retention related to acute illness (e.g. chest infection), trauma (e.g. hip fracture) or surgery (e.g. hernia repair or haemorrhoid surgery) is common and often self-limiting. Sometimes a patient with occult bladder outlet obstruction is precipitated into retention of urine following some other surgical procedure and it may then be necessary to proceed to prostatectomy if spontaneous voiding is to resume.

Clinical features

Acute urinary retention is typically a straightforward diagnosis to make with the patient complaining of an inability to void despite a strong sensation to void with the presence of a palpable bladder typically to the level of the umbilicus or higher. Having made the diagnosis, it is important to consider the underlying cause (e.g. prostatic hyperplasia), and consider any consequences (e.g. renal impairment). For example, there may be a history of progressive LUTS, a history of urethral infection suggesting a stricture, or a history of ureteric colic suggesting a stone.

Examination reveals a distended bladder. The patient should have a digital rectal examination to assess the prostate, and the urethra palpated and meatus examined. Other potential causes may warrant further examination, such as neurological examination. Diagnosis can be confirmed with a portable bladder ultrasound scanner.

The main priority is to relieve the patient's distress by urinary catheterization, after which more detailed history taking and examination may proceed.

Special investigations

- *Creatinine and electrolytes* are measured, looking for evidence of renal impairment.
- *Ultrasound scan* of the urinary tract is indicated to look for hydronephrosis if the creatinine is raised or there was a large residual volume.
- *Serum PSA* may be raised due to retention, infection and catheterization, so any measurement as a test for prostate cancer should be delayed at least 6 weeks.

Treatment

Catheterization is the definitive treatment for the symptoms of acute urinary retention, and patients typically experience relief within minutes. Should the patient have a high residual volume on catheterization (more than one litre) they will need a period of observation to assess for polyuria post catheterization as this may require admission and IV fluid replacement.

Should the creatinine and/or ultrasound scan be abnormal, a urology assessment should be performed prior to removal of the catheter.

Treatment with an α-blocker, such as tamsulosin or alfuzosin, should be offered to the patient before removal of the catheter. Failure of the trial without catheter requires replacement of the catheter; subsequent management may involve surgery, intermittent self-catheterization, or long-term indwelling catheter depending on the fitness of the patient.

Bladder neck obstruction

Bladder neck obstruction may be due to congenital valves in the region of the prostatic urethra and internal meatus, or failure of relaxation of the bladder neck.

Posterior urethral valves

Congenital valves, which usually produce hydronephrosis and retention of urine in childhood. They are usually diagnosed on antenatal ultrasound, and the diagnosis confirmed by micturating cystourethrogram. Early treatment by surgical incision of the valves before renal failure occurs is important.

Failure of bladder neck relaxation

The bladder neck normally relaxes actively during voiding. If this fails to happen, there is functional obstruction, with lower tract obstructive symptoms but without enlargement of the prostate. Bladder neck obstruction can also occur as a consequence of scarring following instrumentation or prostatic surgery.

Treatment

Medical therapy with α-blockers can be offered, and if this fails, endoscopic incision of the bladder neck is considered.

Prostatitis

Acute prostatitis is a bacterial infection of the prostate, usually caused by bacteria entering the prostate from the urinary tract either spontaneously, or after instrumentation of the urinary tract or prostatic biopsy. Infection is usually due to faecal organisms, particularly *Escherichia coli* and *Streptococcus faecalis*.

Non-bacterial prostatitis (chronic pelvic pain syndrome, CPPS) does not have an identifiable cause, although an autoimmune process after prior sensitization, possibly by an infection, may be responsible. Not uncommonly, patients may present with the symptoms in the absence of any inflammation (prostatodynia).

Clinical features

In addition to asymptomatic prostatitis seen histologically in prostatic chippings at the time of resection, the following forms of prostatitis are recognized.

Acute bacterial prostatitis

The patient presents with fever, rigours, perineal pain and difficulty voiding, together with symptoms of a urinary tract infection; acute retention of urine may be evident. In addition, pain on ejaculation and blood in the semen (haematospermia) may be present. Rectal examination reveals an enlarged, exquisitely tender prostate, and occasionally an abscess may be palpable. Epididymitis is a common accompaniment, owing to infection passing along the vas deferens.

A urine culture is taken in attempt to identify the causative organism. Treatment is commenced with an initial 2-week course of ciprofloxacin or oflaxacin antibiotics (with trimethoprim as an alternative first choice if fluoroquinolone antibiotics are contraindicated) which have good penetration into the prostate. The antibiotics are reviewed in light of the sensitivities of the micro-organism grown, but in general a prolonged course (e.g. six weeks) is required.

Chronic pelvic pain syndrome

This is a common insidious problem affecting up to 9% of men. The symptoms are typically pain in the perineum, scrotum, tip of penis or bladder, along with pain on ejaculation or micturition. Symptoms of urinary frequency and a feeling of incomplete emptying are common. Systemic symptoms, such as myalgia and arthralgia, may be present.

The aetiology of the syndrome is unclear; occult infection, an autoimmune process and pelvic muscle abnormality have all been suggested. Treatment options include an empirical course of antibiotics, α-blockers if there are LUTS, and non-steroidal, anti-inflammatory drugs. Investigation for neuropathic pain or psychosocial assessment may be appropriate in some patients.

Prostate cancer

Pathology

Prostate cancer is the most common cancer in men in the UK, with 1 in 8 men being affected in their lifetime. Prostate cancer typically affects those over 50 years of age, and risk increases with age and it is estimated to affect 80% of men aged 80; it is more common to die with the disease than from it. Those with a family history, and those of black race, have the highest lifetime risk (1 in 4).

Macroscopic appearance

The tumour is usually situated in the posterior part of the prostate beneath its capsule and appears as an infiltrating, hard, pale area.

Microscopic appearance

The tumour is almost always an adenocarcinoma. The degree of differentiation is quoted in terms of the Gleason grade,[1] usually from 6 to 10.

Spread

- *Local*: there is invasion of the periprostatic tissues and adjacent organs (i.e. the bladder, urethra, seminal vesicles) and, rarely, invasion around and ulceration into the rectum.

[1]Donald Gleason (1920–2008), Pathologist, Minneapolis, MN, USA. The Gleason grade is a histological score based on the degree of differentiation, such that grade 1 is well differentiated and grade 5 is poorly differentiated. Two scores are given, the first reflecting the dominant pattern in the biopsy, the second reflecting the next most common pattern. Hence the range goes from 2 to 10. Thus a Gleason 4+3 would be a worse prognosis tumour than a 3+2, for example.

- *Lymphatic*: to the iliac and para-aortic nodes.
- *Blood-borne*: especially to the pelvis, spine and skull, usually as osteosclerotic lesions. Secondaries may also be found in the liver and lung.

Clinical features

Prostate cancer may be detected without symptoms on the basis of an elevated PSA and/or an abnormal digital rectal examination, or present with symptoms that are identical to those of benign enlargement. The patient may also present with advanced disease with symptoms from secondary deposits, particularly with pain in the back from vertebral metastases or even with spinal cord compression or cauda equina syndrome.

Rectal examination of the prostate may reveal four different stages (the Tumour component of TNM staging; Figure 45.1).

T1 The prostate feels benign, with no palpable tumour.
　T1a: Incidental finding in ≤5% resected tissue in TURP.
　T1b: Incidental finding in >5% resected tissue in TURP.
　T1c: Tumour identified on prostate biopsy triggered by raised PSA.
T2 A hard nodule in one lobe of the prostate or abolishing the normal sulcus between the two lateral lobes. The tumour is confined to the prostate.
　T2a: Tumour involves half of one lobe or less.
　T2b: Tumour involves more than half of one lobe.
　T2c: Tumour involves both lobes.
T3 A hard mass in the prostate together with infiltration of the tissues on one or both sides of the prostate (**T3a**) or into the seminal vesicles (**T3b**).
T4 A hard mass in the prostate which is fixed to the pelvic side wall and/or is invading the bladder, external sphincter, rectum, levator muscles.

Special investigations

- *PSA concentration* in the blood is usually raised in the presence of prostate cancer (Box 45.1). A PSA over 20 ng/mL suggests disseminated disease. PSA is also useful as a tumour marker to follow the response to treatment.

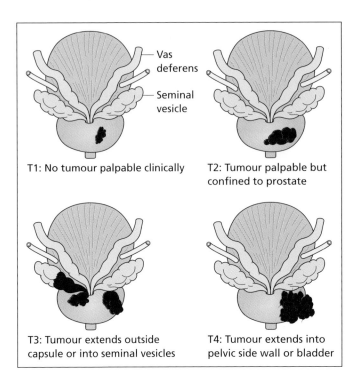

T1: No tumour palpable clinically

T2: Tumour palpable but confined to prostate

T3: Tumour extends outside capsule or into seminal vesicles

T4: Tumour extends into pelvic side wall or bladder

Figure 45.1 The clinical staging of prostatic carcinoma.

Box 45.1 Prostate-specific antigen (PSA)

PSA is an enzyme produced by epithelial cells of the prostate gland, by normal as well as malignant cells. It is may be raised in the following circumstances:

- Increasing age.
- Benign prostatic hyperplasia.
- Ejaculation.
- Prostate biopsy.
- Prostate stimulation, e.g. rectal examination.
- Prostatitis.
- Urethral catheterization.
- Urinary retention.
- Urinary tract infection.
- Vigorous exercise.
- Cycling.
- Prostate cancer.

- *Multiparametric magnetic resonance imaging (mpMRI)* is used increasingly to identify the primary tumour and for staging.
- *Transrectal ultrasound (TRUS) guided prostate biopsy:* TRUS is used to guide needle core biopsies, which are performed systematically through the gland obtaining 10–15 cores. These should confirm the diagnosis and grade of tumour. It is associated with perineal pain, blood in urine, faeces, and semen, and carries a risk of severe sepsis.
- *Bone scan* is indicated if the PSA is greater than 20 ng/mL, or a T3 or T4 tumour, or if there is bone pain or other symptoms suggestive of bony metastases, the presence of which the bone scan will demonstrate.
- *CT scan* to stage the tumour, looking for nodal (iliac and para-aortic) or solid organ metastases (e.g. lung, liver, brain).

The role of PSA in diagnosis

PSA has revolutionized prostate cancer diagnosis since its discovery. PSA is not a cancer-specific marker but an organ-specific marker, meaning it can be elevated without prostate cancer being present in conditions such as BPH, prostatitis, urinary retention and urinary tract infection. Lastly, PSA can be variable with transient rises in PSA which are not sustained on repeat testing. In asymptomatic patients with a normal digital rectal examination, an elevated age-specific PSA on two readings several weeks apart is needed before commencing further investigations for prostate cancer. An abnormal rectal examination in conjunction with an elevated PSA is always an indication for further investigation.

Multiparametric magnetic resonance imaging

Multiparametric MRI (mpMRI) now allows assessment of the prostate using different image acquisition techniques from which the prostate imaging reporting and data system (PI_RADS) score can be used to estimate relative risk of prostate cancer being present. mpMRI allows the identification of suspicious areas within the prostate for targeted biopsy, thus increasing the diagnostic yield of what is a relatively invasive investigation. Hence, mpMRI should be performed before biopsy.

Prostate biopsy

Prostate biopsies have traditionally been taken via the transrectal route with ultrasound guidance under local anaesthesia. More recently, there has been an increased interest in performing biopsies via the transperineal route. This reduces the risk of life-threatening sepsis associated with the transrectal route, which has remained at around 1% even with antibiotic prophylaxis.

Treatment

Treatment is based on the likelihood of tumour confinement to the gland, derived from its degree of histological differentiation (the Gleason grade score), the PSA concentration and the clinical tumour stage (see earlier in this chapter). These have been formulated into a series of Prognostic Groups (CPG, Table 45.1). Equally the patient's overall fitness, their perception of risk and what are acceptable side effects or treatment also play a role in reaching a shared decision, particularly in low-risk localized disease.

Localized disease

The active treatments available for localized disease (Cambridge Prognostic Groups 1 to 3) are as follows:

- Active surveillance.
- Radical Prostatectomy.
- Radical Radiotherapy.

Active surveillance

Active surveillance is designed to avoid harmful side effects from radical treatment in patients with low-risk disease (CPG 1), and to offer an alternative to patients with intermediate disease (CPG 2 and 3) who do not want radical treatment; it is not appropriate for patients with high-risk disease (CPG 4 and 5, see table 45.1). The goal is to keep a patient's prostate cancer under surveillance but in the 'window of curability', and offer curative treatments should the patients disease progress or change.

In the first year, PSA is checked every 3 to 4 months, with digital rectal examination and mpMRI scan at 12 – 18 months. Thereafter, PSA is checked every 6 months, and a rectal examination performed every 12 months, with further mpMRI and prostate biopsies according to local preference, or if indicated by evidence of disease progression. The patient will then be offered one of the radical treatment options.

Table 45.1 Risk stratification for localized or locally advanced prostate cancer

Cambridge Prognostic Group	Level of risk	Prostate-specific antigen		Gleason score		Clinical tumour stage
1	low	<10µg/L	AND	≤6	AND	T1
2		10–20µl/L	OR	3+4	AND	T1 – T2
3	intermediate	10–20µl/L	AND	3+4	AND	T1 – T2
				4+3	AND	T1 – T2
4		>20µl/L	OR	8	OR	T3
5	high	TWO of: PSA>20µg/L	OR	9 to 10	OR	T4

Radical prostatectomy

Radical prostatectomy is typically performed using robotic systems to reduce hospital length of stay. This minimally invasive approach has radically changed how patients are managed after surgery, with some centres discharging patients within 24 hours of their surgery. The procedure involves removing the prostate, seminal vesicles and possibly the pelvic lymph nodes, with anastomosis of the bladder neck to the urethra just distal to the excised prostate. The long-term side effects include erectile dysfunction in half the patients, and urinary incontinence in approximately 13%.

Radical radiotherapy

Radical radiotherapy can be given by external beam or transperineal placement of radio-iodine seeds (brachytherapy) and can be combined with androgen deprivation therapy (ADT) depending on tumour risk. Long-term incontinence rates are lower at 5% as are erectile dysfunction rates at 36%, but the treatment does carry a higher rate of faecal incontinence at 4%. Radiotherapy also carries a small risk of triggering another malignant process in the radiotherapy field.

Watchful waiting

Watchful waiting is part of a strategy for 'managing' prostate cancer and is aimed at people with localized prostate cancer who do not ever wish to have curative treatment, or they are not fit enough to undergo radical treatments. Watchful waiting involves the deferred use of hormone therapy with the objective to maintain quality of life. It avoids the use of surgery or radiation, but implies that curative treatment will not be attempted.

Metastatic prostate cancer

Prostate cancer is often discovered at a stage when it has already spread beyond the prostatic capsule and may well have involved other organs, particularly the bladder base and bones. The mainstay of treatment of advanced disease is androgen deprivation and chemotherapy, with an emphasis on prolonging life and minimizing symptoms.

- *Docetaxel*, which inhibits cell proliferation by stabilizing microtubules within the tumour cells.
- *Gonadotrophin-releasing hormone agonists*, triptorelin, goserelin and leuprorelin, are the mainstay of treatment. They inhibit the release of luteinizing hormone from the anterior pituitary, with consequent reduction of testicular production of testosterone. Initiation of therapy may cause a flare of testosterone production, and hence a flare of disease, so a short 3-week course of anti-androgen therapy (e.g. bicalutamide) is given when treatment commences.
- *Gonadotrophin-releasing hormone (GnRH) antagonist*, e.g. *Degarelix* for the first-line treatment of androgen-dependent advanced prostate cancer. It has a direct mechanism of action that blocks the action of GnRH on the pituitary with no initial surge in gonadotrophin or testosterone levels.
- *Orchidectomy* for prostate cancer is very seldom done nowadays, but can often relieve symptoms and produce dramatic remissions in the course of the disease. It is still offered as an alternative to GnRH agonists.

Palliation produced by hormonal treatment of prostatic cancer suppresses PSA to normal levels for an average of 2 years, after which it slowly rises, with symptoms returning a few months later. When the cancer is refractory to hormone therapy, the average life expectancy decreases significantly. Multiple new treatments have been developed for 2nd line and 3rd line use and overall 5-year survival for metastatic prostate cancer is now 30%.

Radiotherapy may relieve the pain of bony deposits and can also be used for local control to supplement hormonal therapy.

Additional resources

46

The male urethra

Arthur McPhee

Learning objectives

✓ To know the congenital anomalies of the male urethra.
✓ To know the different types of urethral injury and their management.
✓ To know the causes, investigation and treatment of urethral stricture.

Anatomy

The six parts of the male urethra are often subdivided by urologists into anterior and posterior regions, as follows.

The posterior urethra comprises:

- Prostatic urethra, traverses the prostate gland.
- Membranous urethra, passes through the external sphincter and fascial perineal membrane.

The anterior urethra comprises:

- Bulbar urethra passes through the bulb of the penis in the perineum.
- Penile urethra, passing through the penis, often called the spongy urethra since it passes through the corpus spongiosum.
- Sub-meatal urethra, that portion within the glans.
- External meatus visible at the tip of the penis.

Congenital anomalies

Hypospadias

The male urethra is formed by the inrolling of the genital folds, which themselves form the corpus

Ellis and Calne's Lecture Notes in General Surgery, Fourteenth Edition.
Edited by Christopher Watson and Justin Davies.
© 2023 John Wiley & Sons Ltd. Published 2023 by John Wiley & Sons Ltd.
Companion website: www.wiley.com/go/Watson/GeneralSurgery14

spongiosum. If the genital folds fail to develop or fuse completely, the tube is either short or absent. The urethra thus opens onto the ventral surface of the penis anywhere from the perineum up to the glans.

Hypospadias is associated with three abnormalities:

- *Ventral opening of the urethra* on the penis.
- *A hooded foreskin*, due to deficient development of the ventral part of the foreskin.
- *Chordee*, a downward curvature of the penis on erection associated with proximal hypospadias.

Treatment is complex and should be reserved for specialist centres. The essential components of reconstructive surgery include correction of penile chordee, urethroplasty for urethral reconstruction and appropriate skin coverage to obtain a satisfactory cosmetic appearance. The foreskin is utilized as a skin flap; therefore, circumcision before correction of the abnormality is contraindicated.

Epispadias

Epispadias, where the urethra opens dorsally on the penis, is associated with other anterior abdominal wall defects including exstrophy of the bladder as part of the exstrophy-epispadias complex, and occurs more commonly in males. Prenatal screening detects a large proportion of exstrophy patients but epispadias is typically detected at birth.

Surgery to correct this abnormality is again complex and should be performed in specialist centres.

Posterior urethral valves (see also Chapter 45)

A valve-like membrane at the level of the verumontanum. This can obstruct the flow of urine, resulting in chronic retention of urine and uraemia in infants.

Urethral injury and trauma in the male

Urethral injury and trauma may be generally divided into anterior urethral injuries and posterior urethral injuries and then subdivided into those injuries caused by iatrogenic trauma, blunt trauma and those by penetrating trauma.

Anterior urethral injuries

In anterior urethral injuries, the bulbar urethra is the site most commonly affected by blunt trauma, compressing the bulbar urethra against the pubic symphysis and leading to injury/rupture through compression. This can be through straddle injuries, such as falling astride a bicycle cross bar, or blunt force such as a kick to the perineum. Penetrating anterior injuries are rare and are typically associated with other penile, testicular or pelvic injuries.

Iatrogenic injury is unsurprisingly the most common cause of urethral trauma with most injuries being associated with urethral catheterization. These are typically false passages created by forceful insertion of the urinary catheter and incorrect inflation of the retaining balloon within the urethra.

Posterior urethral injuries

Posterior urethral injuries, both blunt and penetrating, are typically associated with significant trauma.

Blunt urethral injuries are almost always as a result of pelvic fractures with the risk increasing with the severity of the fracture, and are most commonly associated with road traffic accidents. Pelvic fracture urethral injuries are again subdivided into partial and complete rupture.

Penetrating posterior urethral injuries are rare and are typically associated with gunshot injuries in which there is a high probability of associated intrabdominal injuries. The associated injuries of posterior urethral trauma in the male can often be life-threatening and will often dictate the patient's initial assessment and management.

Clinical features

The history of injury to the pelvis or perineum should prompt suspicion. There can also be a delay in both signs and symptoms, which can be of delayed onset in relation to the injury itself. The important features are:

- Blood at the external urethral meatus is the 'classic' sign of urethral trauma but the absence of blood does not exclude an injury.
- Urinary retention, in a complete injury.
- Haematuria and pain on voiding (incomplete injury) should also raise suspicion of an injury in the context of trauma.
- Swelling of the penis, scrotum and perineum secondary to urinary extravasation and haematoma.

Digital rectal examination should be performed to exclude rectal injury (blood on glove or palpable defect), which can be present in up to 5% of cases. The presence of a 'high-riding prostate', disconnected from the anterior urethra, is a well-known but unreliable feature.

Special investigations

- *CT scan*, often done as part of a trauma series in patients with pelvic trauma.
- *Retrograde urethrogram*, using dilute water-soluble contrast medium will identify extravasation or loss of continuity, and localize the site of injury. Extravasation with bladder filling suggests incomplete injury, extravasation with no bladder filling is suggestive of complete posterior urethral injury.

Management

Satisfactory management depends on a high index of suspicion leading to early diagnosis.

Anterior urethral injuries

Early management of anterior urethral injuries can be divided into either urinary diversion, via suprapubic or transurethral catheterization, or immediate exploration and reconstruction.

Exploration and reconstruction are reserved for non-life-threatening penetrating injuries and penile-fracture -related injuries. In cases with significant defects or where the presence/risk of infection is very high (e.g. bite wounds), this is done as part of a staged repair.

Urinary diversion is typically performed either through suprapubic catheterization or endoscopic realignment with urethral catheterization. These are typically the interventions of choice in cases of life threating pelvic injury.

Posterior urethral injuries

Management of posterior urethral injury is typically performed in the first instance by an attempt at either urethral catheterization by an experienced clinician or with ultrasound guidance, or open suprapubic catheter insertion. Subsequent early management (2 days to 6 weeks) can either be in the form of an early urethroplasty or early realignment but management of the associated pelvic injuries means that repair beyond 6 weeks ('deferred urethroplasty') is the standard treatment.

Complications

- *Stricture formation* often occurs following injuries to the urethra because of scarring; subsequent repair may be necessary.
- *Impotence* occurs in half the patients, as a consequence of either a pelvic injury involving the terminal branches of the internal iliac arteries or injury to the nerves supplying the penis.

Urethral stricture

Urethral stricture disease can be broadly grouped into anterior urethral stricture and posterior urethral stricture.

Posterior urethral strictures are associated with trauma, as described above, or can be present as a result of previous surgical interventions such as transurethral prostatectomy (TURP) or radical prostatectomy.

Anterior urethral strictures can have many causes:

- *Congenital:* meatal stenosis in hypospadias.
- *Infection/inflammation*:
  a Gonococcal urethritis.
  b Non-specific urethritis, for example *Chlamydia*.
  c Balanitis xerotica obliterans.
- *Trauma*:
  a Blunt trauma, e.g. straddle injury.

- *Iatrogenic*
  a Urethral instrumentation including catheterization.
  b Previous urethral or prostatic surgery.

Clinical features

Typically, the patient with a urethral stricture may complain of difficulty passing urine, with a poor stream and straining to empty his bladder. He is often younger than 50 years (in contrast to men with benign prostatic disease). Patients may also present with urinary infection and acute retention as a consequence of the stricture.

Special investigations

- *Urinary flow rate*: the stricture limits the flow of urine, and measurement of the flow rate shows a flat plateau.
- *Urethrogram* will demonstrate the location and length of the stricture.
- *Urethroscopy* will visualize the stricture and facilitate treatment.

Treatment

Optical urethrotomy or urethral dilatation are common first-line treatments for uncomplicated strictures. Optical urethrotomy has the benefit of being performed under direct vision compared to traditional urethral dilatation. However, newer urethral dilators have been developed with hydrophilic coatings and channels for guidewires so that dilatation can be performed using a Seldinger[1] technique, and are increasingly popular in the acute setting.

Urethral strictures have a high chance of recurrence depending on the length of the stricture and the degree of corporal fibrosis, although 50% will require no further treatment after either optical urethrotomy or urethral dilatation.

Recurrent strictures can be treated by further optical urethrotomy or urethroplasty, with either simple resection of the stricture with end-to-end anastomosis of the ends, or interposition of a graft of buccal mucosa.

The management of acute retention due to urethral stricture is outlined in Chapter 45.

---

[1] Sven Seldinger (1921–1998), Radiologist, Karolinska Hospital, Sweden. The technique involves first passing a wire through the lumen, and then railroading instruments, stents, cannulas, etc. over the wire.

47

The penis

Arthur McPhee

Learning objectives

✓ To understand phimosis, paraphimosis, balanitis and their treatment.
✓ To know about carcinoma of the penis, its presentations and treatment.
✓ To know the causes of erectile dysfunction and its treatment.

Phimosis

Phimosis is narrowing of the preputial orifice, leading to difficulty retracting the prepuce (foreskin); the literal Greek translation is 'muzzling'. It can be divided into physiological, pathological or idiopathic.

Clinical features

The most common symptoms in adults are inability to retract the foreskin or pain during intercourse. In children, the foreskin may balloon and the urinary stream may be reduced to a dribble. Physiological phimosis is very common and typically resolves without intervention as children age.

Treatment

Young children

While non-retractile prepuce is a common presentation in childhood, the natural history of physiological phimosis is that it will resolve with age. Natural history studies have shown around 8% of 6–7-year-olds will have a non-retractile foreskin but this percentage reduces to 1% of 16–17-year-olds. In the absence of

Ellis and Calne's Lecture Notes in General Surgery, Fourteenth Edition.
Edited by Christopher Watson and Justin Davies.
© 2023 John Wiley & Sons Ltd. Published 2023 by John Wiley & Sons Ltd.
Companion website: www.wiley.com/go/Watson/GeneralSurgery14

recurrent infections/balanitis, circumcision is not typically recommended, as the condition can be expected to improve.

Older children and adults

Initial treatment for physiological phimosis is typically with topical steroid cream and stretching exercises. If the symptoms are persistent and troublesome, circumcision is considered the definitive surgical management.

Phimosis caused by scarring after recurrent balanitis is more typically managed with primary circumcision.

Paraphimosis

Paraphimosis results from retracting a tight foreskin proximally over the glans. The foreskin acts as a constricting band, interfering with venous return from the glans, which, therefore, swells painfully. Once swelling starts, it becomes increasingly difficult to replace the foreskin.

Paraphimosis most commonly follows urethral catheterization; the foreskin is retracted over the glans to expose the meatus for cleaning the glans prior to catheter insertion. Once the catheter is inserted, if the foreskin is not replaced promptly, it can constrict the venous return, producing a paraphimosis. Hence it is important to always ensure that the patient's foreskin is pulled forward again after the insertion of an indwelling catheter. Paraphimosis may also occur after an erection.

Treatment

Once a paraphimosis has become established, it can be challenging to reduce. Traditional advice is to apply a swab soaked in 50% dextrose to reduce some swelling by osmosis. This may be followed by direct pressure to the glans for a few minutes to allow the foreskin to be reduced to its normal position. If the patient struggles to tolerate the manual pressure required for reduction, a local anaesthetic penile block can be performed to facilitate this.

Should reduction still prove difficult with local anaesthetic block, the clinician can consider performing the 'Dundee Technique'. With an appropriate local anaesthetic block performed and the area cleaned with anti-septic solution, a 25G needle is used to perform a series of up to 20 punctures in the oedematous foreskin to release the oedema. Once manual pressure has been applied again, oedema should reduce rapidly allowing the foreskin to be reduced to its natural position.

Under rare circumstances where paraphimosis has been present for many hours, a dorsal slit may be required to achieve appropriate resolution. The dorsal slit is used rather than a circumcision as there is a much greater risk of removing too much skin with a circumcision in the presence of distorted anatomy.

After any episode of painful paraphimosis, patients are typically offered circumcision at a later date to prevent recurrence.

Balanitis

Balanitis is an acute inflammation of the foreskin and glans, with possible causes including infection and allergic dermatitis. Management depends on the underlying condition and causative organism. It is important to test the urine for sugar to exclude diabetes, which may predispose to the inflammation, in which case *Candida* may be the infecting organism.

Recurrent balanitis may result in phimosis from scarring.

Treatment

The parents should clean the penis daily with luke-warm water and dry it gently. The foreskin should not be forcibly retracted if it is still fixed, and potential irritants such as soap, bubble bath and baby wipes should be avoided. Nappies should be changed frequently.

- *For suspected allergic dermatitis*, the suspected cause (e.g. soap, bubble bath) should be avoided and 1% hydrocortisone cream applied for up to 14 days.
- *For suspected non-specific dermatitis*, topical 1% hydrocortisone cream and an imidazole cream may be used for up to 4 days.
- *For suspected or confirmed candida balanitis*, a topical imidazole cream for up to 14 days.
- *For suspected or confirmed bacterial balanitis*, oral antibiotics, e.g. flucloxacillin, depending on sensitivities for 7 days.

If there is no improvement after 7 days of treatment, topical hydrocortisone should be stopped (if used) and a swab repeated. Very rarely, and almost exclusively in adults, it will be necessary to perform a biopsy to achieve a diagnosis.

Penile cancer

Pathology

Carcinoma of the penis is uncommon in Europe and the USA (<1 in 100000), but more common in Africa and Asia (19 in 100000). Infant and childhood circumcision is protective with cases being virtually unknown among populations who are circumcised soon after birth. Penile cancer is common in regions with high rates of human papilloma virus (HPV) infection (HPV types 16 and 18 predominantly), with approximately one-third of cases being attributed to HPV-related carcinogenesis. Its viral link explains the higher incidence in the immunosuppressed. Smoking is also associated with penile cancer.

Macroscopic appearance

The premalignant stage is a persistent red patch on the penis progressing to either a papillary growth on the glans or an infiltrating ulcer; the latter is more common.

Microscopic appearance

The lesions are squamous carcinomas, which are usually well differentiated.

Spread

- *Local*: the tumour may fungate under or through the prepuce. Proximal spread along the shaft may destroy the substance of the penis.
- *Lymphatic*: the inguinal lymph nodes are frequently involved, often bilaterally.
- *Blood-borne* spread occurs late and is unusual.

Clinical features

Penile cancer affects the glans in almost half of all cases, followed by the prepuce, and coronal sulcus, with the shaft of penis only rarely being affected. The presentation can range from an area of erythema to a fungating lesion with palpable inguinal lymphadenopathy.

It is common for men to present late, when the tumour has ulcerated through the prepuce or until some of the penis has been destroyed, presumably because of the embarrassment caused by the site of the tumour. Carcinoma of the penis never occludes the urethra and so it does not cause retention of urine.

Treatment

Diagnosis is confirmed by biopsy. Subsequent treatment is dictated by the stage of the tumour. Where the cancer is superficial and has not spread, penile preserving treatment with either topical chemotherapy, laser ablation, glans resurfacing or glansectomy with reconstruction.

Advanced lesions are managed with either partial or total amputation of the penis (penectomy), with inguinal lymph node sampling, or block dissection if the nodes are involved. Radiotherapy may also be required. This operation, although mutilating, does not interfere with micturition because the external sphincter is preserved. After a total amputation of the penis, the patients usually micturate sitting down.

Overall survival is around 75% at five years, but is better for early stage cancers.

Erectile dysfunction

Erectile dysfunction is the inability to achieve, or sustain, an erection sufficient for sexual intercourse.

The prevalence of erectile dysfunction in the adult male population is 20% and is correlated with increasing age.

Erection requires increased arterial flow into the erectile tissue of the penis, together with occlusion of venous outflow. Erection is mediated via efferent parasympathetic fibres from S2, S3 and S4. Reflex erection requires afferent signals via the pudendal nerve, while psychogenic erection requires outflow from the brain via the spinal cord.

Aetiology

Impotence most commonly occurs as a consequence of ageing, such that 70% of 70-year-olds have some difficulty with obtaining an erection (although 70% of 70 year-olds also have sexual intercourse). Aside from ageing, the other causes of erectile impotence are as follows:

Neurogenic

Causes of neurogenic impotence include the following:

- *Congenital*: spina bifida.
- *Spinal causes*: spinal cord injury, spinal cord tumour.
- *Central causes*: hypothalamic injury, cerebral infarction/tumour.
- *Postsurgical causes*: for example, pelvic surgery such as anterior resection, abdominoperineal excision of the rectum and radical prostatectomy, due to damage of the pelvic parasympathetic nerves.

Vascular

Hypertension (and its treatment) is commonly associated with erectile dysfunction. Arterial disease affecting flow in the internal iliac arteries, as may result from aortoiliac disease, can cause impotence and buttock claudication (Leriche's syndrome[1]).

Hormonal

- *Diabetes mellitus*, the most common hormonal cause, probably acting via a diabetic neuropathy. Erectile dysfunction may be a presenting symptom of diabetes in men.

---

[1] René Leriche (1879–1955), Professor of Surgery, successively at Lyon, Strasbourg and Paris, France.

- *Pituitary failure, primary testicular failure, hypothyroidism* and most other endocrine diseases may contribute to impotence.

Pharmacological

Some drugs, in particular antihypertensive agents, tranquillizers and oestrogens, may cause impotence. Alcohol is also a common cause.

Psychogenic

Psychogenic impotence is usually of sudden onset, and the patient continues to have nocturnal erections and erections following masturbation, suggesting there is not a physical cause.

Examination

After a thorough history looking at possible causes, examination should consider the following:

- Penis – malignant or premalignant lesions; penile deformities (e.g. Peyronie's disease).
- Testes – signs of hypogonadism (small testes).
- Gynaecomastia and reduced body hair.
- Rectal examination – large and/or irregular prostate.

Special investigations

A history and examination are conducted to determine the cause. Other investigations include the following:

- *HbA1c estimation* to detect diabetes.
- *hormone screen*: abnormalities in the blood levels of testosterone, follicle-stimulating hormone, luteinizing hormone, prolactin and thyroxine should be excluded.

Treatment

Treatable medical causes are excluded, and hormonal disturbances are corrected when possible. Other treatments include the following.

- *A phosphodiesterase type 5 (PDE5) inhibitor*, such as sildenafil or tadalafil, is taken 1 hour before intercourse. It causes vasodilation of the corpus cavernosum, but is contraindicated in patients on nitrate therapy, for example for ischaemic heart disease, since this combination can result in severe hypotension; a thorough cardiac risk assessment should be performed. Side effects also include nasal congestion, flushing and dyspepsia. PDE5 inhibitors are successful in treating 75% of patients.

  Second line treatments include:

- *Alprostadil* (prostaglandin E1), given by intrapenile injection or by direct intraurethral application.
- *A vacuum condom with constriction ring* or an *intrapenile inflatable prosthesis* may be used.

⦿ Additional resources

Case 118: A foreskin problem in a child
Case 119: An ulcerated prepuce

48

The testis and scrotum

Alexandra J. Colquhoun

Learning objectives

✓ To know the different causes of testicular maldescent and their treatment.

✓ To have knowledge of testicular torsion, how it presents, its differential diagnosis and treatment.

✓ To know the different causes of scrotal lumps, their differing clinical features and treatment, including the diagnosis and management of testicular tumours.

Abnormalities of testicular descent

Embryology

The testis arises from the mesodermal germinal ridge in the posterior wall of the abdominal cavity. It links up with the epididymis and vas deferens, which develop from the mesonephric duct (see Chapter 43). As the testis enlarges, it undergoes caudal migration. By the third month of foetal life, it is in the iliac fossa; by the seventh month, it reaches the inguinal canal; by the eighth month, it has reached the external inguinal ring and by the ninth month, at birth, it has descended into the scrotum. During this descent, a prolongation of peritoneum, called the processus vaginalis, projects into the foetal scrotum; the testis slides behind this and is thus covered in its front and sides by peritoneum. The processus vaginalis becomes obliterated at about the time of birth, leaving the testis

covered by the tunica vaginalis. As expected from the embryology, abnormalities of descent are more common in premature infants (20% incidence) than in full-term infants (2%).

Classification of maldescent

Testicular maldescent can be subdivided according to whether or not the testis followed the normal course of descent.

Ectopic testis (uncommon)

A testis that has strayed from the normal line of descent is termed 'ectopic'. The most common position is in the superficial inguinal pouch, which lies anterior to the external oblique aponeurosis. The testis reaches this site after migrating through the external inguinal ring and then leaves the normal track of descent to pass laterally. Other locations are the groin, the perineum, the root of the penis and the femoral triangle.

Undescended testis (common)

A testis that has followed the normal course of descent but has stopped short of the scrotum is termed an 'undescended' or, more properly, an 'incompletely

Ellis and Calne's Lecture Notes in General Surgery, Fourteenth Edition. Edited by Christopher Watson and Justin Davies. © 2023 John Wiley & Sons Ltd. Published 2023 by John Wiley & Sons Ltd. Companion website: www.wiley.com/go/Watson/GeneralSurgery14

descended testis'. It is a relatively common finding, detected in 1 in 25 boys at birth. The testicle may lie anywhere from the abdominal cavity, along the inguinal canal, to the top of the scrotum. The vast majority are due to a local defect in development. The affected testis is always small and it is probable that this imperfect development impairs descent rather than that the imperfect descent impairs development. The incompletely descended testis is usually accompanied by persistent patency of the processus vaginalis, presenting as a congenital inguinal hernia. Unilateral undescended testes are four times as common as bilateral. The condition of an undescended impalpable testis is termed '*cryptorchidism*', which can be unilateral or bilateral.

Most, if not all, testes that are going to descend do so within the first few months of life. If the testis is not in its normal scrotal position in early childhood, it is very unlikely that it will be capable of spermatogenesis. However, the interstitial (Leydig[1]) cells, which produce testosterone in response to luteinizing hormone, are functional, so that secondary sex characteristics develop normally.

Differential diagnosis: the retractile testis

The most common mistake in diagnosis is to fail to differentiate a true maldescent from a retractile testis. The retractile testis is a normal testis with an excessively active cremasteric reflex, resulting in the testis being drawn up to the external inguinal ring. It is a common condition and often the parents think that the testes have failed to descend; indeed, when the scrotum is palpated the testes may not be felt. However, careful examination will probably reveal the testis at the external inguinal ring or at the root of the scrotum and the testis can, by downward stroking or by gentle traction, be coaxed into the scrotum. A useful trick is to place the child in the squatting position for the examination; this often encourages a retractile testis to descend into the scrotum. It is also worthwhile asking the parents to examine the child when he is relaxed in a warm bath, again, the retractile testis may then slip into its normal position.

[1] Franz Leydig 1821–1908), German Zoologist and Histologist, who also described eponymous cells in fish and crustaceans.

If the testis is easily palpable in the groin and remains easy to feel when the child tenses his abdominal wall muscles, it is lying in the ectopic position and not in the inguinal canal – where it is usually impalpable or, at the most, in a thin boy, detected as a vague, tender bulge.

Treatment

The child with retractile testes is normal; reassurance of the parents is all that is required.

The ectopic or undescended testis must be placed in the scrotum if it is to function as a sperm-producing organ. The optimum age for surgery has been revised in recent times, and current recommendations are for surgery around the age of 6 months. After that age, definite changes in the testis can be seen on microscopy, which may lead to impaired spermatogenesis. The operation, termed 'orchidopexy', consists of mobilizing the testis and its cord, removing the coexisting hernial sac and fixing the testis in the scrotum without tension.

Complications of maldescent

- Defective spermatogenesis, causing sterility if bilateral.
- Increased risk of torsion.
- Increased risk of trauma.
- Increased risk of malignant disease, even if surgical correction is carried out.
- Inguinal hernia – persistence of the processus vaginalis.

Scrotal swelling

Examination

When considering any swelling in the scrotum, the following three questions should be considered in turn (Figure 48.1).

1 *Can you get above the swelling?* If not, the swelling arises from the abdomen and is an inguinoscrotal hernia.
2 *Is it separate from the testis?* If it is, and if it is cystic on transillumination, the swelling is an epididymal cyst.
3 *If it is not separate from the testis, is it cystic or solid?*

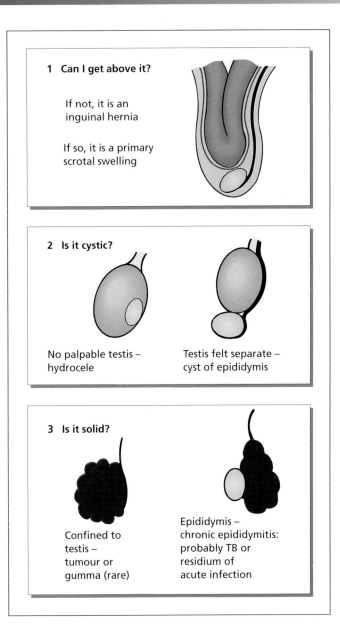

1 **Can I get above it?**

If not, it is an inguinal hernia

If so, it is a primary scrotal swelling

2 **Is it cystic?**

No palpable testis – hydrocele

Testis felt separate – cyst of epididymis

3 **Is it solid?**

Confined to testis – tumour or gumma (rare)

Epididymis – chronic epididymitis: probably TB or residium of acute infection

Figure 48.1 Questions to resolve the differential diagnosis of a scrotal swelling.

a If it is cystic, it is a hydrocele.
b If it is solid, it is very likely to be a testicular cancer.

Special investigation

Ultrasound of the scrotum should clarify the nature of the swelling if there is clinical uncertainty and if a tumour is suspected.

Epididymal cysts

Epididymal cysts are common and due to cystic degeneration of one of the epididymal or para-epididymal structures. They are often multiple, may be bilateral, and produce a swelling in the scrotum that is separate from the testis and should transilluminate.

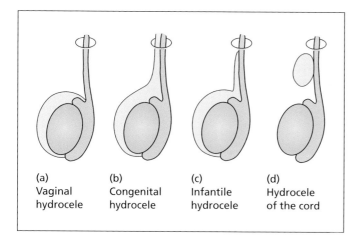

(a)
Vaginal
hydrocele

(b)
Congenital
hydrocele

(c)
Infantile
hydrocele

(d)
Hydrocele
of the cord

Figure 48.2 (a–d) The anatomical classification of hydrocoeles (the ring at the upper end of each diagram represents the internal inguinal ring).

The swelling may be tense and so the cyst may feel hard. The contained fluid may be water-clear or may be milky and contain sperm; hence the old term 'spermatocoele'. There is no way of differentiating clinically between an epididymal cyst and a spermatocoele, and the latter term is best abandoned.

Epididymal cysts are sometimes painful and their bulk may occasionally be troublesome. If they produce significant symptoms, excision may be offered. Aspiration is usually unsuccessful because of recurrence, and is discouraged due to the inherent risk of introducing infection.

Hydrocoele

A hydrocoele is an excessive collection of serous fluid in the processus vaginalis, usually the tunica. Hydrocoeles may be classified as follows.

Primary or idiopathic hydrocoele (Figure 48.2)

This is usually large and tense. There is no disease of the underlying testis. Primary hydrocoeles may be subdivided into the following.

- *Vaginal hydrocoele.* The vaginal hydrocoele is the usual type of hydrocoele surrounding the testis and separated from the peritoneal cavity. The patient presents with a cystic transilluminable swelling in the scrotum. On examination, the testis is difficult to feel and lies at the back of the swelling which, owing to the anatomy of the tunica, encompasses the anterior and lateral portions of the organ.
- *Congenital hydrocoele.* Congenital hydrocoele is associated with a hernial sac, the still patent processus vaginalis. It opens into the peritoneal cavity through a narrow orifice. When elevated, it gradually empties.
- *Infantile hydrocoele.* Infantile hydrocoele extends from the testis to the internal inguinal ring but does not pass into the peritoneal cavity.
- *Hydrocoele of the cord.* Hydrocoele of the cord is rare. It lies in, or just distal to, the inguinal canal, separate from the testis and the peritoneum, and represents a length of patent processus vaginalis in which the upper and lower parts have closed. Diagnosis is confirmed by the simple test of downward traction on the testis, which pulls the hydrocele of the cord down with it. The equivalent in the female is a hydrocoele of the round ligament within the inguinal canal, termed a '*hydrocele of the canal of Nuck*'.[2]

Secondary hydrocoele

A secondary hydrocoele is usually smaller and lax and the fluid collects because of inflammation in the epididymis or testis, or an underlying testicular cancer.

[2] Anton Nuck (1650–1692), Professor of Anatomy and Medicine, Leiden, the Netherlands.

Treatment

Infants

Hydrocoeles in infants should be left alone because most disappear spontaneously. If the hydrocoele persists after the first year, operative treatment is usually advised. The sac is identified and excised, care being taken not to damage any other structures in the cord.

Adults

In young adults, the possibility of tumour should be borne in mind. Ultrasound examination will usually differentiate a normal from an abnormal testis.

Many hydrocoeles are not troublesome, but present because of concern about the nature of the swelling and the possibility of testicular cancer. Reassurance in that situation usually suffices, but if the swelling itself is troublesome, surgery can be offered. If a hydrocoele is aspirated, recurrence is common, and aspiration is seldom helpful. Various surgical options are possible, involving obliteration or excision of the hydrocele sac.

Acute infections of the testis and epididymis

Acute infections usually arise as an ascending infection via the vas deferens, spreading first to the epididymis and then to the testis; occasionally, infection may be blood-borne.

Blood-borne infection

The most common blood-borne agent to infect the testis is the *mumps virus*, the testicular manifestation of which usually follows within a week of the onset of parotid gland enlargement. Occasionally, it may occur in the absence of other manifestations. Diagnosis is confirmed clinically and by the rising level of mumps antibodies in the serum. Young adults are particularly likely to be affected and there may be residual damage to the testis and, if both sides are involved, fertility can be impaired.

Ascending infection

Ascending infection is usually a consequence of a preceding urinary tract infection (e.g. with *Escherichia coli*) or a urethritis or prostatitis from a sexually transmitted organism such as gonorrhoea or *Chlamydia*, which result in epididymitis. Epididymitis may also follow urethral stricture in which straining causes reflux of urine up the vas, or instrumentation of the urethra such as during prostatectomy.

Clinical features

The patient will have a very painful swelling of the epididymis, often with a secondary hydrocoele and constitutional effects (pyrexia, headache and leucocytosis). There may be a history of dysuria, suggesting a urinary tract infection, or urethral discharge, suggesting a sexually transmitted organism. Examination of the urine may reveal the presence of organisms and pus cells, but the urine need not be abnormal. Rectal examination of the prostate may reveal co-existent prostatitis.

Treatment

Treatment is with an appropriate antibiotic given over a prolonged course (4–6 weeks); ciprofloxacin is a typical first-line agent with good specificity for the organisms most often encountered. Patients will need to be fully counselled about ciprofloxacin associated potential collagen-related adverse effects, such as tendon rupture and aortic dissection. If frank abscesses have formed (verified by ultrasound), drainage is required. However, with early adequate treatment, resolution is more likely. The patient will often have residual swelling of the epididymis, which may be rather firm, and differentiation from the tuberculous epididymitis may be difficult unless the history of the previous acute attack of tuberculosis is obtained. When epididymitis arises as a consequence of *Chlamydia* or other sexually transmitted disease, it is important that the sexual partner is also treated. In this situation, doxycycline is the antibiotic of choice.

Differential diagnosis

As with all acutely painful conditions of the testis, torsion must be excluded. If the patient is in their teens, torsion is more likely; if in their twenties and sexually active, epididymitis is more likely. If doubt exists, *urgent* surgical exploration is mandatory.

Chronic infections of the testis

Gumma

Although once common, syphilis of the testis is now a rarity. The testis is enlarged and is clinically difficult to distinguish from a carcinoma. On penicillin therapy, gummas of the testis melt away.

Tuberculosis

This may occur in association with tuberculosis in other parts of the genitourinary tract by ascending infection, but more commonly is a consequence of haematogenous spread.

Clinical features

The patient usually presents with swelling of the epididymis. The vas deferens may be thickened and feel nodular. A cold abscess may develop in relation to the epididymis and rupture through the scrotum, usually posteriorly, resulting in a chronic sinus. The seminal vesicles may be enlarged and palpable on rectal examination.

Diagnosis depends on isolating tubercle bacilli from the urine or biopsy material, and/or evidence of tuberculosis elsewhere.

Treatment

This is the same as for tuberculosis in other situations. If a chronic sinus has developed, unilateral orchidectomy is probably the best form of treatment, as the testis is unlikely to be functional, is a continued source of infection and may lead to spread of the disease elsewhere.

Torsion of the testis

Aetiology

Usually, this is a torsion of the spermatic cord in a congenitally abnormal testis, often maldescended or hanging like a bell clapper within a completely investing tunica vaginalis. Occasionally, true torsion of the testis occurs without involving the cord, when there is an extensive mesorchium between the testis and epididymis. It is probably impossible for torsion to occur in an anatomically completely normal testis. Untreated, the testis undergoes irreversible infarction within a few hours and there is a typical transudation of blood-stained fluid into the tunica vaginalis.

Clinical features

Torsion of the testis is a surgical emergency, which usually occurs in children or adolescents, typically between 12 and 18 years of age, but it can occur in neonates and in men in middle years. There may be a history of mild trauma to the testis or of previous attacks of pain in the testis due to partial torsion and spontaneous untwisting. Cycling, straining, lifting and coitus may be precipitants.

The history is of a sudden onset of severe pain in the groin and lower abdomen, often accompanied by vomiting. The abdominal pain occurs because the nerve supply of the testis is mainly from the T10 sympathetic pathway. Rarely, the pain is limited to the abdomen. Patients with torsion of the right testis have been mistakenly operated on for acute appendicitis because the testis has not been examined with care or, more often, not at all.

Examination of the scrotum reveals a swollen testis, painful to touch, sometimes lying high in the scrotum. Elevation of the hemiscrotum on the side of the pain is said to relieve the pain of epididymitis, but not of torsion, the pain of which may be exacerbated (Prehn's sign[3]).

Differential diagnosis

The differential diagnosis is from acute epididymitis and torsion of a testicular appendage; epididymitis does not come on suddenly.

1 *Epididymitis.* The testis does not lie high in the scrotum, there may be a systemic reaction with pyrexia and leucocytosis and there may be a history of urinary infection with pus cells and organisms in the urine. A useful factor in differential diagnosis is the age of the patient, as torsion of the testis usually occurs before the age of 20 whereas epididymitis usually occurs after that age.
2 *Torsion of a testicular appendage.* Two embryological remnants exist around the testis, the appendix

---

[3] Douglas T Prehn (1901–1974), American Urologist. Described the sign in 1934 while working in a Naval hospital in Brooklyn, New York.

testis and the appendix epididymis, which may themselves twist. They present in a similar fashion to testicular torsion, but on examination the testis does not lie high in the scrotum, and a dark blue pea-like swelling may be visible through the scrotal skin (the so-called 'blue dot sign').

3 *Strangulated inguinal hernia.* Torsion may also mimic a strangulated inguinal hernia.

Colour Doppler ultrasound of the testis may be helpful in diagnosis, provided it can be carried out rapidly by an experienced operator, and only if it does not delay surgical exploration.

Treatment

If there is *any* doubt as to the diagnosis, it is best to explore the testis as soon as possible, because every hour increases the likelihood of irreversible damage to the testis. If still viable, the testis is untwisted and sutured to the tunica vaginalis. If infarcted, it is removed. In every case, fixation of the other testis should be performed at the same time, since any congenital anomaly is likely to be bilateral and torsion of the opposite testis may, therefore, occur.

Varicocoele

This is a condition of varicosities of the pampiniform plexus of veins. It usually occurs on the left, and manifests first in adolescence. It is present in nearly 10% of men, the proportion increasing with age and being higher in infertile men.

Its origin is said to be due to the drainage of the left testicular vein at right angles into the left renal vein, unlike the right testicular vein, which drains obliquely into the inferior vena cava. Patients with varicocoele have absent or incompetent valves at the junction with the left renal vein.

Occasionally, a varicocoele can be secondary to a tumour or other pathological process blocking the testicular vein. The best known example of this is a tumour of the left kidney involving the renal vein and obstructing the drainage of the left testicular vein.

Clinical features

A varicocoele may cause a dragging sensation in the scrotum. It can also be associated with defective spermatogenesis, although surgical correction is not associated with an increased live birth rate. On examination *in the standing position*, the varicose veins within the scrotum feel like a 'bag of worms', but there may be little to feel when the patient lies down.

Treatment

Usually, the varicocoele requires no treatment apart from reassurance that the condition is not likely to give rise to any dangerous complications. If the weight of the varicocoele and testis causes an ache, close-fitting underpants may help. If troublesome, the varicocoele can be cured radiologically by embolizing the left testicular vein; less commonly surgical ligation and division of all the testicular veins that traverse the inguinal canal is required. There is no evidence that treatment of a varicocoele has any effect on male infertility.

Disorders of the scrotal skin

Idiopathic scrotal oedema

Characteristically affecting prepubescent boys, this inflammatory condition is characterized by an erythematous, oedematous swelling of the scrotal skin. It may involve both sides of the scrotum, and can extend into the groins. Unlike torsion, it is painless, and the testis is normal on examination. Spontaneous resolution within a few days is usual.

Fournier's gangrene

Fournier's gangrene,[4] or necrotizing fasciitis of the scrotum, is a result of synergistic infection with several species of bacteria, both aerobic and anaerobic; haemolytic *streptococci*, *staphylococci*, *clostridia* and *E. coli* are common isolates.

The patient is often diabetic and catheterized; there may be a history of minor trauma, perianal abscess or surgery, although there is no obvious precipitating factor in half the cases. The patient develops sudden pain in the scrotum, and rapidly becomes profoundly septic.

---

[4] Jean Alfred Fournier (1832–1914), 'Professeur des maladies cutanées et syphilitiques', Hôpital St Louis, Paris, France.

This is a surgical emergency. Treatment involves high-dose broad-spectrum antibiotics, critical care support and wide debridement of affected skin, with repeated assessment under anaesthesia and further excision if necessary. Due to potential large volume skin loss, combined surgery with a urologist and plastic surgeon is recommended.

Carcinoma of the scrotum

Rare nowadays, this tumour is noteworthy as the first described industrial malignant disease. Percival Pott[5] (1779) noted an association with chimney sweeps, in whom chimney soot acted as a carcinogen when ingrained into the scrotal skin. Later, it was described in workers with mineral oils whose trousers were soaked by the carcinogenic oils.

Presenting as an ulcerating growth, it is usually a squamous carcinoma and is treated by wide excision and block dissection of affected inguinal lymph nodes.

Tumours of the testis

Testicular tumours are the most common solid malignancy in young adult men, although they are relatively uncommon, representing around 1% of malignancies in men.

Aetiology

Undescended and ectopic testes are associated with a three-fold increase in incidence of testicular cancer; that risk is increased if the testis has not been brought to lie in the anatomical position before the age of 13. There is also an increased incidence in patients who are infertile, and those who have had a previous contralateral testicular malignancy (12 times increased risk). Other suggested risk factors include a family history of testicular cancer and hypospadias.

Pathology

There are two main forms of malignant tumours of the testis, seminoma and non-seminomatous germ cell tumours (NSGCTs), of which teratoma is the main

[5] Percival Pott (1714–1788), Surgeon, St Bartholomew's Hospital, London, UK.

type. Rarer tumours include sex-cord tumours and lymphoma, which affects an older age group.

Seminoma

A seminoma arises from cells of the seminiferous tubules, usually occurs between 30 and 40 years of age and is relatively slow growing. Macroscopically, the tumour is solid, appearing rather like a cut potato on section. Microscopically, cells vary from well-differentiated spermatocytes to undifferentiated round cells with clear cytoplasm. Some 10% arise in undescended testes.

Non-seminomatous germ cell tumour

Non-seminomatous germ cell tumours occur in a younger age group, the peak incidence being 20–30 years. They are thought to arise from primitive totipotential germ cells. Macroscopically, it has a markedly cystic appearance and used to be called fibrocystic disease. The cut surface may appear like a colloid goitre, and areas of haemorrhage and infarction are common. Microscopically, the cells are very variable and the tumour may contain cartilage, bone, muscle, fat and other tissues.

Spread

- *Local*: the testis is progressively destroyed by the tumour. Spread through the capsule is unusual, but very occasionally in an advanced case there may be ulceration of the scrotum.
- *Lymphatic*: to the para-aortic nodes via lymphatics accompanying the testicular vein. In advanced cases, there may be enlargement of the supraclavicular nodes, especially on the left side.
- *Blood-borne*: spread from NSGCT occurs relatively early to the lungs and liver. In the seminoma, this tends to occur late in the disease.

Clinical presentation

- As a lump in the testis.
- As a hydrocoele.
- Sometimes as a painful rapidly enlarging swelling, which may be mistaken for orchitis.
- As secondaries, usually metastatic deposits in the lung (presenting as breathlessness), as a mass in the abdomen due to involved abdominal lymph nodes or as a cervical lymphadenopathy.

Tumours of the testis usually present as a painless, swollen testicle, or a lump on a testicle that is hard and may be associated with an overlying secondary hydrocele, which sometimes contains blood-stained fluid. There is often a misleading history of recent trauma, and rarely it may present having undergone torsion.

Occasionally, gynaecomastia may be a presenting feature, owing to the production of paraneoplastic hormones.

Special investigations

- *Scrotal ultrasound* may reveal a solid tumour with or without the presence of a hydrocoele.
- *Tumour markers*: NSGCTs usually produce α-fetoprotein (AFP) and many produce β-human chorionic gonadotrophin (β-HCG); some pure seminomas also produce β-HCG. These are useful not only in making a diagnosis but also in subsequent follow-up.
- *Computed tomography (CT) scans of the chest, abdomen and pelvis* are performed looking for secondary spread in order to stage the disease.

Treatment

If it is suspected that the testicular swelling is due to a tumour, early surgical excision is mandatory. The spermatic cord is exposed through an inguinal incision, occluded by an atraumatic clamp and the testis delivered. The clamp prevents vascular dissemination of tumour cells. Orchidectomy is then performed by ligating the cord and dividing it at the internal ring. The use of intraoperative biopsy to confirm malignancy is now rare, given the accuracy of preoperative scrotal ultrasound scanning. Inguinal, rather than scrotal, exploration is performed to avoid exposure to the scrotal lymphatics, which drain to the inguinal nodes, unlike the spermatic cord, which drains to the internal iliac nodes.

For organ confined disease, adjuvant treatment with chemotherapy is often recommended to treat occult micrometastatic disease. Seminomas are also radiosensitive so adjuvant radiotherapy can be given to the ipsilateral iliac and para-aortic lymph nodes for this pathological disease type.

Patients who have metastatic disease on their staging CT scan are effectively treated with systemic chemotherapy (bleomycin, etoposide and platinum). Patients who exhibit persistent retroperitoneal lymphadenopathy after chemotherapy can be offered retroperitoneal lymph node dissection with curative intent. As chemotherapy is likely to render the patient infertile, prior sperm banking is offered.

Prognosis

Node-negative cases have an extremely good prognosis of nearly 100% 5-year survival. Even with early abdominal lymph node spread, there is still a 95% 5-year survival and, with disseminated disease, long-term survival is often achieved with chemotherapy.

Male infertility

The majority of couples wishing to have children achieve pregnancy within 2 years. However, 1 in 10 couples suffers infertility, with the problem distributed evenly between each partner, with one-third of cases due to factors in both the man and the woman.

Aetiology

Congenital disorder

- *Chromosome abnormality*, for example Klinefelter's syndrome[6] (XXY).
- *Developmental anomaly*, for example testicular maldescent, absent vas deferens.

Physical problems

- *Post-infection*, for example following mumps orchitis or mumps epididymitis.
- *Trauma*, with subsequent atrophy.
- *Neurological*, for example spinal injury, producing erectile and ejaculatory dysfunction.
- *Temperature*, for example varicocele, tight-fitting underpants.
- *Iatrogenic*, for example vasectomy, damage during orchidopexy or hernia repair.

Hormonal

- *Pituitary insufficiency*, for example from a pituitary tumour or craniopharyngioma.
- *Liver failure*, causing increased circulating oestrogens.

---

[6] Harry Fitch Klinefelter (1912–1990), Associate Professor of Medicine, Johns Hopkins Hospital, Baltimore, MD, USA.

Drugs

Chemotherapy and radiotherapy for cancer, including NSGCT or seminoma – patients are offered sperm bank facilities prior to treatment.

Clinical features

A full history and thorough examination are required to exclude obvious contributory pathology. Previous surgery or infection of the testicular apparatus is particularly important, especially as a child. Co-existing diabetes or renal or hepatic failure may contribute to infertility, as can smoking.

Examination should include assessment of hair distribution and general build for evidence of testicular failure (female pattern distribution). Examination of the penis and scrotal contents is particularly important, verifying the course of the vas deferens on each side, the size of the testis and the presence of a varicocoele (with the patient standing). The presence of hypospadias (see Chapter 46) should be noted as this may affect where the sperm are deposited.

Special investigations

Before embarking on investigation, it should be ascertained that coitus is occurring regularly. Invasive tests are withheld until the infertile partner is identified.

- *Semen analysis.* Ideally, this is produced following a period of abstinence of 3 days and is examined within 2 hours. A semen volume over 2 mL, with over 20 million sperm per millilitre, of which 50% are motile at 2 hours, and at least 14% of normal morphology, is acceptable.
- *Hormone assays* in patients with no sperm (azoospermia), or few sperm. Raised prolactin is suggestive of a pituitary tumour. Raised follicle-stimulating hormone levels, with small testes, suggest primary testicular failure.
- *Seminal fructose levels.* Fructose is produced by the seminal vesicles, and is absent in disease of the seminal vesicles and in congenital absence of the vasa deferentia.
- *Transrectal ultrasound* is performed where a low-volume ejaculate is produced to detect ductal obstruction.

Treatment

Non-specific measures

Non-specific measures, if no cause is found, include wearing loose-fitting underpants, avoiding hot baths, and cessation of smoking and excess alcohol intake. Regular intercourse throughout the menstrual cycle is encouraged.

Surgical

Any underlying disease is treated.

- *Vasectomy reversal* is attempted.
- *An epididymal blockage* is corrected.
- *Testicular biopsy* is performed with sperm retrieval only where facilities for sperm storage exist.

The role of varicocoele ligation in the treatment of male infertility is not supported by evidence.

Assisted conception

In vitro fertilization (IVF), in which fertilization of the ovum takes place outside the body, has revolutionized the treatment of infertility.

Complementary techniques include intracytoplasmic sperm injection (ICSI), microsurgical epididymal sperm aspiration, percutaneous epididymal sperm aspiration, percutaneous testicular sperm aspiration and open testicular sperm extraction. Nowadays ICSI, with sperm procurement through one of the above methods, or IVF is the treatment of choice, with birth rates per cycle of treatment of 15–20%.

Since the advent of contraceptive medication, there has been an increase in the age of planned conception with the result that more and more couples are having difficulty in conceiving.

Additional resources

49

Transplantation surgery

Christopher Watson

Learning objectives

✓ To know about organ donation.

✓ To know the different types of organ transplant and their complications.

✓ To know the principles behind organ matching and immunosuppression.

Historical background

Early attempts at organ transplantation were fraught with failure owing to a lack of appreciation of the immune response that resulted in rapid destruction of the transplanted organ. It was not until 1954 that successful replacement of a diseased organ with a transplanted organ occurred, when the immune response was bypassed by performing kidney transplants between identical twins. In 1960, the first immunosuppressive drugs were used with which the immune response could be partly controlled, permitting longer useful function of organs from unrelated donors. In the subsequent decade, regular haemodialysis, and later peritoneal dialysis, became increasingly available, able to support patients with kidney failure while awaiting transplantation. In the 1980s, the more powerful immunosuppressant ciclosporin permitted successful transplantation of the liver, heart, lungs and pancreas, and improved the results of kidney transplantation.

With the advances in immunosuppression, better techniques of organ preservation and improved anaesthetic and intensive care management, organ transplantation to replace diseased organs is now an accepted treatment offering transplant recipients the possibility of long-term survival.

Classification of grafts

- *Autograft*: transplant from one part of the body to another, for example skin graft.
- *Allograft*: between members of the same species, such as human to human; also termed '*homograft*'.
- *Isograft*: between identical twins.
- *Xenograft*: between members of different species, for example pig to human.
- *Structural grafts*: act as a non-living scaffold. Can be of biological origin (e.g. arterial and heart valve grafts) or synthetic (e.g. Dacron vascular prosthesis).

In addition to classifying a graft according to its source, organ grafts are also classified according to where they are implanted relative to the native organ.

- *Orthotopic*: the diseased organ is removed and replaced by the transplanted organ lying in the normal anatomical position, for example heart, lung and liver transplants are usually orthotopic.
- *Heterotopic*: the transplanted organ is placed in a different position from the normal anatomical position, for example kidney and pancreas transplants. The diseased organ is not usually removed.

Ellis and Calne's Lecture Notes in General Surgery, Fourteenth Edition.
Edited by Christopher Watson and Justin Davies.
© 2023 John Wiley & Sons Ltd. Published 2023 by John Wiley & Sons Ltd.
Companion website: www.wiley.com/go/Watson/GeneralSurgery14

This chapter will discuss organ allografts for the functional replacement of diseased organs such as kidney, liver, heart, lungs and pancreas.

Organ donors

There are two potential sources of donor organs.

Living donors

Living donation is possible when removal of either a paired organ (e.g. the kidney) or part of an unpaired organ (e.g. a lobe of the liver or lung) leaves the donor with sufficient residual organ function, and provides an organ or part of an organ for a recipient. Live donation is most common in kidney transplantation, in which the donor can maintain adequate renal function with only one kidney and donate the other to a relative, partner or, less commonly, a friend or stranger. As with any operation, there are risks to the donor, especially of postoperative events such as chest and wound infection, deep vein thrombosis and pulmonary embolism; the risk of death following kidney donation is estimated to be between 1 in 1600 and 1 in 3200. In the UK, a third of all kidney transplants (around 1000 a year) are from living donors.

Donation of a portion of the liver, either to a child or to another adult, involves a major operation and runs the risk of leaving the donor with borderline liver function from the remaining liver lobe. The risk of death following donation of a the right lobe of liver to an adult is estimated at between 1 in 100 and 1 in 200; donation of the smaller left lobe to a child is associated with less risk. Live donation of a lung lobe is also possible, the recipients usually being children.

Deceased donors

There are two types of organ donation from deceased donors.

Donation after brain-stem death (DBD)

Most organs for transplantation come from donors who have sustained a lethal brain injury following a head injury, intracranial haemorrhage or primary brain tumour, and who have been certified dead by 'brain-stem' criteria (see Chapter 17). The organs are removed from the donor in the operating theatre after isolating their vascular pedicles and while the heart is still beating; when circulation ceases, the organs are rapidly cooled by flushing them *in situ* with ice-cold organ preservation solution.

Donation after circulatory death (DCD, or non-heart-beating donation)

When patients have sustained a catastrophic brain injury but do not fulfil the brain-stem criteria for the diagnosis of death, the supervising doctors, in consultation with the next of kin, may nevertheless decide that future treatment is futile. In such circumstances, life-supporting treatment is withdrawn and the patient dies, death being certified by the absence of a circulation. Where there is consent for organ donation, the donor can be transferred to the operating theatre following circulatory arrest and verification of death. The abdomen is rapidly prepared and draped, opened, and the organs rapidly cooled by flushing with ice-cold preservation solution before removal.

Unlike organs from brain-dead donors, organs removed from donors after circulatory death suffer a period of warm ischaemia prior to cooling. During this period, the organs switch from aerobic to anaerobic metabolism, which depletes intracellular energy stores and causes the accumulation of lactic acid. Unchecked, this process rapidly results in cell death as membrane pumps fail and toxic metabolites accumulate. Organs vary in their tolerance of warm ischaemia, with kidneys remaining viable for about 60 min, whereas the liver tolerates less than 30 min. In such cases, the initial function of the organs is inferior to those removed following brain-stem death, but the ultimate function can be satisfactory.

Normothermic regional perfusion

One technique increasingly used to improve the outcomes of organs from DCD donors is to restore a circulation to the abdominal organs *in situ* using an extracorporeal membrane oxygenator circuit, a technique called normothermic regional perfusion. Treatment for 2 hours immediately after death restores cellular energy improving tolerance of ischaemia during storage, as well as affording an opportunity to test organ function. It is associated with better outcomes for the transplanted organs.

Exclusions to organ donation

There are three main reasons why a potential donor may be unsuitable.

1 *Potential transmission of infection.* The transplanted organ could carry with it viral infections such as hepatitis B and C and human immunodeficiency virus, or any bacterial or other infection that was disseminated in the donor. Likewise, donors in whom there is a risk of prion infection such as new-variant Creutzfeldt–Jakob disease are unsuitable.

2 *Potential transmission of cancer.* Malignant disease in the donor can be transplanted into the recipient, where it may become established in the immunosuppressed environment. Therefore, with the exception of primary brain tumours (which rarely spread outside the central nervous system) and superficial non-melanoma skin cancer, active malignancy is a contraindication to organ donation.

3 *Impaired function of donor organ.* If the function of the organ is impaired in the donor, it is unsuitable for transplantation. For example, a heart with severe coronary artery disease is unsuitable, while a donor with polycystic kidneys is an unsuitable kidney donor but may be a suitable heart donor.

Organ preservation

Cold storage

Once removed from the donor, the organs must be maintained in their optimum state prior to transplantation. This is achieved by a combination of (1) cooling the organ to around 4 °C to reduce the metabolic activity and (2) perfusing it with, and storing it in, a preservation solution that contains a pH buffer to counter the lactic acid accumulation and an impermeant to prevent osmotic cell swelling. One such solution is the University of Wisconsin (UW) solution, in which a kidney can be preserved for 36–40 hours, and a liver for up to 13 hours, although in both cases the shortest possible preservation period, or *cold ischaemia time* (the time between cessation of circulation in the donor and restoration of circulation in the recipient), is desirable. No comparable preservation solution

exists for the heart and lungs, and implantation must occur within 4–6 hours to ensure immediate life-sustaining function of these organs.

Hypothermic machine perfusion

Instead of flushing an organ once before storage on ice, an alternative is to constantly pump ice-cold preservation fluid through the organ. This technique is popular for the storage of kidneys, with evidence that it is particularly beneficial for older donor kidneys and others that are more susceptible to cold ischaemia. A variant of this, hypothermic oxygenated perfusion (HOPE) is being increasingly used for donor livers before implantation.

Normothermic machine perfusion

For liver and heart, *ex situ* normothermic perfusion, where the organ is perfused with a red cell-containing solution at normal body temperature, is being used increasingly to prolong storage and evaluate the function of an organ before implantation.

Ex situ lung perfusion is increasingly being used to optimize lungs before implantation. Unlike the other solid organs, adequate tissue oxygenation can be achieved by ventilating the lungs with an oxygen-containing gas; the ability of the lungs to oxygenate an acellular perfusion fluid may then be used as a measure of function. Use of a high-osmolarity perfusate also permits treatment of the pulmonary oedema that is associated with brain death in the donor.

Organ recipients

Patients are considered for transplantation when they are in chronic organ failure without hope of recovery, but still fit enough to withstand the operative procedure. For kidney transplantation, potential transplant recipients should be on or about to start dialysis. Patients with chronic liver disease are placed on the transplant waiting list when their liver disease warrants, such that their risk of death without a transplant is greater than the risk of death following transplantation. For example, in patients with primary biliary cirrhosis, an elevation of serum bilirubin concentration over 100 μmol/L is an indication for transplantation. In acute liver failure, transplantation is indicated if the synthetic function of the liver is severely impaired, as best reflected by the degree of elevation of prothrombin time. The development of predictive indices, such as the model for end-stage liver disease (MELD) or its UK equivalent, UKELD, has helped to predict survival without a transplant to aid in this decision process.

The immunology of organ transplantation

The major histocompatibility complex

When an organ is transplanted, it is recognized as foreign by the host's immune system and the rejection response is initiated. The recognition is mediated by an interaction between host T lymphocytes (T-cells) and histocompatibility antigens on the surface of the allograft (the transplanted organ). The major histocompatibility complex (MHC) is a group of genes that encode molecules (antigens) expressed on the surface of cells. The MHC molecules are of two principal sorts. MHC class I antigens are present on all nucleated cells. MHC class II antigens are present on certain cells (e.g. macrophages, monocytes and dendritic cells), and can be induced to appear on others by the presence of cytokines such as interferon γ (IFN-γ).

The human leucocyte antigen system

The human leucocyte antigen (HLA) system describes the locus on chromosome 6 containing the genes encoding the MHC antigens in the human. HLA-A, -B and -C loci encode class I molecules, whereas class II molecules are encoded by HLA-DP, -DQ and -DR loci. The extensive polymorphism at each locus, in particular the A and B loci, results in differences in the MHC antigens on allografts recognized by the host lymphocytes.

Organ matching

There are three levels of organ matching that can be performed, of which ABO blood group compatibility is required for all transplants. Lymphocytotoxic cross-matching is required in recipients who have previously been exposed to other HLA antigens following previous blood transfusions or transplants or in childbirth, where the possibility of developing anti-HLA antibodies exists. HLA matching is at present restricted to kidneys, where the availability of dialysis enables recipients to wait for an optimally matched kidney, and the better tolerance of cold ischaemia provides the necessary time required move the donor organ between centres to the best matched recipient, and perform a lymphocytotoxic cross-match. This system requires central co-ordination of a large pool of recipients and donors which, in the UK, is based in Bristol.

ABO matching

The existence of preformed ABO antibodies means that the transplanted organs, like blood transfusions, must be ABO compatible. Thus, while a group A recipient can have an organ from either a group A or group O donor, a group O recipient can have only an organ from a donor with blood group O because of the presence of preformed antibodies to group A (and B) antigens. Crossing the ABO barrier results in hyperacute rejection except in the case of the liver, which is relatively resistant to this process. Nevertheless, abiding by the ABO rules is also advisable in liver transplantation since the long-term outcome is better.

Crossing the ABO barrier is possible without hyperacute rejection in certain circumstances. In children, the development of anti-A and anti-B antibodies does not occur usually until after the first year. It has thus been possible to perform ABO-mismatched heart transplants in very young children with excellent results. Some adults also have low titres of ABO antibody, which can be removed immediately prior to an ABO-mismatched kidney transplant from a live donor with good long-term outcomes, even after the antibody reappears.

Lymphocytotoxic cross-match

To detect circulating antibodies in the recipient against donor HLA antigens, a direct lymphocytotoxic cross-match is performed. This involves mixing donor cells (lymphocytes) from peripheral blood, lymph node or spleen with the recipient's serum in the presence of rabbit complement and observing for cytolysis. Alternatively, the presence of anti-donor antibodies can be detected using flow cytometry or special antigen coated beads. Presence of antibodies against donor HLA in the cross-match test is associated with hyperacute rejection; hence, a positive cross-match is a contraindication to transplantation of all organs (except the liver, where it is also advisable but not essential).

MHC matching

In order to minimize the immune response to an organ allograft, the recipient's MHC antigens can be matched to the donor. The best matching, in fact perfect matching, comes from an identical twin. The inheritance of MHC antigens follows Mendelian genetics,[1] and the antigens are co-dominantly expressed with a degree of linkage. Therefore, within a family, there is a one in four chance that two siblings will share the same MHC antigens; a one in two chance of them differing by one haplotype and a one in four chance of them inheriting a completely different set of HLA antigens. One in four living-related sibling donors will thus offer a significant immunological advantage due to complete HLA identity.

Unrelated donor–recipient pairs are also matched with a view to minimizing differences between MHC antigens. Three HLA loci, A, B and DR, are specifically considered. The object of organ matching is to reduce the number of mismatched antigens out of the six possible MHC antigens encoded by the three loci. This strategy has been shown to be beneficial for renal transplantation. Retrospective analysis has also shown a benefit of matching for the survival of heart and lung transplants, but the short preservation time prevents prospective matching.

Rejection

Hyperacute rejection

Patients may develop antibodies to foreign HLA following exposure to them during childbirth, blood transfusion or a previous transplant. When the recipient has preformed antibodies to HLA or ABO blood group antigens on the donor, the recipient antibody (HLA or ABO) binds to the donor cells, activates circulating complement, and results in graft destruction in minutes or hours.

[1] Gregor Mendel (1882–1884), Augustinian priest and scientist, St Thomas's Abbey, Brno, Czech Republic.

Acute rejection

Acute rejection occurs when the amount of immunosuppression is inadequate to prevent the recipient's immune system attacking the graft. Clinically, acute rejection is characterized by a pyrexia, enlargement and tenderness over the transplanted organ, and biochemical dysfunction (a rise in creatinine in a kidney transplant, elevated liver enzymes in a liver transplant). It is confirmed by biopsy of the organ. The most common time for acute rejection is in the first 3 months after transplantation, and it usually responds to a short course of high-dose steroid followed by an increase in baseline immunosuppression.

Chronic rejection

Chronic rejection, more properly termed 'chronic allograft damage', is an insidious process of graft attrition, which generally results in graft loss. It has different names according to the organ concerned, but in all organs it is characterized by a progressive vasculopathy in the graft. The aetiology of the vasculopathy is related to tissue compatibility between donor and recipient, to the immunosuppression, to damage to the graft during the transplant, to hypertension and possibly also to infection of the graft by cytomegalovirus.

Principles of immunosuppressive therapy

Immunosuppressive therapy following organ transplantation is a balance between giving enough drug to prevent rejection, but not too much to make the patient susceptible to opportunist infection. In addition, individual drugs have their own undesirable side effects, which may be reduced by combining drugs with different modes of action and with different side-effect profiles, rather as is done with cancer chemotherapy regimens. A common protocol would be to combine a steroid (e.g. prednisolone) with an anti-nucleotide such as azathioprine or mycophenolate and an inhibitor of T cell activation such as ciclosporin or tacrolimus, often referred to as 'triple therapy'.

Induction therapy. In addition to triple therapy immunosuppression from the outset, it is common to give additional treatment immediately after transplant to enhance the initial immunosuppression. This is termed 'induction therapy', and is either an antibody against all T-cells (e.g. anti-thymocyte globulin) or against activated T-cells (e.g. the CD25 monoclonal antibody basiliximab).

Maintenance therapy. After the initial few months, the incidence of rejection is much less as the graft undergoes a degree of acceptance, so the total amount of immunosuppression may be reduced. This may be achieved either by reducing the dosage of the agents used or by discontinuing one or more of the initial immunosuppressive agents. This is termed 'maintenance immunosuppression'.

Complications of transplantation

Following transplantation, the complications can be divided into early (those occurring in hospital) and late.

Early complications

Early complications may be related to the four components of the transplant procedure.

1 *The surgical operation*, such as bleeding, wound infection, anastomotic breakdown and vascular anastomotic thrombosis.
2 *The quality of the organ*, dependent on the donor organ (in particular the age of the donor), the quality of organ preservation prior to transplant and the duration of ischaemia. A donor organ with a long cold ischaemic time would be expected to perform less well.
3 *The immunological response* of the recipient to the donor (acute rejection).
4 *The effects of immunosuppression.* Initially, high doses of immunosuppression are used, and it is in the early stages that the infective complications of immunosuppression are seen, in particular wound and chest infections; viral infections such as herpes simplex (cold sores) are also common early after transplant.

Late complications

The late complications of transplantation are either immunological, related to the immunosuppression, or the result of recurrent disease.

1 *Immunological complications* include acute and chronic rejection.
2 *Immunosuppressive complications* reflect the difficulty in achieving immunosuppression sufficient to stop rejection, but low enough to stop adverse effects. Such complications include the following:
   a *Drug side effects*, for example nephrotoxicity of ciclosporin and tacrolimus.
   b *Infection* occurs more commonly, particularly opportunist infections such as *Pneumocystis jiroveci* (formerly, *P. carinii*) and cytomegalovirus.
   c *Malignancy*, see later in this chapter.
3 *Recurrent disease.* In some cases, the original disease may recur in the transplanted organ. For example, glomerulonephropathies such as immunoglobulin (Ig)A nephropathy and focal segmental glomerulosclerosis may recur in the transplanted kidney; autoimmune diabetes can recur in a transplanted pancreas; autoimmune liver diseases such as primary biliary cholangitis and sclerosing cholangitis may recur in the transplanted liver, while hepatitis B and C viruses will infect the transplanted liver unless antiviral treatment is given.

Malignancy post-transplant

One of the important complications of transplantation is the increased incidence of malignancy associated with immunosuppression. Viral-associated cancers are particularly common, such as lymphoma (associated with Epstein–Barr virus[2]), and cervical and anal cancers (associated with prior infection with human papilloma virus, HPV). The incidence of non-melanomatous skin cancer is also related to HPV infection, and is around 17-fold more than the normal UK population, and is even higher in Australia where sun exposure is greater; similarly there is an increased incidence of carcinoma of the lip (65-fold higher) and anus (10-fold).

Lymphoma, both Hodgkin's and non-Hodgkin's types, occurs in around 2% of transplant recipients, with the peak incidence in the first 2 years post-transplant.

Recipients of kidney transplants have a much higher incidence of cancer in their native kidneys, possibly related to cystic degeneration of those

---

[2] Michael Anthony Epstein (b. 1921), Professor of Pathology, University of Bristol, Bristol, UK. Yvonne Barr (1932–2016), Virologist, Middlesex Hospital, London, UK.

kidneys. Liver recipients transplanted for alcohol-related liver disease have a high incidence of oropharyngeal cancer, possibly because alcohol intake is a surrogate for other substance abuse including smoking.

While the incidence of most cancers is increased by immunosuppression exposure, a few, most notably breast cancer, are not.

Results of clinical organ transplantation

Kidney transplantation

Kidney transplantation has been a routine treatment for over 50 years, and there are several survivors with transplants functioning for that period. In the UK, over 3000 kidney transplants are performed annually, with over 8000 people on dialysis awaiting transplantation. The shortfall in supply is reflected worldwide.

The kidney is transplanted heterotopically into the iliac fossa, with the donor renal vessels anastomosed to the external iliac vessels of the recipient, and the donor ureter anastomosed to the bladder directly to produce a new ureteric orifice. Unless the recipient's own kidneys are a danger to the recipient (e.g. a source of infection), they are left *in situ*.

As with other organ transplants, results are usually quoted in terms of 1-year and 5-year graft survival, in which the losses in the first 12 months are higher and reflect the early complications, whereas the 5-year figures reflect the rate of chronic losses from recurrent disease or chronic rejection. One-year graft survival following renal transplantation is around 95%, and is over 99% when the kidney resulted from an HLA-identical sibling donation. Thereafter, there is a gradual loss of around 3% per annum, giving a 5-year survival of over 80% (better still for related grafts).

Pancreas transplantation

It has long been thought that transplantation for the treatment of diabetes will eventually involve β-cells or islets, possibly with the help of genetic engineering, but although several hundred islet grafts have so far been attempted in humans, long-term results have been poor. Better short-term and long-term results follow transplantation of the vascularized whole pancreas. However, pancreatic transplantation involves a large operation, the principal complications of which include graft pancreatitis with consequent peritonitis, and graft thrombosis. The favoured technique is to place the pancreas in the iliac fossa anastomosed to the common iliac artery and inferior vena cava (IVC), with the exocrine drainage into a loop of small intestine.

Diabetic nephropathy is the main indication for pancreas transplantation, in which circumstance it is usually combined with a kidney transplant from the same donor. Approximately 80% of pancreas transplants are functioning after 5 years. Combined kidney and pancreas transplantation prolongs life in patients with type 1 diabetes and renal failure compared with kidney transplantation alone, in addition to reducing the number of cardiovascular events and progression of other diabetic complications such as autonomic and peripheral neuropathy.

Liver transplantation

Liver transplantation is the treatment of choice for many forms of fatal liver disease. Patients are offered the operation before they become too sick for what is the most formidable of surgical assaults. The three main indications for liver transplantation are:

1 *Complications of cirrhosis*: hepatocellular carcinoma, recurrent variceal haemorrhage, intractable ascites and poor synthetic function.
2 *Acute hepatic necrosis*, for example paracetamol poisoning.
3 *Metabolic disease*, for example oxalosis (in which kidney grafting may also be required).

Over 90% of liver transplant recipients survive for 1 year, and the 5-year figure is over 80%, with a lower annual loss than kidney transplants after the first year.

Heart, lung and combined heart–lung transplantation

Heart transplantation is a relatively straightforward operative procedure in a unit where open heart surgery is performed. The main indications are atherosclerotic coronary artery disease and cardiomyopathy. Solitary lung transplantation without the heart is more common than combined heart–lung transplantation in which both lungs are transplanted *en bloc* with the heart; in the latter case, only three anastomoses are required, namely aortic, tracheal and right atrial. The most common indications for lung transplantation are primary pulmonary hypertension, chronic obstructive airways disease, pulmonary fibrosis and cystic fibrosis. The survival of recipients of both heart and lung grafts is approximately 70% at 5 years.

Additional resources

Case 123: A renal transplant recipient with a gastrointestinal haemorrhage

Index

Page numbers in *italics* denote figures, those in **bold** denote tables and boxes.

Ellis and Calne's Lecture Notes in General Surgery, Fourteenth Edition.
Edited by Christopher Watson and Justin Davies.
© 2023 John Wiley & Sons Ltd. Published 2023 by John Wiley & Sons Ltd.
Companion website: www.wiley.com/go/Watson/GeneralSurgery14